Cardiology
1993

Cardiology
1993

WILLIAM C. ROBERTS, M.D.

Executive Director
Baylor Cardiovascular Institute
Baylor University Medical Center
Dallas, Texas
Editor-in-Chief, The American Journal of Cardiology

JAMES T. WILLERSON, M.D.
Randall Professor of Medicine and Chairman
Department of Internal Medicine
University of Texas Medical School at Houston
and
Director of Cardiology Research
At The Texas Heart Institute, Houston, Texas
Editor-in-Chief, Circulation

CHARLES E. RACKLEY, M.D.
Professor of Medicine
Division of Cardiology
Department of Medicine
Georgetown University Medical Center
Washington, D.C.

THOMAS P. GRAHAM, JR., M.D.
Professor of Pediatrics
Chief, Division of Pediatrics
Vanderbilt University
Nashville, Tennessee

DEAN T. MASON, M.D.
Physician-in-Chief, Western Heart Institute
Chairman, Department of
Cardiovascular Medicine
St. Mary's Hospital and Medical Center
San Francisco, California
Editor-in-Chief, American Heart Journal

Butterworth–Heinemann
Boston   London   Oxford   Singapore   Sydney   Toronto   Wellington

LC 93-71211

ISBN 07506-9451-3

ISSN 0275-0066

Butterworth–Heinemann
80 Montvale Avenue
Stoneham, MA 02180

10 9 8 7 6 5 4 3 2 1

Printed in the United States of America

Contents

3. Acute Myocardial Infarction and Its Consequences 171

4. Arrhythmias, Conduction Disturbances, and Cardiac Arrest — 247

5. Systemic Hypertension   292

Preface

Cardiology 1993 is the thirteenth book to be published in this series. It contains summaries of 758 articles, all published in 1992. A total of 23 medical journals (Table I) were examined and at least one and usually many articles were summarized from each journal. The number of articles summarized by each of the five authors is listed in Table II. All of Rackley's submissions were from *Circulation;* Mason's from *The American Heart Journal;* and Willerson's from *The Journal of American College of Cardiology*. The contributions of Graham and Roberts were from a variety of medical journals. The summaries from each contributor were submitted to me, organized into the various sections in each of the 10 chapters, and edited.

A book of this type is made possible because of unselfish contributions from several individuals, none of whom is rewarded by authorship. I am enormously grateful to Marjorie Hadsell for typing perfectly the 431 summaries contributed by me; to Angie Esquivel, Leslie Flatt, Azora L. Irby, and Joy Phillips also for typing many summaries; to Karen Oberheim for

TABLE I. *Journals containing articles summarized in* Cardiology 1993.

1. American Heart Journal
2. American Journal of Cardiology
3. American Journal of Hypertension
4. American Journal of Medicine
5. Annals of Internal Medicine
6. Annals of Surgery
7. Annals of Thoracic Surgery
8. Archives of Internal Medicine
9. Archives of Pathology and Laboratory Medicine
10. Arteriosclerosis and Thrombosis
11. British Heart Journal
12. British Medical Journal
13. Chest
14. Circulation
15. Current Problems in Cardiology
16. European Heart Journal
17. Journal of American College of Cardiology
18. Journal of the American Medical Association
19. Journal of Cardiac Surgery
20. Journal of Thoracic and Cardiovascular Surgery
21. Lancet
22. Medicine
23. New England Journal of Medicine

TABLE II. *Contributions of the Five Authors to* Cardiology 1992.

| AUTHOR | CHAPTERS | | | | | | | | | | Totals |
	1	2	3	4	5	6	7	8	9	10	
1) WCR	72	91	76	45	33	26	28	3	13	44	431 (56.86%)
2) JTW	0	33	21	8	1	7	8	1	2	7	88 (11.61%)
3) CER	18	23	12	11	1	6	5	0	1	9	86 (11.34%)
4) TPG, Jr.	0	1	0	5	0	0	1	69	0	1	77 (10.16%)
5) DTM	2	28	14	15	1	8	2	0	5	1	76 (10.03%)
TOTALS	92	176	123	84	36	47	44	73	21	62	758 (100%)
Figures	25	26	26	7	7	8	4	3	6	10	122
Tables	11	5	3	2	1	6	1	1	1	3	34

all her work obtaining permissions and to Barbara Murphy for efficiently coordinating the publishing of the book in Boston.

William C. Roberts, M.D.
Editor

Cardiology
1993

Conversion of Units

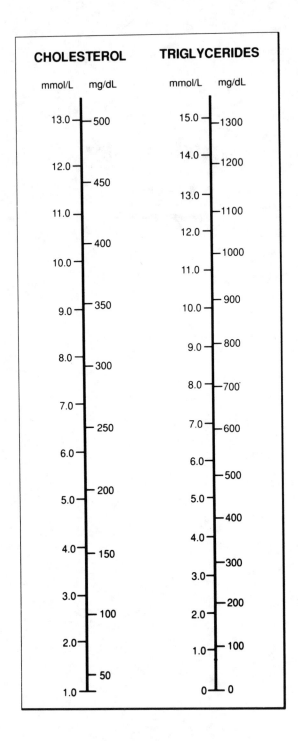

CHOLESTEROL

mmol/L	mg/dL
13.0	500
12.0	450
11.0	400
10.0	
9.0	350
8.0	300
7.0	250
6.0	
5.0	200
4.0	150
3.0	100
2.0	
1.0	50

TRIGLYCERIDES

mmol/L	mg/dL
15.0	1300
14.0	1200
13.0	1100
12.0	1000
11.0	900
10.0	
9.0	800
8.0	700
7.0	600
6.0	500
5.0	400
4.0	300
3.0	200
2.0	
1.0	100
0	0

Cholesterol mg/dL = mmol/L x 38.6

Triglyceride mg/dL = mmol/L x 88.5

Factors Causing, Accelerating, or Preventing Coronary Arterial Atherosclerosis

---

RISK FACTORS—GENERAL

In white men

To assess the combined influence of BP, serum total cholesterol level, and cigarette smoking on death from CAD and to describe how these associations vary with age, Neaton and Wentworth[1] for the Multiple Risk Factor Intervention Trial Research Group examined data on those factors and on mortality for 316,099 men screened for the Multiple Risk Factor Intervention Trial (MRFIT). Vital status of participants has been determined after an average follow-up of 12 years; 6,327 deaths from CAD have been identified. Strong graded relations between serum cholesterol levels above 4.65 mmol/L (180 mg/dL) (Table 1-1, Figure 1-1), systolic BP above 110 mm Hg, and diastolic BP above 70 mm Hg and mortality due to CAD were evident (Figure 1-2). Smokers with serum cholesterol and systolic BP levels in the highest quintiles had CAD death rates that were approximately 20 times greater than nonsmoking men with systolic BP and cholesterol levels in the lowest quintile. Systolic and diastolic BP, serum cholesterol level, and cigarettes per day were significant predictors of death due to CAD in all age groups. Systolic BP was a stronger predictor

TABLE 1-1. *Mean Levels of Serum Cholesterol and Blood Pressure and Percentage of Cigarette Smokers by Age for White Men Screened in the MRFIT.* Reproduced with permission from Neaton, et al.[1]*

Age, y	No. of Men	Mean (±SD) Serum Cholesterol, mmol/L (mg/dL)	Mean (±SD) Systolic BP, mm Hg	Mean (±SD) Diastolic BP, mm Hg	Cigarette Smokers, (%)	Mean (±SD) No. of Cigarettes per Day for Smokers
35-39	65 135	5.33 ± 1.00 (206.1 ± 38.8)	126.3 ± 13.2	81.6 ± 10.0	39.6	26.7 ± 13.2
40-44	69 262	5.52 ± 1.01 (213.3 ± 39.2)	127.5 ± 14.1	83.2 ± 10.2	38.3	27.4 ± 13.3
45-49	74 964	5.63 ± 1.01 (217.6 ± 39.1)	129.7 ± 15.5	84.3 ± 10.5	36.7	27.6 ± 13.4
50-54	73 721	5.66 ± 0.99 (218.9 ± 38.4)	132.4 ± 16.8	84.8 ± 10.6	32.7	26.7 ± 13.4
55-57	33 017	5.67 ± 0.99 (219.1 ± 38.3)	134.9 ± 17.8	84.7 ± 10.7	29.4	25.3 ± 12.9
Total	316 099	5.55 ± 1.01 (214.7 ± 39.1)	129.7 ± 15.6	83.7 ± 10.5	35.9	27.0 ± 13.3

*MRFIT indicates Multiple Risk Factor Intervention Trial; BP, blood pressure.

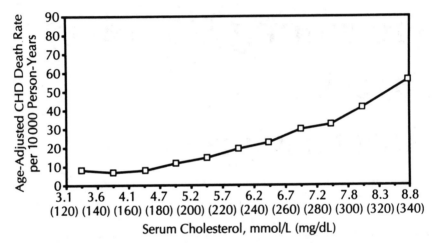

No. Men:	4313	14 118	37 514	58 720	69 343	56 106	37 619	21 577	9429	4200	3160
No. Deaths:	34	104	323	790	1210	1294	1042	761	367	202	200

Fig. 1-1. Age-adjusted coronary heart disease (CHD) death rates per 10000 person-years by level of serum cholesterol for men screened in the Multiple Risk Factor Intervention Trial. Reproduced with permission from Neaton JD and Wentworth D[1]

than diastolic BP. These results, together with the findings of clinical trials, offer strong support for intensified preventive efforts in all age groups.

In symptomatic peripheral arterial disease

Different patterns of risk factors might be related to the involvement of specific vascular districts by atherosclerosis. In this sense, many investigations have addressed CAD, whereas extracoronary atherosclerosis has received less extensive attention. Vigna and co-workers[2] in Padua, Italy, evaluated vascular risk factors, with particular attention to lipid parameters by means of univariate and multivariate analysis in a group of 169 patients (128 men and 41 women; mean ages 58 ± 7 and 62 ± 7 years, respectively) with clinically and angiographically demonstrated athero-

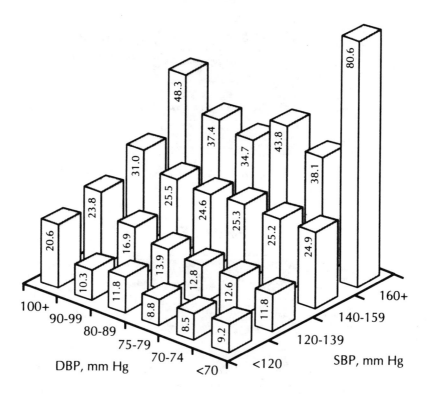

Fig. 1-2. Age-adjusted coronary heart disease death rates per 10000 person-years by level of systolic blood pressure (SBP) and diastolic blood pressure (DBP) for men screened in the Multiple Risk Factor Intervention Trial. Reproduced with permission from Neaton JD and Wentworth D[1]

sclerosis of the supra-aortic trunk and/or lower limbs. Patients with CAD were excluded from this study. The control group consisted of 140 age- and sex-matched individuals. By univariate analysis, smoking was more closely associated with peripheral atherosclerosis, whereas blood pressure was higher in patients with supra-aortic disease. Unrecognized diabetes mellitus was a frequent finding in patients with peripheral disease. The percentage of hyperlipidemias was 4-fold higher in patients than in control subjects, with differences consisting of higher triglycerides and lower HDL concentrations. By discriminant analysis, high correct classification rates were achieved in the various patient subgroups on the basis of variables selected from the statistical function. In male patients with peripheral disease, the variables HDL, smoking, diastolic BP, uric acid, and glucose, yielded a correct classification in 90% of the cases; in female patients, smoking, total cholesterol/HDL, and body mass index gave a correct classification rate of 96% (Figure 1-3). In men with cerebral disease, the selected variables total cholesterol/HDL, diastolic blood pressure, and total cholesterol yielded a correct classification of 91%; in women uric acid, total cholesterol/HDL, and fibrinogen levels produced a correct classification rate of 89%. Risk profiles in atherosclerosis of the supra-aortic trunks and lower limbs seem to differ in relation to gender and circulatory district involved. The importance of lipid parameters, in particular

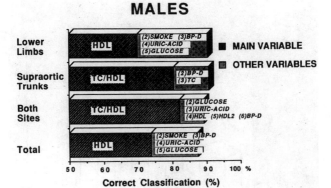

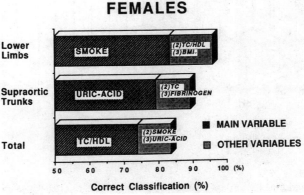

Fig. 1-3. Bar graphs showing variables selected by stepwise multiple discriminant analysis in order of decreasing importance (number in parentheses) and level of correct classification reached through them all and the main one separately. Patients subdivided according to sex and sites of vascular involvement. TC, total cholesterol; HDL, high density lipoprotein cholesterol; HDL2, HDL₂ cholesterol; BMI, body mass index; BP-D, diastolic blood pressure. Reproduced with permission from Vigna, et al.[2]

HDL and total cholesterol/HDL as extracoronary risk factor is further confirmed.

In high-risk pedigrees

Affected members of coronary pedigrees are at markedly increased risk for the development of clinical CAD. In an investigation carried out by Sharp and associates[3] from Salt Lake City, Utah, the relationship between the presence of coronary risk factors and the severity of angiographic CAD in 53 members of high-risk Utah pedigrees was examined. Mean angiographic severity scores were higher in familial hypercholesterolemia or familial low HDL cholesterol pedigrees than in type III hyperlipidemia or familial combined hyperlipidemia pedigrees. One sibling pair with hyperhomocysteinemia had the highest mean angiographic severity scores. Clinical CAD, increasing LDL cholesterol, and decreasing HDL cholesterol were significant predictors of angiographic CAD severity. There appeared to be an interaction between gender and body mass index but not between gender and serum lipids in the prediction of angiographic CAD severity. Results of the present study in members of high-risk Utah pedigrees are consistent with results from other angiographic studies in non-high-risk persons. Of particular interest is the suggested independent predictive value of low HDL cholesterol for angiographic CAD severity in members of high-risk pedigrees.

In low-risk populations (Seventh-Day Adventists)

California Seventh-Day Adventists have lower mortality rates from CAD than other Californians. Associations between traditional risk factor and CAD events have not been reported previously for Adventists. Fraser[4] and coworkers in Loma Linda, California, examined a cohort study that allowed 6 years of follow-up of 27,658 male and female California Seventh-Day Adventists. Data collected included age, sex, physician-diagnosed hypertension and diabetes mellitus, body height, weight, previous and current cigarette smoking habits, and current exercise habits. Incident cases of definite AMI and definite fatal CAD were diagnosed according to recognized criteria. Both stratified and proportional hazards analyses demonstrated that in this low-risk population, the above traditional coronary risk factors exhibit their usual associations with risk of CAD events. It was noted that exercise had a strong negative association with fatal CAD events but no association with risk of AMI. Conversely, obesity was much more clearly associated with AMI than with fatal events. The importance of the risk factors was similar in both sexes, except that the effect of cigarette smoking seemed more pronounced in women. The epidemiology of CAD in this low-risk California population appears to be at least qualitatively similar to that seen in other groups. There was evidence that the effects of exercise and obesity may differ depending on whether fatal CAD and AMI is the end point.

BLOOD LIPIDS

Cholesterol awareness

Data from the 44 states and the District of Columbia which participated in the CDC's Behavioral Risk Factor Surveillance System (BRFSS) during 1990, were analyzed by unidentified authors.[5] The BRFSS is a random-digit-dialed monthly telephone survey of persons aged ≥18 years. Respondents were asked whether they had ever had their cholesterol levels checked and, if so, whether they were told their cholesterol levels. Persons who reported having been told their levels were asked to state their levels; respondents who reported a level from 100–450 mg/dL were considered to know their levels. The results were weighted to account for the age, race, and sex distribution of each state population. In 1990, the percentage of adults who reported having had their cholesterol checked ranged from 48% in the District of Columbia to 70% in Rhode Island (median = 63%). The percentage of adults who had been told their cholesterol levels ranged from 29% in the District of Columbia to 58% in Washington and New Hampshire (median 48%), and those who knew their levels ranged from 12% in the District of Columbia to 37% in Rhode Island and New Hampshire (median = 29%).

To determine whether cholesterol-related knowledge and behavior and plasma cholesterol levels were stable until the inception of large-scale national interventions in the mid to late 1980s, whether they subsequently improved, and whether these levels varied by subgroups, Frank and associates[6] from Palo Alto, California, collected data from 4,173 adults aged 25–74 years in 2 cities (San Luis Obispo and Modesto, California) of the Stanford Five-City Project. Five separate, community-based surveys were conducted in 1979–1980, 1981–1982, 1983–1984, 1985–1986, and 1989–1990. Cholesterol-related knowledge and behavior and plasma cholesterol levels improved in both cities after the early 1980s. Those who were more educated, female, older, or nonsmokers had significantly higher knowledge and behavior scores, and those who were younger, less educated, or normotensive had significantly lower plasma cholesterol levels. Improvements in this population's cholesterol-related knowledge and behavior and plasma cholesterol levels began in 1985–1986, suggesting that the extensive cholesterol interventions that began in the middle 1980s in the United States created positive cholesterol-related changes at the community level.

In young military cadets in Spain

Casasnovas and associates[7] from Zaragoza, Spain, studied 572 young cadets from their local military academy in 2 different situations. On admission to the academy, apparently at a mean age of 20 years, when physical activity was very intense (A) and after 8 months, by which time they had all received identical diets and physical activity was considerably reduced (B). On both occasions they were asked about their smoking habits and their personal and family histories. Their height and weight were recorded and a sample of venous blood was taken to determine the lipid, biochemical and hematological profiles. The authors found that more smokers had a family history of sudden death or AMI than the non-smokers. The smokers also showed a lower HDL cholesterol level (54 ± mg/dl ± SD) than the non-smokers (59 ± 11) and a higher level of triglycerides (75 ± 25 mg/dl) than the non-smokers (65 ± 21 mg/dl). The lipid profile of the whole population showed a significant deterioration in the second extraction (B): the total cholesterol increased from 146 ± 3 mg/dl (in A) to 166 ± 28 mg/dl (in B), the LDL cholesterol increased from 75 ± 26 mg/dl (in A) to 95 ± 27 mg/dl (in B), the HDL cholesterol decreased from 61 ± 12 mg/dl (in A) to 58 ± 11 mg/dl (in B) and the triglycerides increased from 55 ± 18 mg/dl (in A) to 68 ± 23 mg/dl (in B). The lipid profile of the military cadets is less favorable in situation B with moderate physical exercise than in A with intensive physical activity. Young smokers show a less favorable lipid profile and an increased white cell count, hematocrit and hemoglobin value when compared with non-smokers.

In the elderly

The Bronx Aging Study is a 10-year prospective investigation of very elderly volunteers (mean age at study entry, 79 years; range, 75–85 years) designed to assess risk factors for dementia and coronary and cerebrovascular (stroke) diseases. Entry criteria included the absence of terminal illness and dementia. Zimetbaum and associates[8] from Bronx, New York, analyzed 350 subjects from the Bronx Aging Study who had at least 2 lipid and lipoprotein determinations. Overall, more than a third of subjects showed at least a 10% change in lipid and lipoprotein levels between the initial and final measurements (Table 1-2). Moreover, mean levels for women were consistently different than those for men, and because of this finding subjects were classified into potential-risk categories based on the changes observed by using their sex-specific lipid and lipoprotein distributions. The incidences of cardiovascular disease, dementia, and death were compared between risk groups. Proportional-hazards analysis showed that in men a consistently low HDL cholesterol level (≤30 mg/dl) was independently associated with the development of AMI, cardiovascular disease, or death. For women, however, a consistently elevated LDL cholesterol level (≥171 mg/dl) was associated with AMI. Thus, low HDL cholesterol remains a powerful predictor of CAD risk for men even into old age, while elevated LDL cholesterol continues to play a role in the development of AMI in women. The findings suggest that an unfavorable lipoprotein profile increases the risk of cardiovascular morbidity and mortality even at advanced ages for both men and women.

To assess the proportion of community-dwelling adults aged ≥65 years who are eligible for referral for lipoprotein analysis and intervention according to the National Cholesterol Education Program (NCEP) guidelines, Manolio and associates[9] for the Cardiovascular Health Study Collaborative Research Group performed a cross-sectional study based on examinations and questionnaires collected in 1989 and 1990 in 4 communities in the USA. A sample of 4,810 men and women aged 65 to 100 randomly selected and recruited from the Health Care Financing Administration Medicare eligibility lists for the 4 communities were studied. The subjects were not institutionalized, they were not wheelchair-bound, they were not currently receiving therapy for cancer, they were not currently taking lipid-lowering medications, and they had not eaten in the 9 hours prior to drawing blood for the cholesterol studies. Total cholesterol levels were <5.17 mmol/L (200 mg/dL) in 37% of participants, 5.17 to 6.19 mmol/L (200 to 239 mg/dL) in 39%, and 6.20 mmol/L (240 mg/dL) or greater in 24% (Figure 1-4, Table 1-3). Compared with their counterparts, older participants, especially those over 80 years of age, were more likely to have levels below 5.17 mmol/L, as were men, nonwhites, and those with CAD or 2 or more CAD risk factors. Based on this screening measurement, 2,174 participants were eligible for lipoprotein analysis, 80% were eligible for dietary or drug therapy using NCEP guidelines. Overall, 46% of Cardio-

TABLE 1-2.   *Baseline Distribution of Lipid and Lipoproteins by Gender. Reproduced with permission from Zimetbraum, et al.*[8]

	Mean	Median	75%	Tertile		
				1st	2nd	3rd
HDL cholesterol						
Men	38.1±12.1	37	45	0–30	31–40	≥41
Women	46.5±13.8	46	55	0–40	41–50	≥51
LDL cholesterol						
Men	140.5±37.4	139	159	0–130	131–150	≥151
Women	157.8±39.2	157	184	0–150	151–170	≥171
Triglycerides						
Men	137.9±69.4	120	172	0–101	102–153	≥154
Women	134.7±77.4	111	161	0–95	96–137	≥138
Cholesterol*						
Men	206.8±40.2	203	228	0–220	≥221	
Women	234.2±44.3	235	263	0–250	≥251	

All values are in milligrams per deciliter.
*Cholesterol levels were divided into two groups by using only one cut point, following the example of the National Cholesterol Education Program guidelines, but specific to the gender distribution of the Bronx Aging Study.

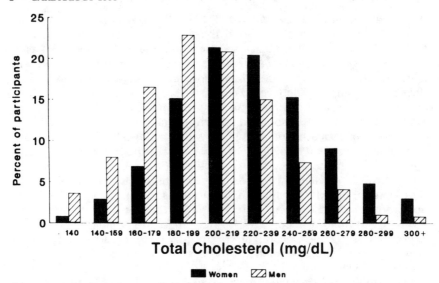

Fig. 1-4. Comparison of total cholesterol levels in men and women participating in the Cardiovascular Health Study. To convert data to mmol/L, multiply by 0.02586. Reproduced with permission from Manolio, et al.[9]

TABLE 1-3. *Characteristics of Cardiovascular Health Study Participants in Relation to Total Cholesterol Levels and Proportion Needing Lipoprotein Analysis. Reproduced with permission from Manolio, et al.*[9]

Characteristic	Patients	Total Cholesterol Levels			Proportion Needing Lipoprotein Analysis*
		< 5.17 mmol/L	5.17 to 6.19 mmol/L	≥ 6.20 mmol/L	
	n	←———————— % ————————→			%(95% CI)
Age, *y*					
65 to 69	1673	34	39	27	47 (45 to 50)
70 to 74	1492	36	40	25	47 (44 to 49)
75 to 79	987	38	40	22	45 (42 to 49)
80 to 84	472	40	40	20	43 (38 to 47)
≥ 85	186	48	34	18	40 (33 to 47)
Gender					
Men	2092	51	36	13	41 (38 to 43)
Women	2718	26	42	33	50 (48 to 52)
Race					
White	4555	36	39	24	46 (45 to 48)
Non-white	255	45	35	20	42 (36 to 48)
Education, *y*					
≤ 12	2689	36	39	25	49 (47 to 51)
> 12	2121	38	40	23	42 (40 to 44)
Definite coronary heart disease					
Absent	3813	36	40	24	42 (41 to 43)
Present	1006	40	36	23	60 (57 to 63)
Two risk factors					
Absent	2350	32	41	27	33 (31 to 35)
Present	2460	41	37	21	59 (57 to 61)
Coronary heart disease or two risk factors					
Absent	1979	31	42	27	27 (25 to 29)
Present	2831	41	37	22	59 (57 to 61)

* The Adult Treatment Panel has recommended that lipoprotein analysis be done in all patients with high cholesterol levels confirmed by repeat measurement, as well as in those with borderline-high levels confirmed by repeat measurement plus definite coronary heart disease or two risk factors.

vascular Health Study (CHS) participants were eligible for lipoprotein analysis and 36% for intervention by NCEP guidelines, based on a single cholesterol measurement. A substantial proportion of older adults in this community sample were eligible for lipoprotein analysis and intervention.

Cardiovascular disease is the leading cause of death and disability in older people. There is little information about the distributions of risk factors in older populations. In order to describe the distribution and correlates of lipoprotein lipids in people >65 years old, Ettinger and co-workers[10] in Winston-Salem, North Carolina, measured lipoprotein lipid concentrations in 2,106 men and 2,732 women who were participants in the Cardiovascular Health Study, a population-based epidemiological study. Distributions of lipids by age and sex and bivariate and multivariate relations among lipids and other variables were determined in cross-sectional analyses. The total cholesterol to HDL cholesterol ratios were: male 4.5 and female 4.1. Triglycerides, total cholesterol and LDL cholesterol concentrations were lower with increasing age, the last more evident in men than in women. Total triglyceride concentration was possibly associated with obesity (in women), central fat patterning, glucose intolerance, use of beta blockers (in men), and use of estrogens (in women) and negatively associated with age, renal function alcohol use, and socioeconomic status. In general, HDL cholesterol had opposite relations with these variables, except that estrogen use was associated with higher HDL cholesterol concentrations. LDL cholesterol concentration was associated with far fewer variables than the other lipids but was negatively associated with age in men and women and positively correlated with obesity and central fat patterning and negatively correlated with renal function and estrogen use in women. There were no differences in total cholesterol and LDL cholesterol concentrations among participants with and without prevalent CAD and stroke, but triglyceride concentration was higher and HDL cholesterol lower in men with both CAD and stroke and in women with CAD. Cholesterol and cholesterol/HDL ratio were lower and HDL cholesterol higher than previously reported values in older people, suggesting that lipid risk profiles may be improving in older Americans. Triglyceride and HDL cholesterol concentrations, and to a lesser extent LDL cholesterol, were associated with potentially important modifiable factors such as obesity, glucose intolerance, renal function, and medication use.

In the Edinburgh population

A higher than expected number of violent deaths and suicides in coronary prevention trials has provoked interest in the possibility that low serum cholesterol concentrations are associated in the general population with personality characteristics predisposing to aggressive and suicidal behavior. Fowkes and associates[11] from Edinburgh, UK, investigated this possibility in the Edinburgh Artery Study. They measured serum lipid concentrations in blood samples taken from fasting subjects and assessed personality characteristics on the Bedford Foulds Personality Deviance Scales in a random sample of 1,592 men and women aged 55–74 years, selected from age-sex registers of 10 general practices in Edinburgh. Serum cholesterol concentration was not significantly associated with aggression in men, but it was associated in multivariate analysis (though not univariate analysis) with denigratory attitudes towards others among women. However, serum triglyceride concentration was related, especially in men, to hostile acts and domineering attitude independently of age, total and HDL cholesterol, cigarette smoking, and alcohol consumption. Subjects taking part in prevention trials have higher triglyceride concentrations than the general population and the relation between serum triglyceride concentration and aggression merits further investigation.

Usefulness of one measurement

Hetland and associates[12] from Glostrup, Denmark, investigated how well a single or double measurement of serum total cholesterol represents the spontaneous, future level in a particular person. The spontaneous fluctuations in serum total cholesterol levels in 169 healthy early post-menopausal women were followed during the course of 12 years. The initial measurement and the long-term level of serum total cholesterol were highly related. The long-term level (calculated for each woman as the area under the curve of serum total cholesterol versus time) was not statistically significantly different from the initial level (mean difference: 0.036 ± 0.046 mmol/L [mean ± SEM], NS). The initial serum total choles-terol level was then used to classify each woman into a high or a low cholesterol group, according to the current recommendations. The pre-dictive value of an initial total cholesterol value in the high level (≥ 6.2 mmol/L) group was 84%, when compared with the long-term level. The predictive value of an initial total cholesterol level below 6.2 mmol/L was 80%. No improvement in these parameters was found when the average of the initial 2 (or 3, when the difference exceeded 9.9 mmol/L) measure-ments were used as the baseline value. The fluctuations in serum total cholesterol levels were mainly due to short-term variations. For screening purposes, 1 measurement of serum total cholesterol do not improve the predictability of future cholesterol levels. The data also suggest that, at least in postmenopausal women with an elevated level of serum total cholesterol, 1 should proceed immediately to lipoprotein analysis for further risk assessment.

Very high high-density lipoprotein

Little is known about individuals who have very high values of serum HDL cholesterol with the exception of those who have very rare genetic conditions, such as familial hyperalphalipoproteinemia or hypobetalipo-proteinemia. During 60 months of testing for HDL cholesterol, Weitzman and Vladutiu[13] found 46 individuals (of whom 43 were women) who had an HDL cholesterol ≥100 mg/dl (range 100–238 mg/dl). Sixteen individuals were treated with estrogens or rantidine or were alcoholic, and several had evidence of CAD. The authors concluded that very high levels of HDL cholesterol can be found in the general population but mostly in women and that it was often related to environmental causes such as the use of H_2-blockers, estrogens, and alcohol. The finding of very elevated HDL cholesterol levels in serum is probably not always due to a genetic con-dition and does not always signify absence of CAD and increased life expectancy.

Lipoprotein (a)

A fine review of lipoprotein(a) was provided by Rader and Brewer[14] in the February 16, 1992, *Journal of the American Medical Association*. The authors concluded that it might be useful to determine plasma LP(a) in patients with or at risk for premature atherosclerotic cardiovascular disease, especially if pharmacologic therapy for elevated LDL cholesterol or other dyslipoproteinemia is indicated. In such cases, the authors rec-ommended that strong consideration should be given to including nico-tinic acid as part of the pharmacologic regimen. The authors cautioned that drugs still need to be developed that are targeted specifically against

LP(a), and prospective trials are still needed to confirm the efficacy of reducing LP(a) in preventing CAD.

Sorrentino and associates[15] from Chicago, Illinois, measured plasma lipoprotein(a) protein levels prior to coronary angiography in 127 white and 111 black patients. Each angiogram was given a total CAD score based on the number and severity of atherosclerotic coronary narrowings. White and black patients had no differences in total plasma cholesterol, HDL cholesterol, LDL cholesterol, or triglycerides. Black patients had higher lipoprotein (a) protein levels than white patients (8.6 versus 4.0 mg/dL). The extent and severity of CAD was the same in both white and black patients. White and black patients with CAD had higher lipoprotein (a) levels than patients without CAD (4.37 versus 1.99 mg/dL). In both groups, there was a weak but significant positive correlation between lipoprotein (a) protein levels and CAD score. Thus, lipoprotein(a) is higher in patients with CAD. Black patients have higher plasma lipoprotein(a) protein levels than white patients and a comparable degree of CAD.

Averna and associates[16] from Palermo, Italy, evaluated plasma lipid, apoprotein and Lp(a) levels in patients with severe CAD undergoing CABG and related these parameters to the involvement of 1 or more coronary arteries by severe narrowing. Seventy-seven males and seventy-seven car-diovascular disease-free controls, matched for sex, age, and body weight were studied. Higher triglyceride and apo B levels with lower HDL-choles-terol and apo A-I levels were found in CABG patients in comparison with the controls. Lp(a) levels were slightly, but not significantly, increased. Moreover CABG patients presented a significantly higher prevalence of HDL-cholesterol levels below 35 mg dl^{-1} (49.3% vs 22.1%) and Lp(a) levels above 70 mg/dl (10.4% vs 1.3%) than the controls. When patients were divided according to the number of coronary arteries involved, no signifi-cant difference was found, with a trend to increase in Lp(a) mean levels and in prevalence of Lp(a) levels above 30 and 70 mg/dl in more severely diseased patients. These results suggest that patients with severe CAD undergoing CABG show low HDL-cholesterol levels with high triglyceride levels. Moreover Lp(a) levels above 70 mg dl^{-1} are highly associated with severe CAD.

Although serum lipoprotein(a) is an independent risk factor for athero-sclerosis in the general population and lipoprotein(a) levels are increased in hemodialysis patients, and association of LP(a) with the risk of clinical events attributed to atherosclerosis has not been established in the chronic hemodialysis patient population. Cressman and co-investiga-tors[17] in Cleveland, Ohio, determined the association between lipopro-tein(a) levels and the risk of clinical events of presumed atherosclerotic etiology in a prospective study of an outpatient hemodialysis population. LP(a) was measured by radioimmunoassay in a baseline cardiovascular disease risk assessment in a consecutive series of 129 hemodialysis pa-tients. The relation between baseline lipoprotein(a) and clinical events of presumed atherosclerotic etiology was determined during 48 months of follow-up. Hemodialysis patients had a median LP(a) concentration that was approximately 4 times as high as the median concentration in normal controls and twice as high as the levels in controls with angiographic evidence of CAD. Baseline LP(a) levels were no different in participants with or with no history of a previous clinical event at the time of the baseline examination. Baseline LP(a) concentration and a history of ath-erosclerotic clinical events were associated with clinical events during the period of follow-up. In contrast, baseline serum total cholesterol, triglyceride, HDL cholesterol, LDL cholesterol, age, gender, race, or duration of hemodialysis were unrelated to this risk in the prospective study. Stepwise multiple logistic regression analysis demonstrated that serum LP(a) concentration and the presence of a previous clinical event were the only independent contributors to the risk of a clinical event during the period of follow-up. LP(a) is an independent risk factor for clinical events attributed to atherosclerotic cardiovascular disease in patients receiving chronic hemodialysis treatment of end-stage renal disease.

Studies in patients undergoing liver transplantation suggest that LP(a) is synthesized in the liver. To determine the influence of liver disease on lipoprotein(a) concentrations, Feely and associates[18] from Dublin, UK, compared concentrations of LP(a) in patients with varying degrees of severity of hepatic disease, controls, and patients with established CAD. Thirty patients with histologically diagnosed cirrhosis were matched for age and sex with healthy controls and patients with established CAD, all with normal liver function. Cirrhosis was secondary to chronic alcohol intake in 24 patients, to chronic active hepatitis in 5, and hemochromatosis in 1. The LP(a) concentrations were raised in the patients with established CAD and reduced in the patients with cirrhosis. A low concentration of LP(a) may be 1 reason why patients with cirrhosis are less prone to have CAD (Figure 1-5).

Prognostic value of apolipoproteins

Kwiterovich and associates[19] from Baltimore, Maryland, examined the predictors of premature CAD in 203 patients (99 men aged ≤50 years, and 104 women aged ≤60 years) undergoing elective diagnostic coronary angiography. Age, cigarette smoking, hypertension, obesity, diabetes, positive family history of premature CAD, and plasma levels of total cholesterol, triglyceride, lipoproteins (i.e., very low, intermediate-, LDL-, and HDL and their subfractions [HDL$_2$ and HDL$_3$], and lipoprotein [a]) and apolipoproteins (apo A-1, apo A-2 and apo B, respectively) were examined using univariate analyses and multivariate logistic regression. In men, age, smoking, and plasma triglyceride and apo A-1 levels were independently associated with CAD (Figure 1-6). In women, smoking and plasma apo B levels were the strongest variables independently associated with CAD. It is concluded that the "nontraditional" risk factors (plasma apo A-1 and apo B levels) are better predictors of premature CAD than are plasma lipoproteins and that smoking is the strongest of the traditional nonlipid risk factors.

Some studies have suggested that measurements of apolipoproteins may be valuable in the clinical assessment of susceptibility to CAD, over and above the lipoprotein levels. Only a few of these studies have been prospective in nature and further knowledge is therefore needed to clarify the issue. Sigurdsson and associates[20] from Reykjavik, Iceland, estimated the independent prognostic value of apolipoproteins (apo-B, apo-A1 and apo[a]) with regard to CAD from a prospective survey among 1,332 randomly selected Icelandic men, aged 45 to 72 years, participating in a health survey from 1979 to 1981. The group was followed for 8.6 years, and during that period 104 men had fatal or nonfatal AMI. The Cox's proportional hazards model was used to estimate the significance of independent variables. The results of multivariate analysis showed that apo(a) was a significant independent risk factor (odds ratio 1.22 for 1 SD), but apo-A1 was a stronger negative risk factor (odds ratio 0.70 for 1 SD). Apo-B was a highly significant risk factor in a univariate analysis, but not in a multivariate analysis when serum cholesterol was included. Previous

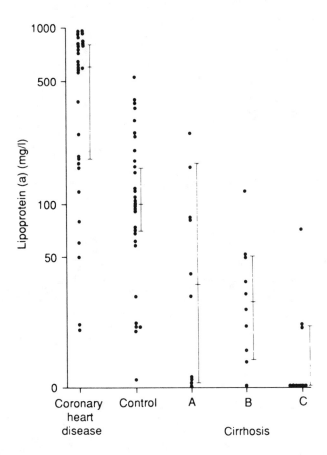

Fig. 1-5. Lipoprotein(a) concentrations (median and 95% confidence intervals) in matched patients with coronary heart disease, controls, and patients with varying degrees of cirrhosis (Child's stage A-C), Coronary heart disease>control>cirrhosis (p<0.01) Reproduced with permission from Feely, et al.[18]

population surveys in Iceland have confirmed the importance of cigarette smoking, cholesterol, triglycerides, and BP as risk factors for CAD. The present results illustrate additional importance of apo-A1 and apo(a) concentrations in predicting CAD among Icelandic men, whereas apo-B did not contribute anything further to the prediction than serum total cholesterol.

Usefulness of parental levels in identifying children with hypercholesterolemia

It was hypothesized that healthy children with high cholesterol levels may have parents who exceed acceptable cholesterol levels established by the National Cholesterol Education Program. Accordingly, Benuck and associates[21] from Chicago, Illinois, evaluated 160 families (320 parents, 263 children aged 3 to 10 years) for total cholesterol and other risk factors. Before the study, almost half of the parents had not had serum total cholesterol measured. The odds ratio for a child having a total cholesterol ≥5.17 mmol/L (200 mg/dl) was 13.6:1 (confidence interval 5.7 to 32.5) for

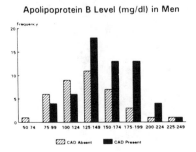

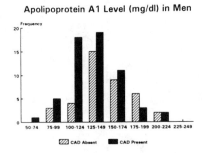

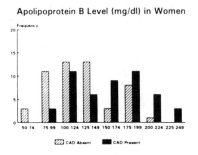

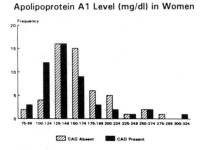

Fig. 1-6. The distribution of plasma levels of apolipoproteins B (left) and A-1 (right) in men (top) and women (bottom) with (black bars) and without (crossed-hatched bars) coronary artery disease (CAD). Reproduced with permission from Kwiterovich, et al.[19]

a child with at least 1 parent having cholesterol ≥6.20 mmol/L (240 mg/dl) versus a child whose parents had low total cholesterol. Testing only children who had at least 1 parent with a total cholesterol ≥5.17 mmol/L (200 mg/dl) had a sensitivity of 98% for detecting children's total cholesterol ≥5.17 mmol/L. It is concluded that parental total cholesterol is useful in identifying children with high total cholesterol levels. Pediatricians may identify a large number of parents with hypercholesterolemia not previously recognized.

Relation of hypertriglyceridemia to coronary artery disease

Grundy and Vega[22] from Dallas, Texas, analyzed 2 different views to explain the link between hypertriglyceridemia and CAD. First, triglyceridemia-rich lipoproteins, particularly VLDL, may be directly atherogenic (Figure 1-7). Or second, the metabolic consequences of hypertriglyceridemia may account for the triglyceride-CAD relation (Figure 1-8). These consequences include an increase in postprandial lipoproteins, large VLDL particles, small, dense LDL particles, low levels of HDL cholesterol, and possibly a procoagulant state. The appropriate treatment of hypertriglyceridemia depends on which of these views is nearer the truth. If triglyceride-rich lipoproteins are directly atherogenic, then the preferred therapy would be hepatic hydroxymethylglutaryl coenzyme A reductase inhibitors, which lower both VLDL and LDL levels. On the other hand, if the link to atherogenesis is through the metabolic consequences of hypertriglyceridemia, the appropriate therapy would be to directly lower serum triglyceride levels, as with niacin or a fibric acid. Thus, discovery of the mechanism of the connection between triglycerides and CAD is crucial for developing a rational therapy.

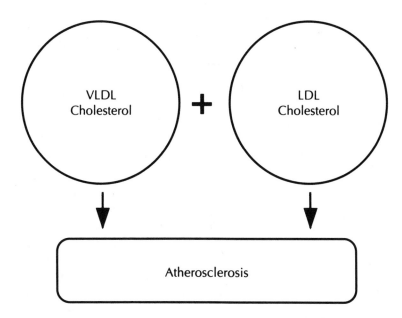

Fig. 1-7. One view of the relationship of serum triglycerides to atherosclerosis (and coronary heart disease). According to this view, cholesterol of triglyceride-rich very-low-density lipoprotein (VLDL) has a similar atherogenic potential to low-density lipoprotein (LDL) cholesterol. Consequently, the VLDL + LDL cholesterol may be a better indicator of coronary heart disease risk than LDL alone. Reproduced with permission from Grundy SM and Vega GI.[22]

Effects of drugs

To examine the available published reports on commonly prescribed drugs and their effects on blood lipid and lipoprotein levels, Henkin and associates[23] from Birmingham, Alabama, searched English-language articles from 1975–1990 and found more than 500 articles for inclusion in their analysis. Articles were selected on the basis of appropriateness of design to demonstrate significant results. The studies were classified according to type (observational or interventional), length of follow-up, and type of controls. Quantitative analysis of lipid, lipoprotein, and apoprotein changes induced by drugs was computed as the percentage of change observed during the course of the study (interventional) or compared with the controls at a given time (observational) (Figure 1-9) (Table 1-4). Steroid hormones that have strong progestogenic and androgenic properties, retinoids, cyclosporine A, and phenothiazines are potentially atherogenic. Steroid hormones with dominant estrogenic properties, several anticonvulsants, biguanides, high-dose ketoconazole, and aminosalicyclic acid are potentially antiatherogenic. Corticosteroids appear to elevate all the lipoprotein cholesterol levels. Oral estrogens, retinoids, and corticosteroids also can elevate triglyceride levels. Other drugs with questionable effects on lipoprotein metabolism are reviewed. Although the long-term implications of drug-induced lipoprotein changes are still undefined, physicians need to consider these effects in clinical practice.

To evaluate the differential effects of B-blockers on serum lipids and apolipoproteins in normolipidemic and dyslipidemic hypertensive pa-

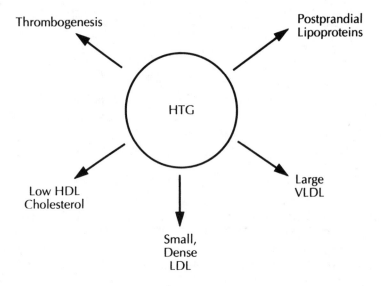

Fig. 1-8. Possible atherogenic processes accompanying hypertriglyceridemia. These include increased postprandial lipoproteins, increased levels of large very-low-density lipoprotein (VLDL) particles, the presence of small, dense low-density lipoprotein (LDL) particles, low high-density lipoprotein (HDL)-cholesterol levels, and changes in the coagulation system that may predispose to thrombogenesis. All of these secondary changes may heighten risk for coronary artery disease. HTG indicates hypertriglyceridemia. Reproduced with permission from Grundy SM and Vega GL.[22]

tients, Vyssoulis and associates[24] from Athens, Greece, studied 330 patients with mild to moderate essential hypertension 1 month after placebo therapy and 6 months after monotherapy with propranolol (n = 53), atenolol (n = 66), metoprolol (n = 58), pindolol (n = 53), or celiprolol (n = 100). Serum total cholesterol, triglycerides, HDL cholesterol, LDL cholesterol, and apolipoproteins (Apo) A, and B were measured at baseline and study end. A total of 136 (41.2%) patients were considered normolipidemic (pretreatment LDL cholesterol <160 mg/dl[1]) and 194 (59%) were considered dyslipidemic (LDL cholesterol >160 mg/dl). Changes in total cholesterol differed between normolipidemics and dyslipidemics with propranolol (+13% in normolipidemics vs −0.5% in dyslipidemics), atenolol (+7% vs p−2%), metoprolol (+9% vs −4%), and celiprolol (+9% vs −4%); none of these changes between normolipidemic and dyslipidemic patients were statistically significant. LDL cholesterol changes differed the most, with propranolol (+35% vs −1%), atenolol (+15% vs −4%), metoprolol (+12% vs −6%), pindolol (+12% vs −13%), and celiprolol (+3% vs −16%). No overall differences between normolipidemic and dyslipidemic patients were observed for triglycerides and APO A, while changes in Apo B differed to a degree with propranolol (+23% vs +18%), atenolol (−1% vs +4%), metoprolol (+13% vs +1%), pindolol (+14% vs −7%), and celiprolol (−10% vs −8%). Patient age did not influence overall serum lipid changes. It is concluded that older non-cardioselective B-blockers, such as propranolol, have significant dyslipidemic effects, particularly in normolipidemic hypertensive patients. Cardioselective B-blockers, such as atenolol and metoprolol and non-selective agents with partial

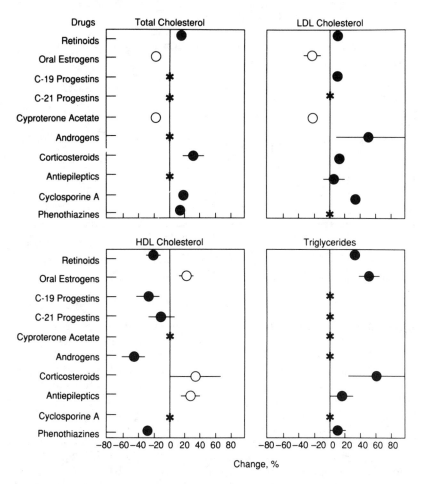

Fig. 1-9. Summary of the estimated lipid and lipoprotein levels associated with selected nonantihypertensive drugs. Asterisks indicate no significant average effect; horizontal lines, the range of changes described in clinical trials; open circles, the median of these changes that might be interpreted as antiatherogenic; closed circles, the median of these changes that might be interpreted as atherogenic; LDL, low-density lipoprotein; and HDL, high-density lipoprotein. Reproduced with permission from Henkin, et al.[23]

agonist activity such as pindolol, have milder effects. Newer cardioselective ß-blockers with partial agonist activity, such as celiprolol, have favorable lipid effects, particularly in dyslipidemic hypertensive patients.

Effects of testosterone

To investigate the role of physiologic levels of testosterone in the control of lipoproteins in healthy men, Bagatell and associates[25] from Seattle, Washington, and La Jolla, California, performed a double-blind, randomized study of 15 healthy men aged 20–36 years. The authors induced acute, reversible hypogonadism in 5 normal men by administering daily subcutaneous injections of the gonadotropin-releasing-hormone (GnRH) antagonist, Nal-Glu, for 6 weeks. Another group of 5 normal men received Nal-Glu plus weekly injections of testosterone enanthate, 100

TABLE 1-4. *Various Drugs Reported to Affect Lipoprotein Levels.* Reproduced with permission from Henkin, et al.[23]

Agents	Total Cholesterol	LDL	HDL	VLDL	Triglyceride
Amiodarone[118,119]	↑	–	–	–	↑
Antacid[120-122]	↓	↓	↓ –	–	–
Ascorbic acid[123-128]	–	–	–	–	–
Aspirin[129-132]	–	–	–	–	↓ –
Biguanides[133-137]	↓	↓	–	–	↓
Cimetidine†/ranitidine[138-141]	–	–	↑ –	–	–
Interferons[142]	↓	↓	↓	↑	↑
Ketoconazole (high-dose)[143,144]	↓	↓	–	–	–
Neomycin[145,146]	↓	↓	–	–	–
Nicotinic acid/nicotinamide[159]‡	–	–	–	–	–
Nonsteroidal anti-inflammatory drugs[147,148]	–	–	–	–	–
Aminosalicylic acid[149,150]	↓	↓	–	–	↓
Sulfonylureas[151-158]	–	–	–	–	–

*LDL indicates low-density lipoprotein; HDL, high-density lipoprotein; VLDL, very-low-density lipoprotein; dashes, no substantial change, inconsistent results, or insufficient data; up arrow, increase; and down arrow, decrease.
†Only cimetidine showed increased high-density lipoprotein levels in some studies.
‡When used as a vitamin or as the amide derivative (nicotinamide), nicotinic acid has little effect on lipoprotein levels. However, in pharmacological doses, niacin increases high-density lipoprotein levels and reduces low-density lipoprotein and triglyceride levels.

mg/wk., thereby maintaining normal serum testosterone levels. Five additional men received placebo injections. Plasma lipids, including HDL subfractions HDL_2 and HDL_3, apoprotein A1, and serum levels of gonadotropins, estradiol, and testosterone were measured before, during, and after treatment. At the end of the treatment period, HDL cholesterol levels in men receiving Nal-Glu increased by 26%. Levels of HDL_2, HDL_3, and apoprotein A1 increased by 63%. Total cholesterol increased by 12%. LDL cholesterol and triglyceride concentrations did not change. No statistically significant changes occurred in any lipid measurement in men receiving Na1-Glu plus androgen replacement or placebo. Experimental hypogonadism induced by administration of a GnRH antagonist results in a statistically significant increase in HDL cholesterol, including HDL_2 and HDL_3. These effects are most likely due to decreased androgen levels because they are reversed by administration of antagonist together with testosterone. The results imply that androgen levels in the normal adult male range have a suppressive effect on HDL cholesterol concentration and may contribute to the increased risk for CAD in men.

Effects of cancer and chemotherapy

To assess cardiovascular risk factors over time in patients who received chemotherapy for disseminated testicular cancer and were apparently cured, Gietema and associates[26] from Groningen and Bilthoven, The Netherlands, studied 57 consecutive patients aged 16 to 43 years (mean 28) who received cisplatin-containing chemotherapy between 1978 and 1985. Serum total cholesterol and HDL cholesterol levels, body mass index (BP, kidney function, and hormonal status were monitored during follow-up after chemotherapy (follow-up 56–143 months [mean 88]). The body mass index and cholesterol values obtained 4 to 6 years after chemotherapy were compared with values from a sample of healthy, age-matched Dutch men; the cholesterol level was also compared with that of 31 patients treated with orchidectomy for stage I disease. The mean cholesterol level in patients at the start of chemotherapy was 3.96 ± 0.98 mmol/L [153 ±

38 mg/dL], increasing 4 to 6 years later to 6.12 ± 1.20 mmol/L [237 ± 46 mg/dL]); 49 of 57 patients had an elevated LDL cholesterol level (>3.4 mmol/L [130 mg/dL]), with a mean level of 4.47 ± 1.05 mmol/L [173 ± 41 mg/dL]. Compared with a sample of healthy Dutch men, the chemotherapy group had an elevated cholesterol level. At 4 to 6 years, the mean HDL cholesterol level was 0.76 ± 0.18 mmol/L [29 ± 7 mg/dL], which was low compared with that of the healthy Dutch men. The mean body mass index for all patients was 2.8% higher than expected 4 to 6 years after chemotherapy but was not higher than expected 7 to 10 years after chemotherapy. In addition to other known late side effects of chemotherapy in patients with testicular cancer, hypercholesterolemia and overweight might represent risk factors for cardiovascular disease in such patients, especially in those who are younger.

Buchwald[27] from Minneapolis, Minnesota, reasoned that prevention of tumor cell growth can be achieved by restricting either cholesterol availability or cholesterol synthesis. In-vivo and cell-culture experiments have shown that lowering the plasma cholesterol concentrations or intervening in the mevalonate pathway with 3-hydroxy-3-methylglutaryl (HMG) CoA reductase inhibitors decreases tumor growth. Currently prescribed doses of HMG-C-A reductase inhibitors given orally or continuously by an implantable infusion pump could achieve tumor therapeutic tissue concentrations of these agents. Buchwald's hypothesis is that cholesterol inhibition can inhibit tumor cell growth, can act as an adjuvant to cancer chemotherapy, and, possibly, can prevent carcinogenesis.

Effects on thromboxane biosynthesis

Increased platelet thromboxane A_2 production has been described in type IIa hypercholesterolemia. To verify the relevance of these capacity-related measurements to the actual rate of thromboxane A_2 biosynthesis in vivo, Davi and colleagues[28] in Rome, Italy studied the urinary excretion of its major enzymatic metabolites in 46 patients with type IIa hypercholesterolemia and 20 age-matched controls. Urinary 11-dehydro-thromboxane B_2 and 2,3-*dinor*-thromboxane B_2 were measured by previously validated radioimmunoassays. The excretion rate of 11-dehydro-thromboxane B_2 was significantly higher in patients than in controls, with metabolite excretion >2 standard deviations of the normal mean in 74% of the patients. Urinary thromboxane B_2 was significantly correlated with the threshold aggregating concentration of collagen and arachidonate and with agonist-induced platelet thromboxane B_2 production in vitro. Moreover, a statistically significant correlation was found between 11-dehydro-thromboxane B_2 excretion and total plasma cholesterol (Figure 1-10). The enzyme 3-hydroxy-3-methylglutaryl coenzyme A reductase inhibitor simvastatin (20 mg/day for 6 months) significantly reduced cholesterol levels by 22–28% and urinary thromboxane B_2 excretion by 32–42% in 10 patients. However, the reduction in the latter did not correlate with the reduction in the former and may have resulted from a nonspecific effect of simvastatin. Moreover, selective inhibition of platelet cyclooxygenase activity by low-dose aspirin was associated with cumulative inhibition of thromboxane B_2 excretion by approximately 70% in 6 patients. Thromboxane A_2 biosynthesis is enhanced in the majority of patients with type IIa hypercholesterolemia; this is, at least in part, a consequence of abnormal cholesterol levels, as suggested by the correlation between the 2. Low-dose aspirin can largely suppress increased metabolite excre-

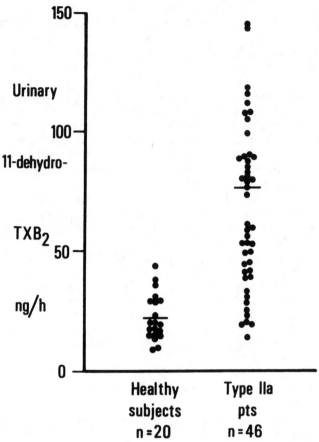

Fig. 1-10. Graph shows urinary excretion rates of 11-dehydro-thromboxane (TX)B$_2$ in healthy subjects and patients (pts) with type IIa hypercholesterolemia. Dots represent individual measurements; horizontal bar represents mean value for each group. Reproduced with permission from Davi, et al.[28]

tion, thus suggesting that it reflects thromboxane A$_2$-dependent platelet activation in vivo.

Relation to blood rheology

Recent studies have suggested that several hemostatic factors, leukocyte count, and plasma viscosity are predictive of CAD. Detailed analyses on lifestyle correlates, in particular plasma lipids and lipoproteins, of determinants of blood rheology have not been reported from epidemiologic studies. Koenig and co-workers[29] in Ulm, Germany, studied the relation between determinants of blood rheology and components of lipoproteins in a large sample of a population aged 25–64 years. The rheological parameters investigated were plasma viscosity, hemoglobin, and total serum protein; the lipoprotein variables included cholesterol, HDL, and the apoproteins A-I, A-II, and B. Covariables considered for possible confounding effects were age, body mass index, smoking behavior, alcohol consumption, and hypertension. Plasma viscosity was found to have a positive linear association with total cholesterol and apoprotein B, and a small negative linear association with HDL cholesterol and with apoprotein A-I. Polynomial regression showed a strong quadratic relation with HDL cholesterol in men, whereas no other variable revealed an appreciable deviation from linearity. The covariables had only a small, if any, confounding effect. Total serum protein, after control for the covariables, appeared to be associated only with total cholesterol. No association was found with hemoglobin. The investigators concluded that rheological mechanisms may be involved in the pathogenesis of ischemic syndromes in hyperlipidemias. However, the finding that in particular men with very low HDL cholesterol exhibit increased plasma viscosity cannot be explained in pure rheological terms but may be, at least in part, the result of concomitant hypertriglyceridemia. This was not assessed in this study.

Effects of mental stress and postural change

Serum lipid levels vary widely within individuals, but the causes of these fluctuations are poorly understood. One area of research concerns elevations in cholesterol concentration in response to emotional stress. In a laboratory-based experiment, Muldoon and associates[30] from Pittsburgh, Pennsylvania, compared the effects of acute mental stress and postural change (standing) on serum cholesterol concentration. In addition, plasma volume was indirectly monitored to determine whether cholesterol changes with mental stress, if present, were a function of hemoconcentration. Twenty-sic men attended 2 laboratory sessions, each consisting of baseline (30 minutes), task (20 minutes), and recovery (30 minutes) periods. Subjects rested in the supine position during the baseline and recovery periods. During the task period of 1 session, subjects performed a mental task (Stroop test and mental arithmetic); during the other session, the subjects stood for the task period. Both mental stress and standing elicited significant elevations in heart rate, BP, and plasma catecholamine concentrations, relative to the baseline and recovery periods. Both the mental and orthostatic tasks also significantly increased serum cholesterol concentration (by 0.10 and 0.57 mmol/L [3.7 and 21.9 mg/dL], respectively), as well as hemoglobin level and hematocrit. Cholesterol elevations with standing were reversible, while those resulting from mental stress persisted through the recovery period. When values were corrected for concomitant hemoconcentration, no net change in serum cholesterol level occurred during either task. Acute mental stress can produce rapid elevations in serum cholesterol concentration. It can also increase hemoglobin concentration and hematocrit (i.e., reduce plasma volume). Therefore, increases in serum cholesterol level after acute mental stress are analogous to those with standing and may reflect hemoconcentration rather than altered lipoprotein metabolism.

Effects of coffee

To determine the effect of filtered-coffee consumption on plasma lipoprotein cholesterol levels in healthy men, Fried and associates[31] from Baltimore, Maryland, performed a randomized control trial with an 8-week washout period followed by an 8-week intervention period during which men were randomly assigned to drink 720 mL/d of caffeinated coffee, 360 mL/d of caffeinated coffee, 720 mL/d of decaffeinated coffee, or no coffee. One hundred healthy male volunteers were studied. Men who consumed 720 mL of caffeinated coffee daily had mean increases in plasma levels of total cholesterol (0.24 mmol/L), LDL cholesterol (0.17

mmol/L), and HDL cholesterol (0.08 mmol/L). No significant changes in these plasma lipoprotein levels occurred in the other groups. Compared with the group who drank no coffee, the group who drank 720 mL/d of caffeinated coffee had increases in plasma levels of total cholesterol (0.25 mmol/L), LDL cholesterol (0.15 mmol/L), and HDL cholesterol, which appears to be due to increases of both LDL and HDL cholesterol levels.

In persons with coronary artery disease

To examine the concentration of serum lipoproteins and the association of their genetic variation with the occurrence of CAD, Nieminen and associates[32] from Helsinki, Finland, determined composite serum lipoprotein profiles including lipoprotein (a) (Lp[a]), apolipoprotein (apo) E phenotypes, and apo B Xba I genotypes in patients with angiographically verified CAD (CAD+ group, n = 111) and in subjects without angiographic evidence of CAD (CAD− group, n = 46) (Table 1-5). In addition, the authors determined the concentrations of serum lipids, lipoproteins, and apolipoproteins in 96 healthy controls. Both CAD− and CAD+ groups had lower concentrations of apos A-I and A-II but higher concentrations of serum total and very LDL triglyceride and very LDL cholesterol than did healthy controls. The mean concentrations of serum total and LDL cholesterol and the median values of Lp(a) were similar in the CAD+ and CAD− groups, both having higher concentrations of LDL cholesterol and apo B than the healthy controls. Irrespective of gender, patients with CAD had significantly lower serum HDL cholesterol than did those without CAD (1.48 ± 0.40 versus 1.16 ± 0.29 mmol/l). In women, the mean serum total and very LDL triglyceride concentration was also higher in the CAD+ than in the CAD− group. The frequency of the apo E4 allele (e4) was significantly higher in the CAD+ group (0.293) than in the CAD-group (0.174). The frequencies of the 2 apo B alleles, X1 (Xba I restriction site absent) and X2 (Xba I restriction site present), were similar in the 2 groups. Stepwise discriminant analysis revealed that in men, serum

TABLE 1-5. *Concentrations of Serum Lipids, Lipoproteins, and Apolipoproteins A-I, A-II, and B and Lipoprotein(a) in Patients With (CAD+) and Without (CAD−) Coronary Artery Disease and in Random Controls. Reproduced with permission from Nieminen, et al.[32]*

	Random controls			CAD− patients			CAD+ patients		
Constituent	Male (n=61)	Female (n=35)	All (n=96)	Male (n=23)	Female (n=23)	All (n=46)	Male (n=100)	Female (n=11)	All (n=111)
Serum cholesterol (mmol/l)	5.9±1.01	5.8±1.19*	5.9±1.07*	6.30±1.07	6.13±1.23	6.22±1.14	6.20±1.12	6.75±1.36	6.25±1.15
VLDL cholesterol (mmol/l)	0.33±0.28†,‡	0.19±0.14†,‡	0.28±0.25‡,§	0.63±0.67	0.34±0.21*	0.49±0.52‡	0.69±0.41	0.71±0.44	0.69±0.41
LDL cholesterol (mmol/l)	4.01±0.95*	3.89±1.1*	3.97±1.00‖	4.19±0.97	4.17±1.05	4.18±1.00	4.35±0.97	4.78±1.12	4.39±0.97
HDL cholesterol (mmol/l)	1.53±0.38‡	1.71±0.32†	1.59±0.37‡	1.38±0.38‖	1.60±0.40*	1.48±0.40‡	1.15±0.28	1.26±0.31	1.16±0.29
Serum triglyceride (mmol/l)	1.31±0.71†,‡	1.07±0.35†,¶	1.23±0.61‡,§	2.24±2.44	1.33±0.46‖	1.80±1.82‡	2.33±1.30	2.47±1.14	2.35±1.28
VLDL triglyceride (mmol/l)	0.74±0.60†,‡	0.46±0.22†,‡	0.64±0.51‡,§	1.50±2.06	0.72±0.34‖	1.12±1.53‡	1.61±1.14	1.57±1.05	1.60±1.13
Apo B (mg/dl)	101±25§,‖	90±22†,‡	97±25‡,§	135±40*	113±28	124±36	116±32	138±45	118±34
Apo A-I (mg/dl)	129.5±18.3‡,§	145.2±9.4†,‡	135.3±20.1‡,§	110.6±20.6*	124.9±22.4	117.6±22.4‡	101.0±19.7	115.7±21.5	102.5±20.3
Apo A-II (mg/dl)	35.4±6.0†,‡	35.7±7.4*,†	35.5±6.5‡,§	29.9±7.6*	29.8±6.3	29.8±6.9‖	26.2±5.1	30.6±5.6	26.6±5.3
Lp(a) (mg/dl)	152	111	149	101	222	148	128	177	135
	(16–861)	(16–919)	(16–919)	(16–590)	(16–1,327)	(16–1,327)	(16–3,133)	(31–2,230)	(16–3,133)

Values are mean ±SD. Lp(a) is given as a median, and the figures in parentheses indicate the range of Lp(a) concentration.
CAD, coronary artery disease; VLDL, very low density lipoprotein; LDL, low density lipoprotein; HDL, high density lipoprotein; Apo, apolipoprotein; Lp(a), lipoprotein(a).
*p<0.05, ‖p<0.01, ‡p<0.001 for differences from respective figures in patients with CAD.
¶p<0.05, †p<0.01, §p<0.001 for differences from respective figures in patients without CAD.

HDL cholesterol had the highest power to discriminate for CAD. In addition, the concentration of plasma apo B levels and the occurrence of apo E phenotypes were independently associated with CAD in men. In women, the only independent factor associated with CAD after adjustment for B-blocker and diuretics usage was the concentration of serum triglycerides.

Genetic lipoprotein disorders have been associated with premature CAD. Genest and co-workers[33] in Boston, Massachusetts, determined the prevalence of such factors in 102 kindreds (n = 603 subjects) in whom the proband had significant CAD documented by angiography before the age of 60 years. Fasting plasma cholesterol, triglyceride, LDL, apolipoprotein (apo) B, and lipoprotein (a) [Lp(a)] values above the 90th percentile and HDL cholesterol and apo A-I below the 10th percentile of age- and sex-specific norms were defined as abnormal. An abnormality was noted in 74% of probands compared with 38% in age-matched controls, with a low HDL cholesterol level (hypoalphalipoproteinemia) being the most common abnormality in 39% of cases. In these kindreds, 54% had a defined phenotypic familial lipoprotein or apolipoprotein disorder. The following frequencies were observed: Lp(a) excess, 19%; hypertriglyceridemia with hypoalphalipoproteinemia, 15%; combined hyperlipidemia, 14%; hyperapobetalipoproteinemia 5%; hypoalphalipoproteinemia, 4%; hypercholesterolemia 3%; hypertriglyceridemia, 1%; decreased apo lipoprotein A-I only, 1%. Overall, 54% of the probands had a familial dyslipidemia; unclassifiable lipid disorders were found in 3%. No identifiable familial dyslipidemia was noted in 43% of kindreds of those; nearly half (45%) had a sporadic lipid disorder. Parent-offspring and proband-spouse correlations for these biochemical variables revealed that lipoprotein and apolipoprotein levels are in part genetically determined, with Lp(a) showing the highest degree of parent-offspring correlation. These data indicated that more than half of patients with premature CAD have a familial lipoprotein disorder, with Lp(a) excess, hypertriglyceridemia with hypoalphalipoproteinemia, and combined hyperlipidemia with hypoalphalipoproteinemia being the most common abnormalities.

Lipid and lipoprotein profiles of CAD patients have usually not included data on HDL cholesterol, except in small groups, and have not included information on women. Both aspects are meaningful in the evaluation of patients for risk classification and for the importance of HDL cholesterol in dictating further evaluation. In the screening phase of a clinical trial, the investigators in the Bezafibrate Infarction Prevention Study Group[34] in Tel Hashomer, Israel obtained lipid and lipoprotein levels under Centers for Disease Control-standardized procedures in more than 6,700 men and 1,500 women ages 42–70 years. Mean total cholesterol was higher in women but changed little with age. Mean HDL cholesterol, however, progressively increased with age for both sexes (34 at age <50 years to 38 mg/dl at age 65 or older in men, and from 41 to 45 mg/dl for respective age groups in women). Triglycerides were lower in elderly groups, particularly in men. The number of previous infarctions, severity of CHF, and severity of angina were negatively correlated with mean HDL cholesterol in a dose-response manner, whereas the association with mean triglyceride was inverted, creating a mirror image of that observed with HDL cholesterol. More than half of patients with total cholesterol <200 mg/dl exhibited HDL cholesterol levels consistent with the accepted "high risk" range of <35 mg/dl, whereas an increasing percentage of desirable HDL cholesterol level was found with increasing levels of total cholesterol. These results provide previously unavailable information on the lipid profile of female patients and appear to strongly establish the case for obtaining all three standard blood lipid determinations (for instance, total cholesterol, HDL cholesterol, and triglycerides) in coronary patients as well as in the framework of detecting and classifying individuals at high risk for CAD.

Patients with CAD are at considerable risk for subsequent cardiovascular events. Although hyperlipidemia accentuates the risk, predictors of subsequent events with CAD and desirable total cholesterol have not been assessed. Miller and colleagues[35] in Baltimore, Maryland, performed a survival analysis in a subset of 740 consecutive patients who underwent diagnostic coronary arteriography between 1977 and 1978. Eighty-three men and 24 women with angiographically documented CAD and desirable total cholesterol (<5.2 mmol/l) were followed for subsequent cardiovascular events, including AMI and cardiovascular death. Over a 13-year period, 75% of CAD subjects with reduced HDL cholesterol developed a subsequent cardiovascular event compared with 45% of those with HDL cholesterol ≥0.9 mmol/l. A Kaplan-Meier analysis revealed significantly greater survival from cardiovascular end points in patients with baseline levels of HDL cholesterol ≥0.9 mmol/l (Figure 1-11). After 11 variables were tested, an age-adjusted Cox proportional-hazards model identified 2 pairs of independent predictors of subsequent cardiovascular events: they were a LV EF <35% and reduced HDL cholesterol in the first model and LV EF <35% and total cholesterol:HDL ratio ≥5.5 in the second model. Low HDL cholesterol (or high total cholesterol:HDL cholesterol) is strongly predictive of subsequent cardiovascular events in subjects with CAD, despite desirable total cholesterol. As such, identification of this potentially modifiable risk factor should be actively pursued in this high-risk subgroup.

Rubins and associates[36] from Boston, Massachusetts, Milwaukee, Wisconsin, and Minneapolis, Minnesota, obtained lipid profiles in 255 men

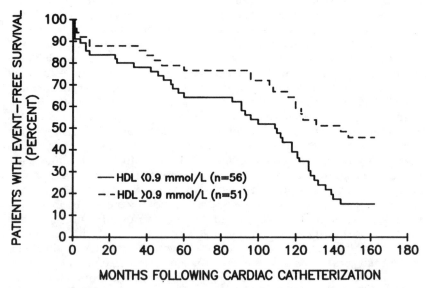

Fig. 1-11. Kaplan-Meier survival analysis comparing coronary artery disease patients with desirable total cholesterol and baseline high density lipoprotein (HDL) <0.9 mmol/l or ≥0.9 mmol/l. Peto and Peto's log-rank test indicates significant differences in event-free survival between the groups. Z = − 2.80; p = 0.005. Reproduced with permission from Miller, et al.[35]

(mean age 65 ± 9 years) with CAD in 3 Veterans Affairs medical centers. Desirable levels of lipids were defined according to National Cholesterol Education Program guidelines as follows: LDL cholesterol levels <130 mg/dL; HDL cholesterol levels ≥35 mg/dL, and triglyceride levels <2.83 mmol/L. Seventy-six percent of the group had 1 or more abnormalities on lipid profile: 51% had high LDL cholesterol levels with or without abnormalities of HDL cholesterol and/or triglyceride levels; 22% had low HDL cholesterol levels with desirable levels of LDL cholesterol, and 3% had hypertriglyceridemia without any cholesterol abnormalities. Normal lipid profiles were significantly more prevalent in subjects over the age of 65 years than in younger patients (40% vs 14%). These data suggest that (1) a high proportion of men with CAD have dyslipidemia, including 50% with LDL cholesterol level elevations. For these men, the potential benefits of therapeutic intervention have been documented in clinical trials, although the cost-efficiency of wide-scale treatment has not been determined; (2) isolated hypertriglyceridemia is rare in this population; and (3) low HDL cholesterol levels in association with desirable LDL cholesterol levels are present in more than one-fifth of male patients with CAD.

Drexel and associates[37] from Zurich, Switzerland, obtained plasma lipid profiles, including HDL subfractions HDL_2 and HDL_3 in 115 men undergoing coronary angiography to assess the relation of lipid levels to CAD. CAD was present in 87 patients (76%) and absent in 28 (24%). The largest difference between the 2 groups was observed for HDL_2 cholesterol, with a mean of 0.13 mmol/liter (5 mg/dl) in patients with CAD compared with 0.25 mmol/liter (10 mg/dl) in those without CAD. Smaller differences were found for HDL_3 (1.02 mmol/L [39 mg/dl] vs 1.19 mmol/liter [46 mg/dl]) and HDL (1.15 vs 1.42 mmol/L [45 vs 55 mg/dl]) cholesterol, and apolipoprotein A-1 (1.37 vs 1.50 g/liter) and plasma triglycerides (1.79 vs 1.38 mmol/L [159 vs 122 mg/dl]). No significant difference was found for plasma and LDL cholesterol, and apolipoprotein B levels. Simple regression analysis revealed that the most powerful independent variable associated with the extent of CAD was HDL_2 cholesterol. Stepwise multiple regression analysis proved HDL_2 cholesterol was reasonably well correlated with HDL cholesterol, but less so with plasma apolipoprotein A-1. The data add to the growing body of information demonstrating an important association of HDL (and more specifically HDL_2) with CAD in men.

Assman and Schulte[38] from Munster, Germany, assessed the incidence of atherosclerotic CAD in 4,559 male participants aged 40–64 years from the Prospective Cardiovascular Munster study over a 6-year follow-up period. During this time, 186 study participants developed atherosclerotic CAD (134 definite non-fatal AMIs and 52 definite atherosclerotic CAD deaths including 21 sudden cardiac deaths and 31 fatal AMIs). Univariate analysis revealed a significant association between the incidence of atherosclerotic CAD and HDL cholesterol and triglycerides (Tables 1-6 and 1-7). The relation to HDL cholesterol remained after adjustment for other risk factors. By contrast, the relation between the incidence of atherosclerotic CAD and triglycerides disappeared if, in a multivariate analysis by means of a multiple logistic function, cholesterol or HDL cholesterol were taken into account (Figures 1-12 and 1-13). However, the data suggested that hypertriglyceridemia is a powerful additional coronary risk factor, when excessive triglycerides coincide with a high ratio of plasma LDL cholesterol to HDL cholesterol (>5.0). Even though the prevalence of this subgroup was only 4.3%, it included a quarter of all atherosclerotic CAD events observed.

TABLE 1-6. *Mean Values of Age-Standardized Factors for Male Participants (aged 40 to 65 years) in the PROCAM Study, With (CAD +) and Without (CAD −) Development of Atherosclerotic CAD Within Six Years. Reproduced with permission from Assman, et al.*[38]

Variable	CAD− (n = 4,221)	CAD+ (n = 186)	p Value
Cholesterol (mg/dl)	222.9 (41.0)	251.8 (47.3)	<0.001
HDL cholesterol (mg/dl)	45.2 (11.8)	39.5 (10.6)	<0.001
LDL cholesterol (mg/dl)*	147.1 (35.9)	176.2 (39.5)	<0.001
Triglycerides (mg/dl)†	134.5	163.0	<0.001
Systolic blood pressure (mm Hg)	132.7 (18.9)	139.4 (21.2)	<0.001
Diastolic blood pressure (mm Hg)	86.3 (11.1)	89.5 (12.7)	<0.01
Body mass index (kg/m²)	26.3 (3.0)	26.7 (2.9)	<0.05
No. of cigarette smokers	1317 (31.2%)	98 (52.7%)	<0.001

*n = 4,086 in CAD− subjects, and n = 177 in CAD+ subjects.
†Geometric mean.
Values are mean ± standard deviation (in brackets) unless otherwise indicated.
CAD = coronary artery disease; HDL = high-density lipoprotein; LDL = low-density lipoprotein; PROCAM = Prospective Cardiovascular Münster study.

TABLE 1-7. *Incidence of Atherosclerotic Coronary Artery Disease (n = 186) Within Six Years of Initial Examination in Tertiles of Age-Standardized Factors for Male Participants aged 40 to 65 Years (n = 4,407) in the PROCAM Study. Reproduced with permission from Assman, et al.*[38]

Variable	Tertile Cut-Off Points	CAD Incidence (%) in: Lower Tertile	Middle Tertile	Upper Tertile	p Value
Cholesterol (mg/dl)	<205 and >239	2.1	3.4	7.2	<0.001
HDL cholesterol (mg/dl)	<39 and >48	7.7	2.7	2.6	<0.001
LDL cholesterol (mg/dl)*	<132 and >162	1.7	2.8	8.0	<0.001
Triglycerides (mg/dl)	<105 and >166	2.8	3.9	6.0	<0.001
Systolic blood pressure (mm Hg)	<124 and >138	3.1	3.6	5.7	<0.001
Body mass index (kg/m²)	<25.0 and >27.2	3.3	4.2	5.3	<0.05

*n = 4,263; 177 incidences of atherosclerotic coronary artery disease.

Studies in non-human animals indicate a possible role for lipid oxidation in the development of atherosclerosis. Regenstrom and associates[39] from Stockholm, Sweden, investigated whether there was a relation between the ability of LDL cholesterol to resist oxidation in vitro and the severity of CAD. Thirty-five unselected male survivors (mean age 40 ± 4 years) survivors of AMI underwent angiography, and LDL was isolated from that plasma by density gradient ultracentrifugation. In-vitro LDL susceptibility to oxidation was assessed by determination of the lag phase for the formation of conjugated dienes in the presence of copper ions. An inverse relation was found between lag phase and quantitative esti-

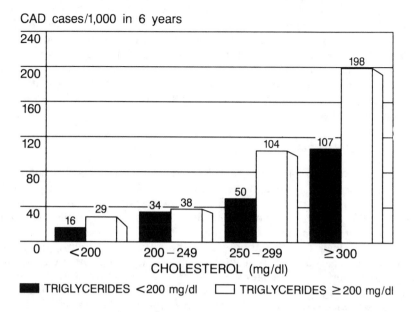

Fig. 1-12. Incidence of coronary artery disease (CAD)/1,000 subjects over a 6-year period according to triglycerides and cholesterol levels. Reproduced with permission from Assmann G and Schulte H.[38]

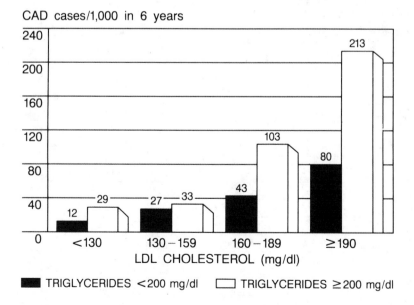

Fig. 1-13. Incidence of coronary artery disease (CAD)/1,000 subjects over a 6-year period according to triglycerides and low-density lipoprotein (LDL) cholesterol levels. Reproduced with permission from Assmann G and Schulte H.[38]

mates of global coronary atherosclerosis. Multivariate analysis indicated that the lag phase for oxidative modification of LDL and LDL cholesterol concentration correlated independently with severity of coronary atherosclerosis. The lag phase for oxidation of LDL was also related to the triglyceride content of the LDL fraction. The finding that susceptibility to LDL oxidation is associated with severity of coronary atherosclerosis may indicate that lipid oxidation promotes premature coronary atherosclerosis and that individuals with an LDL enriched in triglycerides are at particular risk.

Relation to mortality

To examine the relation between plasma total cholesterol concentration and mortality from major causes of death, Smith and associates[40] from London, UK, studied 17,718 male civil servants aged 40 through 64 years at the time of study entry between 1967 and 1969 (Table 1-8). The main outcome measure was mortality from major cause groups. There were 4,022 deaths in the cohort over the 18 years of follow-up. Total mortality increased with cholesterol level, although mortality in the small group with very low cholesterol levels (5% of study population) was nonsignificantly higher than that of the remainder of the lowest quintile cholesterol group. Coronary heart disease mortality increased with increasing cholesterol concentration from the lowest levels. The cancer mortality rate in the group below the fifth centile of the cholesterol distri-

TABLE 1-8. *Age-Adjusted Mortality Rates (per 1000 Person-Years) by Plasma Cholesterol Concentration.* Reproduced with permission from Smith, et al.*[40]

Cause of Death (ICD-8 Codes)	No. of Deaths	Plasma Cholesterol Concentration, mmol/L					χ^2 for Trend (1 df)	Relative Hazard for 1 SD (1.21 mmol/L) Decrease in Cholesterol Level (95% CI)
		<3.34	3.34-4.50	4.51-5.14	5.15-5.92	>5.92		
All cause	4022†	13.78	13.29	14.23	14.05	15.83	15.56‡	0.93‡(0.90-0.95)
Cardiovascular (390-458)	2114	5.17	6.60	6.76	7.61	9.66	61.31‡	0.83‡(0.80-0.86)
Coronary heart disease (410-414)	1542	3.60	4.38	4.55	5.62	7.80	92.69‡	0.78‡(0.74-0.81)
Stroke (430-438)	263	0.76	0.94	1.03	1.00	0.85	0.01	0.99 (0.93-1.06)
Other cardiovascular	309	0.81	1.29	1.18	0.99	1.02	0.79	1.01 (0.90-1.14)
Cancer and other neoplasms (140-239)	1247	5.40	4.24	4.84	4.23	4.23	0.96	1.02 (0.97-1.08)
Digestive (150-159)	379	1.72	1.33	1.40	1.27	1.29	0.78	1.05 (0.95-1.17)
Esophagus (150)	37	0.06	0.12	0.13	0.09	0.20	1.41	0.77 (0.57-1.04)
Stomach (151)	97	0.37	0.37	0.38	0.39	0.24	1.45	1.10 (0.90-1.36)
Colon (153)	117	0.37	0.51	0.40	0.32	0.44	0.34	1.10 (0.91-1.33)
Rectum (154)	40	0.23	0.07	0.20	0.20	0.08	0.00	0.95 (0.70-1.30)
Liver (155-156)	19	0.17	0.06	0.06	0.06	0.06	0.65	1.23 (0.77-1.97)
Pancreas (157)	62	0.51	0.19	0.22	0.17	0.23	0.61	1.17 (0.90-1.52)
Lung (162)	432	2.21	1.53	1.79	1.36	1.41	6.94§	1.09 (0.99-1.20)
Prostate (185)	92	0.06	0.29	0.38	0.35	0.36	1.97	0.85 (0.69-1.04)
Bladder (188)	47	0.23	0.17	0.22	0.16	0.13	0.80	1.03 (0.76-1.38)
Kidney (189)	27	0.23	0.07	0.09	0.11	0.09	0.01	1.07 (0.73-1.58)
Nervous system (191-192)	46	0.00	0.08	0.19	0.19	0.20	5.22‖	0.76‖(0.58-0.99)
Unspecified primary (195-199)	57	0.25	0.15	0.20	0.18	0.26	1.58	0.83 (0.64-1.06)
Hematopoietic (200-207)	98	0.37	0.37	0.32	0.39	0.28	0.26	1.06 (0.87-1.30)
Lymphomas (200-203)	55	0.21	0.19	0.12	0.27	0.18	0.12	0.95 (0.73-1.24)
Leukemia (204-207)	43	0.17	0.18	0.20	0.12	0.10	1.34	1.24 (0.90-1.71)
Smoking-related neoplasm¶	731	3.81	2.50	2.93	2.25	2.53	2.67	1.04 (0.96-1.13)
Nonsmoking-related neoplasm	516	1.59	1.73	1.91	1.98	1.71	0.18	1.00 (0.92-1.09)
Non-CVD, non-neoplasm	648	3.15	2.43	2.58	2.18	1.88	8.84‖	1.12§(1.03-1.21)
Respiratory (460-519)	336	1.91	1.36	1.47	1.06	0.82	15.72‡	1.25‡(1.11-1.40)
Bronchitis etc (490-493)	95	0.71	0.32	0.45	0.36	0.18	5.24‖	1.35§(1.08-1.68)
Pneumonia (480-486)	176	1.04	0.74	0.73	0.44	0.53	7.50§	1.18‖(1.01-1.39)
Other respiratory	65	0.17	0.31	0.28	0.26	0.11	3.03	1.28 (0.98-1.66)
Digestive (520-577)	72	0.44	0.31	0.24	0.23	0.20	2.74	1.10 (0.87-1.40)
Liver and pancreas (570-577)	32	0.21	0.14	0.07	0.16	0.06	1.68	1.31 (0.90-1.90)
Other digestive (520-569)	40	0.23	0.17	0.17	0.07	0.14	1.12	0.96 (0.70-1.32)
Accidents and violence (800-999)	90	0.28	0.35	0.27	0.31	0.32	0.01	1.02 (0.83-1.26)
Suicide (950-959)	36	0.13	0.14	0.11	0.15	0.09	0.46	1.19 (0.90-1.57)
Other accidents and violence	54	0.15	0.21	0.17	0.16	0.23	0.19	0.93 (0.72-1.21)

*ICD-8 indicates *International Classification of Diseases, Eighth Revision*; CI, confidence interval; CVD, cardiovascular disease.
†Includes 13 men whose specific cause of death was not known.
‡P< .001.
§P< .01.
‖P< .05.
¶Smoking-related neoplasms *ICD-8* codes include 140-150, 157, 161, 162, 188, 189, and 195-199.

bution was higher than in the remainder of the cohort for lung, pancreas, liver, and all smoking-related cancers. Only for lung cancer was there a consistent inverse trend with cholesterol level. Rates of mortality due to non-neoplastic respiratory disease were inversely related to cholesterol level. Health state at the time of examination and socioeconomic position were related to cholesterol concentration—subjects in lower employment grades, with disease at baseline, with a history of recent unexplained weight loss, or who had been widowed had lower initial cholesterol levels. These associations largely accounted for the relationships between cholesterol level and noncardiovascular mortality. The inverse associations between plasma cholesterol concentration and mortality from certain causes of death seen in cohort studies could be because the participants with low cholesterol levels possess other characteristics that place them at an elevated risk of death.

With increased efforts to lower serum cholesterol levels, it is important to quantify associations between serum cholesterol level and causes of death other than CAD, for which an etiologic relationship has been established. For an average of 12 years, Neaton and associates[41] of the Multiple Risk Factor Intervention Trial followed for an average of 12 years, 350,977 men aged 35 to 57 years who had been screened for the Multiple Risk Factor Intervention Trial after a single standardized measurement of serum cholesterol level and other CAD risk factors; 21,499 deaths were identified. A strong, positive, graded relationship was evident between serum cholesterol level measured at initial screening and death from CAD. This relationship persisted over the 12-year follow-up period. No association was noted between serum cholesterol level and stroke. The absence of an association overall was due to different relationships of serum cholesterol level with intracranial hemorrhage and nonhemorrhagic stroke. For the latter, a positive, graded association with serum cholesterol level was evident. For intracranial hemorrhage, cholesterol levels less than 4.14 mmol/L (<160 mg/dL) were associated with a 2-fold increase in risk. A serum cholesterol level less than 4.14 mmol/L (<160 mg/dL) was also associated with a significantly increased risk of death from cancer of the liver and pancreas; digestive diseases, particularly hepatic cirrhosis; suicide; and alcohol dependence syndrome. In addition, significant inverse graded associations were found between serum cholesterol level and cancers of the lung, lymphatic, and hematopoietic systems, and chronic obstructive pulmonary disease. No significant associations were found of serum cholesterol level with death from colon cancer, with accidental deaths, or with homicides. Overall, the inverse association between serum cholesterol level and most cancers weakened with increasing follow-up but did not disappear. The association between cholesterol level and death due to cancer of the lung and liver, chronic obstructive pulmonary disease, cirrhosis, and suicide weakened little over follow-up.

Relation to heart rate

Prospective epidemiological studies indicate that elevated heart rate may carry increased risk for CAD. Little is known about the relation between heart rate and serum lipid and lipoprotein concentrations in the general population. Bønaa and Arnesen[42] in Tromsø, Norway assessed anthropometric and life-style determinants of heart rate and examined the association between heart rate and serum lipid and lipoprotein concentrations in a cross-sectional study of 9,719 men and 9,433 women

12–59 years old. Stratified and multivariate analyses were used to detect possible modification of effect and to control for confounding variables. Heart rate was positively associated with male sex and smoking, decreased with body height and physical activity, and showed a U-shaped relation to body mass index. In both sexes, there was a significant progressive increase in age-adjusted levels of total cholesterol, non-HDL cholesterol, and triglycerides and a decrease in HDL cholesterol with heart rate. Men with heart rate >89 beats per minute had 15% higher non-HDL cholesterol and 36% higher triglyceride levels than men with heart rate <60 beats per minute. The corresponding differences in women were 13% and 22%. The associations remained significant when anthropometric and life-style factors were controlled for. The slopes relating total and non-HDL cholesterol level to heart rate were steeper with advancing age. Increases in heart rate correlated with higher levels of atherogenic serum lipid fractions in the general population. Alterations in aortic impedance and/or autonomic influences may underlie these associations.

Relation to arterial calcific deposits

Megnien and co-investigators[43] in Paris, France, studied the prevalence of coronary calcifications and extracoronary plaques in patients with asymptomatic hypercholesterolemia. Ultrafast computed tomography for coronary calcification and echographic assessment of carotid, aortic, and femoral plaques were performed in 111 hypercholesterolemic men: 65% had coronary calcification, 72% had extracoronary plaque. The 2 lesions were associated as: 1) compared with subjects without coronary calcification, those with calcification had a higher prevalence of aortic and femoral plaque and of 2 diseased sites; 2) the prevalence of coronary calcification was higher in the presence than in the absence of aortic or femoral plaque and higher in 2 and 3 diseased sites than in no diseased site; 3) the calcium score was higher in the presence than in the absence of carotid, aortic, or femoral plaque, higher in 2 and 3 diseased sites than in no diseased sites, and higher in 2 than in 1 diseased site; and 4) the calcium score correlated with femoral plaque. Overall, the presence of 2 or 3 diseased extracoronary sites versus no or 1 diseased site showed a power of 78% for predicting coronary calcification. Coronary calcium score correlated with age and triglycerides. The close relation between coronary calcium and extracoronary plaques suggests that echography of extracoronary arteries could aid in the screening of coronary atherosclerosis in high-risk, asymptomatic individuals.

In peripheral arterial disease

The role of lipoprotein disturbances in the development of peripheral vascular disease has not been sufficiently clarified. Senti and co-workers[44] in Barcelona, Spain studied the relations of IDL, apoprotein B, apoprotein E, and other lipoproteins in 102 men with peripheral vascular disease and 100 healthy men who formed a control group. Patients with peripheral vascular disease had significantly higher levels of serum triglycerides, VLDL cholesterol, VLDL triglycerides, VLDL proteins, IDL cholesterol, and IDL triglycerides and lower levels of HDL than controls. Serum cholesterol and triglycerides were normal in 30 patients who had significant increases in IDL triglycerides and significant decreases in HDL cholesterol compared with the 47 controls, who had normal cholesterol and triglyceride levels. Patients with more severe distal involvement showed higher cholesterol and triglycerides carried by IDL and a greater reduction in HDL cholesterol. Smoking patients with peripheral vascular disease showed increased VLDL cholesterol and VLDL triglycerides and lower HDL concentrations. Apo E polymorphism in the study population did not differ from that reported for other European populations. Alleles E2 and E4 had a major impact on serum triglycerides and VLDL lipids in the study patients with peripheral vascular disease. Lipoprotein disturbances are a major risk factor for peripheral vascular disease. IDL abnormalities play an important role in the development and severity of peripheral vascular disease and should also be considered a vascular risk factor in normocholesterolemic and normotriglyceridemic patients.

THERAPY OF HYPERLIPIDEMIA

Diet—general

The "Western" diet, sex, and apolipoprotein E polymorphism have been implicated as codeterminants of lipid levels. In a retrospective analysis, Cobb and co-investigators[45] in New York, New York, evaluated the combined impact of dietary fat, sex, and apolipoprotein E phenotype on lipoprotein levels in 67 subjects fed 2 contrasting, metabolically controlled diets: one a "Western" diet, with a low polyunsaturated to saturated fatty acid ratio and the other a "therapeutic" diet, with a high polyunsaturated/saturated ratio. The high saturation diet compared with the low saturation diet exerted a far stronger predictive influence on lipoprotein concentrations than apolipoprotein E phenotype, sex, or the latter two factors combined. Apolipoprotein E phenotype alone was associated with a stepwise increase in low density lipoprotein cholesterol, such that 3/2<3/3<4/3 on either the low or the high polyunsaturated/saturated diets. On the low saturation diet only, sex was shown to be a significant predictor of HDL cholesterol levels, with women greater than men, and the associated LDL/HDL ratio with men greater than women. On the high saturation diet, women displayed a dramatic fall in HDL cholesterol, effectively raising the LDL/HDL ratio to equivalency with men and obliterating the sex influence seen with the low saturation diet. Controlled for dietary fat, apolipoprotein E and sex exerted independent, additive effects on lipoprotein levels on the low saturation diet only. Only the apolipoprotein E phenotype remained predictive on the high polyunsaturated to saturation diet. Women of the apolipoprotein E 3/2 phenotype stand to benefit the least from a high polyunsaturated/saturated diet because of reduction in the more "protective" HDL cholesterol, whereas men of the 4/3 phenotype showed the greatest improvement in the LDL/HDL ratio.

Singh and associates[46] from Moradabad, India, designed a study to test the efficacy of the administration of fruits and vegetables for 12 weeks as an adjunct to a prudent diet in decreasing blood lipids in 310 (intervention group A) and 311 (control group B) patients with risk factors of CAD in a parallel, single-blind fashion. At entry to the study, sex, mean age, body weight, body mass index, systolic and diastolic BP, and blood lipoproteins were comparable between both groups. Tasty fruits and vegetables were given to patients to eat before major meals for better nutrient adherence and adequacy. Dietary intakes were determined by questionnaires and by weighing of fruit and vegetable intake. Fruits and vegetables decreased total cholesterol level by 6.5% and LDL cholesterol level by 7.3% in group A, whereas the levels were unchanged in group B. The HDL cholesterol levels that decreased during the diet stabilization period in both groups, increased by 5.6% in group A after 12 weeks. Serum triglycerides also decreased (7%) more in group A than B. Fasting blood glucose decreased by 6.9% in group A and by 2.6% in group B. The combined effect of a fat-modified diet plus fruits and vegetables was greater than these changes. Because tasty fruits were taken by the patients before meals (when they are hungry) and are easily available at reasonable cost in our marketing and buying capacity, the compliance was excellent.

Lack of response to a cholesterol-lowering diet can be caused by physiological nonresponsiveness, inadequate knowledge, or inability to change dietary habits (poor compliance). Henkin and associates[47] from Birmingham, Alabama, evaluated the dietary compliance of hyperlipidemic individuals who received intensive initial dietary education and follow-up, and who showed an initial reduction of their plasma cholesterol levels. One hundred and five individuals with fasting cholesterol levels of 5.17 mmol/L (200 mg/dL) or greater received intensive education and follow-up on the American Heart Association Step I diet during an initial 12-week period. The participants provided 3-day dietary records every week, and fasting lipoprotein analysis was performed biweekly. Six months after termination of this period, the subjects were requested to return for a follow-up evaluation of their lipoprotein profile and dietary adherence. Seventy-three (70%) of the subjects returned for a follow-up evaluation of lipoprotein cholesterol levels. Of these, 42 (58%) had a 10% or greater average initial decrease in total cholesterol levels at weeks 3 and 4 ("baseline"), and they were considered to be "high responders." At the 6-month follow up, the average plasma cholesterol level in these responders remained 6.4% below that at entry level, but it had increased by 19% compared with baseline values (6.30 mmol/L [244 mg/dL] vs 5.43 mmol/L [210 mg/dL], respectively). Corresponding significant increases at 6 months were found in HDL cholesterol (8%), LDL cholesterol (16%), and very LDL cholesterol (66%) levels. Analysis of dietary histories revealed that dietary cholesterol and percent calories from fat increased significantly, but remained within the recommended guidelines. The increase in percent calories from saturated fat (from 10.0% ± 0.5% to 14.4% ± 1.0% [mean ± SEM]) deviated markedly from these guidelines. The results suggest the long-term compliance to the reduction of dietary saturated fat remains a problem, even in individuals who receive intensive initial training and show an early favorable response.

Vegetarian soy diet

Nephrotic patients with persistent proteinuria also have various lipid abnormalities that may promote atherosclerosis and more rapid progression of renal disease. D'Amico and associates[48] from Milan, Italy, aimed to find out whether dietary manipulation can correct the hyperlipidemia found in these patients. After a baseline control period of 8 weeks on their usual diets, 20 untreated patients with chronic glomerular diseases, stable long-lasting severe proteinuria (5.9 [SD 3.4] g/24 h) and hyperlipidemia (mean serum cholesterol 8.69 [3.34] mmol/l) ate a vegetarian soy diet for 8 weeks. The diet was low in fat (28% of total calories) and protein (0.71 [0.36] g/kg ideal body weight daily), cholesterol free, and rich in monosaturated and polyunsaturated fatty acids (polyunsaturated/saturated ratio 2.5) and in fiber (40 g/day). After the diet period the patients resumed their usual diets for 8 weeks (washout period). During the soy-diet period there were significant falls in serum cholesterol (total LDL, and HDL) and apolipoproteins A and B, but serum triglyceride concentrations did not change. Urinary protein excretion fell significantly. The concentrations of all lipid fractions and the amount of proteinuria tended to return towards baseline values during the washout period. The authors do not know whether the favorable effect of this dietary manipulation on proteinuria was due to the qualitative or quantitative modifications of dietary protein intake or was a direct consequence of the manipulation of dietary lipid intake.

Nuts

Although dietary factors are suspected to be important determinants of CAD risk, the direct evidence is relatively sparse. The Adventist Health Study is a prospective cohort investigation of 31,208 non-Hispanic white California Seventh-Day Adventists. Fraser and associates[49] from Loma Linda, California, obtained extensive dietary information at baseline, along with the values of traditional CAD risk factors. These were related to risk of definite fatal CAD or definite nonfatal AMI. Subjects who consumed nuts frequently (>4 times per week) experienced substantially fewer definite fatal CAD events and definite nonfatal AMIs, when compared with those who consumed nuts less than once per week (Figure 1-14). These findings persisted on covariate adjustment and were seen in almost all of 16 different subgroups of the population. Subjects who usually consumed whole wheat bread also experienced lower rates of definite nonfatal AMI and definite fatal CAD when compared with those who usually ate white bread. Men who ate beef at least 3 times each week had a higher risk of definite fatal CAD, but this effect was not seen in women or for the nonfatal AMI end point. The data strongly suggest that the frequent consumption of nuts may protect against risk of CAD events.

Water soluble dietary fiber

Guidelines for the use of water-soluble dietary fibers (WSDF) in the dietary management of elevated plasma cholesterol are not well-established. Consequently, Haskell and associates[50] from Stanford, Los Altos, and San Francisco, California, conducted 4 studies to explore the plasma lipid lowering effects of a variety of WSDF. Studies were randomized, double-blind, placebo-controlled trials involving healthy men and women (plasma cholesterol >5.17 mmol/liter; >200 mg/dl). Study duration ranged from 4 to 12 weeks. The WSDF acacia gum yields a low viscosity, palatable beverage when mixed in water. However, despite its WSDF classification, acacia gum consumed for 4 weeks as the sole WSDF source (15 g of WSDF/day) or primary source in a WSDF mixture (17.2 g of WSDF/day; 56% derived from acacia gum) did not produce a significant lipid-lowering effect versus placebo. When 15 g of WSDF/day consisting of psyllium husk, pectin, and guar and locust bean gums (medium viscosity) was consumed for 4 weeks, significant reductions in cholesterol resulted (total cholesterol 8.3%, LDL cholesterol 12.4% that were comparable to changes achieved with 10 g of WSDF/day from high-viscosity guar gum. The magnitude of the lipid-lowering effect was related to intake of WSDF ranging from 5 to 15 g/day (LDL cholesterol +0.8% [placebo], −5.6% [5 g/day], −6.8% [10 g/day], −14.9% [15 g/day]; for trend). The effects of WSDF on plasma lipids were similar for men and women.

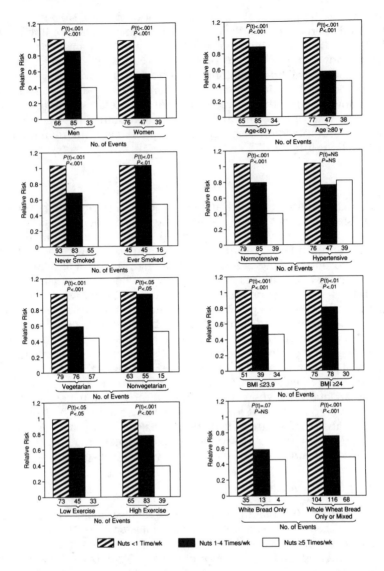

Fig. 1-14. Age- and sex-stratified analyses of associations between the consumption of nuts and definite coronary heart disease events in different subgroups of the population in the Adventist Health Study. *P*(t) is the *P* value for a test of trend; *P* is the *P* value for the overall test of difference between categories. NS indicates not significant; BMI, body-mass index. Reproduced with permission from Fraser, et al.[49]

Guava fruit

There is evidence that inclusion of high fiber foods such as oats, fruits and vegetables in the diet can decrease fat intake and modulate blood lipids. To test this hypothesis, Singh and associates[51] from Moradabad, India, administered guava fruit preferably before meals in a foods-to-eat approach to 61 group A and 59 group B patients with essential hypertension in a randomized and single-blind fashion for 12 weeks. At entry into the study, mean age, male sex, mean body mass index, percentages of risk factors and mean levels of blood lipids were comparable between groups A and B. Adherence to guava consumption was assessed by questionnaires and weighing of guava intake by 24-hour recall after 12 weeks of follow-up. Nutrient intakes including saturated and total fat were significantly decreased; carbohydrates, total and soluble fiber and vitamins and mineral intakes were significantly higher in group A than in group B at 12 weeks. There was a significant net decrease in serum total cholesterol (9.9%), triglycerides (7.7%) and BP (9.0/8.0 mm Hg) with a significant net increase in HDL cholesterol (8.0%) after 12 weeks of guava fruit substitution in group A than in group B. By adding moderate amounts of guava fruit in the usual diet, changes in dietary fatty acids and carbohydrates may occur, providing significant amounts of soluble dietary fiber and antioxidant vitamins and minerals without any adverse effects.

Oat products

To test the a priori hypothesis that consumption of oats will lower the blood total cholesterol level and to assess modifiers and confounders of this association, Ripsin and colleagues[52] from multiple medical centers reviewed a computerized literature search (MEDLINE) and the Quaker Oats Co identified published and unpublished trials as of March 1991. The trials were included if they were randomized and controlled, if a formal assessment of diet and body weight changes occurred, and, if raw data were not received, if there was enough information in the published report to perform calculations. Twenty trials were identified. Using the methods of Der Simonian and Laird, a summary effect size for change in blood total cholesterol level of -0.13 mmol/L (-5.9 mg/dL) (-0.19 to -0.017 mmol/L [-8.4 to -3.3 mg/dL]) was calculated for the 10 trials meeting the inclusion criteria. The summary effect size for trials using wheat control groups was -0.11 mmol/L (-4.4 mg/dL) (-0.21 to -0.01 mmol/L [8.3 to -0.38 mg/dL]). Calculation of Keys scores demonstrated that substituting carbohydrates for dietary fats and cholesterol did not account for the majority of blood cholesterol reduction. Larger reductions were seen in trials in which subjects had initially higher blood cholesterol levels (≥ 5.9 mmol/L [≥ 229 mg/dL]), particularly when a dose of 3 g or more of soluble fiber was employed. This analysis supports the hypothesis that incorporating oat products into the diet causes a modest reduction in blood cholesterol level.

Fast foods

Five of every 10 dollars spent on restaurant food in the USA is spent at a fast-food restaurant. Each person in the USA spends an average of $250 a year on fast foods. Over 160,000 fast-food restaurants are available in the USA and $70,000,000,000 (10 zeros) are spent at them each year. The fast-food restaurants outnumber the traditional restaurants in the USA. McDonald's, the largest of the fast-food chains, has over 11,000 outlets and a new one goes up somewhere in the world every 15 hours. McDonald's is the largest owner of commercial real estate in the world, and they employ over 500,000 persons. One of 5 persons in the USA visits a fast-food restaurant everyday, and 4 of 5, every month. More than half of the fast-food business is done at drive-through windows. Fast-food restaurants are located in hospitals, zoos, military bases, college campuses (including dormitories), museums, airports, naval ships and boats (Mississippi River), bus stations, amusement parks, private-office and state-government buildings, and department stores. Mobile (restaurants on wheels) fast-food restaurants visit neighborhoods, playgrounds, and beaches. Menus are being diversified. McDonald's now offers more than 40 items. The top 15 fast-food chains spent $1,217,000,000 on advertising in 1989, directing many of their ads to children. Survey after survey shows that parents let their children make restaurant choices. When children under age 17 eat at a restaurant in the USA, 83% of the time it is at a fast-food chain. The above information, reviewed by Roberts[53] from Bethesda, Maryland, comes from the second edition of the FAST-FOOD GUIDE published in 1991 and written by Michael F. Jacobson, PhD, Executive Director, Center for Science in the Public Interest, and Sarah Fritschner, a nutritionist and the food editor of the Louisville Courier-Journal. Like their first edition, which appeared in 1986, this new book details the amounts of calories, fat, sodium, sugar, and other "nutrients" in the foods and liquids sold by the 15 largest fast-food chains in the USA. When Jacobson and Fritschner wrote their 1986 book, virtually all fast-food chains were resistant to supplying them with the ingredients of the products sold. For their 1991 book, in contrast, most chains freely supplied them the ingredients of the products. From 1986 to 1991, the 5-year period between the 2 editions of the 2 fast food books, most, but not all, of the fast-food chains decreased the calorie, fat and sodium contents of their foods. Several switched from beef fat to vegetable shortening for all frying, and 1 switched from coconut oil (92% saturated) to a less saturated vegetable shortening for all frying. McDonald's became the first chain to offer 1% low-fat milk and breakfast cereals. Frozen and non-fat yogurt was introduced by McDonald's and Baskin-Robbins. Wendy's dropped completely the Triple Cheeseburger from its menus. This hamburger/cheeseburger was number 1 for calories (1,040), fat (15 teaspoons), and sodium (1,848 mg) in 1986. Today's worst is Carl's Jr. Double Western Bacon Cheeseburger which contains 1,030 calories, 14 teaspoons of fat and 1,810 mg of sodium (Table 1-9). Several (Arby's, Dunkin' Donuts, and Hardee's) either switched to cholesterol free or to a lower calorie mayonnaise. Despite these type changes, the saturated fat and cholesterol contents of the fast-food products remain far too high. Most changes, however, are in the right direction, and many others can be expected by the time the Jacobson/Fritschner third edition appears.

Drug review

An excellent review of drug therapy of hyperlipidemia was written by Prihoda and Illingworth[54] from Portland, Oregon, and it appeared in the September 1992 issue of *Current Problems in Cardiology*.

Estrogen replacement

To examine the effects of estrogen replacement on lipids and angiographically defined CAD in postmenopausal women, Hong and associates[55] from Washington, D.C., obtained lipid profiles in 90 consecutive postmenopausal women undergoing diagnostic coronary angioplasty (Table 1-10). Eighteen women (20%) were receiving estrogen and 72 (80%) were not. CAD (defined as ≥25% luminal diameter narrowing in a major coronary artery) was present in only 22% of women (4 of 18) receiving estrogen and in 68% (49 of 72) who were not, with an odds ratio of 0.13. Mean HDL cholesterol level was significantly higher (63 ± 6 vs 48 ± 2) and mean total/HDL cholesterol ratio significantly lower in women receiving estrogen than in those who were not (4.2 ± 0.5 vs 5.1 ± 0.2). The other

TABLE 1-9. *Hamburgers and Cheeseburgers. Reproduced with permission from Roberts, et al.*[53]

Company/Product	Calories	Fat (tsp)	Sodium (mg)	Gloom
McDonald's Hamburger	255	2	490	16
Hardee's Hamburger	270	2	490	16
Burger King Hamburger	272	3	505	18
Jack in the Box Hamburger	267	3	556	18
McDonald's McLean Deluxe	320	2	670	18
McDonald's Cheeseburger	305	3	710	22
Hardee's Real Lean Deluxe	340	3	650	22
Burger King Cheeseburger	318	3	661	24
Burger King Burger Buddies	349	4	717	26
Burger King Hamburger Deluxe	344	4	496	27
Dairy Queen Single Hamburger with Cheese	365	4	800	29
McDonald's Quarter Pounder	410	5	650	31
Carl's Jr. Carl's Original Hamburger	460	5	810	31
Hardee's Big Twin	450	6	580	33
Dairy Queen Double Hamburger	460	6	630	37
Wendy's Double Hamburger	520	6	710	39
Jack in the Box Double Cheeseburger	467	6	842	40
Burger King Double Cheeseburger	483	6	851	40
McDonald's Big Mac	500	7	890	41
Hardee's Big Deluxe Burger	500	7	760	42
Hardee's Quarter-Pound Cheeseburger	500	7	1,060	42
McDonald's Quarter Pounder with Cheese	510	7	1,090	43
Burger King Bacon Double Cheeseburger	515	7	748	45
Wendy's Big Classic	570	7	1,085	48
Burger King Whopper	614	8	865	49
Jack in the Box Jumbo Jack	584	8	733	50
Hardee's Bacon Cheeseburger	610	9	1,030	54
Wendy's Big Classic with Cheese	640	9	1,345	56
Carl's Jr. Western Bacon Cheeseburger	730	9	1,490	59
Burger King Whopper with Cheese	706	10	1,177	61
Dairy Queen DQ Homestyle Ultimate Burger	700	11	1,110	63
Wendy's Double Big Classic	750	10	1,295	64
Burger King Double Whopper	844	12	933	72
Wendy's Double Big Classic with Cheese	820	12	1,555	72
Burger King Double Whopper with Cheese	935	14	1,245	83
Jack in the Box Ultimate Cheeseburger	942	16	1,176	88
Carl's Jr. Double Western Bacon Cheeseburger	1,030	14	1,810	91

Befriend your arteries by choosing small burgers and skipping the "special sauces." Cheeseburgers provide some calcium, but skim milk, yogurt, and green vegetables are much better, lower calorie sources.

The "Gloom" rating was designed by Jacobsen and Fritschner to give a quick summary of a food's or a meal's overall nutritional value. The formula for the Gloom rating provides 0.9 point/g of polyunsaturated oil; 1.1 point/g of highly saturated animal fat; 0.1 point/g of refined sugar or corn syrup; 1 point/20 mg of cholesterol; and 1 point/133 mg of sodium. This sum is then multiplied by a number ranging from 0.5 to 1.5 depending on the food's nutrient density, which is the ratio of nutrients/calorie (based on protein, calcium, iron, vitamin A, and vitamin C). For example, the multiplier would be 1 if a food contained 100% of the FDA of each of the 5 nutrients. Reprinted with permission of the publisher.

lipid values were similar in both groups. On multiple logistic regression analysis, absence of estrogen use was the most powerful independent predictor of the presence of CAD, with total/HDL cholesterol ratio as the only other variable selected. Thus, among 90 consecutive postmenopausal women undergoing diagnostic coronary angiography, estrogen replacement therapy was associated with an 87% reduction in the prevalence of CAD, and those receiving estrogen had a significantly higher mean HDL cholesterol level and lower mean total/HDL cholesterol ratio.

A committee of the American College of Physicians[56] prepared guide-

TABLE 1-10. *Mean Lipid Values of Study Groups. Reproduced with permission from Hong, et al.*[55]

	Estrogen (n = 18)	No Estrogen (n = 72)
Total cholesterol (mg/dl)	225 ± 51	222 ± 42
Low-density lipoprotein cholesterol (mg/dl)	131 ± 42	151 ± 42
High-density lipoprotein cholesterol (mg/dl)	63 ± 25	48 ± 17*
Triglycerides (mg/dl)	165 ± 144	147 ± 42
Total/high-density lipoprotein cholesterol	4.2 ± 0.5	5.1 ± 0.2**

*p <0.01; **p <0.05 vs estrogen group.
Values are mean ± standard deviation.

lines for counseling postmenopausal women about preventive hormone therapy. This article, which appeared in the 15 December 1992 issue of *Annals of Internal Medicine*, is highly recommended. The general recommendations of the committee are as follows: (1) All women, regardless of age, should consider preventive hormone therapy. (2) Women who have had a hysterectomy are likely to benefit from estrogen therapy. There is no reason to add progestin to the hormone regimen in such women. (3) Women who have CAD or who are at increased risk for CAD are likely to benefit from hormone therapy. If such women have a uterus, a progestin should be added to the estrogen therapy unless careful endometrial monitoring is performed. (4) The risks of hormone therapy may outweigh its benefits in women who are at increased risk for breast cancer. (5) For other women, the best course of action is not clear.

Cholestyramine

Participants in the Lipid Research Clinics Coronary Primary Prevention Trial, a randomized, cholesterol-lowering trial comparing cholestyramine (N = 1907) vs placebo (N = 1899) treatment in 35- and 59-year-old asymptomatic hypercholesterolemic men, conducted between 1973 and 1983, were followed up by the Lipid Research Clinics investigators annually from 1985 until 1989.[57] Post-trial treatment was not provided. Eleven predefined hypotheses pertaining to possible benefits and adverse effects of in-trial cholestyramine treatment were tested by standard statistical comparisons of the 2 original Coronary Primary Prevention Trial treatment groups (cholestyramine and placebo). Similar increasing proportions of cholestyramine and placebo used cholesterol lowering drugs post-trial. After 13.4 years of in-trial plus post-trial follow-up, there were 13 (143 vs 156) fewer deaths in the cholestyramine group than in the placebo group (Figure 1-15). Although not statistically significant, the mortality hazard ratio (0.89) was similar to that in other cholesterol-lowering trials. This trend, a result of reduced CAD mortality (Figure 1-16) occurred despite a post-trial narrowing of the in-trial cholestyramine-placebo difference in CAD incidence from 32 (155 vs 187) to 16 (268 vs 284). The cholestyramine and placebo groups had similar 13.4-year mortality rates from cancer,

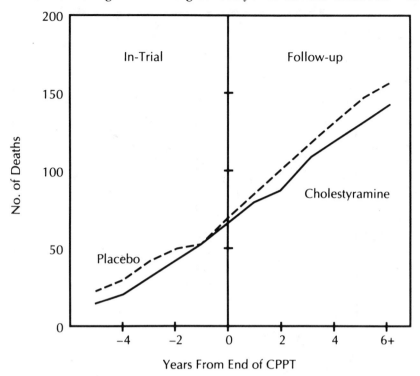

Fig. 1-15. Annual cumulative mortality for men who received cholestyramine (solid line) and placebo (dashed line) during the Coronary Primary Prevention Trial (CPPT). Each surviving participant's follow-up time is measured from the date of his scheduled CPPT close-out visit. A close-out date of June 18, 1983 (the mean close-out date for CPPT survivors), or the date of death (for deaths occurring between June 18 and August 27, 1983) was used for the 136 men who died without completing a CPPT close-out visit. Thus, post-trial deaths are associated with positive and in-trial deaths with negative (or zero) values of the abscissa. Reproduced with permission from Lipid Research Clinics Investigators.[57]

other medical causes, and trauma and similar cancer incidence rates. However, 13.4-year incidences of benign colorectal tumors (50 vs 34), cancer of the buccal cavity and pharynx (8 vs 2), gallbladder disease (68 vs 53), and gallbladder surgery (58 vs 40) were non-significantly increased in the cholestyramine group. Overall, 6 years of post-Coronary Primary Prevention Trial follow-up have not provided conclusive evidence of benefit or long-term toxicity of cholestyramine treatment beyond that evident at the cessation of the trial.

Colestipol

Recommended doses of bile-acid binding resins have an established hypocholesterolemic effect, but data on responses to low doses, especially in women and subjects with moderate hypercholesterolemia, are sparse. Superko and associates[58] from multiple USA medical centers performed a double-blind, placebo-controlled, randomized trial of 3 low doses of colestipol hydrochloride in men with moderate hypercholesterolemia. Men and women with plasma LDL cholesterol concentrations 4 mmol/l (155 mg/dl) and triglyceride concentrations 2.82 mmol/l (250 mg/dl) were recruited for the study. Eligible patients (54 women and 98 men) were placed on the American Heart Association step I diet 6 weeks before

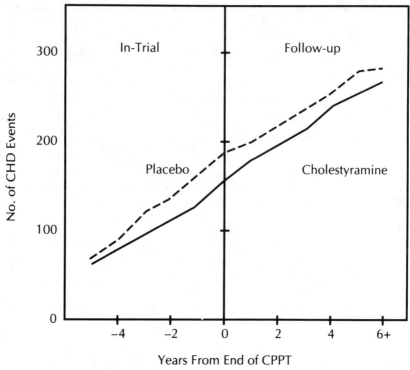

Fig. 1-16. Annual cumulative coronary heart disease (CHD) incidence for men who received cholestyramine (solid line) and placebo (dashed line) during the Coronary Primary Prevention Trial (CPPT). Follow-up time (abscissa) is represented as in Fig. 1-15. Reproduced with permission from Lipid Research Clinics Investigators.[57]

randomization. Participants were subsequently assigned to 1 of 4 drug treatment groups (placebo, and 5, 10 and 15 g/day of colestipol in 2 divided doses) for an additional 12 weeks. Of the 152 patients randomized, 141 completed all aspects of the study. For the treatment groups—placebo, and 5, 10 and 15 g of colestipol—LDL cholesterol reductions (mmol/l) were observed respectively (n = 141): 0.10 ± 0.49 (2.7%), 0.65 ± 0.41 (16.3%), 0.98 ± 0.36 (22.8%) and 1.17 ± 0.47 (27.2%). Similar changes were observed in total cholesterol and apolipoprotein B concentrations. The apolipoprotein B/LDL cholesterol ratio increased significantly with increasing colestipol dosage. Modest but insignificant changes in plasma triglyceride levels occurred, and HDL cholesterol levels remained unchanged. A dose of 5 g/day colestipol achieved 51% of the LDL cholesterol reduction noted with 15 g/day. Low-dose colestipol therapy is effective in the treatment of patients with moderate hypercholesterolemia. The proportionally greater LDL cholesterol reduction in moderate compared with severe hypercholesterolemia was confirmed by examination of the Lipid Research Clinics' Coronary Primary Prevention Trial data set.

Niacin

Levy and associates[59] from New Orleans, Louisiana, assessed the efficacy of sustained release niacin therapy in CAD patients with HDL cholesterol <35 mg/dl with 82% of the 34 consecutive men having values <30 mg/dl. Therapy with sustained release niacin was begun at a dose of 500 mg twice daily with meals and was increased to 3 times daily after 1 to 2 weeks and then was increased as tolerated to 1,000 mg 3 times daily with meals after 4 to 6 weeks of treatment. The average dose used in the 3-month treatment period was 2.4 g/day (range 1,000 to 3,000 mg). All patients had been treated with nonpharmacologic therapy, including exercise and weight reduction for ≥3 months before instituting niacin therapy. Lipid values were compared at baseline and after 3 months of niacin therapy. The results of the trial are summarized in Tables 1-11 and 1-12.

Niacin is available in both unmodified and in time-release preparations. The latter were developed in attempts to minimize the skin-flushing reaction that affects virtually all users and may limit acceptance. Adverse effects on the liver from both unmodified and time-release preparations have been recognized for many years. Rader and associates[60] from Washington, D.C., reviewed publications on the hepatic toxicity of both types of niacin preparations. Adverse reactions in 6 patients resulted from the exclusive use of unmodified niacin and in 2 patients from the exclusive use of time-release preparations. In 10 additional patients, adverse reactions developed after an abrupt change from unmodified to time-release preparations. Many of these patients were ingesting time-release niacin at doses well above the usual therapeutic doses currently recommended. Signs of liver toxicity developed in less than 7 days in 4 of these 10 patients. In doses that achieve equivalent reductions in serum lipids, hepatic toxicity

TABLE 1-11. *Lipid Changes with Sustained-Release Niacin in Coronary Patients with Very Low Levels of High-Density Lipoprotein Cholesterol (n = 34). Reproduced with permission from Lauie, et al.*[59]

Lipids	Baseline	3-Month Niacin	% Change	p Value
Total cholesterol (mg/dl)	196 ± 38	174 ± 43	−11	<0.005
Triglycerides (mg/dl)	205 ± 84	201 ± 78	−2	NS
HDL cholesterol (mg/dl)	26 ± 4	33 ± 6	+30	<0.0001
LDL cholesterol (mg/dl)	142 ± 53	114 ± 34	−20	<0.01
LDL/HDL	5.7 ± 2.6	3.6 ± 1.2	−37	<0.0001

HDL = high-density lipoprotein; LDL = low-density lipoprotein; NS = not significant.

TABLE 1-12. *Comparison of Niacin Effects in Patients with "Isolated" Low High-Density Lipoprotein Cholesterol Versus Those with Hypertriglyceridemia. Reproduced with permission from Lauie, et al.*[59]

Lipid Values	Isolated Low HDL (n = 19)				Hypertriglyceridemia (n = 10)			
	Baseline	3-Month Niacin	% Change	p Value	Baseline	3-Month Niacin	% Change	p Value
Total cholesterol (mg/dl)	189 ± 28	170 ± 42	−10	=0.08	192 ± 46	175 ± 48	−9	NS
Triglycerides (mg/dl)	163 ± 51	180 ± 77	+10	NS	310 ± 47	238 ± 80	−23*	=0.05
HDL cholesterol (mg/dl)	25 ± 4	32 ± 6	+27	<0.002	27 ± 5	38 ± 3	+41	<0.0001
LDL cholesterol (mg/dl)	120 ± 22	114 ± 31	−5	NS	156 ± 80	101 ± 25	−35†	=0.05
LDL/HDL	5.0 ± 1.3	3.7 ± 1.2	−26	<0.01	6.2 ± 4.1	2.7 ± 0.7	−56†	<0.02

*p · 0 05, †p · 0 02 compared with isolated low HDL group

occurred more frequently with time-release preparations than with un-modified preparations. An awareness of toxicity associated with ingestion of high doses of time-release niacin preparations is important because of their widespread availability and the potential for self-prescribed, un-monitored use.

Gemfibrozil

Manninen and colleagues[61] in Helsinki, Finland, studied the joint effect of baseline triglyceride and lipoprotein cholesterol levels on the incidence of cardiac end points in the trial group of the Helsinki Heart Study, a 5-year randomized coronary primary prevention trial among dyslipidemic middle-aged men (n = 4081). The relative risks were calculated using Cox proportional hazards models with a dummy variable technique that allows simultaneous study of subgroup combinations from the placebo and treatment groups. In the placebo group, the LDL cholesterol/HDL cholesterol ratio was the best single predictor of cardiac events. This ratio in combination with the serum triglyceride level revealed a high-risk subgroup: subjects with LDL/HDL ratio ≥5 and triglyceride ≥2.3 mmol/l had a relative risk of 3.8 compared with those with LDL/HDL ratio equal ≤5 and triglyceride concentration ≤ that 2.3 mmol/l. In subjects with triglyceride concentration >2.3 mmol/l and LDL/HDL ratio ≤5, rela-tive risk was close to unity, whereas in those with triglyceride levels ≤2.3 mmol/l and LDL/HDL ratio >5, relative risk was 1.2. The high-risk group with LDL/HDL ratio >5 and triglyceride level >2.3 mmol/l profited most from treatment with gemfibrozil, with a 71% lower incidence of coronary heart disease events than the corresponding placebo subgroup. In all other subgroups, the reduction in CAD incidence was substantially smaller. Serum triglyceride concentration has prognostic value, both for assessing CAD risk and in predicting the effect of gemfibrozil treatment, especially when used in combination with HDL and LDL.

Koskinen and associates[62] from Helsinki, Finland, compared the effi-cacy of 3 formulations and 2 dosage regimens of gemfibrozil in 322 dyslipi-demic (non-HDL cholesterol level, ≥5.2 mmol/L [≥200 mg/dL]) middle-aged male and postmenopausal female patients in a 1-year open-label trial. Of the patients studied, 109 received the standard 1200-mg dose of gemfibrozil, ie, 2 300-mg capsules twice daily; 107 received 1 600-mg tablet twice daily; and 106 received a single dose of 900 mg of gemfibrozil in 2 450-mg tablets in the evening. The 3 treatment groups showed equal changes in each lipoprotein measure studied, ie, in serum levels of triglyc-erides, total cholesterol, LDL and HDL cholesterol, HDL subfractions HDL_2 and HDL_3, and apolipoproteins A-I, A-II, and B. When the therapeutic responses were analyzed separately in men (n = 219) and women (n = 103), significantly greater decreases in serum levels of total triglycerides, LDL cholesterol, and apolipoprotein B, and a significantly greater increase in HDL_3 cholesterol level and apolipoprotein A-I/B ratio, were seen in the women. When the study population was divided into smokers (n = 80) and nonsmokers (n = 242), the changes were similar in all lipoprotein measures except HDL_3 cholesterol level, in which a significantly greater increase was seen in the nonsmokers. This study showed that gemfibrozil is as effective, or more so, in dyslipidemic postmenopausal women as in dyslipidemic middle-aged men, and that smoking does not abolish its lipid-regulating effects. Importantly, a daily dose of 900 mg was found to be as effective as the standard dose of 1200 mg.

Lovastatin

Lovastatin produces consistent dose-related reductions in plasma levels of LDL cholesterol along with variable decreases in triglycerides and increases in high HDL cholesterol. Patient characteristics from the Expanded Clinical Evaluation of Lovastatin study were examined by Shear and co-investigators[63] in Bluebell, Pennsylvania, to determine their association with the magnitude of lovastatin-induced changes in these lipids and lipoproteins. After baseline period consisting of dietary therapy, 8,245 patients with moderate hypercholesterolemia were randomized to 5 groups that received 48 weeks of treatment with either placebo or daily doses of lovastatin ranging from 20 to 80 mg. By use of linear statistical models, 20 different patient characteristics were examined for modification of the dose-dependent responses observed. For LDL cholesterol, the following were associated with enhanced lowering (percent changes are placebo-corrected, adjusted mean changes from baseline for the 80-mg/day lovastatin group): full drug compliance versus 80% compliance; and age of 65 versus 45 years for women; white race versus black race; and 4.5-kg weight gain versus 4.5-kg weight loss. Similar relations for enhanced triglyceride lowering were found with older age and weight gain. Patients with initially low HDL cholesterol and high triglycerides had enhanced responses for these parameters; placebo-corrected percent changes at 80 mg/day were −27.4% for triglycerides and +12% for HDL cholesterol. Overall, patient characteristics had very little impact of clinical importance on the dose-dependent LDL cholesterol lowering found with lovastatin. In patients with initially high levels of triglycerides and low levels of HDL cholesterol, the elevation of HDL cholesterol produced by lovastatin appears to be enhanced.

Familial defective apolipoprotein B-100 is an autosomal dominant disorder associated with hypercholesterolemia in which an aminoacid substitution in apoprotein B-100 leads to LDL particles which have defective binding to the LDL receptor. All known patients are heterozygous, and their plasma contains normal and poorly binding LDL particles. Illingworth and associates[64] from Portland, Oregon, and San Francisco, California, treated 12 hypercholesterolemic patients from 10 unrelated families with familial defective apolipoprotein B-100 with lovastatin. In 6 patients treated with 20 mg lovastatin daily, LDL cholesterol decreased by 21.5% (from 6.23 to 4.89 mmol/l) whereas it fell by 32.1% (from 6.99 to 4.81 mmol/l) in 9 patients who received 40 mg daily. These results indicate that the hypercholesterolemia of familial defective apolipoprotein B-100 may respond to treatment with statins.

Lovastatin vs gemfibrozil

D'Agostino and associates[65] from Boston, Massachusetts, performed a randomized, multi-center, double-blind, perspective, 18-week comparison of lovastatin with gemfibrozil to compare the efficacy and tolerability in adults with types IIa and IIb primary hypercholesterolemia. Sixty men and 44 women aged 24 to 78 years participated in the trial. Each treatment group of 52 patients was closely matched by the randomization procedure. All participants met national cholesterol education program guidelines for evaluation and treatment. In all, 94 (90%) completed the 18 weeks of study. After 18 weeks of diet-plus-active treatment, lovastatin decreased serum total cholesterol and LDL cholesterol significantly better than gemfibrozil (adjusted mean decreases were 63 vs 35 mg/dl for total cholesterol and 67 vs 28 mg/dl for LDL) (Figure 1-17). Gemfibrozil was more effective than lovastatin in increasing HDL cholesterol (8 vs 5 mg/dl adjusted mean HDL cholesterol increases) after 18 weeks. No significant differences in the adjusted mean ratio of total to HDL cholesterol were noted, but the lovastatin group had a significantly greater adjusted mean reduction in the ratio of LDL to HDL cholesterol (1.8 vs 1.3). The gemfibrozil group achieved significantly greater reductions in VLDL cholesterol and triglycerides compared with the lovastatin group (adjusted mean decreases were 14 vs 1 mg/dl for VLDL cholesterol and 71 vs 15 mg/dl for triglycerides). After 18 weeks of lovastatin therapy, 49% of patients achieved goal LDL cholesterol, whereas only 9% of those who took gemfibrozil achieved this goal.

McKenney and associates[66] from Richmond, Virginia, compared the

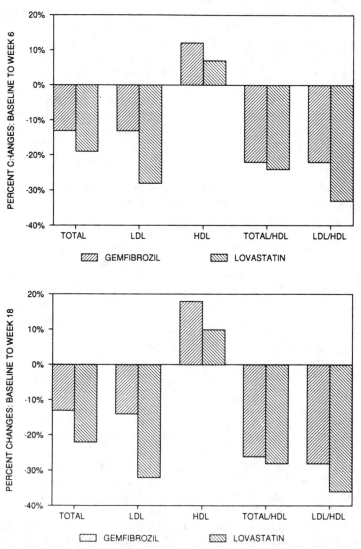

Fig. 1-17. Percent changes from baseline for treatment groups. HDL = high-density lipoprotein; LDL = low-density lipoprotein. Reproduced with permission from Agostino, et al.[65]

efficacy of gemfibrozil and lovastatin in the treatment of patients with an elevated LDL cholesterol level and a low HDL cholesterol level. After at least 6 weeks of cholesterol-lowering diet, 17 patients who had a mean baseline LDL cholesterol level >160 mg/dL (4.14 mmol/L) and an HDL cholesterol level <40 mg/dL (<1.03 mmol/L) received gemfibrozil 600 mg twice daily and lovastatin 20 mg twice daily, each for 6 weeks according to a randomized, cross-over, double-blind research design. Lovastatin and gemfibrozil reduced LDL cholesterol levels 34% and 9% and raised HDL cholesterol levels 15% and 18%, respectively (Figure 1-18). Thus, lovastatin is more effective in lowering LDL cholesterol levels and is as effective as gemfibrozil in increasing HDL cholesterol levels in these patients.

Lovastatin + gemfibrozil

Glueck and associates[67] from Cincinnati, Ohio, in a retrospective, observational study assessed safety and efficacy of long-term (21 months/patient), open-label, gemfibrozil-lovastatin treatment in 80 patients with primary mixed hyperlipidemia (68% of whom had atherosclerotic vascular disease). Because ideal lipid targets were not reached (LDL cholesterol <130 mg/dl, HDL cholesterol >35 mg/dl, or total cholesterol/HDL cholesterol <4.5 mg/dl) with diet plus a single drug, gemfibrozil (1.2 g/day)-lovastatin (primarily 20 or 40 mg) treatment was given. Follow-up visits were scheduled with 2-drug therapy every 6 to 8 weeks, an average of 10.3 visits per patient, with 741 batteries of 6 liver function tests and 714 creatine phosphokinase levels measured. Only 1 of the 4,446 liver function tests (0.02%), a gamma glutamyl transferase, was ≥3 times the upper normal limit. Of the 714 creatine phospokinase levels, 9% were high; only 1 (0.1%) was ≥3 times the upper normal limit. With 2-drug therapy, mean total cholesterol decreased 22% from 255 to 200 mg/dl, triglyceride levels decreased 35% from 236 to 154 mg/dl, LDL cholesterol decreased 26%

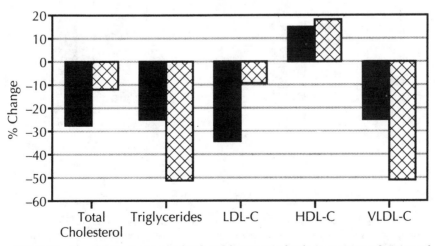

Fig. 1-18. Percentage changes in lipid and lipoprotein levels in patients administered gemfibrozil (hatched bars) and lovastatin (black bars). LDL-C indicates low-density lipoprotein cholesterol; HDL-C, high-density lipoprotein cholesterol; and VLDL-C, very-low-density lipoprotein cholesterol. Reproduced with permission from McKenney, et al.[66]

from 176 to 131 mg/dl, and the total cholesterol/HDL cholesterol ratio decreased 24% from 7.1 to 5.4. Myositis, attributable to the drug combination and symptomatic enough to discontinue it, occurred in 3% of patients, and in 1% with concurrent high creatine phosphokinase (769 U/liter); no patients had rhabdomyolysis or myoglobinuria. Gemfibrozil-lovastatin treatment mandates careful clinical follow-up with serial creatine phosphokinase and liver function tests in reliable patients who (1) do not respond optimally to 1-drug therapy, (2) are well informed about possible myositis, and (3) are prepared to discontinue 2-drug therapy at earliest onset of myositis symptoms. Within this frame of reference, combined gemfibrozil-lovastatin treatment is safe and effective, reducing total and LDL cholesterol, triglycerides, and the total cholesterol/HDL cholesterol ratio to levels at which regression of CAD may occur.

Simvastatin vs pravastatin

The European Study Group[68] enrolled a total of 291 patients with primary hypercholesterolemia (total plasma cholesterol 6.20 mmol/liter) in an open, randomized, parallel, comparative study of simvastatin and pravastatin. All patients started or continued a standard lipid lowering diet for 6 weeks before entry into the 4-week placebo baseline period. There were 145 patients who received simvastatin and 146 patients who received pravastatin, both at the commonly recommended starting dose of 10 mg once daily, for a treatment period of 6 weeks. Concentrations of total cholesterol in plasma were reduced by 23% with simvastatin, and by 16% with pravastatin (Figure 1-19). Concentrations of LDL cholesterol in

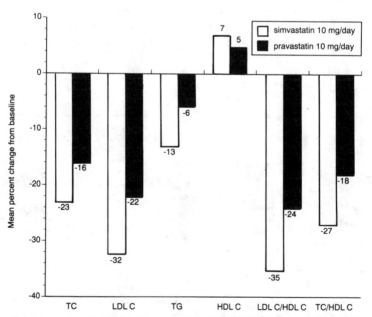

Fig. 1-19. Mean change (%) from baseline in plasma lipid concentrations (median for triglycerides [TG]). All changes were significant (p≤0.01) except for triglycerides with pravastatin (p≤0.05). Between-group differences for all parameters were statistically significant (p≤0.01) except for triglycerides (p≤0.05) and high density lipoprotein cholesterol (HDL C) (p=0.06). LDL C = low-density lipoprotein cholesterol; TC = total cholesterol. Reproduced with permission from European Study Group.[68]

plasma were reduced by 32 and 22%, and HDL cholesterol concentrations were increased by 7 and 5% with simvastatin and pravastatin, respectively. Plasma triglyceride concentrations were reduced by 13% with simvastatin and by 6% with pravastatin. Adverse experiences were similar between treatment groups and both drugs were well tolerated. In each treatment group, 3 patients were withdrawn from the study for clinical adverse experiences; 1 patient in the pravastatin group required a reduction in dose to 5 mg/day because of insomnia. At the commonly recommended starting dose for each, simvastatin had a significantly greater lipid-lowering effect than pravastatin. Both drugs were well tolerated.

Pravastatin vs cholestyramine

To compare the efficacy and safety of cholestyramine versus pravastatin, Betteridge and associates[69] from 8 medical centers in the UK performed a double blind, double dummy, placebo controlled study with 3 parallel groups involving 128 patients aged 18–70 years with heterozygous familial hypercholesterolemia. The main outcome measures were total plasma cholesterol, triglyceride, lipoprotein subfractions, and biochemical and hematological safety parameters. Pravastatin (40 mg/day) led to a 25% reduction in total plasma cholesterol concentration and a reduction in LDL cholesterol concentration of 30%. Cholestyramine (24 g/day) led to similar reductions in concentrations of total cholesterol (23%) and LDL cholesterol (31%). No consistent changes occurred in HDL cholesterol values with either compound. Plasma triglyceride concentrations showed a small rise (18%) on resin therapy. No serious adverse drug reactions occurred during the study. Pravastatin seems to be a highly effective, well tolerated drug for severe hypercholesterolemia. Patients chosen for this study were recruited on the basis that they could tolerate a full dose of cholestyramine, and in this situation cholestyramine was also highly effective in lowering plasma LDL cholesterol concentrations.

Calcium carbonate

In recent years several studies have noted that oral calcium treatment was associated with a reduction in serum cholesterol levels. Bell and associates[70] from Minneapolis, Minnesota, examined calcium carbonate for its ability to lower serum cholesterol levels in hypercholesterolemic patients. Fifty-six patients with mild to moderate hypercholesterolemia were examined in this randomized, double-blind, placebo-controlled crossover study. Patients were treated with a low-fat, low-cholesterol diet targeted at the American Heart Association Step-1 diet for 8 weeks before and while receiving placebo or calcium carbonate (9.98 mmol [400 mg] of elemental calcium) 3 times daily with meals for 6 weeks. Patients were then crossed over to the alternate treatment for an additional 6-week period. Compared with placebo, calcium carbonate achieved a 4.4% reduction in the LDL cholesterol level, and a 4.1% increase in the HDL cholesterol level. The ratio of LDL cholesterol to HDL cholesterol significantly decreased by 6.5% with calcium carbonate treatment. Calcium carbonate treatment did not significantly affect BP or serum levels of triglycerides, lipoprotein Apo B, or calcium. Relative urinary saturation ratios of calcium oxalate levels were unchanged during calcium carbonate therapy. Compliance with diet and treatment was excellent and no significant adverse effects were noted. Thus, calcium carbonate was a modestly effective and well-tolerated adjunct to diet in the management of mild to moderate hypercholesterolemia.

Partial ileal bypass

The Program on the Surgical Control of the Hyperlipidemias (POSCH) provided the clearest and the most convincing evidence supporting the beneficial effects of cholesterol lowering in hypercholesterolemic survivors of AMI. In POSCH, 78 of the 838 patients (9.3%) were women, with 32 randomized to the diet-control group and 46 to the diet plus partial ileal bypass (Figure 1-20) surgery-intervention group. Buchwald and associates[71] from Minneapolis, Minnesota, summarized the results of this intervention in the women. At 5 years, the mean percent change from baseline was −24% for total plasma cholesterol, −36% for LDL cholesterol, and 9% for HDL cholesterol (Figure 1-21). Because of the small number of women, no statistically significant changes in clinical event rates were observed between the control and the surgery groups. A com-

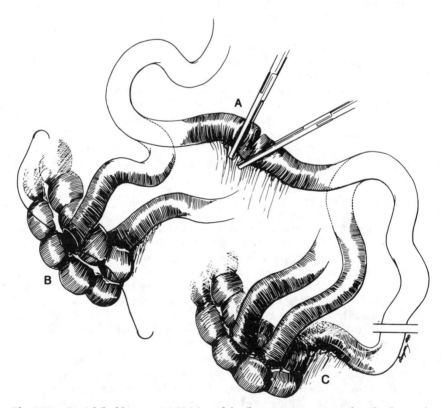

Fig. 1-20. Partial ileal bypass. (A) Division of the ileum 200 cm proximal to the ileocecal valve or one third of the total small bowel length proximal to the ileocecal valve if the total small intestinal length is greater than 600 cm. (B) End-to-side anastomosis of the proximal segment into the anterior taenia of the cecum, 6 cm distal to the appendiceal stump. (C) Tacking of the closed distal segment to the anterior taenia of the cecum midway between the anastomosis and the appendiceal stump. Reprinted with permission from Buchwald H, Stoller DK, Campos CT, Matts JP, Varco RL. Partial ileal bypass for hypercholesterolemia: 20- to 26-year follow-up of the first 57 consecutive cases. Ann Surg 1990; 212:318–331.

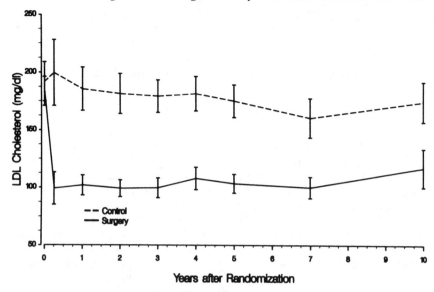

Fig. 1-21. Low-density lipoprotein cholesterol levels (mg/dL) in the control and surgery groups in the POSCH women. Values are mean ± 2 SEM. The difference between the groups at each follow-up interval was significant (p<0.001). Reproduced with permission from Buchwald, et al.[71]

parison of 162 coronary arteriography film pairs in the POSCH women, between baseline and 3, 5, 7, and 10 years, consistently showed less disease progression in the surgery group. Because the lipid and coronary arteriography findings in the POSCH women paralleled these findings in the total POSCH population and in the POSCH men, and because the arteriography changes in POSCH have previously been demonstrated to be statistically significant surrogate end points for certain clinical events and predictors of overall and atherosclerotic CAD mortality rates, the authors concluded that the lipid modification achieved in the POSCH women by partial ileal bypass reduced their atherosclerosis progression. The POSCH findings in women support the aggressive treatment of hyperlipidemia in the general management of atherosclerosis in women.

Aphresis

A subgroup of patients with familial hypercholesterolemia (FH) respond inadequately to standard diet and drug therapy, and are therefore at high risk for the premature development or progression of CAD. Gordon and associates[72] for the Liposorber Study Group representing multiple medical centers evaluated LDL cholesterol and lipoprotein (a) removal in a multicenter, controlled trial with a new LDL aphresis procedure (Liposorber LA-15 System). The study comprised patients with FH who had not responded adequately to diet and maximal drug therapy. There were 54 patients with heterozygous FH (45 randomized to treatment and 9 control subjects) and 10 with homozygous FH (all of whom received LDL aphresis). The study included 3 6-week treatment phases and a 4-week rebound phase. Treatments were administered at 7- to 14-day intervals. Mean acute reduction in LDL cholesterol were 76% in heterozygous FH patients and 81% in homozygous ones. Time-averaged levels of LDL cholesterol were reduced 41% (243 to 143 mg/dl) in heterozygous

FH patients and 53% (447 to 210 mg/dl) in homozygous ones. The substantial acute reduction of lipoprotein (a) (means: 65%, heterozygous FH; 68%, homozygous FH) has not been reported with other therapies. The Liposorber LA-15 System represents an important therapeutic option in FH patients who respond inadequately to diet and drug therapy.

Effects on life expectancy and morbidity

To evaluate the lifetime benefits of reducing total serum cholesterol levels to prevent CAD, Grover and associates[73] from Montreal, Canada, developed a CAD primary prevention computer model to estimate the benefits associated with life-time risk-factor modification. The authors validated the model by comparing the computer estimates with the observed results of 3 primary CAD prevention trials. Men and women age 35 to 65 years who are free of CAD, with total serum cholesterol levels ranging from 5.2 to 7.8 mmol/L (200 to 300 mg/dL), with or without additional CAD risk factors. Serum cholesterol reduction through dietary modification or diet and medications were interventions. Changes in life expectancy and the delay of symptomatic CAD were the main outcome measures. The computer forecasts for CAD end points closely matched the observed results of the Lipid Research Clinics Trial, the Helsinki Heart Study, and MRFIT. The authors then applied the computer model to low-risk and high-risk men and women with total serum cholesterol levels between 5.2 and 7.8 mmol/L (200 and 300 mg/dL) and estimated that, after reducing serum cholesterol levels 5% to 33%, the average life expectancy would increase by 0.03 to 3.16 years. The authors also forecast that the average onset of symptomatic CAD would be delayed among these patient groups by 0.06 to 4.98 years. The authors concluded that this computer model accurately estimates the results of clinical trials and can be used to forecast the changes in life expectancy and morbidity (the development of CAD) associated with specific CAD risk reduction interventions. The wide variation surrounding these estimates underscores the need to better define which groups of individuals will gain the most from cholesterol reduction.

DIABETES MELLITUS

To examine prospectively the association between regular exercise and the subsequent development of non-insulin-dependent diabetes mellitus (NIDDM), Manson and associates[74] from Boston, Massachusetts, studied 21,271 US male physicians participating in the Physicians' Health Study, aged 40 to 84 years and free of diagnosed diabetes mellitus, myocardial infarction, cerebrovascular disease, and cancer at baseline. Morbidity follow-up was 98% complete and there was five years of follow-up. At baseline, information was obtained about frequency of vigorous exercise and other risk indicators. During 105 141 person-years of follow-up, 285 new cases of NIDDM were reported. The age-adjusted incidence of NIDDM ranged from 369 cases per 100,000 person-years in men who engaged in vigorous exercise less than once weekly to 214 cases per 100,000 person-years in those exercising at least 5 times per week (Figure

1-22). Men who exercised at least once per week had an age-adjusted relative risk of NIDDM of 0.64 compared with those who exercised less frequently. The age-adjusted relative risk of NIDDM decreased with increasing frequency of exercise: 0.77 for once weekly, 0.62 for 2 to 4 times per week, and 0.58 for 5 or more times per week. A significant reduction in risk of NIDDM persisted after adjustment for both age and body-mass index. Further control for smoking, hypertension, and other coronary risk factors did not alter these associations. The inverse relation of exercise to risk of NIDDM was particularly pronounced among overweight men. Exercise appears to reduce the development of NIDDM even after adjusting for body-mass index. Increased physical activity may be a promising approach to the primary prevention of NIDDM.

To determine the influence of control of diabetes mellitus on serum lipoprotein (a) concentrations, Ramirez and associates[75] from Dallas, Texas, compared lipoprotein (a) concentrations between a normal control group, a group of diabetic patients with glycated hemoglobin (HbA_{1c}) <8%, and a group of patients with diabetes mellitus with HbA_{1c} of 8% or higher. The study included 95 normal controls and 93 diabetic subjects (49 with insulin dependent diabetes and 44 with non-insulin dependent diabetes mellitus). No difference in the lipoprotein (a) distribution was noted between diabetic men and women. No correlation was observed between lipoprotein (a) levels and total cholesterol, LDL cholesterol, and triglyceride levels. Lipoprotein (a) levels are elevated in poorly controlled diabetic patients. Increased levels of lipoprotein (a) may be a contributing factor to the high risk for atherosclerosis observed in diabetic patients.

Patients who have insulin-dependent diabetes mellitus and nephropathy have an excess of cardiovascular disease. Familial factors may in part

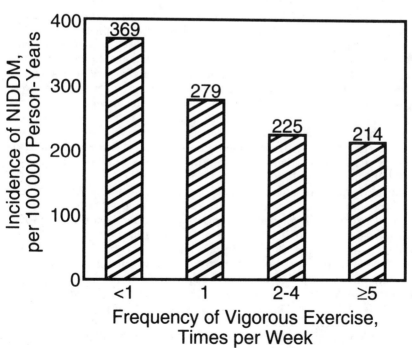

Fig. 1-22. Age-adjusted incidence rates of non-insulin-dependent diabetes mellitus (NIDDM) according to frequency of vigorous exercise (X^2, trend [1 df] = 13.1; P<.001). Reproduced with permission from Manson, et al.[74]

account for this phenomenon. Earle and associates[76] from London, UK, identified 61 white patients under 65 years of age with insulin-dependent diabetes who had nephropathy, and then matched them with 61 diabetic patients without nephropathy. The authors determined the prevalence of cardiovascular disease in the parents of these patients with the use of information obtained from death certificates or from the World Health Organization questionnaire for cardiovascular disease. The rates of ascertainment of information were 96% (n = 117) for the parents of diabetic patients with nephropathy and 95% (n = 116) for the parents of patients without nephropathy. Cardiovascular disease was more often a direct cause of death among the parents of diabetic patients with nephropathy (40% vs. 22%), and the combined morbidity and mortality from cardiovascular disease in this group was greater than that in the parents of diabetic patients without nephropathy (31% vs. 14%). The age-adjusted and sex-adjusted relative risk of cardiovascular disease in this group of parents was 2.9 (95% confidence interval, 1.5 to 5.5). Moreover, a paternal history of cardiovascular disease was associated with a significantly increased risk of nephropathy in the diabetic patient after the analysis was adjusted for age, sex, and duration of diabetes. Among the diabetic patients with nephropathy, those who had had a cardiovascular event were much more likely to have a family history of cardiovascular disease (odds ratio, 6.2) than those who had not had such an event. Among patients with insulin-dependent diabetes, a parental history of cardiovascular disease is significantly associated with the development of nephropathy and, among those with nephropathy, increases the likelihood of cardiovascular disease.

Barrett-Connor[77] from La Jolla, California, compared plasma androgen levels in 44 men with untreated, non-insulin-dependent diabetes mellitus and 88 age-matched men who had normal glucose tolerance test. Men with diabetes had significantly lower plasma levels of free (4.96 nmol/L compared with 5.58 nmol/L) and total testosterone (14.7 nmol/L compared with 17.4 nmol/L), dihydrotestosterone (428 pg/mL compared with 533 pg/mL), and dehydroepiandrosterone sulfate (DHEA-S) (1.92 umol/L compared with 2.42 umol/L) than nondiabetic men. They also had significantly lower HDL cholesterol and significantly higher triglyceride levels. Differences were not explained by obesity, alcohol use, or cigarette habit. Overall, the total testosterone level, but not the free testosterone level, was positively correlated with the HDL cholesterol level and negatively correlated with the triglyceride level. Similar associations were seen in analyses restricted to the men without diabetes. Lower levels of endogenous androgens are seen in older diabetic men, and low androgen levels are associated with diabetic dyslipidemia.

Barnard and associates[78] from Los Angeles, California, investigated the effects of an intensive, 3-week, dietary and exercise program on hyperinsulinemia, systemic hypertension, hypertriglyceridemia and obesity. The group was divided into diabetic patients (non-insulin-dependent diabetes mellitus [NIDDM], n = 13), insulin-resistant persons (n = 29) and those with normal insulin, ≤10 uU/ml (n = 30). The normal groups had very small but statistically significant decreases in all of the risk factors. The patients with NIDDM had the greatest decreases. Insulin was reduced from 40 ± 15 to 27 ± 11 uU/ml, BP from 142 ± 9/83 ± 3 to 132 ± 7/71 ± 3 mm Hg, triglycerides from 353 ± 76 to 196 ± 31 mg/dl and body mass index from 31.1 ± 4.0 to 29.7 ± 3.7 kg/m². Although there was a significant weight loss for the group with NIDDM, resulting in the decrease in body mass index, 8 of 9 patients who were initially overweight were still overweight at the end of the program, and 5 of the 8 were still obese (body mass index >30 kg/m²), indicating that normalization of body weight is not a requisite for a reduction or normalization of other risk factors. Insulin was reduced from 18.2 ± 1.8 to 11.6 ± 1.2 uU/ml in the insulin-resistant group, with 17 of the 29 subjects achieving normal fasting insulin (<10 uU/ml). BP was reduced from 129 ± 4/84 ± 3 to 124 ± 5/78 ± 2 mm Hg, while triglycerides were reduced from 204 ± 17 to 162 ± 15 mg/dl. Body mass index was reduced from 32.6 ± 5.3 to 31.2 ± 5.1 kg/m², with only 4 of 24 who were overweight reaching a normal weight.

Overweightness and body fat distribution

Overweight in adults is associated with increased morbidity and mortality. In contrast, the long-term effect of overweight in adolescence on morbidity and mortality is not known. Must and associates[79] from Boston, Massachusetts, and Allendale, Michigan, studied the relation between overweight and morbidity and mortality in 508 lean or overweight adolescents aged 13 to 18 years of age who participated in the Harvard Growth Study of 1922 to 1935. Overweight adolescents were defined as those with a body-mass index that on 2 occasions was greater than the 75th percentile in subjects of the same age and sex in a large national survey. Lean adolescents were defined as those with a body-mass index between the 25th and 50th percentiles. Subjects who were still alive were interviewed in 1988 to obtain information about their medical history, weight, functional capacity, and other risk factors. For those who had died, information on the cause of death was obtained from death certificates. Overweight in adolescent subjects was associated with an increased risk of mortality from all causes and disease-specific mortality among men, but not among women (Figure 1-23). The relative risks among men were 1.8 for mortality from all causes and 2.3 for mortality from CAD. The risk of morbidity from CAD and atherosclerosis was increased among men and women who had been overweight in adolescence. The risk of colorectal cancer and gout was increased among men and the risk of arthritis was increased among women who had been overweight in adolescence. Overweight in adolescence was a more powerful predictor of these risks than overweight in adulthood. Overweight in adolescence predicted a broad range of adverse health effects that were independent of adult weight after 55 years of follow-up.

The hypothesis that body fatness modifies the relation between dietary cholesterol and 25-year CAD mortality was examined by Goff and associates[80] from Houston, Texas, Wageningen, The Netherlands, and Chicago, Illinois, in a cohort of 1,792 middle-aged men employed by the Western Electric Company in Chicago. Relative risks of coronary death associated with a 225 mg/day greater intake of dietary cholesterol for men with a subscapular skinfold thickness ≤14, 15–20, and ≥21 mm were 1.44, 1.07, and 0.95, respectively, after adjustment for age; serum total cholesterol level; systolic BP; cigarette smoking; family history of cardiovascular disease; evidence of major organ system disease at baseline; and intake of saturated fatty acids, polyunsaturated fatty acids, energy, and ethanol. Adjusted relative risks associated with a 15-mm greater subscapular skinfold thickness for men with a dietary cholesterol intake 649, 650–799, and 800 mg/day were 1.76, 1.64, and 1.00, respectively. Fatter men apparently did not benefit from a diet lower in cholesterol, while men who ate a diet high in cholesterol apparently did not benefit from leanness. These results support the hypothesis that body fatness modifies the relation between dietary cholesterol and coronary mortality, perhaps because

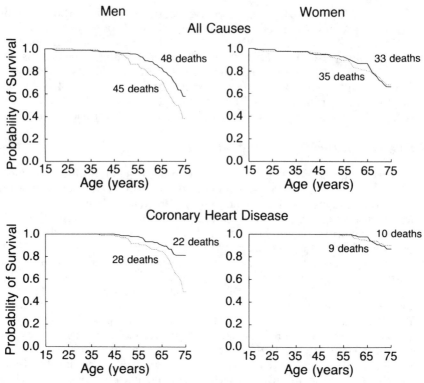

Fig. 1-23. 1. Mortality from All Causes and Mortality from Coronary Heart Disease According to Weight in Adolescence. The solid line represents the lean group, and the broken line the overweight group. Reproduced with permission from Must et al.[79]

leaner men are more responsive than fatter men to the effects of dietary cholesterol on the concentration of LDL cholesterol.

Zamboni and associates[81] from Verona, Italy, evaluated the relation between body fat distribution and severity of CAD. The study sample comprised 33 patients with angiographically demonstrated CAD and 10 angiographically normal control subjects. Body fat distribution was estimated by computed tomography and degree of coronary narrowings by angiographic score. Body weight, body mass index and total and subcutaneous abdominal adipose tissue areas showed no statistical differences in the 2 groups; visceral abdominal adipose tissue area and the visceral to subcutaneous abdominal adipose tissue area ratio were significantly higher in patients with CAD. There was a significant correlation between visceral fat and triglycerides, apoprotein B and sum of glucose and insulin during glucose oral tolerance test. Sum of insulin during glucose oral tolerance test, visceral abdominal adipose tissue area and visceral/subcutaneous abdominal adipose tissue area ratio correlated significantly with severity of CAD, as evaluated by coronary score in all subjects and in CAD patients alone. Stepwise multiple regression analysis using the coronary score as the dependent variable and anthropometric and metabolic parameters as independent variables shows that in all subjects and in CAD patients alone, visceral/subcutaneous abdominal adipose-tissue area ratio entered the regression first and the sum of insulin during glucose oral tolerance test second. The results suggest that visceral abdominal adipose tissue area and visceral to subcutaneous abdominal adipose tissue area ratio may be cardiovascular risk factors.

Cigarette smoking

Cigarette smoking is associated with increases in plasma triglycerides and decreases in plasma HDL cholesterol. These changes not only increase risk of CAD but also are secondary to resistance to insulin-stimulated glucose uptake or hyperinsulinemia. To see whether there is a relation between cigarette smoking and insulin-mediated glucose uptake, Facchini and associates[82] from Stanford and Palo Alto, California, measured plasma lipid and lipoprotein concentrations, plasma glucose and insulin response to an oral glucose challenge, and insulin-mediated glucose uptake in 40 matched healthy volunteers (20 non-smokers, 20 smokers). Smokers had significantly higher mean VLDL triglycerides (0.66 [0.10] vs 0.39 [0.03] mmol/l) and cholesterol (0.45 [0.06] vs 0.23 [0.04] mmol/l) concentrations and lower HDL cholesterol concentrations (1.16 [0.05] vs 1.51 [0.08] mmol/l). Although plasma glucose concentrations in response to the oral glucose load were similar in the 2 groups, plasma insulin response of the smokers was significantly higher. Finally, smokers had higher steady-state plasma glucose concentrations in response to a continuous infusion of glucose, insulin, and somatostatin (8.4 [0.2] vs 5.0 [0.3] mmol/l), despite similar steady-state plasma insulin concentrations. The findings show that chronic cigarette smokers are insulin resistant, hyperinsulinemic, and dyslipidemic compared with a matched group of nonsmokers, and may help to explain why smoking increases risk of CAD.

Activated platelets have been implicated in both acute thrombus formation and atherogenesis. Because smoking is a risk factor for cardiovascular disease in men and women and male smokers have biochemical evidence of increased platelet activation, Rångemark and colleagues[83] in Gothenburg, Sweden studied whether smoking augments platelet activity in women as well. Data on smoking habits and a urinary sample were obtained from 125 healthy female nonsmokers and an equal number of smokers, stratified by age in 5 groups from 18 to 59 years old. Urinary samples were analyzed with gas chromatography/mass spectrometry for the metabolites of thromboxane A_2, reflecting platelet activity, and prostacyclin, representing platelet/vessel wall interaction. Urinary thromboxane in smokers was higher than in nonsmokers, increasing with the number of cigarettes smoked per day and with age. In nonsmokers, there was no difference in thromboxane A_2 between the age groups. Urinary prostacyclin in smokers was higher than that in nonsmokers and decreased with age in nonsmokers but not in smokers. There was no difference in thromboxane A_2 between previous smokers and lifelong nonsmokers. The elevated thromboxane A_2 in women who smoke cigarettes indicates an increased platelet activity that is dependent on smoking intensity. In parallel, prostacyclin is augmented, suggested that platelet/vessel wall interaction is stimulated. Quitting smoking is an effective means to restore platelet function. The investigators proposed that the observed increase in platelet activity in women who smoke cigarettes may be related to subsequent development or cardiovascular disease and that quitting smoking should be considered a high-priority medical target also in this sex.

Coffee consumption

Myers and Basinski[84] from Toronto, Canada, determined if coffee consumption is associated with an increased risk of developing CAD by examining 11 published articles between 1966 and August, 1992, all of which examined a possible link between coffee consumption and CAD. The coronary events for subjects consuming little or no coffee (≤1 cup per day) were compared with event rates for those consuming greater amounts of coffee. The studies exhibited heterogeneity of results. The typical odds ratios and 95% confidence intervals across studies were estimated by logistic regression analysis. Coffee intake from 1 to 4 cups per day was not associated with any increase in CAD occurrence compared with 1 cup or less per day (odds ratio, 1.01). The odds ratios for 4 to 6 and 6 cups or more per day compared with up to 1 cup per day were 1.01 and 1.09, respectively. There is no association between coffee consumption and the occurrence of CAD. This conclusion holds in the absence of adjustment for other coronary risk factors.

Alcohol consumption

Several epidemiological studies have shown light-to-moderate alcohol consumption to have a net protective effect on the incidence of CAD. Major components of this effect, both positive and negative, may be explored using models that include both alcohol and variables expected to mediate the observed alcohol effect. Langer and co-workers[85] in San Diego, California, examined such modeling in a cohort of men of Japanese descent followed in the Honolulu Heart Program and observed that about half of the observed protection against CAD afforded by moderate alcohol consumption was mediated by an increase in HDL cholesterol. An additional 18% of this protection was attributable to a decrease in LDL cholesterol, but was counterbalanced by a 17% increase in risk due to increased systolic blood pressure. The explanation for the residual 50% benefit attributable to alcohol is unknown but may include interference with thrombosis. The results in this population replicate those in the Lipid Research Clinics cohort studied earlier with the same analytic technique. The consistency of these findings across populations, along with the demonstration of reasonable biological pathways for this effect of alcohol, provides strong support for the hypothesis that light-to-moderate alcohol intake is protective against CAD in men.

In most countries, high intake of saturated fat is positively related to high mortality from CAD. The situation in France is paradoxical in that there is a high intake of saturated fat but low mortality from CAD. This paradox may be attributable in part to high wine consumption. Renaud and De Lorgeril[86] from Bron Cedex, France, reviewed epidemiological studies which indicate that consumption of alcohol at the level of intake in France (20–30 g per day) can reduce risk of CAD by at least 40%. Alcohol is believed to protect from CAD by preventing atherosclerosis through the action of HDL cholesterol, but serum concentrations of this factor are no higher in France than in other countries. Re-examination of previous results suggest that, in the main, moderate alcohol intake does not prevent CAD through an effect on atherosclerosis, but rather through a hemostatic mechanism. Data from Caerphilly, Wales, shows that platelet aggregation, which is related to CAD, is inhibited significantly by alcohol at levels of intake associated with reduced risk of CAD. Inhibition of platelet reactivity by wine (alcohol) may be 1 explanation for protection from CAD in France, since pilot studies have shown that platelet reactivity is lower in France than in Scotland.

Moderate alcohol consumption has been reported to provide protection against CAD. Seppa and associates[87] from Tampere, Finland, studied serum lipid values in 380 men, including 184 controls (37 teetotalers and 147 moderate drinkers), 90 heavy drinkers, and 106 alcoholics. Total cholesterol values were significantly lower among alcoholics than controls (mean ± SEM, 5.43 ± 0.15 mmol/L [210 ± 5.8 mg/dL] vs 6.01 ± 0.08 mmol/L [232 ± 3.1 mg/dL]), and their HDL cholesterol values were higher (1.66 ± 0.07 mmol/L [64 ± 2.7 mg/dL] vs 1.14 ± 0.02 mmol/L [44 ± 0.8 mg/dL]) (Figure 1-24). Accordingly, there was a highly significant difference in the HDL/total cholesterol ratio (0.32 ± 0.13 vs 0.19 ± 0.01). Heavy drinkers had significantly higher total cholesterol values than controls (6.30 ± 0.13 mmol/L [244 ± 5.0 mg/dL] vs 6.01 ± 0.08 mmol/L [232 ± 3.1 mg/dL]); the same was true of HDL cholesterol values (1.25 ± 0.07 mmol/L [48 ± 2.7 mg/dL] vs 1.14 ± 0.02 mmol/L [44 ± 0.8 mg/dL]). No significant difference was found in the HDL/total cholesterol ratio between controls and heavy drinkers or between teetotalers and moderate drinkers. Therefore, moderate alcohol intake apparently does not change HDL/total cholesterol ratio; if moderate drinking is protective against CHD, the mechanism is probably not via lipids.

To study the association between alcohol consumption and death from CAD and to determine the extent to which the association can be explained by the HDL cholesterol level, Suh and associates[88] for the Multiple Risk Factor Intervention Trial Research Group performed a cohort study involving men enrolled in the Multiple Risk Factor Intervention Trial (MRFIT). Men (n = 11,688) at high risk for developing CAD but without clinical evidence of it were studied. More than 90% of the men were white and the average age was 46 years. Five percent of the men abstained from alcohol during the trial, 81% consumed fewer than 21 alcoholic drinks per week, and 14% consumed >21 alcoholic drinks per week. Average alcohol intake over 7 years was calculated for MRFIT participants who were alive at the end of the trial and who had at least 3 follow-up records of alcohol consumption. Post-trial mortality during a 3.8-year period was assessed. The adjusted relative risk for death from CAD for each increase of 7 drinks per week was 0.89, with an apparent dose-response relationship. The average HDL level was associated with the average alcohol intake in a least-squares regression model (Figure 1-25). When the average HDL level was included in the proportional hazards model for mortality from CAD, the absolute value of the coefficient for average drinks per week declined 45%, yielding an adjusted relative risk for each additional 7 drinks per week of 0.94. It is concluded that in middle-aged men who are light to moderate drinkers, the inverse association between alcohol consumption and death from CAD can be explained,

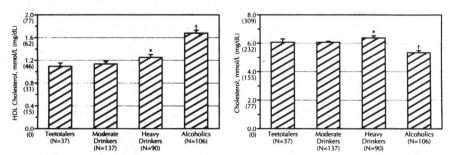

Fig. 1-24. Serum high-density lipoprotein (HDL) (left) and total cholesterol (right) values (mean ± SEM) in teetotalers, moderate drinkers, heavy drinkers, and alcoholics. Comparison of moderate drinkers with teetotalers; comparison of heavy drinkers and alcoholics with the control group consisting of teetotalers and moderate drinkers. Asterisk indicates P<.05; dagger, P<.001. Reproduced with permission from Seppa, et al.[87]

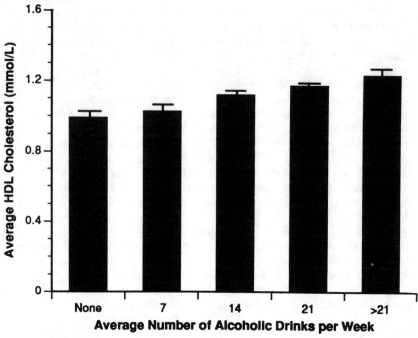

Fig. 1-25. Average high-density lipoprotein cholesterol level and alcohol consumption. HDL = high-density lipoprotein. Reproduced with permission from Suh, et al.[88]

in large part, by the HDL cholesterol level, which increases with alcohol consumption. However, alcohol consumption cannot be recommended because of the known adverse effects of excess alcohol use.

MISCELLANEOUS TOPICS

Chlamydia pneumonia infection

To investigate in the prospective Helsinki Heart Study whether chronic Chlamydia pneumonie infection, indicated by elevated antibody titers against the pathogen, chlamydial lipopolysaccharide-containing immune complexes, or both, is a risk factor for CAD, Saikku and associates[89] from Helsinki and Tampere, Finland, randomized participants in the Helsinki Heart Study to receive either gemfibrozil (2,046 patients) or placebo (2,035 patients) and collected serum samples at 3-month intervals from all patients during the 5-year clinical trial. One hundred and forty cardiac events, namely fatal and nonfatal AMI and/or sudden cardiac death occurred during the follow-up period. Serum samples from 103 case patients obtained 3 to 6 months before cardiac endpoint were matched with those from controls for time point, locality, and treatment. Samples were tested for markers of chronic chlamydial infection. Immunoglobulin A (lgA) and G (lgG) antibodies to C. pneumonia were measured using the microimmunofluorescence method. Lipopolysaccharide-containing immune complexes were measured using 2 antigen-specific enzyme immunoassays, the lipopolysaccharide-capture and immunoglobulin M (lgM)-capture methods. Using a conditional logistic regression model, odds ratios for the development of CAD were 2.7 for elevated lgA titers, 2.1 for the presence of immune complexes, and 2.9 for the presence of both factors. If the authors adjusted for other CAD risk factors such as age, hypertension, and smoking, the corresponding values would be 2.3, 1.8, and 2.6, respectively. The results suggest that chronic C. pneumonia infection may be a significant risk factor for the development of CAD.

Leukocyte count

To examine the relation of white blood cell (WBC) count to the development of cardiovascular disease, including CAD, stroke, peripheral arterial disease, and congestive heart failure, Kannel and associates[90] from Boston and Framingham, Massachusetts, analyzed 1,393 men and 1,401 women from the Framingham Offspring Study who were free of cardiovascular disease at the onset of the study and who were age 30 to 59 years at baseline. There were 180 cardiovascular events in the men and 80 in the women. The WPC count correlated most strongly with the number of cigarettes smoked per day, hematocrit, and vital capacity. Among non-smoking men with WBC counts within the normal range, the age-adjusted WBC count was significantly associated with cardiovascular disease and CAD incidence. For each 1.0×10^9/L-cell difference in WBC count, the cardiovascular disease risk increased 32%. In women, each 1.0×10^9/L-cell increment in WBC count was associated with a 17% increase in cardiovascular disease risk, but only in smokers, and the relation was not statistically significant after adjustment for relevant risk factors. The degree of elevation of WBC count within the normal range is a marker for increased risk of cardiovascular disease that is partially explained by cigarette smoking.

Mänttäri and associates[91] from Helsinki, Finland, investigated the role of an elevated serum leukocyte count as a coronary risk factor in dyslipidemic middle-aged men (n = 420) participating in the Helsinki Heart Study, a coronary primary prevention trial. Baseline serum leukocyte count was significantly higher, 6.93×10^9/L in patients with cardiac events, than in controls, 6.26×10^9/L. This association was time-dependent, however, since the difference was not significant for events occurring during the second half of the 5-year study. Using nonsmokers in the lowest serum leukocyte count tertile as the reference sample, the relative risks in the highest serum leukocyte count tertile were 1.86 for nonsmokers and 3.07 for smokers. Logistic regression analysis including smoking disclosed an independent contribution of elevated serum leukocyte count for CAD. It was concluded that elevated leukocyte count was a coronary risk factor even in a dyslipidemic population.

Physical activity

Aging is associated with an increased risk of women dying from CAD as well as from all causes combined. Alterations in the major biological risk factors for early CAD and all-cause mortality are frequently seen in aging. Owens and colleagues[92] in Pittsburgh, Pennsylvania tested the hypothesis that high levels of physical activity could protect against age-associated changes in biological risk factor levels. In the Healthy Women Study, 507 women were evaluated at study entry and 3 years later. Weekly physical activity level was measured at each examination via the Paffenbarger Physical Activity Questionnaire. During the 3-year period, women increased significantly in weight, bp, levels of total and LDL cholesterol, triglycerides, and insulin and decreased significantly in levels of total HDL cholesterol and HDL$_2$. Consistent with the study hypothesis, women who reported higher levels of activity at baseline had less weight gain over time. Furthermore, women who increased their activity during the 3-year interval had the smallest increases in weight and tended to have the smallest decreases in total HDL cholesterol and HDL$_2$ cholesterol. The changes in lipids due to activity were largely independent of changes in body weight.

References

1. Neaton JD, Wentworth, D: Serum cholesterol, blood pressure, cigarette smoking, and death from coronary heart disease: Overall findings and differences by age for 316,099 white men. Arch Intern Med 1992 (Jan);152:56–64.

2. Vigna G, Bolzan M, Romagnoni F, Valerio G, Vitale E, Zuliani G, Fellin R: Lipids and Other Risk Factors Selected by Discriminant Analysis in Symptomatic Patients With Supra-Aortic and Peripheral Atherosclerosis. Circulation 1992 (June);85:2205–2211.

3. Sharp SD, Williams RR, Hunt SC, Schumacher MC: Coronary risk factors and the severity of angiographic coronary artery disease in members of high-risk pedigrees. Am Heart J 1992 (February);123:279–290.

4. Fraser G, Strahan T, Sabate J, Beeson W, Kissinger D: Effects of Traditional Coronary Risk Factors on Rates of Incident Coronary Events in a Low-Risk Population. The Adventist Health Study. Circulation 1992 (August);86:406–413.

5. Cholesterol screening and awareness—Behavioral risk factor surveillance system, 1990. MMWR 1992 (Sept 11);669, 675–678.

6. Frank E, Winkleby MA, Fortmann SP, Rickhill B, Farquhar JW: Improved cholesterol-related knowledge and behavior and plasma cholesterol levels in adults during the 1980s. JAMA 1992 (Sept 23/30);268:1566–1572.

7. Casasnovas JA, Lapetra A, Puzo J, Pelegrin J, Hermosilla T, De Vicente J, Garza F, Del Rio A, Giner A, Ferreira IJ: Tobacco, physical exercise and lipid profile. Euro Heart J 1992 (Apr);13:440–445.

8. Zimetbaum P, Frishman WH, Ooi WL, Derman MP, Aronson M, Gidez LI, Eder HA: Plasma lipids and lipoproteins and the incidence of cardiovascular disease in the very elderly: The Bronx Aging Study. Arteriosclerosis and Thrombosis 1992 (Apr);12:416–423.

9. Manolio TA, Furberg CD, Wahl PW, Tracy RP, Borhani NO, Gardin JM, Fried LP, O'Leary DH, Kuller LH: Eligibility for cholesterol referral in community-dwelling older adults: The cardiovascular health study. Ann Intern Med 1992 (Apr 15);116:641–649.

10. Ettinger W, Wahl P, Kuller L, Bush T, Tracy R, Manolio T, Borhani N, Wong N, O'Leary D, for the CHS Collaborative Research Group: Lipoprotein Lipids in Older People, Results From the Cardiovascular Health Study. Circulation 1992 (September);86:858–869.

11. Fowkes FGR, Leng GC, Donnan PT, Deary IJ, Riemersma RA, Housley E: Serum cholesterol, triglycerides, and aggression in the general population. Lancet 1992 (Oct 24);340:995–998.

12. Hetland ML, Haarbo J, Christiansen C: One measurement of serum total cholesterol is enough to predict future levels in healthy postmenopausal women. Am J Med 1992 (Jan);92:25–28.

13. Weitzman JB, Vladutiu AO: Very high values of serum high-density lipoprotein cholesterol. Arch Pathol Lab Med 1992 (Aug);116:831–836.

14. Rader DJ,, Brewer HB Jr: Lipoprotein(a): Clinical approach to a unique atehrogenic lipoprotein. JAMA 1992 (Feb 26);267:1109–1112.

15. Sorrentino MJ, Vielhauer C, Eisenbart JD, Fless GM, Scanu AM, Feldman T: Plasma lipoprotein (a) protein concentration and coronary artery disease in black patients compared with white patients. Am J Med 1992 (Dec);93:658–662.

16. Averna MR, Barbagallo CM, Ocello S, Doria O, Davi G, Scafidi V, Albiero R, Notarbartolo

A: Lp(a) levels in patients undergoing aorto-coronary bypass surgery. Eur Heart J 1992 (Oct);13:1405–1409.

17. Cressman M, Heyka R, Paganini E, O'Neil J, Skibinski C, Hoff H: Lipoprotein(a) Is an Independent Risk Factor for Cardiovascular Disease in Hemodialysis Patients. Circulation 1992 (August);86:475–482.

18. Feely J, Barry M, Keeling PWN, Weir DG, Cooke T: Lipoprotein(a) in cirrhosis. Br Med J 1992 (Feb 29);304:545–546.

19. Kwiterovich PO Jr, Smith HH, Bachorik PS, Derby CA, Pearson TA: Comparison of the plasma levels of apolipoproteins B and A-1, and other risk factors in men and women with premature coronary artery disease. Am J Cardiol 1992 (Apr 15);69:1015–1021.

20. Sigurdsson G, Baldursdottir A, Sigvaldason H, Agnarsson U, Thorgeirsson G, Sigfusson N: Predictive value of apolipoproteins in a prospective survey of coronary artery disease in men. Am J Cardiol 1992 (May 15);69:1251–1254.

21. Benuck I, Gidding SS, Donovan M, Traisman ES, Traisman HS: Usefulness of parental serum total cholesterol levels in identifying children with hypercholesterolemia. Am J Cardiol 1992 (Mar 15);69:713–717.

22. Grundy SM, Vega GL: Two different views of the relationship of hypertriglyceridemia to coronary heart disease: Implications for treatment. Arch Intern Med 1992 (Jan);152:28–34.

23. Henkin Y, Como JA, Oberman A: Secondary dyslipidemia: Inadvertent effects of drugs in clinical practice. JAMA 1992 (Feb 19);267:961–968.

24. Vyssoulis GP, Karpanou EA, Pitsavos CE, Skoumas JN, Palelogos AA, Toutouzas PK: Differentiation of B-blocker effects on serum lipids and apolipoproteins in hypertensive patients with normolipidemic or dyslipidemic profiles. Eur Heart J 1992 (Nov);13:1506–1513.

25. Bagatell CJ, Knopp RH, Vale WW, Rivier JE, Bremner WJ: Physiologic testosterone levels in normal men suppress high-density lipoprotein cholesterol levels. Ann Intern Med 1992 (June 15);116:967–973.

26. Gietema JA, Sleijfer DT, Willemse PHB, Koops HS, Van Ittersum E, Verschuren WMM, Kromhout D, Sluiter WJ, Mulder NH, De Vries EGE: Long-term follow-up of cardiovascular risk factors in patients given chemotherapy for disseminated nonseminomatous testicular cancer. An of Intern Med 1992 (May 1);116:709–715.

27. Buchwald: Cholesterol inhibition, cancer, and chemotherapy. Lancet 1992 (May 9);339:1154–1156.

28. Davi G, Averna M, Catalano I, Barbagallo C, Ganci A, Notarbartolo A, Ciabattoni G, Patrono C: Increased Thromboxane Biosynthesis in Type IIa Hypercholesterolemia. Circulation 1992 (May);85:1792–1798.

29. Koenig W, Sund M, Ernst E, Mraz W, Hombach V, Keil U: Association Between Rheology and Components of Lipoproteins in Human Blood, Results From the MONICA Project. Circulation 1992 (June);85:2197–2204.

30. Muldoon MF, Bachen EA, Manuck SB, Waldstein SR, Bricker PL, Bennett JA: Acute cholesterol responses to mental stress and change in posture. Arch Intern Med 1992 (Apr);152:775–780.

31. Fried RE, Levine DM, Kwiterovich PO, Diamond EL, Wilder LB, Moy TF, Pearson TA: The effect of filtered-coffee consumption on plasma lipid levels: Results of a randomized clinical trial. JAMA 1992 (Feb 12);267:811–815.

32. Nieminen MS, Mattila KJ, Aalto-Setala A, Kuusi T, Kontula K, Kauppinen-Makelin R, Ehnholm C, Jauhiainen M, Valle M, Taskinen MR: Lipoproteins and their genetic variation in subjects with and without angiographically verified coronary artery disease. Arteriosclerosis and Thrombosis 1992 (Jan);12:58–69.

33. Genest J, Martin-Munley S, McNamara J, Ordovas J, Jenner J, Myers R, Silberman S, Wilson P, Salem D, Schaefer E: Familial Lipoprotein Disorders in Patients With Premature Coronary Artery Disease. Circulation 1992 (June);85:2025–2033.

34. The Bezafibrate Infarction Prevention Study Group: Lipids and Lipoproteins in Symptomatic Coronary Heart Disease, Distribution, Intercorrelations, and Significance for Risk Classifications in 6,700 Men and 1,500 Women. Circulation 1992 (September);86:839–848.

35. Miller M, Seidler A, Kwiterovich PO, Pearson TA: Long-term Predictors of Subsequent Cardiovascular Events With Coronary Artery Disease and "Desirable" Levels of Plasma Total Cholesterol. Circulation 1992 (October);86:1165–1170.

36. Rubins HB, Schectman G, Wilt TJ, Iwane MK: Distribution of lipid phenotypes in community-living men with coronary heart disease: High prevalence of isolated low levels of high-density lipoprotein cholesterol. Arch Intern Med 1992 (Dec)152:2412–2416.

37. Drexel H, Amann FW, Rentsch K, Neuenschwander C, Luethy A, Khan SI, Follath F: Relation of the level of high-density lipoprotein subfractions to the presence and extent of coronary artery disease. Am J Cardiol 1992 (Aug 15);70:436–440.

38. Assmann G, Schulte H: Relation of high-density lipoprotein cholesterol and triglycerides to incidence of atherosclerotic coronary artery disease (the PROCAM experience). Am J Cardiol 1992 (Sept 15);70:733–737.

39. Regenstrom J, Nilsson J, Tornvall P, Landou C, Hamsten A: Susceptibility to low-density lipoprotein oxidation and coronary atherosclerosis in man. Lancet 1992 (May 16);339:1183–1186.

40. Smith GD, Shipley MJ, Marmot MG, Rose G: Plasma cholesterol concentration and mortality: The Whitehall study. JAMA 1992 (Jan 1);267:70–76.

41. Neaton JD, Blackburn H, Jacobs D, Kuller L, Lee DJ, Sherwin R, Shih J, Stamler J, Wentworth D, Multiple Risk Factor Intervention Trial Research Group: Serum cholesterol level and mortality findings for men screened in the multiple risk factor intervention trial. Arch Intern Med 1992 (July);152:1490–1500.

42. Bønaa K, Arnesen E: Association Between Heart Rate and Atherogenic Blood Lipid Fractions in a Population, The Tromsø Study. Circulation 1992 (August);86:394–405.

43. Megnien J, Sene V, Jeannin S, Hernigou A, Plainfosse M, Merli I, Atger V, Moatti N, Levenson J, Simon A, and the PCV METRA Group: Coronary Calcification and Its Relation to Extracoronary Atherosclerosis in Asymptomatic Hypercholesterolemic Men. Circulation 1992 (May);85:1799–1807.

44. Senti M, Nogues X, Pedro-Botet J, Rubies-Prat J, and Vidal–Barraquer F: Lipoprotein Profile in Men with Peripheral Vascular Disease Role of Intermediate Density Lipoproteins and Apoprotein E. Phenotypes. Circulation 1992 (January);85:30–36.

45. Cobb M, Teitlebaum H, Risch N, Jekel J, Ostfeld A: Influence of Dietary Fat, Apolipoprotein E Phenotype, and Sex on Plasma Lipoprotein Levels. Circulation 1992 (September);86:849–857.

46. Singh RB, Rastogi SS, Niaz MA, Ghosh S, Singh R, Gupta S: Effect of fat-modified and fruit- and vegetable-enriched diets on blood lipids in the Indian diet heart study. Am J Cardiol 1992 (Oct 1);70:869–874.

47. Henkin Y, Garber DW, Osterlund LC, Darnell BE: Saturated fats, cholesterol, and dietary compliance. Arch Intern Med 1992 (June);152:1167–1174.

48. D'Amico G, Gentile MG, Manna G, Fellin G, Ciceri R, Cofano F, Petrini C, Lavarda F, Perlolini S, Porrini M: Effect of vegetarian soy diet on hyperlipidemia in nephrotic syndrome. Lancet 1992 (May 9);339:1131–1134.

49. Fraser GE, Sabate J, Beeson WL, Strahan TM: A possible protective effect of nut consumption on risk of coronary heart disease: The Adventist health study. Arch Intern Med 1992 (July);152:1416–1424.

50. Haskell WL, Spiller GA, Jensen CD, Ellis BK, Gates JE: Role of water-soluble dietary fiber in the management of elevated plasma cholesterol in healthy subjects. Am J Cardiol 1992 (Feb 15);69:433–439.

51. Singh RB, Rastogi SS, Singh R, Ghosh S, Niaz MA: Effects of guava intake on serum total and high-density lipoprotein cholesterol levels and on systemic blood pressure. Am J Cardiol 1992 (Nov 15);70:1287–1291.

52. Ripsin CM, Keenan JM, Jacobs DR, Elmer PJ, Welch RR, Van Horn L, Liu K, Turnbull WH, Thye FW, Kestin M, Hegsted M, Davidson DM, Davidson MH, Dugan LD, Demark-Wahnefried W, Beling S: Oat products and lipid lowering: A Meta-analysis. JAMA 1992 (June 24);267:3317–3325.

53. Roberts WC: More on fast foods and quick plaques. Am J Cardiol 1992 (July 15);70:268–270.

54. Prihoda JS, Illingworth DR: Drug therapy of hyperlipidemia. Current Problems in Cardiology 1992 (Sept).

55. Hong MK, Romm PA, Reagan K, Green CE, Rackley CE: Effects of estrogen replacement therapy on serum lipid values and angiographically defined coronary artery disease in postmenopausal women. Am J Cardiol 1992 (Jan 15);69:176–178.

56. American College of Physicians: Guidelines for counseling postmenopausal women about preventive hormone therapy. An Intern Med 1992 (Dec 15);117:1038–1048.

57. Lipid Research Clinics Investigators: The lipid research clinics coronary primary prevention trial: Results of 6 years of post-trial follow-up. Arch Intern Med 1992 (July);152:1399–1410.

58. Superko HR, Greenland P, Manchester RA, Andreadis NA, Schectman G, West NH, Hunninghake D, Haskell WL, Probstfield JL: Effectiveness of low-dose colestipol therapy in patients with moderate hypercholesterolemia. Am J Cardiol 1992 (July 15);70:135–140.

59. Lavie CJ, Mailander L, Milani RV: Marked benefit with sustained-release niacin therapy in patients with "isolated" very low levels of high-density lipoprotein cholesterol and coronary artery disease. Am J Cardiol 1992 (Apr 15);69:1083–1085.

60. Rader JI, Calvert RJ, Hathcock JN: Hepatic toxicity of unmodified and time-release preparations in niacin. Am J Med 1992 (Jan);92:77–82.

61. Manninen V, Tenkanen L, Koskinen P, Huttunen JK, Manttari M, Heinonen OP, and Frick MH: Joint Effects of Serum Triglyceride and LDL Cholesterol and HDL Cholesterol Concentrations on Coronary Heart Disease Risk in the Helsinki Heart Study Implications for Treatment. Circulation 1992 (January);85:37–45.

62. Koskinen P, Kovanen PT, Tuomilehto J, Manninen V: Gemfibrozil also corrects dyslipidemia in postmenopausal women and smokers. Arch Intern Med 1992 (Jan);152:90–96.

63. Shear C, Franklin F, Stinnett S, Hurley D, Bradford R, Chremos A, Nash D, Langendorfer A: Expanded Clinical Evaluation of Lovastatin (EXCEL) Study Results, Effect of Patient Characteristics on Lovastatin-Induced Changes in Plasma Concentrations of Lipids and Lipoproteins. Circulation 1992 (April);85:1293–1303.

64. Illingworth DR, Vakar F, Mahley RW, Weisgraber KH: Hypocholesterolemic effects of lovastatin in familial defective apolipoprotein B-100. Lancet 1992 (Mar 7);339:598–600.

65. D'Agostino RB, Kannel WB, Stepanians MN, D'Agostino LC: A comparison between lovastatin and gemfibrozil in the treatment of primary hypercholesterolemia. Am J Cardiol 1992 (Jan);69:28–34.

66. McKenney JM, Barnett MD, Wright JT Jr, Proctor JP: Comparison of gemfibrozil and lovastatin in patients with high low-density lipoprotein and low high-density lipoprotein cholesterol levels. Arch Intern Med 1992 (Sept);152:1781–1787.

67. Glueck CJ, Oakes N, Speirs J, Tracy T, Lang J: Gemfibrozil-lovastatin therapy for primary hyperlipoproteinemias. Am J Cardiol 1992 (July 1);70:1–9.

68. European Study Group: Efficacy and tolerability of simvastatin and pravastatin in patients with primary hypercholesterolemia (Multicountry Comparative Study). Am J Cardiol 1992 (Nov 15);70:1281–1286.

69. Betteridge DJ, Bhatnager D, Bing RF, Durrington PN, Evans GR, Flax H, Jay RH, Lewis-Barned N, Mann J, Matthews DR, Miller JP, Reckless JPD, Sturley R, Taylor KG, Winder AF: Treatment of familial hypercholesterolemia: United Kingdom lipid clinics study of pravastatin and cholestyramine. Br Med J 1992 (May 23);304:1335–1338.

70. Bell L, Halstenson CE, Halstenson CJ, Macres M, Keane WF: Cholesterol-lowering effects of calcium carbonate in patients with mild to moderate hypercholesterolemia. Arch Intern Med 1992 (Dec);152:2441–2444.

71. Buchwald H, Campos CT, Matts JP, Fitch LL, Long JM, Varco RL, POSCH Group: Women in the POSCH Trial: Effects of aggressive cholesterol modification in women with coronary heart disease. Ann Surg 1992 (Oct);216:389–400.

72. Gordon BR, Kelsey SF, Bilheimer DW, Brown DC, Dau PC, Gotto AM Jr, Illingworth DR, Jones PH, Leitman SF, Prihoda JS, Stein EA, Stern TN, Zavoral JH, Zwiener RJ: Treatment of refractory familial hypercholesterolemia by low-density lipoprotein apheresis using an automated dextran sulfate cellulose adsorption system. Am J Cardiol 1992 (Oct 22);70:1010–1016.

73. Grover SA, Abrahamowicz M, Joseph L, Brewer C, Coupal L, Suissa S: The benefits of treating hyperlipidemia to prevent coronary heart disease: Estimating changes in life expectancy and morbidity. JAMA 1992 (Feb 12);267:816–822.

74. Manson JE, Nathan DM, Krolewski AS, Stampfer MJ, Willett WC, Hennekens CH: A prospective study of exercise and incidence of diabetes among US male physicians. JAMA 1992 (July 1);268:63–67.

75. Ramirez LC, Arauz-Pacheco A, Lackner C, Albright G, Adams BV, Raskin P: Lipoprotein (a) levels in diabetes mellitus: Relationship to metabolic control. An Intern Med 1992 (July 1);117:42–47.

76. Earle K, Walker J, Hill C, Viberti GC: Familial clustering of cardiovascular disease in

patients with insulin-dependent diabetes and nephropathy. NEJM 1992 (Mar 5);326:673–677.

77. Barrett-Connor E: Lower endogenous androgen levels and dyslipidemia in men with non-insulin-dependent diabetes mellitus. An Intern Med 1992 (Nov 15);117:807–811.

78. Barnard RJ, Ugianskis EJ, Martin DA, Inkeles SB: Role of diet and exercise in the management of hyperinsulinemia and associated atherosclerotic risk factors. Am J Cardiol 1992 (Feb 15);69:440–444.

79. Must A, Jacques PF, Dallal GE, Bajema CJ, Dietz WH: Long-term morbidity and mortality of overweight adolescents: A follow-up of the Harvard Growth Study of 1922 to 1935. N Engl J Med 1992 (Nov 5);327:1350–1355.

80. Goff DC Jr, Shekelle RB, Katan MB, Gotto AM Jr, Stamler J: Does body fatness modify the association between dietary cholesterol and risk of coronary death? Results from the Chicago Western Electric study. Arteriosclerosis and Thrombosis 1992 (July)12:755–761.

81. Zamboni M, Armellini F, Sheiban I, De Marchi M, Todesco T, Bergamo–Andreis IA, Cominacini L, Bosello O: Relation of body fat distribution in men and degree of coronary narrowings in coronary artery disease. Am J Cardiol 1992 (Nov 1);70:1135–1138.

82. Facchini FS, Hollenbeck CB, Jeppesen J, Chen YDI, Reaven GM: Insulin resistance and cigarette smoking. Lancet 1992 (May 9);339:1128–1130.

83. Rångemark C, Benthin G, Granström EF, Persson L, Winell S, Wennmalm Å: Tobacco Use and Urinary Excretion of Thromboxane A$_2$ and Prostacyclin Metabolites in Women Stratified by Age. Circulation 1992 (November);86:1495–1500.

84. Myers MG, Basinski A: Coffee and coronary heart disease. Arch Intern Med 1992 (Sept);152:1767–1772.

85. Langer RD, Criqui MH, Reed DM: Lipoproteins and Blood Pressure as Biological Pathways for Effect of Moderate Alcohol Consumption on Coronary Heart Disease. Circulation 1992 (March);85:910–915.

86. Renaud S, De Lorgeril M: Wine, alcohol, platelets, and the French paradox for coronary heart disease. Lancet 1992 (June 20);339:1523–1526.

87. Seppa K, Sillanaukee P, Pitkajarvi T, Nikkila M, Koivula T: Moderate and heavy alcohol consumption have no favorable effect on lipid values. Arch Intern Med 1992 (Feb);152:297–300.

88. Suh I, Shaten J, Cutler JA, Kuller LH: Alcohol use and mortality from coronary heart disease: The role of high-density lipoprotein cholesterol. An Intern Med 1992 (June 1);116:881–887.

89. Saikku P, Leinonen M, Tenkanen L, Linnanmaki E, Ekman MR, Manninen V, Manttari M, Frick MH; Huttunen JK: Chronic chlamydia pneumonia infection as a risk factor for coronary heart disease in the Helsinki heart study. An Intern Med 1992 (Feb 15);116:273–278.

90. Kannel WB, Anderson K, Wilson PWF: White blood cell count and cardiovascular disease: Insights from the Framingham study. JAMA 1992 (Mar 4);267:1253–1256.

91. Manttari M, Manninen V, Koskinen P, Huttunen JK, Oksanen E, Tenkanen L, Heinonen OP, Frick MH: Leukocytes as a coronary risk factor in dyslipidemic male population. Am Heart J 1992 (April);123:873–877.

92. Owens J, Matthews K, Wing R, Kuller L: Can Physical Activity Mitigate the Effects of Aging in Middle-Aged Women? Circulation 1992 (April);85:1265–1270.

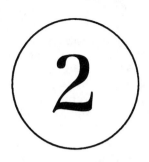

Coronary Artery Disease

MISCELLANEOUS TOPICS

USA incidence and mortality

The incidence of CAD has not been as well characterized among women as it has among men. In an anonymously authored report in the *Morbidity and Mortality Weekly Report* of July 24, 1992, data was presented on age-specific incidence of CAD and the risks associated with cigarette smoking, diabetes mellitus, systemic hypertension, serum total cholesterol, body mass, and age using data from the Epidemiologic Follow-up Study of the First National Health and Nutrition Examination Survey (NHEFS).[1] NHEFS is the first prospective cohort study of a representative sample (N = 14,407) of the noninstitutionalized US adult population. During 1971–1975, members of the First National Health and Nutrition Examination Survey (NHANES I) cohort completed an extensive interview regarding demographic characteristics and medical history and received a standardized physical examination. During 1982–84, 1986, and 1987 the NHEFS attempted to trace and re-interview NHANES I participants aged ≥25 years during the baseline examination. Death certificates and records of hospitalizations also were obtained. As of 1987, >96% of the initial study participants either had been contacted at least once or had died. Present analysis was limited to persons without CAD at baseline as ascertained through self-report and physical examination. The report was limited to the 12,402 white participants. Rates were calculated as incidence densities; each person could contribute person-years of follow-up to >1 age category (e.g., a 42-year-old person who was followed for 11 years contributed 3 years to the 25–44-year age group and 8 years to the 45–54-year age group). The mean length of follow-up for CAD incidence was 12.4 years. The age-adjusted CAD incidence rate for men was 110/10,000 person-years; for women, the rate was 64/10,000 person-years. Within each age group, men had a higher rate of CAD incidence (Figure

2-1). While the rate generally increased by the same amount with age for men aged 25–74 years, the rate of increase of CAD incidence among women accelerated after age 65 years. Men were more likely than women to be first diagnosed with an acute form of CAD. Death was the incident CAD event among 18.6% of men compared with 12.5% of women. AMI was diagnosed in 41.3% of incident CAD vents among men and 29.7% of incident events among women.

Since the mid-1960s, national death rates for CAD have been decreasing for both sexes. The proportional decrease, however, has been greater among men than women, even though the decline began first among women. During that time, women in other developed countries (e.g., Finland and Sweden) have had larger proportional reductions in CAD mortality than men, even though in these countries, as in the USA, men aged 40–69 years have been at least 2.5 times more likely to die from CAD than women.

In 1989 approximately 500,000 persons died from CAD in the USA. Age adjusted CAD death rates for the US population aged ≥35 years declined 24%—from 588 per 100,000 in 1980 to 449 per 100,000 in 1988.[2] Although CAD death rates declined more rapidly for men than women and for whites than for blacks, they declined for each of the 4 race-sex groups (Figure 2-2). The average annual decline (as estimated) was 3.7% for white men, 3.1% for black men, 2.9% for white women, and 2.2% for black women. During the 9 year period, overall rates of CAD mortality were highest in the northeast, followed by the midwest, the south, and the west. Throughout the 9 year period, CAD death rates declined in each of the 50 states and the District of Columbia for both men and women. The annual median rate of decline among the states was 3.0% for women and 3.8% for men.

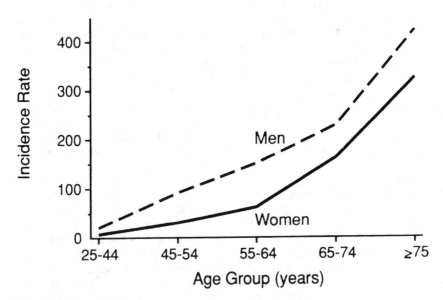

*Per 10,000 person-years.
†Because of the small number of persons of other races in the sample, this includes only the 12,402 white participants.

Fig. 2-1. Coronary heart disease incidence rate,* by sex and age group—Epidemiologic Follow-up Study of the First National Health and Nutrition Examination Survey, 1982–84, 1986, and 1987†. Reproduced from MMWR.[2]

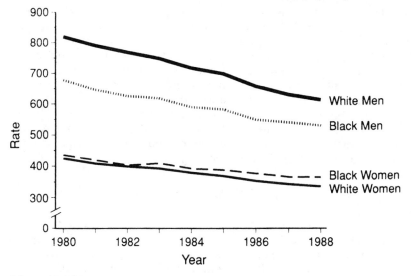

*Per 100,000 population, adjusted to the 1980 U.S. standard population.

Fig. 2-2. Age-adjusted death rates* for ischemic heart disease among adults aged 35 years, by race and sex—United States, 1980–1988. Reproduced with permission from MMWR.[2]

Gender bias in referral and outcome

To determine whether a gender bias exists in referral for CABG among patients with catheterization-documented CAD, Bickell and associates[3] from Chapel Hill and Durham, North Carolina, performed a historical cohort study (1969–1984) involving 5,795 patients with catheterization-documented CAD. The surgical referral patterns of men and women grouped by risk of cardiac death and by treatment effectiveness were evaluated. Time trends were evaluated for three periods: 1969–1974, 1975–1979, and 1980–1984. Overall, when no adjustment was made for baseline risk for cardiac death, no statistical difference was found between men and women regarding referral for surgery (46% compared with 44%, respectively). When an adjustment was made for such risk, the male-to-female odds ratio for surgical referral was 1.28 among patients with a low risk for cardiac death. This effect was most evident in the 1980 to 1984 period (odds ratio, 1.73). In the high-risk group, the odds ratio was 0.84 with little change occurring during the study. Men were more likely to be referred for surgery when surgery offered the least survival benefit relative to medical therapy (odds ratio, 1.29). This effect was most pronounced in the 1980 to 1984 period (odds ratio, 1.63). Women are less likely than men to be referred for CABG among patients with a low risk for cardiac death, in whom surgery offers little or no survival benefit over medical treatment. Women are at least as likely as men to be referred for CABG among more symptomatic and more severely diseased patients, in whom surgery offers the greatest survival benefits.

One third of all deaths in women in the USA each year are attributable to CAD. Gender differences exist in the course and management of patients with CAD. Few randomized trials have been conducted in women to evaluate effective therapeutic strategies. Eysmann and Douglas[4] reviewed gender-related outcomes with coronary revascularization and reperfusion therapies. English-language journal articles and reviews on the subject of women with CAD or gender-specific responses to CAD management, from 1970–1992, were identified. The studies selected included only randomized controlled trials for topics related to thrombolysis, and articles considered to contribute significantly to the topic of women with CAD in the case of angioplasty and CABG. Thrombolysis in AMI reduces mortality in men and women, although women may have a reduced mortality benefit compared with men (Table 2-1). Angioplasty and the newer interventional devices result in greater procedural morbidity but similar if not better long-term outcomes in women. Women may have a greater mortality rate than men with CABG, although studies suggest that outcome after bypass surgery may depend more on coronary size and preoperative risk factors than on gender itself.

Second opinion for angiography

Graboys and associates[5] from Boston, Massachusetts, performed a study to assess the feasibility of carrying out a second-opinion trial for patients urged to undergo coronary angiography and to assess the long-range outcome of such patients denied that procedure. The case series included patients referred for a second opinion as to need for coronary angiography. The patients were followed up by questionnaire, telephone call, and center visits. One hundred and seventy-one patients with CAD (144 men, average age 60 years; range, 36–88). Three patients became unavailable for follow-up during a mean of 46 months. One hundred and thirty-four (80%) of the 168 patients were judged not to require angiography; it was recommended in 6. In 28 (16%) recommendation was deferred pending further studies. At a mean follow-up of 46.5 months among the 168 patients, there were 7 cardiac deaths (annualized cardiac mortality of 1.1%); 19 patients experienced a new AMI (1.7% annualized rate), while 27 patients (4.3%) were judged to have developed unstable angina. Twenty-six patients (15.4%) ultimately underwent either coronary bypass or angioplasty. In a large fraction of medically stable patients with coronary disease who are urged to undergo coronary angiography, the procedure can be safely deferred. While there may be a limitation in terms of generalizing this experience to all patients with CAD, the authors reasonably concluded that an estimated 50% of coronary angiography currently being undertaken in the USA is unnecessary, or at least could be postponed.

TABLE 2-1. *Mortality by Gender in Thrombolysis Trials. Reproduced with permission from Eysmann, et al.*[4]

| Study* | No. of Subjects | | Thrombolysis Group | | | Control Group | | | Reduction in Mortality Rate, % (Thrombolysis Group) | |
	Women	Men	Treatment	Mortality Rate, % Women	Men	Treatment	Mortality Rate, % Women	Men	Women	Men
ISIS-2[15]	3945	13 125	Streptokinase and aspirin	12.2	6.7	Placebo	17.5	12.0	31	45
GISSI-1[16]	2313	9398	Streptokinase	18.5	8.8	Standard care	22.6	10.6	19	17
GISSI-1 (12-mo follow-up)[17]	2310	9386	Streptokinase	28.3	14.5	Standard care	31.3	16.0	10	10
ASSET[18]	1151	3854	Recombinant tissue-type plasminogen activator and heparin	8.6	6.8	Placebo and heparin	10.9	9.4	21	28
European Working Party[19]	133	597	Streptokinase	20.3	18.1	Heparin	26.6	26.2	24	31
WWT (12-mo follow-up)[21]	34	216	Intracoronary streptokinase	13.3	7.5	Standard care	21.0	13.4	37	44
WWT[20]	59	309	Streptokinase	2.9	7.0	Standard care	16.0	8.6	82†	19†

*ISIS-2 indicates International Study of Infarct Survival, part 2; GISSI-1, Gruppo Italiano per lo Studio della Streptochi-nasi nell'Infarto Miocardico, part 1; ASSET, Anglo-Scandinavian Study of Early Thrombolysis; and WWT, Western Washington Trial.
†P=.08 for women vs men.

Snow shoveling

Sheldahl and colleagues[6] in Milwaukee, Wisconsin, and Pinehurst, North Carolina, evaluated the effect of age and CAD on responses to snow shoveling. Sixteen men with asymptomatic CAD and relatively good functional work capacity, 13 older normal men and 12 younger normal men shoveled snow at a self-paced rate. Oxygen consumption, heart rate, and BP were determined. In nine men with CAD, LVEF was evaluated with an ambulatory radionuclide recorder. Oxygen consumption during snow shoveling differed among groups; it was lowest in those with CAD, intermediate in older normal men and highest in younger normal men. Percent peak treadmill oxygen consumption and heart rate with shoveling in the three groups ranged from 60% to 68% and 75% to 78%, respectively. LVEF and frequency of arrhythmias during shoveling were similar to those during treadmill testing. Thus, snow shoveling increases the rate of energy expenditure in relation to each man's peak oxygen consumption; older and younger normal men and asymptomatic men with CAD paced themselves at similar relative work intensities; the work intensity selected represents hard work but was within commonly recommended criteria for aerobic exercise training. Arrhythmias and LVEFs were similar to those associated with dynamic exercise.

Plaque composition in juvenile diabetes mellitus

Mautner and associates[7] from Bethesda, Maryland, determined the composition of atherosclerotic plaques in 331 5-mm segments of the 4 major (LM, LAD, LC, and right) epicardial coronary arteries of 8 patients with juvenile (mean age at onset, 9 years; mean age at death, 29 years) diabetes mellitus by computerized planimetric analysis. Analysis of all coronary segments disclosed that the plaques consisted primarily of dense (53%) and cellular (38%) fibrous tissue. Pultaceous debris (7%), foam cells (1.2%) and calcific deposits (0.7%) occupied a small percentage of the plaques. Thus, 91% of the coronary plaques in these young diabetic patients consisted of fibrous tissue and nearly all of the remaining 9% consisted of lipid deposits. Analysis of composition according to degrees of cross-sectional luminal narrowing revealed marked increases in dense fibrous tissue (from 31 to 74%), pultaceous debris (from 3 to 12%), and calcific deposits (from 0% to 3%) as the cross-sectional area narrowing increased from ≤25% to >75% (Figure 2-3). Compared with older patients with fatal CAD, the patients with juvenile diabetes had more dense fibrous tissue and pultaceous debris and less calcific deposits.

In cocaine users

To evaluate the spectrum of CAD in cocaine users, Om and associates[8] from Richmond, Virginia, obtained coronary angiograms from 33 patients (26 men and 7 women, mean age 37 years) with a history of cocaine use and cardiac symptoms were retrospectively reviewed. Clinical indications for coronary angiograms included chest pain (n = 28), congestive failure (n = 4) and complete heart block (n = 1). Coronary angiograms were reviewed independently by 2 angiographers unaware of patient's clinical status. Thirteen patients (40%) had normal coronary angiograms, and 20 (60%) had CAD; 7 (21%) had mild CAD (≤70% diameter stenosis), and 13 (40%) had significant CAD (>70% diameter stenosis). Of 13 patients with significant CAD, 7 had 1-vessel, 4 had 2-vessel and 2 had 3-vessel CAD.

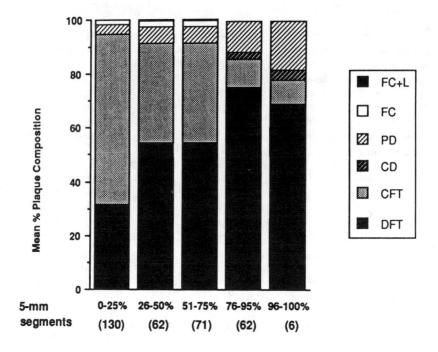

Fig. 2-3. Graph showing mean coronary arterial plaque composition in each of the 5 categories of cross-sectional area narrowing. The number of total 5-mm segments for each coronary artery is shown in parentheses. Abbreviations as in Figure 2. Reproduced with permission from Mautner, et al.[7]

There wase enzymatic evidence of AMI in 12 of 33 patients (36%); all 12 had CAD (10 with significant and 2 with mild CAD). Mean age and number of risk factors (serum total cholesterol, cigarette smoking, systemic hypertension, diabetes mellitus, family history of CAD, and obesity) in patients with CAD (mild or significant) and with normal coronary angiograms were not statistically different. LVEF was normal in 15 patients (45%) and depressed in 18 (55%). All patients with CAD and low EFs (n = 12) had regional wall motion abnormalities, whereas all those with normal coronary arteries and low EFs (n = 6) had global hypokinesia.

Coronary aneurysms in Kawasaki disease

Akagi and associates[9] from Toronto, Canada, reviewed a total of 583 children with Kawasaki disease of whom 14% had coronary artery involvement. The mean age at onset was 3 ± 2.5 years and follow-up was for a mean period of 4 ± 4 years. Giant aneurysms (maximum diameter ≥8 mm) were found in 22 children, moderate-sized aneurysms (≥4 to <8 mm) in 44 and dilation lesions (<4 mm) in 14. Myocardial infarction occurred in 9 (1.5%) all of whom had giant aneurysms. The persistence rate for aneurysms was 72% at 1 year and 41% at 5 years of follow-up. In multivariate analysis, the regression of an aneurysm was significantly related to the severity of lesions, initial treatment, and gender. Although >80% of small or moderate-sized aneurysms regressed within 5 years, giant aneurysms did not regress during the follow-up period. In patients who received immune globulin therapy, coronary lesions tended to resolve more rapidly than those treated with salicylate therapy alone, probably because 91% of the lesions in the former were small or moderate. These authors indicate that severity of coronary artery involvement during the initial stages of Kawasaki disease influences the regression of these lesions and that immune globulin therapy should improve outcome by reducing the prevalence of severe lesions.

DETECTION

By simple clinical parameters

Hubbard and associates[10] from Rochester, Minnesota, examined the ability of clinical and resting electrocardiographic variables to provide useful estimates of the probability of 3-vessel or LM CAD. The study group consisted of 680 patients with symptomatic CAD who underwent exercise equilibrium radionuclide angiography and coronary angiography within 6 months. Sixteen clinical and electrocardiographic variables were examined by logistic regression analysis. The independently predictive variables were then used to develop convenient graphic estimates of the probability of 3-vessel or LM disease and to classify patients into high risk (>35%), intermediate-risk (15–35%), or low-risk (<15%) groups. Five variables were independently predictive of LM or 3-vessel disease: age, typical angina, diabetes, gender, and both history and electrocardiographic evidence of a prior AMI. A single graph was constructed that displayed the probability of severe CAD as a function of a 5-point cardiac risk scale, which incorporated these variables. Two hundred sixty-two patients (39% of the study group) were classified as high risk; 127 of these patients (48%) had 3-vessel or LM disease. An additional 96 patients were classified as low risk; 9 of these patients (9%) had 3-vessel or LM disease. Five clinical variables that were obtained on an initial patient assessment can provide useful estimates of the likelihood of severe CAD.

Diagonal earlobe crease

Tranchesi and associates[11] from Sao Paulo, Brazil, evaluated the association between the presence of diagonal earlobe creases (ELC) and CAD. One thousand four hundred twenty-four patients (760 men and 664 women, aged 30 to 80 years) were examined for the presence of ELC and classified into 2 groups: group I control—1,086 consecutive patients who denied symptoms of myocardial ischemia and were admitted to a general hospital for other reasons; group II CAD—338 patients with documented CAD (presence of ≥70% coronary diameter stenosis at angiography). ELC was present in 304 patients (28%) in group I and 220 (65%) in group II. The patients were stratified in age groups to isolate the influence of age because the prevalence of ELC and CAD increased with advancing age. This association remained statistically significant in all decades, except for patients aged >70 years (Figure 2-4). To further remove the confounding effect of different age and sex distributions between the groups, a direct adjustment of the ELC prevalence was performed. When adjusted for age and sex, the prevalence of creases was still 58% higher in patients with CAD than in control subjects. The presence of ELC was also related to the extent of CAD as measured by the number of major arteries nar-

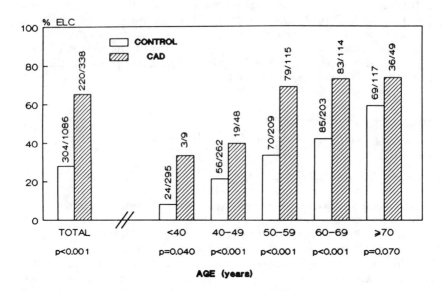

Fig. 2-4. Prevalence of the diagonal earlobe creases (ELC) in patients with and without coronary artery disease (CAD) in the age strata. Reproduced with permission from Tranchesi, et al.[11]

rowed. The observed sensitivity of the sign for the diagnosis of CAD was 65%, the specificity 72%, the positive predictive value 42% and the negative predictive value 87%.

Fluoroscopic coronary calcium

Loecker and associates[12] in San Antonio, Texas, and Rochester, Minnesota, compared the presence of fluoroscopically detected coronary artery calcium with angiographic evidence of CAD in asymptomatic male military aircrew undergoing noninvasive cardiac screening tests and coronary arteriography for occupational indications. Among 1,466 men screened with coronary fluoroscopy, 613 underwent coronary arteriography because of one or more abnormal noninvasive test results. The mean age of all subjects screened was 40 ± 5 years. Significant CAD ≥50% diameter stenosis was found in 104 of the 613 patients with arteriograms (17% disease prevalence). Overall sensitivity and specificity for coronary artery calcification detection of significant CAD based only on those subjects undergoing arteriography were 66% and 78%, respectively. For measurable disease, sensitivity was 61% and specificity 86%. Positive and negative predictive results were 38% and 92%, respectively, for significant CAD. For measurable disease, positive and negative predictive values were 69% and 81%, respectively. In asymptomatic young men, a fluoroscopic examination negative for coronary artery calcification indicated a low risk of significant CAD, whereas a positive test result with calcification present substantially increased the likelihood of angiographically significant CAD.

Treadmill exercise

Bobbio and associates[13] determined the difference in accuracy between 2 frequently published noninvasive indicators of severity of CAD, including exercise-induced ST segment depression and heart rate-adjusted ST segment depression. The study was designed as a survey of consecutive patients undergoing exercise electrocardiography and coronary angiography. A total of 2,270 patients without prior AMI or cardiac valvular disease referred for angiography from 8 institutions in 3 countries were studied. Four hundred and one of these patients had triple vessel or LM CAD. The sensitivities of exercise-induced ST depression and heart rate-adjusted ST segment depression in detecting triple vessel or LM CAD were, respectively, 75% and 78% with specificities of 64%. The small increase in the accuracy of the heart rate-adjusted ST segment depression was evident only at peak exercise heart rates below the median value of 132 beats/min, where the sensitivities of ST segment depression related to exercise and heart rate-adjusted ST segment depression were 73% and 76%, respectively. The results were consistent at all 8 participating institutions. The increase in accuracy achieved by dividing exercise-induced ST segment depression by heart rate is small and limited almost exclusively to those patients with a low exercise heart rate. Therefore, this method need not be generalized to all methods of heart rate adjustment.

Multiple lead systems are shown to have a higher sensitivity than that of single leads for detecting CAD during exercise testing, but the value of ST-segment depression isolated to the inferior leads is questionable. To ascertain the diagnostic accuracy of inferior limb lead II compared with that of precordial lead V_5, Miranda and associates[14] from Irvine, California, and Budapest, Hungary, performed a retrospective analysis of 173 men (108 in a training population and 65 in a validation cohort). All patients had a standard exercise test and underwent diagnostic coronary angiography within 15 days of the exercise test (range 1 to 65). Sixty-three patients had ≥1 coronary stenoses ≥70%, or left main lesion ≥50%, whereas 45 patients in the training population did not. Exclusion criteria were female sex, LV hypertrophy, left BBB or resting ST-segment depression on the baseline electrocardiogram, previous AMI or revascularization procedures, and any significant valvular or congenital heart disease. Lead V_5 had a better combination of sensitivity (65%) and specificity (84%) than that of lead II (sensitivity 71%, specificity 44%) at a single cut point, and this improved specificity was substantial. Receiver-operating characteristic curve analysis also revealed that lead V_5 was markedly superior to lead II over multiple cut points. In fact, the area under the lead II curve was not significantly >0.50, suggesting that for the identification of CAD, isolated ST-segment depression in lead II is unreliable. In patients with normal electrocardiograms, precordial lead V_5 is a better marker for CAD during exercise testing than is limb lead II. Exercise-induced ST-segment depression isolated to the inferior leads is of little value.

It is generally believed that exercise-induced hypotension is the result of severe LM or triple-vessel CAD. Since this is not invariably so, and since most studies were performed in men, Watson and associates[15] from Tucson, Arizona, determined the frequency of and the significance of exercise-induced hypotension in a more general population. The treadmill exercise tests of 4,850 consecutive patients performed at a university medical center over a period of 7.5 years were reviewed. To identify patients for further analysis, a hypotensive BP response was initially defined (1) as a progressive fall in systolic BP, (2) as a failure of the systolic BP to rise more than 5 mm Hg during exercise, or (3) as an initial rise followed by a fall below the resting standing systolic BP. The incidence of exercise-induced hypotension so defined was <2%. Exercise-induced hypotension occurred in 2 patterns. An early hypotension response was defined as a fall in systolic BP of more than 10 mm Hg, associated with symptoms or ST-segment depression, during the first 5 minutes of exercise or as a progressive fall in systolic BP of at least 20 mm Hg. Most patients (9 of 10) with an early hypotensive response had severe CAD. The late hypotension pattern was characterized by an initial rise, followed by a fall in the systolic BP with continued exercise. Only half of the patients with this pattern had significant CAD, and half of the patients had other causes for exercise-induced hypotension. A late hypotensive response was 6 times more frequent than an early hypotensive response. This study identified 2 patterns of exercise-induced hypotension. Early, almost always due to severe CAD, and late, 6 times more common than early in which only half were due to CAD. Causes of a late hypotensive response to exercise that were not due to severe CAD included valvular heart disease, orthostatic hypotension, cardiomyopathy, idiopathic causes, and drugs. Drugs that contributed to a late exercise-induced hypotension response were diuretics, vasodilators, and negative inotropic agents.

Hypotension during exercise testing has been considered a marker of extensive CAD and poor prognosis. Iskandrian and associates[16] from Philadelphia, Pennsylvania, examined the mechanism of hypotension in 25 CAD patients who developed hypotension during treadmill exercise testing (mean decrease in systolic BP 33 ± 13 mm Hg) (group 1) and was compared with the results of 25 CAD patients who had a normal systolic BP response to exercise (mean increase 53 ± 15 mm Hg) (group 2). The 2 groups were comparable in age, sex, extent of CAD, previous AMI, LVEF, history of hypertension and cardiac medications. Exercise heart rate (121 ± 23 vs 133 ± 25 beats/min) and duration (6 ± 2 vs 7 ± 3 minutes) were comparable. ST-segment depression occurred in 44% of patients in group 1 and in 52% in group 2, and angina during exercise occurred in 60% of both groups. Single-photon emission computed tomographic thallium images were abnormal in 24 patients (96%) in group 1 and in 20 patients (80%) in group 2. Percent thallium abnormality was 19 ± 12% in group 1, and 18 ± 14% in group 2, and the severity of thallium abnormality was 710 ± 510 in group 1, and 510 ± 500 in group 2. Ischemia involving the inferior/posterior segments was seen in 68% of patients in group 1 and in 60% in group 2. Increased lung thallium uptake was seen in 48% of both groups. Thus, exercise-induced hypotension cannot be explained by the extent of CAD or ischemia; it is probably due to ischemic activation of mechanoreceptors, a mechanism similar to those of other types of neurally mediated hypotension.

Hambrecht and associates[17] from Heidelberg, Germany, compared maximal hemodynamic and ventilatory responses using cycle and treadmill ergometer in 52 asymptomatic patients with angiographically proved CAD. Moreover, test sensitivity with respect to ST-segment depression and typical angina pectoris were compared between exercise modes used. Exercise tests were performed on different days in randomized order. In 42 patients, exercise-induced myocardial ischemia, expressed as a fraction of LV circumference, was assessed by thallium-201 scintigraphy. The main finding of this study was a significantly higher maximal oxygen uptake (1.87 ± 0.4 vs 2.2 ± 0.5 L/min), heart rate (148 ± 19 vs 158 ± 18 beats/min) and rate-pressure product (28 ± 5 · 10³ vs 31 ± 5 · 10³) during treadmill walking than during cycling. Therefore, stress-induced AMI was significantly more extensive after treadmill walking (31 ± 37° vs 45 ± 40°). Moreover, there were significantly more patients with signs of AMI (ST-segment depression or typical angina pectoris, or both) during treadmill than during cycle ergometry (35 vs 25 patients). However, lactate levels measured at peak exercise (4.07 ± 2.0 vs 4.38 ± 1.9 mmol/liter) and 3 minutes into the recovery period (5.60 ± 2.2 vs 5.80 ± 2.2 mmol/liter) were comparable between both methods, indicating no significant difference in anaerobic energy production. These findings suggest that walking on a treadmill represents an exercise method with a greater ability than cycling to detect CAD.

In a Veterans Affairs Medical Center, Long Beach, California, Ribisl and associates[18] studied 107 men to determine whether patterns and severity of CAD could be predicted by means of standard clinical and exercise test data. The authors found significant differences in clinical, hemodynamic, and electrocardiographic measurements among patients with progressively increasing disease severity determined by angiography. Left main CAD produced responses significantly different from those of 3-vessel CAD only when accompanied by a 70% or greater narrowing of the right coronary artery. Discriminant function analysis revealed that the maximum amount of horizontal or downsloping ST depression in exercise and/or recovery was the most powerful predictor of disease severity, with 2-mm ST depression yielding a sensitivity of 55% and a specificity of 80% for prediction of severe CAD (3-vessel disease plus LM disease). Patients with increasingly severe CAD also demonstrated a greater frequency of abnormal hemodynamic responses to exercise.

Exercise echocardiography

Quinones and co-workers[19] in Houston, Texas, performed exercise echocardiography and thallium 201 single-photon emission computed tomography in 292 patients being evaluated for CAD. Pretreadmill and posttreadmill echocardiographic images of diagnostic quality were obtained in 289 patients, and the LV was divided into anterior, inferior, and lateral regions. Any wall motion or perfusion abnormality observed within each region was classified as totally reversible, fixed or partially reversible. Exercise echocardiography and emission tomography were normal in 137 patients and abnormal in 118 (88% agreement). Equal numbers of regional abnormalities were detected by one test when missed by the other. The 2 tests had an 82% agreement in detecting the same type of finding within the regions analyzed. Emission tomography detected more reversible abnormalities than echocardiography, whereas echocardiography detected more fixed abnormalities than emission tomography. Regions with a fixed abnormality by echocardiography frequently showed partial reversibility of a perfusion defect by emission tomography. Nearly one third of regions with fixed perfusion defects by emission tomography demonstrated normal resting function or reversible abnormalities by echocardiography. Sensitivity for CAD by angiography in 112 patients was similar for the two test, ranging from 58% and 61% for 1-vessel CAD to 94% for 3-vessel CAD. The specificities for echocardiography and emission tomography were 88% and 81%, respectively. Exercise echocardiography had a diagnostic accuracy comparable to that of emission tomography for the detection of regional abnormalities produced by significant CAD. A greater number of abnormal regions were detected with the combined use of both tests.

Marwick and colleagues[20] in Cleveland, Ohio, examined the results of 179 posttreadmill stress echocardiograms in 150 consecutive patients who also underwent cardiac catheterization and in 29 normal individuals at low risk for CAD. Among the 114 patients who had significant coronary stenosis at angiography, 96 had an abnormal exercise echocardiogram; the overall sensitivity was 84%. False negative results correlated with the patient only doing submaximal exercise, single-vessel disease and moderate (50% to 70% diameter) coronary artery stenoses. After the exclusion of seven patients performing submaximal exercise, the sensitivity was 90%. In 54 patients without prior AMI performing maximal exercise, the sensitivity was 87%, highest in patients with multivessel CAD (96%) and lower in those with single-vessel CAD (79%). After the exclusion of patients with nondiagnostic results, due either to submaximal stress or the presence of electrocardiographic changes at rest, exercise echocardiography had a higher sensitivity than did exercise electrocardiography (87% vs 63%). In 36 patients without significant CAD, exercise echocardiography had an overall specificity of 86%. After the exclusion of patients with a nondiagnostic test, exercise echocardiography had a specificity of 82% compared with 74% for exercise electrocardiography. Similarly, among the 29 normal subjects, 93% had a normal exercise echocardiogram and 97% had a normal exercise electrocardiogram. Age, gender, body weight and image quality did not significantly influence the accuracy of exercise echocardiography. Thus, this study confirms the high sensitivity and specificity of exercise echocardiography in detecting CAD. The technique has the highest accuracy when patients achieve >85% of age-predicted maximal HRs and when there is more disease in multiple arteries. Exercise echocardiography improved on the ability of exercise electrocardiography alone to suggest the presence of CAD.

Coronary echocardiography

Sawada and associates[21] in Indianapolis, Indiana, have used transthoracic echocardiographic examination of the proximal left coronary system in 59 patients with dilated cardiomyopathy to determine if the technique distinguishes between ischemic and nonischemic dilated cardiomyopathy. With use of annular array transducers and digital image processing, echocardiographic visualization of the coronary arteries was successful in 55 (93%) of 59 patients. As assessed by coronary angiography, 32 patients had ischemic cardiomyopathy and 27 had nonischemic cardiomyopathy. Twenty-seven (87%) of the 32 patients who had coronary artery disease and 24 (89%) of the 27 patients with nonischemic cardiomyopathy were correctly identified. The accuracy of coronary echocardiography was 86% in the entire group and 93% when patients with inadequate studies were excluded. All subjects with ischemic cardiomyopathy had evidence of disease by coronary echocardiography or segmental wall motion abnormalities. Multivariate analysis permitted correct classification of 93% of all subjects based on the results of the coronary echocardiogram, evaluation of segmental wall motion, and a history of prior AMI. The correct diagnosis was made in 86% when the results of coronary echocardiography were excluded from analysis using all echocardiographic and clinical variables. Therefore, transthoracic coronary echocardiography may be performed with a high degree of success in patients with dilated ventricles and the technique can distinguish between ischemic and nonischemic dilated cardiomyopathy.

Exercise thallium-201 scintigraphy

Christian and associates[22] from Rochester, Minnesota, examined the ability of exercise thallium-201 tomographic imaging to predict the presence of LM or 3-vessel CAD in 688 patients who underwent both exercise thallium-201 testing and coronary angiography. Significant differences existed for multiple variables between patients with (n = 196) and without (n = 492) severe LM or 3-vessel CAD (Table 2-2). Logistic regression analysis identified 4 variables as independently predictive of LM or 3-vessel CAD. These variables were the magnitude of ST-segment depression with exercise, the number of visually abnormal short-axis thallium-201 segments, the presence or absence of diabetes mellitus, and the change in systolic BP with exercise. Using these variables, patients were classified by nomograms into low-, intermediate- and high-probability groups. Patients at high probability (n = 205) had a 52% prevalence of 3-vessel or LM CAD, whereas those at low probability (n = 170) had only a 12% prevalence. Only 53 patients (29%) with 3-vessel or LM CAD had perfusion abnormalities in all 3 coronary territories. Clinical and exercise parameters provide important independent information in the identification of LM or 3-vessel CAD by exercise thallium-201 tomographic imaging, because thallium scintigraphy alone is suggestive of extensive CAD in few patients.

Thallium reinjection immediately after stress-redistribution imaging identifies ischemic but viable myocardium in as many as 50% of the regions characterized by conventional redistribution imaging as irreversibly injured. Dilsizian and co-investigators[23] in Bethesda, Maryland, had previously shown that some regions in which irreversible defects persist despite reinjection remain metabolically active, and hence viable, by positron emission tomography. In the current study, the investigators determined whether the severity of reduction in thallium activity within

TABLE 2-2. *Clinical, Exercise and Thallium-201 Variables Significantly Associated with Three-Vessel or Left Main Coronary Artery Disease. Reproduced with permission from Christian, et al.[22]*

| | Left Main or 3-Vessel Disease | | |
Variable	Present (n = 196)	Absent (n = 492)	p Value
Clinical			
Age (yr)	64 ± 9	62 ± 10	<0.05
Diabetes mellitus (%)	27	14	<0.001
Hypertension (%) (>140/90 mm Hg)	57	46	<0.01
Exercise			
Duration (METs)	6.9 ± 2.2	7.3 ± 2.3	<0.02
Magnitude of ST depression	1.5 ± 1.6	0.9 ± 1.3	<0.0001
Peak exercise heart rate (beats/min)	121 ± 24	126 ± 25	<0.01
Change in systolic blood pressure (mm Hg)	22 ± 31	35 ± 24	<0.0001
Exercise systolic blood pressure × heart rate	19,351 ± 6,290	21,501 ± 6,454	0.0001
Thallium-201			
Cardiac enlargement (%)	40	26	<0.001
Increased pulmonary uptake (%)	27	19	<0.05
No. of abnormal segments			
Postexercise	7.2 ± 3.9	5.2 ± 3.8	<0.0001
Delayed	4.4 ± 3.4	3.2 ± 3.4	<0.0001
Postexercise − delayed	2.8 ± 2.8	2.0 ± 2.4	0.0001
Abnormal coronary distributions			
Postexercise	1.9 ± 0.9	1.4 ± 0.9	0.0001
Delayed	1.2 ± 0.8	0.9 ± 0.8	0.0009
Postexercise − delayed	0.7 ± 0.8	0.5 ± 0.7	0.009

irreversible defects on redistribution images and the magnitude of change in regional thallium activity after reinjection can further discriminate viable from nonviable myocardium in such defects. The investigators studied 150 patients with CAD by exercise thallium tomography using the rest-reinjection protocol. The three sets of images (stress, redistribution, and reinjection) were then analyzed quantitatively. The increase in regional thallium activity from redistribution to reinjection was computed, normalized to the increase observed in a normal region, and termed "differential uptake." Of the 175 myocardial regions designated to have irreversible thallium defects on conventional 3–4 hour redistribution images, 132 had only mild-to-moderate reduction in thallium activity and 43 had severe reduction in thallium activity. Thallium reinjection resulted in enhanced relative activity in 60 of 132 (45%) of the mild-to-moderate irreversible defects and 22 of 43 (51%) of the severe irreversible defects, leaving roughly half of these defects remaining irreversible after reinjection. However, in regions that appeared to remain irreversible despite reinjection, the magnitude of differential uptake differed between mild-to-moderate and severe irreversible defects. All regions with mild-to-moderate defects demonstrated >50% differential uptake after reinjection. In contrast, all except 2 regions with severe irreversible defects demonstrated differential uptake of <50%. Fifteen patients also underwent positron emission tomography at rest with ^{18}F-fluorodeoxyglucose and ^{15}O-water. ^{15}F-fluorodeoxyglucose uptake was present in 91% of regions with mild-to-moderate reduction in thallium activity, and the results of differential uptake and ^{18}F-fluorodeoxyglucose data were concordant in 81% of these regions. These data indicated that the magnitude of thallium uptake after reinjection differed between mild-to-moderate and severe irreversible defects on standard 3–4 hour redistribution images. The substantial differential uptake of thallium (>50%) after reinjection in mild-to-moderate defects, even when relative thallium activity does not increase appreciably, coupled with preserved metabolic activity by positron emission tomography, supported the concept that such mild-to-moderate irreversible defects represent viable myocardium.

Delonca and associates[24] from Geneva, Switzerland, reviewed the records of 68 patients with right BBB and 66 patients with left BBB, who had undergone thallium-201 exercise scintigraphy and coronary arteriography, to determine the sensitivity, specificity, and positive and negative predictive values of thallium-201 imaging for the detection of CAD in the presence of intraventricular conduction abnormalities. In patients with right BBB the sensitivity, specificity, and positive and negative predictive values were, respectively, 83%, 89%, 79%, and 92% for the anteroseptal region and 83%, 84%, 83%, and 84% for the inferoposterior region. In patients with left BBB these values were, respectively, 94%, 33%, 36%, and 93% for the anteroseptal region and 77%, 90%, 81%, and 88% for the inferoposterior region. In this second group defects limited to the septal region were a good predictor of false positive scintigrams (9/10 cases), but if apical defects used as the sole criterion for detecting lesions in the LAD improved the specificity to 85%, the sensitivity was greatly reduced (35%). It was concluded that exercise scintigraphy is a reliable method for detection of coronary lesions in patients with right BBB and in patients with left BBB and inferoposterior perfusion defects, but it is unable to discriminate between normal subjects and patients with CAD in the presence of left BBB and anteroseptal perfusion defects. In addition, limited septal defects are highly suggestive of false positive scintigrams in this latter group of patients.

Adenosine thallium-201 scintigraphy

In an investigation by O'Keefe and associates[25] from Kansas City, Missouri, 340 consecutive patients (mean age 69 ± 9 years) were evaluated with adenosine tomographic thallium-201 scintigraphy for suspected CAD. Minor side effects occurred in 91% of patients. Out of 28 patients (8%) with potentially serious side effects, 28 had significant A-V block (second-degree 24 patients; third-degree 4 patients; syncope occurred in 2 patients). Acute bronchospasm and severe refractory angina pectoris occurred in 1 patient each. All side effects were transient and without sequelae. Coronary angiography was carried out in 121 patients within 9 days of adenosine thallium imaging. The predictive accuracies of adenosine thallium imaging for identifying and localizing ischemia to a specific coronary distribution were: LAD 88%, LC 84%, right coronary 88%. The predictive accuracy of adenosine thallium imaging in patients with left BBB was 91%, and was higher than the 71% predictive accuracy noted in 39 patients who underwent exercise thallium testing. It was concluded that adenosine thallium-201 myocardial scintigraphy was 1) highly accurate for the detection and localization of significant CAD; 2) it was more accurate at detecting ischemia in patients with left BBB than exercise thallium testing, and 3) subjective side effects were common and were of no diagnostic importance; transient A-V block occurred occasionally.

Adenosine vs exercise thallium-201 scintigraphy

Gupta and associates[26] for the Multicenter Adenosine Study Group from Omaha, Nebraska, evaluated pharmacologic stress with dipyridamole in patients undergoing thallium-201 myocardial perfusion imaging. Adenosine may be a coronary vasodilator of choice for myocardial perfusion imaging because of its very short half-life and potent vasodilator effect. Fifty-one healthy subjects and 93 patients with suspected CAD constituted the study group. In this multicenter study, the comparative safety and diagnostic efficacy of single-photon emission computed tomography (SPECT) thallium-201 imaging during adenosine-induced coronary hyperemia was compared with exercise treadmill stress. There was a mean increase in heart rate of 37% and a mean decrease in diastolic blood pressure of 5% during the adenosine infusion of 140 μg/kg per minute for 6 minutes. Adenosine infusion was well tolerated in 95% of the patients. Side effects occurred in seven subjects (5%). None of the patients experienced a life-threatening complication. The sensitivity, specificity and predictive accuracy for detecting CAD with quantitative analysis were 83%, 87%, and 84% for adenosine SPECT and 82%, 80%, and 81% for exercise SPECT studies, respectively. Most false negative results with adenosine, as well as exercise SPECT studies, occurred in patients with single vessel CAD. The results of adenosine SPECT imaging are concordant with exercise SPECT imaging. Therefore, adenosine SPECT thallium-201 imaging provides a safe and accurate imaging method for the detection of CAD relatively noninvasively.

Nishimura and associates[27] in Houston, Texas studied the relative values of pharmacologic and exercise stress during thallium-201 single-photon tomography. Both exercise and adenosine myocardial perfusion imaging were used in a study group consisting of 175 subjects: 55 health volunteers and 120 patients with suspected CAD were evaluated. All subjects had two thallium tomographic studies performed 30 days apart, one during intravenous administration of adenosine as 140 μg/kg per min for 6 minutes and one during exercise stress. All images were computer quantified and interpreted without knowledge of the stress test performed. Agreement on the presence of normal or abnormal tomograms by adenosine and exercise scintigraphy occurred in 83% by visual analysis and by 86% by computer quantification. Agreement on localization of the perfusion defect to a specific coronary vascular territory varied from 83% to 91% but was highly significant (p < 0.0001). There was a good correlation between quantified perfusion defect size by adenosine and exercise, but the values for defect size were significantly greater by adenosine scintigraphy. There were frequent side effects following administration of adenosine, but these were transient and ceased spontaneously in most subjects within 1 to 2 minutes after discontinuation of the infusion. Therefore, adenosine thallium-201 scintigraphy provides diagnostic information similar to that obtained with exercise, although values for defect sizes are greater with adenosine stress.

Dipyridamole-thallium imaging

Lette and associates[28] from Quebec, Canada, performed preoperative cardiac risk assessment using 23 clinical parameters, 7 multivariate clinical scoring systems, and quantitative dipyridamole-thallium imaging in 360 patients to postoperative AMI and cardiac death after *noncardiac surgery*. There were 30 postoperative and an additional 13 cumulative long-term cardiac events after an average follow-up of 15 months. Clinical descriptors were not useful in predicting the outcome of individual patients. The postoperative and long-term cardiac event rates were 1% and 3.5%, respectively, in patients with normal scans or fixed perfusion defects, and 17.5% and 22% in patients with reversible defects (Figure 2-5). Using quantitative indices reflecting the amount of jeopardized myocardium, patients could be stratified by dipyridamole imaging into multiple scintigraphic subsets, with corresponding postoperative and 1-year coronary morbidity and mortality rates ranging from 0.5% to 100%. Thus, postoperative and long-term cardiac events cannot be predicted clinically, whereas quantitative dipyridamole imaging accurately identifies high-risk patients who require preoperative coronary angiography.

Computed tomography

Simons and associates[29] in Rochester, Minnesota, determined the relation between coronary artery calcification detected by ultrafast computed tomographic scanning and histopathologic CAD. Thirteen consecutive perfusion-fixed autopsy hearts from eight males and five females ranging in age from 17 to 83 years were scanned by ultrafast computed tomographic scanning in contiguous 3-mm tomographic sections. The major epicardial arteries were dissected free, positioned longitudinally and scanned again in cross section. Coronary artery calcification in a coronary artery segment was defined as the presence of one or more voxels with a computed tomographic density >130 Hounsfield units. Each epicardial coronary artery was sectioned longitudinally, stained and measured with a planimeter for quantitation of cross-sectional and atherosclerotic plaque areas at 3-mm intervals, corresponding to the computed tomographic scans. A total of 522 paired coronary computed tomographic and histologic sections were studied. There were direct relations between ultrafast computed tomography scanning coronary artery calcium burden and atherosclerotic plaque area and percent lumen area stenosis. The range

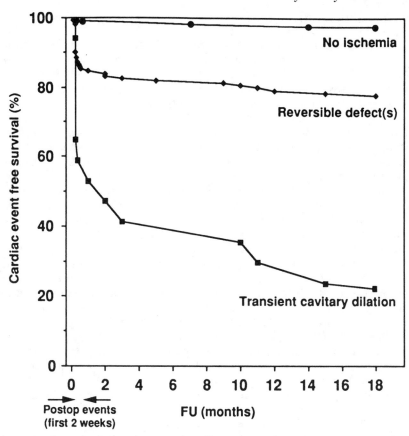

Fig. 2-5. Proportion of patients who remained cardiac event-free with normal scans or fixed defects (upper curve), reversible perfusion defect(s) (middle curve), and transient dipyridamole-induced left ventricular cavitary dilatation (lower curve). Patients with normal scans or fixed defects have an excellent prognosis; patients with reversible defect(s) are at an increased risk but clearly cannot be labeled as high risk. For patients with transient dipyridamole-induced left ventricular cavitary dilatation, the postoperative cardiac event rate is high, and most patients who survive the surgery eventually sustained a cardiac event on long-term follow-up, usually within the first 3 months after the surgery. Reproduced with permission from Letle, et al.[28]

for plaque area or percent lumen stenosis, or both, associated with a given calcium burden was broad. Three hundred thirty-one coronary artery segments showed no calcification by computed tomography. Although atherosclerotic disease was found in several corresponding pathologic specimens, >97% of these noncalcified segments were associated with nonobstructive disease. If no calcium was found in an entire coronary artery, all corresponding CAD was found to be nonobstructive. Ultrafast computed tomographic scanning had a sensitivity and specificity of 59% and 90%, respectively, and a negative and positive predictive value of 65% and 87%, respectively. A direct correlation was found between total calcium burden calculated from tomographic scans of the heart as a whole and scans of the arteries obtained in cross section. Thus, detection of coronary calcium by ultrafast computed tomographic scanning is predictive of the presence of CAD, but the use of this technique to define the extent of CAD may be limited.

Intravascular ultrasound

Catheter-based intracoronary ultrasound has proven useful both in detecting and quantitating CAD, but the ultrasound appearance of young, angiographically normal, coronary arteries has not been well defined. St. Goar and co-workers[30] in Stanford, California, examined 25 subjects with intracoronary ultrasound within 1 month of cardiac transplantation. Mean age of the donor hearts was 28 years. Measurements of an index of intimal thickening were obtained at 4 left anterior descending coronary artery sites in each patient. All study patients had angiographically normal coronary arteries. Ultrasound in 14 subjects demonstrated a three-layered appearance of the coronary vessel wall with a mean intimal index of 0.16. The other 10 subjects, including all donors under the age of 25 years, had coronary vessel wall layers too thin to be imaged separately at the 30-MHz sound frequency. Five subjects had ultrasound evidence of focal intimal thickening greater than 500 μm. The donors of these hearts each had risk factors for CAD. Two subjects died within 5 weeks of their ultrasound study. Histological measurements of the vessel wall layers were similar to the corresponding ultrasound values. This study provides a reference for the intravascular ultrasound appearance of young adult coronary arteries and confirms that young subjects with antiographically normal arteries have a range of coronary intimal thickening, which includes occasional evidence of focal, early atheromatous lesions.

Coronary artery calcium is invariably associated with atherosclerosis and has been linked to an increased risk of coronary events. Ultrafast computed tomography (CT) has been used to document the presence and relative quantity of coronary calcium. The use of the self-reported coronary risk factors to identify persons with coronary calcium as documented by ultrafast CT screening was examined in 458 men and 139 women aged 26 to 81 years (88% asymptomatic) by Goel and associates[31] from Irvine and Brea, California. All subjects underwent ultrafast CT scanning, and received a questionnaire and underwent an interview regarding medical and risk factor history. Total calcium score was calculated as the sum of lesion-specific scores, each calculated as the product of density ≥130 Hounsfield units and area ≥0.51 mm². The prevalence of coronary calcium increased significantly by age group, and the greater the number of risk factors present, the greater the likelihood of calcium. From multiple logistic regression, age, male sex, and history of smoking were independently associated with the probability of detectable calcium. Among asymptomatic subjects, an association with hypercholesterolemia was also seen. The results demonstrate that cardiovascular risk factors can help in identifying the likelihood of coronary calcium.

Quantitative angiography

At present, there is extensive knowledge on the clinical course of CAD, whereas data on the underlying anatomical changes and their relation to clinical events are still limited. Lichtlen and co-workers[32] in Hanover, Germany investigated progression and regression of CAD prospectively over 3 years in 230 patients with mild to moderate disease by applying quantitated, repeated coronary angiography. Minimal stenotic diameters, segment diameters, and percent stenoses were analyzed by the computer-assisted Coronary Angiography Analysis System. Progression was defined either as an increase in percent stenosis of preexisting stenoses by ≥20% including occlusions or as formation of new stenoses ≥20% and new occlusions in previously angiographically "normal" segments. At first angiography, the investigators found 838 stenoses ≥20% and 135 occlusions in the 4 major coronary branches. At second angiography, 82 of the preexisting stenoses had progressed, 15 of them up to occlusion. In addition, there were 144 newly formed stenoses and 10 new occlusions. Hence, 25 of all stenoses had become occluded. Altogether, 129 patients showed progression: 68 with new lesions only, 27 with preexisting lesions, and 34 with both types. Regression was present in 29 stenoses and 28 patients. The incidence of new AMI was low, with 3 originating from occluding preexisting stenoses and 1 from new stenoses; hence, only 4 of the 25 new occlusions led to AMI. Risk factor analysis showed that cigarette smoking correlated significantly with the formation of new lesions, whereas total cholesterol correlated with the further progression of preexisting stenoses but not with the incidence of new lesions. In patients with mild to moderate CAD, the angiographic progression is slow but exceeds regression. Progression is predominantly seen in the formation of new coronary stenoses and less in growth of preexisting ones. Most stenoses were of a low degree, clinically not manifest including those going into occlusion and leading to AMI. Progression was influenced by risk factors, especially cigarette smoking and high cholesterol levels.

In peripheral vascular disease

To determine the incidence and significance of intraoperative and postoperative myocardial ischemia and their relation to preoperative ischemia and postoperative cardiac events in patients undergoing peripheral arterial surgery, Raby and associates[33] from Boston, Massachusetts, studied 115 patients undergoing elective vascular surgery who met predefined eligibility criteria and were believed to have acceptable cardiac risk as assessed by independent cardiologists. Ambulatory electrocardiographic monitoring preoperatively, intraoperatively, and up to 72 hours postoperatively was performed. Preoperative clinical characteristics and laboratory data were collected. Predefined adverse cardiac events were identified by an investigator who was "blinded" to monitoring results. Monitor recordings were interpreted for ST-segment depression by investigators blinded to patient information. Intraoperative ischemia was present in 21 patients (18%), and postoperative ischemia was present in 35 (30%). There were 16 postoperative cardiac events. The relative risk of suffering a cardiac event was 2.7 in patients with intraoperative ischemia and was 16 in patients with postoperative ischemia. Preoperative ischemia closely correlated with intraoperative and postoperative ischemia. Preoperative and postoperative ischemia preceded cardiac events in 14 of 16 patients. Preoperative ischemia appears to identify high-risk patients, and subsequent perioperative monitoring detects silent ischemia that commonly precedes clinical events and that may be treatable with anti-ischemia therapy.

PROGNOSTIC INDICES

Chest pain in the emergency room

To evaluate the long-term prognosis of patients with acute chest pain, Lee and associates[34] from Boston, Massachusetts, collected prospective clinical data and long-term follow-up data (mean 30 ± 9 months) for 1,956 patients who presented to the emergency department of an urban teaching hospital with this chief complaint. During follow-up of the 1,915 patients who were discharged alive from the emergency department or hospital, there were 113 (6%) cardiovascular deaths. No differences were detected in the post-discharge cardiovascular survival rates after 3 years of experience with patients who were discharged from the emergency department with a known prior diagnosis of angina or AMI (89%) and patients who had been admitted and found to have AMI (85%), angina (87%), or other cardiovascular diagnoses (87%). Patients who were discharged from either the hospital or the emergency department without cardiovascular diagnoses had an excellent prognosis. Multivariate Cox regression analysis identified 5 independent correlates of cardiovascular mortality after discharge: age, prior history of CAD, ischemic changes on the emergency department electrocardiogram, CHF and cardiogenic shock. These findings indicate that the postdischarge cardiovascular mortality of patients with chest pain who are discharged from the emergency department with a known history of CAD is similar to that of admitted patients with angina or AMI. These data suggest that the same types of prognostic evaluation strategies that have been developed for admitted patients with CAD should also be considered when such patients present to the emergency department but are not admitted.

Effect of gender in black patients

Liao and associates[35] from Maywood, Illinois, evaluated the influence of gender on the prognosis of CAD among black patients. The study included 1,719 consecutive black patients (780 men and 939 women) who had any one of the following events: cardiac catheterization for presumed CAD, hospitalization for AMI, or CABG. Hospital and operative mortality rates following AMI and CABG were similar between the 2 sexes. The relative risks for cardiac death in women vs men were 0.88, 0.79, and 0.79 for CAD, AMI, and CABG, respectively, after adjusting for age, history of diabetes, hypertension, angina pectoris and AMI, number of narrowed coronary arteries, and EF (Figure 2-6). Compared with patients of the same sex with normal angiograms, relative risk estimates were 5.0, 10.1, and 6.3 for women and were 1.8, 4.0, and 2.0 for men in the same 3 groups of patients, respectively. Survival with CAD in black women is similar to that observed in black men, but relative to members of the same sex without CAD, the prognosis for women is considerably worse than for men.

With left main narrowing

In early reports, coronary arteriography in patients with LM CAD had a substantial risk, but recent reports suggest that arteriography in these subjects is now associated with a low mortality. Boehrer and associates[36] from Dallas, Texas, performed a study to examine the periprocedure mortality in patients with LM CAD undergoing catheterization to compare the periprocedure mortality in these patients with that in subjects with less CAD and to identify the variables associated with pericatheterization mortality in this patient cohort. Of 4,009 patients undergoing elective coronary arteriography from 1978 to 1992, 176 had LM CAD. Of the 10 deaths during or within 24 hours of catheterization, 5 occurred in these 176 subjects. This periprocedure mortality of 2.8% in patients with LM

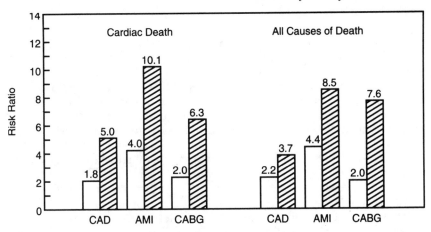

Fig. 2-6. Multivariate-adjusted risk ratios for cardiac and all causes of death in patients with angiographically confirmed coronary artery disease (CAD), acute myocardial infarction (AMI), and coronary artery bypass grafting (CABG) vs patients with normal angiograms, by sex. Open bars indicate men; hatched bars, women. Reproduced with permission from Liao, et al.[35]

CAD was >20 times that of those without LM CAD (0.13%). In comparison with the 171 patients with LM CAD who survived, the 5 who died were older (67 ± 8 vs 58 ± 12 years), and had more severe LM CAD (92 ± 10% vs 72 ± 16%) and a lower cardiac index (1.9 ± 0.4 vs 2.6 ± 0.7 liters/min/m²). Thus, even in the 1980s and early 1990s, patients with LM CAD have a high pericatheterization mortality, especially those who are older and have severe LM CAD.

Loss of painless myocardial ischemia

During exercise radionuclide ventriculography, many patients with CAD have painless myocardial ischemia defined as an abnormal LVEF response without accompanying angina pectoris. To see if complete suppression of such exercise-induced painless ischemia by anti-ischemic medication implies a better prognosis in medically treated CAD, Lim and associates[37] from London, UK, studied 34 patients with repeat testing at 4 weeks receiving regular conventional therapy that rendered angina no worse than class I. With such therapy, painless ischemia was abolished in 12 patients (group I) and persisted in 22 (65%), (group II). Both groups were similar in age, number of diseased vessels, proportion with previous myocardial infarction, exercise EF, and degree of exercise-induced painless ischemia at baseline. At 9 months, adverse events had occurred in 11 patients (2 patients with AMI, 4 with unstable angina, 2 with angioplasty and 3 with bypass surgery). Only 1 of 12 patients (8%) in group I had experienced events compared with 10 of 22 (45%) in group II (chi-square, 5.4). Thus, the relative risk of adverse events in patients whose painless ischemia was abolished was only 18% of that in patients in whom it was persistent. These results suggest that (1) the abolition of exercise-induced painless ischemia by conventional symptom-dictated medical therapy confers a better short-term prognosis in medically treated CAD, and (2) therapeutic efficacy may need to be assessed by titration against ischemia and not against angina.

Premature departure from work force

Work disability is common in patients with CAD and adversely affects both economic well-being and quality of life. Mark and colleagues[38] in Durham, North Carolina, constructed a model to predict premature departure from the work force of patients with CAD and to validate this model prospectively in an independent cohort of patients. The investigators enrolled 1,252 CAD patients referred for diagnostic cardiac catheterization who were less than age 65, employed, and without prior PTCA or CABG. Medical, functional, psychological, economic, and job-related variables were measured at the time of baseline diagnostic cardiac catheterization, and all patients were followed for 1 year. Three hundred twelve patients underwent PTCA within 60 days of catheterization, and 449 had CABG within 60 days of catheterization. The remaining 491 patients were treated with initial medical therapy. Logistic regression was used to develop a multivariable model for predicting 1-year work status in the training sample patients. This model was then validated in the independent prospective test sample. Eight factors were independent predictors of departure from the work force: lower initial functional status (as assessed by the Duke Activity Status Index), followed by older age, black race, presence of CHF, lower education level, presence of extracardiac vascular disease, poorer psychological status, and lower job classification. Standard clinical variables provided only 20% of the total predictive information available from the model about follow-up work outcomes, whereas functional measures provided 27%, and demographic and socioeconomic measures provided 45%. After adjustment for baseline imbalances, there was no significant difference in 1-year return-to-work rates among the patients receiving initial PTCA or CABG therapy versus initial medical therapy. Patients with CAD who are at high risk for premature departure from the work force can be accurately identified from a combination of medical and nonmedical risk factors. The model developed in this study provides a tool to identify patients at high risk for premature loss from the work force. Such patients may benefit from special multidimensional intervention programs designed to preserve work status. These data show that revascularization with either PTCA or CABG is not, by itself, sufficient to accomplish this goal.

Echocardiographic predictors

Galderisi and associates[39] from Bethesda, Maryland, Boston, Massachusetts, and Burlington, Vermont, examined echocardiographic predictors of clinical outcome in subjects from the Framingham Heart Study with overt CAD. The study population consisted of 185 men and 147 women with CAD who underwent M-mode echocardiography and were followed for a mean of 3.90 years. At baseline, 37 men (18.4%) and 16 women (10.9%) had reduced fractional shortening, 43 men (23.2%) and 28 women (19%) had LV dilatation, and 76 men (41%) and 76 women (51.7%) had LV hypertrophy. During the follow-up period new cardiovascular disease events (coronary disease, stroke, transient ischemic attack, claudication, heart failure and deaths from cardiovascular disease) occurred in 60 men (32%) and 58 women (39%). With use of age-adjusted proportional hazards analyses, LV mass/height in men and LV end-diastolic diameter in women were predictors of new cardiovascular disease events. Cardiovascular risk was also associated with LV end-systolic diameter in both sexes. Reduced fractional shortening alone and in combination with LV dilatation was associated with the incidence of new cardiovascular disease outcomes in men. In women, cardiovascular risk was increased with LV hypertrophy, high LV wall thickness, high LV end-systolic diameter and a combination of low fractional shortening and LV dilatation. Thus, M-mode echocardiography has prognostic value in identifying subjects with CAD who are at increased risk for new morbid or fatal events.

Exercise thallium-201 scintigraphy

The prognostic value of exercise thallium-201 myocardial perfusion imaging has not been studied in an elderly population (aged ≥70 years). Hilton and associates[40] from St. Louis, Missouri, retrospectively analyzed 120 consecutive patients aged 70 or over undergoing Bruce protocol exercise stress with quantitative planar thallium-201 scintigraphy, followed clinically for a mean of 36 ± 12 months after testing. The patients had a 10% cardiac event rate (6 cardiac deaths from arrhythmia or CHF, and 5 fatal and 1 nonfatal AMI). There were no exercise stress-related complications. Survival without cardiac events was associated with greater exercise duration (5.6 ± 2.4 vs 3.1 ± 2.4 minutes) and peak exercise heart rate (131 ± 18 vs 120 ± 19 beats/min). Univariate variables associated with higher cardiac event rates included: (1) peak exercise ≤stage I (18 vs 6%); (2) maximal ST-segment depression ≥2 mm (27 vs 6%); and (3) presence of a fixed or reversible thallium-201 perfusion defect (18 vs 2%). Multivariate stepwise logistic regression analysis identified the combination of peak exercise ≤stage I and any thallium-201 perfusion defect as the most powerful predictor of subsequent cardiac events. Thus, exercise thallium-201 scintigraphy in elderly patients is safe and provides important prognostic information. Based on the peak Bruce protocol exercise stage achieved and presence or absence of a thallium-201 perfusion defect, most elderly patients (64%) can be stratified into very low- and high-risk groups with annual cardiac events rates of <1 and >15%, respectively.

Dipyridamole thallium-201 scintigraphy

Shaw and associates[41] in St. Louis, Missouri, utilized intravenous dipyridamole myocardial perfusion imaging in patients ≥70 years of age with suspected CAD to determine the predictive value of intravenous dipyridamole thallium-201 imaging for subsequent cardiac death or nonfatal AMI. Among 348 patients, 207 were symptomatic and 141 were asymptomatic. Fifty-two percent of the asymptomatic group had documented CAD. During 23 ± 15 months of follow-up, there were 52 cardiac deaths, 24 nonfatal AMIs and 42 revascularization procedures (PTCA in 20 and CABG in 22). Clinical univariate predictors of a cardiac event included previous AMI, CHF symptoms, hypercholesterolemia and diabetes. The presence of a fixed, reversible or combined thallium-201 defect was significantly associated with the occurrence of cardiac death or AMI during follow-up. Cardiac death or nonfatal AMI occurred in only 7 (5%) of 150 patients with a normal dipyridamole thallium-201 study. Stepwise logistic regression analysis of clinical and radionuclide variables revealed that an abnormal dipyridamole thallium-201 study was the single best predictor of cardiac events. Previous AMI and symptoms of CHF at presentation were also independent clinical predictors of cardiac death or AMI. Thus, dipyridamole thallium-201 myocardial imaging is a powerful independent non-invasive technique for predicting prognosis in elderly patients.

Positron emission tomography

Eitzman and colleagues[42] in Ann Arbor, Michigan, determined the prognostic significance of perfusion-metabolism imaging in patients undergoing positron emission tomography for myocardial viability assessment. Positron emission tomography using nitrogen-13 ammonia and [18]fluorodeoxyglucose to assess myocardial blood flow and metabolism has been shown to predict improvement in wall motion after CABG. The prognostic implications of metabolic imaging in patients with advanced CAD have not been studied. Eighty-two patients with advanced CAD and impaired LV function had positron emission tomographic imaging between August, 1988 and March, 1990 to assess myocardial viability after CABG. Forty patients underwent successful revascularization. Patients who exhibited evidence of metabolically compromised myocardium by positron emission tomography as evidenced by decreased blood flow with preserved metabolism who did not undergo subsequent CABG were more likely to experience AMI, death, cardiac arrest or late revascularization due to development of new symptoms than were the other patients groups. Decreased flow and metabolism in segments of previous AMI did not affect outcome in patients with or without subsequent CABG. Those with a compromised myocardium who did not undergo revascularization were more likely to have an improvement in functional class than were patients with preoperative positron emission tomographic findings of matched decreases in flow and metabolism. Therefore, positron emission tomographic myocardial viability imaging appears to identify patients at increased risk of having adverse cardiac event or death. Patients with impaired LV function and positron emission tomographic evidence for jeopardized myocardium appear to have the most benefit from a revascularization procedure.

After non-cardiac surgery

To determine the 2-year cardiac prognosis of high risk patients undergoing noncardiac surgery and to determine the predictors of long-term adverse cardiac outcome, Mangano and associates[43] for the Study of Perioperative Ischemia Research Group studied a consecutive sample of 444 patients with or at high risk for CAD who had undergone elective noncardiac surgery and were discharged from the hospital in stable condition. The main outcome measures were cardiac death, AMI, unstable angina pectoris, progressive angina requiring CABG or PTCA, and new unstable angina requiring hospitalization. Forty-seven patients (11%) had major cardiovascular complications during a 728-day (median) follow-up period: 24 had cardiac death; 11, nonfatal AMI; 6, progressive angina requiring CABG or coronary angioplasty; and 6, new unstable angina requiring hospitalization. Thirty percent of outcomes occurred within 6 months of surgery and 64% within 1 year. Five independent predictors of long-term outcome were identified. Three predictors reflected the preexisting chronic disease state: (1) the presence of known vascular disease; (2) a history of CHF; and (3) known CAD. Two predictors reflected acute postoperative ischemic events: (1) AMI/unstable angina and (2) myocardial ischemia. Patients surviving a postoperative in-hospital AMI had a 28-fold increase in the rate of subsequent cardiac complications within 6 months following surgery, a 15-fold increase within 1 year, and a 14-fold increase within 2 years. Seventy percent of all long-term adverse outcomes were preceded by in-hospital postoperative ischemia that occurred at least 30 days (median, 282 days) before the long-term event. The development of CHF or VT (without ischemia) during hospitalization was not associated with adverse long-term outcome. The incidence of long-term adverse cardiac outcomes following noncardiac surgery is substantial. At increased risk are patients with chronic cardiovascular disease; at highest risk are patients with acute perioperative ischemic events.

To identify predictors of postoperative myocardial ischemia in patients scheduled to undergo major noncardiac surgery, Hollenberg and associates[44] for the Study of Perioperative Ischemia Research Group obtained clinical, laboratory and physiological data prospectively before and during surgery in a consecutive sample of 474 men at high risk for or with CAD who were scheduled to undergo major noncardiac surgery to identify potential univariate predictors of postoperative myocardial ischemia, which then were entered into multivariate logistic models. Continuous 2-lead electrocardiograms before, during, and after surgery were used to identify episodes of myocardial ischemia. Five major preoperative predictors of postoperative myocardial ischemia were identified: (1) LV hypertrophy by electrocardiogram; (2) history of systemic hypertension; (3) diabetes mellitus; (4) definite CAD; and (5) use of digoxin. The risk of postoperative myocardial ischemia increased progressively with the number of predictors present: in 22% of patients with no predictors, in 31% with 1 predictor, in 46% with 2 predictors, in 70% with 3 predictors, and in 77% with 4 predictors. Patients subgroups who are at high risk for developing postoperative myocardial ischemia and who might benefit the most from intensive Holter monitoring in the postoperative period now can be identified preoperatively.

UNSTABLE ANGINA PECTORIS

Silent myocardial ischemia

Romeo and colleagues[45] in Rome and Catania, Italy, assessed the long-term prognostic significance of total ischemic time (silent plus painful ischemia) and silent ischemia in patients with unstable angina whose condition stabilized with medical therapy. Seventy-six patients were studied. All patients underwent Holter ambulatory electrocardiographic monitoring for ≥48 hours beginning within the first 12 hours of the hospital stay. Forty-three patients (Group A) had a total ischemic time ≥60 minutes, whereas 33 patients (Group B) had a total ischemic time <60 minutes. More than 78% of the ischemic episodes in patients in Group A and 62% of those in Group B were silent. Nine patients in Group A and 6 in Group B had only silent episodes. Patients in Group A frequently showed three-vessel CAD (65% vs 18%), angiographic findings of subtotal occlusion of the coronary arteries (77% vs 42%) and ischemic alterations in the resting electrocardiogram (51% vs 30%). During a 6-week follow-up period, 15 patients in Group A and 8 in Group B had AMIs, 9 patients in Group A and 4 in Group B required CABG, and 10 patients in Group A and 4 in Group B died of cardiac causes. Multivariate analysis showed three-vessel CAD to be the most important predictor of cardiac mortality and morbidity followed by total ischemic time ≥60 minutes and by LV dysfunction. The presence of silent ischemia was not shown to be an independent predictor of long-term morbidity and mortality. Therefore, patients with unstable angina and a total ischemic time ≥60 minutes frequently have silent ischemic episodes on Holter electrocardiographic monitoring, a greater extent of coronary atherosclerosis and ischemia alterations on the resting electrocardiogram. The long-term prognosis of patients with unstable angina whose condition stabilized with medical therapy depends on the extent of CAD and on the longer duration of total ischemic time but not on the presence of silent ischemia.

Left ventricular dysfunction

The relation between coronary artery narrowings on angiogram and associated segmental LV dysfunction in patients with unstable angina pectoris is unclear. Warner and associates[46] from Richmond, Virginia, evaluated 52 patients with angina occurring at rest who underwent cardiac catheterization within 3 days of the last episode of pain and had no enzymatic evidence of myocardial necrosis. Coronary artery narrowings deemed responsible for the ischemic episodes were analyzed with regard to the artery involved, maximal diameter of the narrowing, presence of thrombus, and complex appearance. Time to catheterization, age, sex, and electrocardiographic evidence of ischemia were also noted. Segmental LV dysfunction in the territory supplied by the "culprit lesion" was present in 58% of patients. It occurred significantly more often with narrowing location in the LAD coronary artery, and was less frequent with narrowing in the LC and ramus coronary arteries. Ischemic electrocardiographic changes were more sensitive in predicting LV dysfunction with culprit lesion location in the LAD or right coronary artery. LV dysfunction could not be predicted by any other parameter analyzed. It is concluded that postischemic LV dysfunction occurs frequently in rest angina, especially when the severest narrowing is in the LAD coronary artery.

Lymphocyte activation

Blood clotting activation is an important component of the inflammatory response; the outbursts of unstable angina are usually associated with increased thrombin formation and coronary mural thrombosis. To investigate 1) whether monocyte activation is responsible for the enhanced thrombin formation during bursts of unstable angina and 2) what mechanism(s) might be responsible for monocyte activation, Neri Serneri and colleagues[47] in Florence, Italy, studied patients with unstable angina, stable effort angina, left ventricular thrombosis, and control subjects, measuring plasma fibrinopeptide A levels and the capacity of monocytes to express procoagulant activity and of lymphocytes to modulate this expression. Patients with unstable angina and patients with ventricular thrombosis had significantly higher plasma fibrinopeptide A levels than patients with effort angina and control subjects. Only monocytes from unstable angina patients expressed significantly increased procoagulant activity characterized as tissue factor-like activity. When 14 patients with unstable angina were restudied 8–12 weeks later, they showed neither elevated fibrinopeptide A plasma levels nor monocyte procoagulant activity. In unstable angina patients, there was a correlation between fibrinopeptide A and procoagulant activity. For expression of procoagulant activity by monocytes, both an incubation of at least 2 hours with lymphocytes and direct monocyte-lymphocyte contact were needed. In reconstitution and cross-mixing experiments, only lymphocytes from patients with active unstable angina induced the expression of procoagulant activity by monocytes from both control and patient groups. The results demonstrate that the increased thrombin formation in unstable angina patients is due to the expression of tissue factor-like activity by activated monocytes.

Serum troponin T

Cardiac troponin T is a regulatory contractile protein not normally found in blood. Its detection in the circulation has been shown to be a sensitive and specific marker for myocardial cell damage. Hamm and associates[48] from multiple European medical centers screened 109 patients with unstable angina (25 with accelerated or subacute angina and 84 with acute angina at rest) for serum creatine kinase activity, creatine kinase isoenzyme MB activity, and troponin T every 8 hours for 48 hours after admission to the hospital. The outcomes of interest during the hospitalization were death and AMI. Troponin T was detected (range, 0.20 to 3.64 ug per liter; mean, 0.78; median, 0.50) in the serum of 33 of the 84 patients (39%) with acute angina at rest. Only 3 of these patients had elevated creatine kinase MB activity (2 were positive for troponin T, and 1 was negative). Of the 33 patients who were positive for troponin T, 10 (30%) had AMI (3 after CABG), and 5 of these died during hospitalization. In contrast, only 1 of the 51 patients with angina at rest who were negative for troponin T had an AMI, and this patient died. Thus, 10 of the 11 patients with AMIs had detectable levels of troponin T; only 1 had elevated creatine kinase MB activity. Troponin T was not detected in any of the 25 patients with accelerated or subacute angina, and none of these patients died. Cardiac troponin T in serum appears to be a more sensitive indicator of myocardial-cell injury than serum creatine kinase MB activity, and its detection in the circulation may be a useful prognostic indicator in patients with unstable angina.

Coronary angioscopy

Disruption of an atherosclerotic plaque in a coronary artery followed by the formation of a thrombus is believed to be the cause of unstable angina and AMI. Although thrombotic therapy is efficacious in patients with AMI, it is far less effective in patients with unstable angina. Mizuno and associates[49] postulated that there might be differences in the composition of the coronary-artery thrombi in unstable angina and in AMI. To investigate the appearance of coronary-artery thrombi, Mizuno and associates performed percutaneous transluminal coronary angioscopy in 15 patients with unstable angina and in 16 with AMI. Angioscopy was performed within 48 hours after an episode of pain at rest in the patients with unstable angina and within 8 hours of onset in those with AMI. Angioscopy revealed coronary thrombi in all but 2 patients (1 in each group). Of the 29 patients with thrombi, those with unstable angina were frequently observed to have grayish-white thrombi (10 of 14, 17%), but none were seen in the 15 patients with AMI. By contrast, reddish thrombi were observed in all 15 patients with AMI who had thrombi, but in only 4 of the 14 patients with unstable angina and thrombi. As assessed by coronary angiography, occlusive thrombi occurred frequently in patients with AMI (13 of 16 patients) but were not seen in any of the 15 patients with unstable angina. Coronary-artery thrombi play an important part in the pathogenesis of unstable angina and AMI. However, the appearance of the thrombi is different in 2 conditions, possibly reflecting differences in the composition or age of the thrombi or the presence or absence of blood flow in the artery. This difference may account for the contrasting results of thrombolytic therapy.

Thrombolysis

Because coronary thrombosis is important in the pathogenesis of unstable angina and correlates with in-hospital events, Freeman and co-workers[50] in Toronto, Canada, hypothesized that thrombolytic therapy would decrease cardiac events. The investigators randomized 70 patients with unstable angina to tissue-type plasminogen activator with an initial dose followed by infusion for 9 hours or placebo. All patients received full doses of intravenous heparin for 96 hours and aspirin. The primary end points of the study were in-hospital death, AMI and urgent revascularization. Three secondary end points were also evaluated. Myocardial perfusion was assessed with resting planar thallium scintigraphy 90 minutes after initiation of therapy. Silent ischemia was assessed with 48-hour Holter monitoring for ST shift beginning at time of initiation of drug therapy. PTCA was performed at 18 hours and analyzed quantitatively to assess the stenosis responsible for unstable angina, the presence of intraluminal filling defects consistent with intracoronary thrombus, and stenosis morphology and severity. There was no difference in total in-hospital cardiac events between patients receiving thrombolytic and those receiving placebo. Resting thallium defects were larger in the patients receiving thrombolytic than in those receiving placebo, and this difference persisted when corrected for previous AMI. Although the numbers of patients with ST shift were similar, the duration of ST shift was significantly longer in the patients receiving thrombolytic therapy than with placebo. The frequency of intracoronary thrombi in patients with stenoses >50% was significantly less in patients treated with thrombolytic therapy as compared with placebo, but there was no significant difference in minimal lesion cross-sectional area or ulceration index of the culprit artery. The investigators concluded that a prolonged infusion of tissue-type plasminogen activator in unstable angina reduces intracoronary thrombi but does not significantly decrease in-hospital cardiac events.

The clinical effect of a low-dose rapid-infusion intravenous regimen was assessed by Chaudhary and associates[51] from Christ Church, New Zealand, using human recombinant tissue-type plasminogen activator (rt-PA) in unstable angina pectoris. Fifty patients with unstable angina pectoris were randomly assigned to blinded treatment with either placebo (24 patients) or low-dose (20 mg bolus, 30 mg infusion over 1 hour) intravenous rt-PA (26 patients). Before randomization, all patients were treated with aspirin, twice-daily subcutaneous heparin, and maximally tolerated anti-anginal therapy. Of the 50 patients assigned, 26 received rt-PA and the outcome was successful in 15 (58%) (angina settled, no AMI or urgent intervention) compared with 9 (38%) successful outcomes in the 24 who received placebo. Angina remained refractory in 8 (31%) of the rt-PA group and in 13 (54%) of the placebo group. Urgent interventions were required in 6 patients (23%) who received rt-PA and in 11 patients (46%) who received placebo. Three patients in each group sustained an AMI within 72 hours of entering the trial and there were 3 deaths (1 in the active treatment group, 2 in placebo group) within 2 weeks of the trial. Administration of intravenous rt-PA was not associated with any complications. Low-dose rt-PA administration in patients with unstable angina was associated with a tendency to stabilization of anginal symptoms and a reduction in the need for urgent intervention. However, these trends did not achieve statistical significance.

Barr and co-investigators[52] in Maastricht, the Netherlands, in the unstable angina study using *eminase,* studied 159 patients in a double-blind, placebo-controlled multicenter trial. Patients without a previous AMI, with a typical history of unstable angina, and electrocardiographic abnormalities indicative of ischemia were included. After baseline angiography, study medication (anistreplase or placebo) was given. Angiography was repeated after 12 to 28 hours. A significant decrease occurred in diameter stenosis between the first and second angiogram in the anistreplase group compared with the placebo group (11% versus 3%). This difference was caused by reopening of occluded vessels in the thrombolytic group. No beneficial clinical effects of thrombolytic treatment were found. Bleeding complications were significantly higher in patients who received thrombolytic therapy (21 vs 7 patients). Thus, angiographic but no clinical improvement after thrombolytic therapy with anistreplase was found in patients with unstable angina with an excess of bleeding complications. Therefore, thrombolytic therapy cannot be recommended in patients diagnosed as having unstable angina.

Lipoprotein(a) [Lp(a)] is a LDL-like particle whose apolipoprotein B (apo B) moiety is disulfide-linked to apo(a), a plasminogen-like inhibitor of fibrinolysis in vitro. Hegele and colleagues[53] in Ontario, Canada, hypothesized that plasma concentrations of Lp(a) are acutely affected by intravenous tissue-type plasminogen activator. Patients with unstable angina were randomized to receive either intravenous tissue-type plasminogen activator or placebo. Tow-way ANOVA using repeated measures revealed a significant effect of tissue-type plasminogen activator on concentrations of Lp(a). There was a 48% fall in Lp(a) from baseline concentrations in the tissue-type plasminogen activator group at 12 hours but not at 72 hours. Lp(a) in the placebo group was unchanged. Hegle concluded that tissue-type plasminogen activator produces a sharp and substantial but reversible reduction in plasma Lp(a). These data suggest that Lp(a) concentration is not as static in vivo and might be acutely modifiable through some mechanism that induces its removal from the freely circulating state.

To compare the clinical benefit of intravenous *urokinase* with that of conventional antithrombotic therapy in preventing the progression of unstable angina to new AMI, intractable angina, or death within the first 96 hours after hospitalization, Schreiber and co-investigators[54] in Royal Oak, Michigan, randomized 149 patients with unstable angina to 1 of 2 intravenous thrombolytic strategies. Forty-nine patients received 3 million units urokinase intravenously over 90 minutes plus intravenous heparin (group A); 47 patients received unblinded 3 million units urokinase intravenously plus 325 mg aspirin orally daily (group B); and 53 patients received placebo thrombolytic infusion plus full-dose heparin (group C). The primary end point of this trial was 96-hour clinical status. There were no significant differences in the baseline characteristics of age, previous AMI, hypertension, diabetes, tobacco use, or previous CABG among the 3 groups. Despite an excess of minor untoward reactions for the urokinase groups, there was no significant differences with respect to major bleeds. At 96 hours after presentation, no significant difference emerged in the incidence of new cardiac events: new AMI developed in

10% of group A, 6% of group B, and 4% of group C; intractable angina occurred in 6% of group A, 11% of group B, and 9% of group C. There were no deaths. All 3 groups encountered a similar incidence of overall cardiac events. Although trial enrollment was to extend to 600 patients, interim analysis led to early cessation of enrollment due to a negative trend in respect to outcome after thrombolysis. High-dose intravenous urokinase followed by either heparin or aspirin can be safely administered to a broad, unselected group of patients with unstable angina. This study suggests that no clinical advantage is conferred by urokinase, with either adjunctive antithrombotic therapy over standard heparin therapy alone, when given relatively late after admission for unstable angina.

Return after stopping heparin

Heparin is an effective, widely used treatment for unstable angina pectoris. Among patients enrolled in a double-blind, randomized, place-bo-controlled trial comparing intravenous heparin, aspirin, both treat-ments, and neither during the acute phase of unstable angina, Theroux and associates[55] from Montreal, Canada, encountered patients in whom unstable angina was reactivated after heparin was discontinued. The study population included 403 of the original 479 patients in the trial who had completed 6 days of blinded therapy without refractory angina or AMI. After the discontinuation of therapy, clinical events, including reactivation of unstable angina and AMI occurring within 96 hours after hospitalization, were closely monitored. Early reactivation occurred in 14 of the 107 patients who received heparin alone, as compared with only 5 patients in each of the other 3 study groups (Figure 2-7). These reactivations required urgent intervention (thrombolysis, angioplasty, or CABG) in 11 patients treated with heparin alone, but in only 2 patients in the other groups combined. Four of the 6 patients who had an AMI during a reactivation of their disease were in the heparin group. Reactiva-tions in this group occurred in a cluster a mean (± SD) of 9.5 ± 5 hours after the discontinuation of the study drug but were randomly distributed over the initial 96 hours in the other 3 groups. Although heparin is benefi-cial in treating unstable angina, the disease process may be reactivated within hours of the discontinuation of this drug. Concomitant therapy with aspirin may prevent this withdrawal phenomenon.

Five-drug medical therapy

A group of 125 patients with unstable angina were studied by Grambow and Topol[56] from Cleveland, Ohio, over a 5-year period to define the frequency of refractory unstable angina in the current era of 5-drug medi-cal therapy with intravenous heparin, aspirin, nitrates, calcium antago-nists and B blockers. All patients had >20 minutes of chest pain at rest with reversible electrocardiographic changes occurring in the absence of AMI. Patients were considered refractory only if chest pain continued despite treatment with maximal 5-drug therapy. At the time of transfer to the center, 65 patients continued to have ischemic chest pain at rest and were considered "medically refractory" by their referring physicians. A more aggressive medical regimen was used, and 54 patients (83%) were rendered chest pain-free. Of the 11 truly refractory patients (8.8%), coronary arteriography revealed an increased likelihood of LM or 3-vessel CAD (7 of 11 vs 26 of 114). In-hospital treatment strategies for the 114 patients stabilized with medical therapy included continued medical

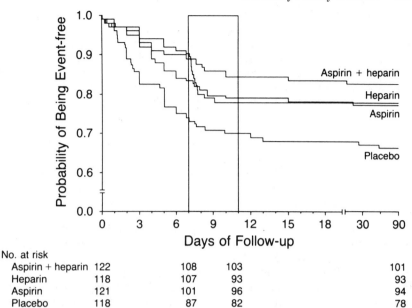

Fig. 2-7. Kaplan-Meier Event-free Curves for Patients in the Four Study Groups. The curves cover the study period of seven days, which included the double-blind administration of the study drugs; a 96-hour period early after drug discontinuation, from day 7 to day 11 (indicated by the rectangle); and a follow-up period extending through three months. The time of drug discontinuation was adjusted to day 7 for all patients for comparability. The rate of attrition in the heparin group after the discontinuation of the study drug was important, but not when aspirin was administered concomitantly with heparin. Reproduced with permission from Theroux, et al.[55]

therapy (n = 37), coronary angioplasty (n = 46) and CABG (n = 31). The rate of AMI or death in patients managed medically was 3%. Coronary angioplasty in medically stabilized patients was complicated by an abrupt closure rate of 26%, and a 17% rate of AMI, death or need for emergency CABG grafting had a 9% rate of AMI or death. Unstable angina truly refractory to current, maximal medical therapy is infrequent (8.8%). However, the refractory group is vulnerable to adverse angioplasty results and cardiac events.

Coronary angioplasty

To assess the results of a conservative coronary angioplasty strategy in patients with unstable angina pectoris, Stammen and associates[57] from Leuven, Belgium, reviewed the records of 1,421 consecutive patients without previous AMI undergoing a first PTCA between 1986 and 1990. Of these patients, 631 had unstable and 790 had stable angina pectoris. Only after an intense effort to medically control symptoms, the unstable patients underwent PTCA at an average of 15.4 days (range 1 to 76) after hospital admission. Primary clinical success was achieved in 91.7% of patients with unstable and in 94.4% of those with stable angina pectoris. In-hospital mortality rates were 0.3 and 0.1%, respectively. Nonfatal in-hospital event rates for AMI, cerebrovascular accident and coronary bypass surgery were only slightly higher in patients with unstable angina pectoris; however, the difference from the stable group was significant when all events were combined (9 vs 5.9%). During 6-month follow-up, no significant difference in adverse events was found between the groups. The respective rates for the unstable and stable groups were 0.4 and 0.2% for death, 5.5 and 5.1% for major nonfatal events, and 17.7 and 20.1% for repeat PTCA. These results suggest that use of a conservative PTCA strategy in the treatment of patients with unstable angina pectoris results in favorable and similar immediate and 6-month outcomes compared with those in patients with stable angina pectoris.

STABLE ANGINA PECTORIS

Left ventricular dysfunction

LV function and the electrocardiogram of 55 patients with CAD and angina were monitored by Taki and associates[58] from Boston, Massachusetts, for a mean of 3.2 ± 1.9 hours with an ambulatory LV function monitor. During the monitoring interval, patients performed daily activities such as sitting, walking, climbing stairs, and eating. Sixty episodes of transient reduction in EF of >5% lasting >60 seconds were observed in 24 patients; 13 episodes were associated with typical angina, but 47 were asymptomatic. Asymptomatic episodes had a shorter duration of ventricular dysfunction (116 ± 49 vs 189 ± 113 seconds), and smaller increases in relative end-diastolic and end-systolic volumes (end-diastolic 0.9 ± 5.4% vs 4.6 ± 4.9%, and end-systolic 21 ± 11% vs 35 ± 20%) than did symptomatic ones. When a subset of patients with both symptomatic and asymptomatic episodes were analyzed, similar results were observed: in asymptomatic episodes, duration was shorter (82 ± 31 vs 200 ± 110 seconds), EF decrease was smaller (−7.3 ± 2.6% vs −11.0 ± 4.7%), and end-systolic volume increase was smaller (23 ± 12% vs 37 ± 19%). The data suggest that asymptomatic transient LV dysfunction is less severe and of shorter duration in patients with angina pectoris.

Effect of heart rate on ischemia

Panza and associates[59] in Bethesda, Maryland, investigated the role of increases in heart rate in the development of ischemic episodes recorded during ambulatory ECG monitoring in patients with stable CAD and attempted to establish the importance of such increases in determining the frequency of ambulatory myocardial ischemia. Fifty-four patients (42 men and 12 women with a mean age of 61 years) with proved CAD who had ≥1 mm ST segment depression during exercise testing underwent an exercise treadmill test and a 48 hour period of ambulatory electrocardiogram monitoring. The exercise ischemic threshold was determined as the heart rate at the onset of ST segment depression during exercise testing. During monitoring, 48 (89%) of the 54 patients had at least one episode of ST segment depression. The majority of ischemic episodes were preceded by an increase in heart rate ≥10 beats/min. The most significant increase occurred during the 5 minute period before the onset of the episode. An ischemic episode occurred 80% of the times the heart rate reached the exercise ischemic threshold. A strong correlation was observed between the number of times the exercise ischemic threshold was reached during monitoring and the number and duration of ischemic episodes. Therefore, increase in heart rate that exceed the exercise ischemic threshold are frequently observed at the onset of episodes of ambulatory myocardial ischemia in patients with stable CAD.

Platelet hyperaggregability

Platelet aggregation is believed to contribute to the precipitation of acute ischemic syndromes. Because physical activity has been proposed as 1 possible trigger in converting a patient with chronic CAD to 1 with an acute ischemic syndrome, Diodati and co-workers[60] in Bethesda, Maryland, examined the hypothesis that platelets become activated when coronary blood flow velocities (and thereby shear stress) increase across an atherosclerotic bed. During catheterization, 82 patients (36 with left CAD, 12 with only right CAD, and 34 with normal coronary arteries) had measurement of whole blood platelet aggregation performed on blood samples obtained simultaneously from the coronary sinus and aorta at rest, 2 minutes after onset of rapid atrial pacing, and 10 minutes after pacing was terminated. There was no arteriovenous difference in platelet aggregation under resting conditions in patients with versus those without CAD. Atrial pacing in patients with left CAD caused an increase in platelet aggregation in the coronary sinus blood but not in arterial blood. This increase was transient and returned nearly to baseline 10 minutes after termination of pacing. Patients with nonsignificant left CAD, those with normal coronary arteries, and patients with significant CAD only in the right coronary artery did not show any changes in either the coronary sinus or arterial blood with atrial pacing. There is no evidence of platelet activation across a normal or an atherosclerotic coronary bed at rest. When coronary blood flow increases in the presence of significant ($\geq$50%) narrowing of epicardial coronary arteries, however, platelets are activated and aggregate more easily. This mechanism may play a role in the precipitation of acute ischemic syndromes in patients with CAD.

Aspirin

Clinical trials have demonstrated a prophylactic role for aspirin in AMI and in unstable angina pectoris. The Swedish Angina Pectoris Aspirin Trial (SAPAT) is the first prospective study of aspirin in stable angina. Juul-Moller and associates[61] for the Swedish SAPAT Group randomized 2,035 patients double-blindly to treatment with aspirin 75 mg daily or placebo. All patients were treated with *sotalol* for control of symptoms. The median duration of follow-up was 50 months. Compared with the placebo + sotalol group, the aspirin + sotalol group had a 34% (81 vs 124 patients) reduction in primary outcome events (AMI and sudden death) and the reduction observed in secondary outcome events (vascular events, vascular death, all cause mortality, stroke) ranged from 22% to 32%. Treatment withdrawal caused by adverse events occurred in 109 patients in the aspirin + sotalol group; major bleeds, including hemorrhagic stroke, occurred in 20 and 13 patients, respectively. The addition of a low dose of aspirin to sotalol treatment showed significant benefit in terms of cardiovascular events, including a significant reduction in the incidence of first AMI in patients with symptoms of stable angina pectoris.

Nifedipine

Parmley and colleagues[62] evaluated the influence of nifedipine on the circadian pattern of angina and silent ischemia in patients with chronic stable angina at 118 sites in the United States and in 207 patients in the Nifedipine Gastro-Intestinal Therapeutic System Circadian Anti-ischemic Program. To be eligible for participation, patients were required to have at least two episodes of angina a week and at least two episodes of myocardial ischemia during 48 hour ambulatory electrocardiographic monitoring. Beta-blockers were continued in those patients already receiving them. In this 7 to 10 week single-blind placebo withdrawal study, a 1 week placebo run-in was followed by up to 5 weeks of single-blind titration with nifedipine, a 4 week efficacy phase with an established dose, and a final single 2 week placebo withdrawal period. Ambulatory electrocardiogram monitoring was performed at the end of each placebo phase and at the end of the efficacy phase with a digital monitoring device that was validated in a pilot study. Overall, nifedipine significantly reduced the weekly number of anginal episodes from 5.7 to 1.8 and the number of ischemic events from 7.3 to 4 reported during the 48 hour monitoring periods with a significant increase in both during the placebo withdrawal period. The baseline circadian pattern of ischemia showed an early morning peak and a secondary peak in the afternoon. Nifedipine significantly reduced ischemia during the 48 hour period when administered as monotherapy or in combination with a beta-blocker. The primary side effect of nifedipine was edema, which was dose related. Thus, nifedipine reduced the number of anginal and ischemic episodes when given alone or in combination with a beta-blocker in patients with stable angina.

Angioplasty vs bypass

In an investigation performed by Mulcahy and associates[63] from London, UK, to assess the effects of standard therapeutic interventions on the total ischemic burden, 86 patients with stable angina underwent 48 hours of ambulatory ST segment monitoring and treadmill exercise testing before and at a mean of 10 weeks after CABG (group 1, n = 46) or PTCA (group 2, n = 40). There were 72 male and 14 female patients with a mean age of 56 years. All patients had documented CAD (24 single-vessel; 28 2-vessel; 34 3-vessel disease). Both groups were characteristically similar apart from more severe CAD and more previous myocardial infarctions in group 1. Groups with CABG and PTCA had significant prolongation of exercise time after intervention (group 1: 7.6 to 9.8 minutes; group 2: 8.1 to 10 minutes), and both interventions led to a significant reduction in ischemic responses to exercise. During a total of 7643 hours of ST segment monitoring, 253 episodes of ischemia were recorded in 3768 hours before and 44 ischemic episodes in 3875 hours after intervention. Both interventions reduced the mean frequency of ischemia per 24 hours (group 1: 1.24 to 0.22 episodes per 24 hours; group 2: 1.9 to 0.3 episodes per 24 hours). The resting electrocardiographic findings were improved as a result of the interventions in 28% (n = 24) of patients. Both CABG and PTCA are effective in improving exercise capacity and reducing the total ischemic burden.

Coronary artery bypass grafting

The 18-year effect of CABG compared with medical therapy on survival, incidence of AMI and relief of angina was evaluated in 686 randomized patients with stable angina in the Veterans Affairs Cooperative Study of CABG, West Haven, Connecticut.[64] The primary treatment comparisons were made according to intent to treat; 44% of the entire medical cohort had CABG during a median follow-up of 17 years. Overall 18-year survival rates were 33% for medicine compared with 30% for surgery. Survival rates for high-risk patients without LM CAD, which had shown a significant advantage for surgical therapy up to 11 years, were 23% medicine versus 24% surgery for patients with 3-vessel CAD and impaired LV function, and 22% versus 25% for those with multiple clinical risk factors. For patients with 2-vessel CAD, who had significantly better survival with medical therapy at 11 years, rates were similar at 18 years in the 2 treatment groups (34% medicine vs 30% surgery). Cumulative 18-year AMI rates (fatal plus nonfatal) were 41% in medical and 49% in surgical patients. Nonfatal infarction rates were lower with medical than with surgical therapy (32% vs 44%), but fatal infarction rates were similar (14% medicine vs 13% surgery). The combined rate of AMI or death was also lower with medical therapy (75% vs 82%). In contrast, surgery reduced mortality after AMI by 35% at 10 years but only by 13% at 18 years. The percent of medical and surgical patients who were angina-free was 3% versus 22% at 1 year and 4% versus 12% at 5 years, compared with rates of 6% versus 5% at 10 years and 3% versus 4% at 15 years. The benefits of CABG on survival, symptoms, and post infarction mortality were transient and lasted fewer than 11 years. The benefits began to diminish after 5 years, when graft closure accelerated. Surgery was effective in reducing mortality only for patients with a poor natural history. Low-risk patients, who had a good prognosis with medical therapy, derived no survival benefit with surgical therapy at any time during the follow-up period. Regardless of risk, surgery also did not reduce the incidence of AMI or the combined incidence of infarction or death.

SILENT MYOCARDIAL ISCHEMIA

Naka and colleagues[65] from Nagano-ken, Japan, studied patients with and without diabetes with respect to the prevalence of silent myocardial ischemia, by means of treadmill exercise testing and coronary angiography. Results of treadmill exercise testing showed ischemic ST depression in 41 of the 132 diabetic patients (mean age 61 ± 4 years) and in 42 of the 140 nondiabetic control subjects (mean age 60 ± 8 years). Coronary angiography was performed in 36 of 41 diabetic patients and 34 of 42 consenting nondiabetic control individuals with positive results of treadmill exercise tests. Among treadmill-positive individuals, diabetic patients had a prevalence of silent myocardial ischemia that was 2.2 times higher than that in nondiabetic control individuals. Diabetic patients who received insulin had a 2.6 times higher prevalence of silent myocardial ischemia than those who did not. Similarly, diabetic patients with retinopathy had a 2.5 times higher prevalence of silent myocardial ischemia than those without it.

Nyman and associates[66] from Linköping, Sweden, studied the prognostic value of silent ischemia during a symptom-limited predischarge exercise test in 740 men after an episode of unstable angina or non-Q wave myocardial infarction. The 51% of patients with ST depression at the exercise test had a higher rate of myocardial infarction or death after 1 year (18%) compared with those without ST depression (9%). This increased risk was not influenced by the presence or absence of pain at the exercise test: 18% in patients with painful ischemia and in those with silent ischemia. However, ST depression combined with pain at the exercise test predicted a higher incidence of class III or IV angina at follow-up (44% compared with 17% in the group with asymptomatic ST depression). Because revascularization in addition to alleviating symptoms also enhances the prognosis in certain groups of patients, selections for coronary angiography and possible revascularization should not be made only on the basis of symptoms but also on the presence of myocardial ischemia, whether symptomatic or not.

Kurita and associates[67] from Saitama, Japan, sought to clarify whether plasma beta-endorphin and bradykinin affects the pathophysiology of myocardial ischemia and the perception of cardiac pain, by studying 35 patients with CAD with treadmill testing and 48-hour Holter electrocardiographic monitoring to measure their pain thresholds. Patients were divided into 2 groups during exercise testing: group 1 (n = 19) who had ST segment depression, and group 2 (n = 16) who had chest pain. Both groups were then compared with 12 age-matched control individuals. Pain thresholds were measured after Holter electrocardiographic monitoring, and blood samples were drawn before and immediately after exercise. No statistical differences were noted between groups 1 and 2 with regard to the severity of myocardial ischemia as assessed by ST segment depression or exercise tolerance time. The frequency of the episodes of silent myocardial ischemia in group 1 was found to be significantly higher than that in group 2. The duration of the episodes of silent myocardial ischemia in group 1 was 42 minutes (range 3 to 343 minutes), which was significantly longer than that in group 2 (12 minutes; range 0 to 74). The pain threshold in group 1 was a statistically higher value than that in group 2. Although the resting plasma beta-endorphin level in group 1 was not statistically significantly different from values in either group 2 or the control group, during exercise the plasma beta-endorphin levels in both group 1 and the control group were significantly elevated in comparison with their resting levels. The resting plasma bradykinin level in group 2, on the other hand, was significantly higher than those values in group 1 and the control group. Similarly during exercise the plasma bradykinin level increased in all 3 groups, but after exercise this increase was sustained only in group 2. These results suggest that plasma beta-endorphin and bradykinin appear to possess factors that influence the perception of angina pain.

Quyyumi and associates[68] in Bethesda, Maryland, evaluated the prognostic value of radionuclide measurements of LV function at rest and during exercise specifically examining the relationship between LV function at rest and exercise-induced ischemia assessed by radionuclide ventriculography and by ambulatory electrocardiographic monitor. Among the 155 patients with CAD studied, 88% had LV dysfunction with exercise, defined as failure of the ejection fractions to increase by >4% with exercise, and 33% of patients had LV dysfunction at rest with LV ejection fractions <45%. Fifty-two percent of these patients had transient episodes of ST segment depression during 48 hour ambulatory electrocardiographic monitoring. Exercise-induced LV dysfunction during radionuclide ventriculography was very sensitive (94%) in detecting patients with ischemic episodes during ambulatory electrocardiographic monitoring. However, only 55% of patients with exercise-induced LV dysfunction had ST segment depression during ambulatory ECG monitoring. Patients with LV dysfunction at rest had a lower prevalence of transient episodes of ST segment depression (31%) than did patients with normal LV function at rest (62%). The relation between prognostically important variables during exercise radionuclide ventriculography and the number and duration of transient episodes of ST segment depression was examined. By multivariate regression analysis, only the change in LV ejection fraction with exercise was independently related to the number and duration of episodes of ST segment depression. Therefore, myocardial ischemia during daily life detected by ST segment monitoring correlates poorly with radionuclide ventriculographic measurements of ischemia.

On exercise testing after an episode of unstable angina pectoris or non Q-wave AMI, a proportion of patients show ST-segment depression, indicating myocardial ischemia, but do not report concomitant symptoms of angina. Treatment of such "silent" ischemia aims mainly to reduce the risk of subsequent cardiac events. Nyman and associates[69] of the Research Group on Instability in Coronary Artery Disease in Southeast Sweden studied the effect of low-dose aspirin in patients with myocardial ischemia defined at the predischarge test as silent (though patients might have had symptomatic ischemia at other times) or symptomatic. Seven hundred forty men with unstable CAD aged 70 years or less underwent symptom-limited exercise testing before hospital discharge; 144 showed ST depression without pain and 230 ST depression with simultaneous chest pain. Of the silent ischaemia group, 67 were randomly assigned placebo and 77 aspirin (75 mg daily); the corresponding numbers in the symptomatic group were 125 and 105. Angina symptoms were less common in the silent than in the symptomatic ischemia group both before inclusion and during follow-up, and a greater proportion of the silent ischemia group were included because of myocardial infarction. In both ischemia groups aspirin treatment reduced the risk of subsequent myocardial infarction or death by 3 months' follow-up (silent 4% of aspirin-treated vs 21% of placebo-treated patients; symptomatic 9% vs 18%); at 12 months' follow-up a significant benefit of aspirin was still apparent in the silent ischemia group (9% vs 28%) but not in the symptomatic group (13% vs 22%). Low-dose aspirin reduced the risk of subsequent myocardial infarction at least as well in silent as in symptomatic myocardial ischemia. Since improvement of outlook is the main treatment objective in symptom-free patients, aspirin should be a mainstay of their treatment.

VARIANT ANGINA PECTORIS AND CORONARY SPASM

Since coronary artery spasm has been suggested as a mechanism leading to the development of fixed atherosclerotic coronary obstruction, Kaski and co-workers[70] in London, England studied 10 patients with typical Prinzmetal's variant angina in whom the disease remained active for 5 years and in whom occlusive coronary spasm occurred reproducibly at the same arterial site during repeat coronary arteriography (25 months after initial angiography). At initial evaluation, 4 patients had significant one-vessel CAD, and 6 had nonsignificant disease. Spasm developed at stenotic sites in 9 patients and at an angiographically normal site in 1 patient. The progression of coronary disease was assessed in 62 segments: 10 spastic and 52 nonspastic, using computerized arteriography. Mean diameters were not significantly different at first and second arteriograms. Stenosis progression (from 65% diameter reduction to total occlusion) occurred in 1 patient at a spastic site and in 2 at nonspastic sites. Complicated stenoses suggestive of plaque fissuring were not observed during the study. Thus in patients with chronic Prinzmetal's variant angina without AMI, stenosis progression was not frequently observed at spastic sites despite the recurrence of focal coronary spasm over relatively long periods of time.

Risk factors for pure coronary spasm are not known. Clinical observations have pointed to cigarette smoking, a known risk factor for obstructive CAD. Caralis and co-workers[71] in St. Louis, Missouri, conducted a case-neighborhood control study of premenopausal women, a population segment with the lowest prevalence of obstructive CAD. The cases were 21 premenopausal women (age range, 36–41 years) with angiographically proven coronary spasm. All coronary arteriograms were analyzed by 2 independent experienced cardiologists on two occasions. There were no differences between analyses; all cases had normal baseline coronary angiogram except for 2, who had less than 20% coronary luminal stenosis in segments other than the site of the focal vasospasm. All cases had normal hemodynamics at rest, normal LV function, and were in sinus rhythm. Ascertainment of the cases was done by angiographic demonstration of focal coronary spasm spontaneously or by ergonovine provocation. Six cases developed spontaneous coronary spasm before catheter engagement, and in 15, coronary spasm was induced by ergonovine provocation. Each case was asked to name as many as possible female neighborhood acquaintances of similar age and racial background who were willing to answer the same standardized questionnaire. The same standardized questionnaire was completed for each case and each control (n = 63). The standardized questionnaire was designed to obtain information on health characteristics, habits, socioeconomic status, and education. Only cigarette smoking was significantly more prevalent among coronary spasm cases. Cigarette smokers were 13 cases (62%) and 11 controls (18%). These findings suggest that there is a very strong association between cigarette smoking and pure coronary spasm in young women.

Coronary artery spasm plays an important role in acute ischemic events, and it has a close relation with coronary atherosclerosis. Nobuyoshi and associates[72] from Kitakyushu, Japan, attempted to determine the *most significant risk factor for coronary artery spasm*. Among 3000 consecutive patients who underwent coronary cineangiography for ergonovine maleate testing, 330 with typical angina pectoris (group 1) and 294 with old myocardial infarction (group 2) were studied. Each group was divided into 3 or 4 subgroups according to the presence of fixed organic stenosis or a positive reaction to ergonovine maleate (coronary artery spasm). The relationship between coronary artery spasm and 8 coronary risk factors was examined: age, sex, hypertension, diabetes mellitus, smoking, and serum cholesterol, uric acid, and HDL levels. The proportion of smokers in the subgroups with coronary artery spasm was significantly higher than in the subgroups without coronary artery spasm. There was no correlation between smoking and fixed organic stenosis. According to the results of multiple regression analysis, there was a positive correlation between smoking and coronary artery spasm and between serum HDL levels and coronary artery spasm. Thus it was concluded that smoking is the most significant risk factor in discriminating between patients with and without coronary artery spasm.

As part of a long-term study of sudden cardiac death, Myersburg and associates[73] from Miami, Florida, collected data on arrhythmias, coronary anatomy, and *responses to ergonovine testing* to provoke coronary artery spasm among survivors of out-of-hospital cardiac arrest who had no flow-limiting coronary artery narrowings, prior myocardial infarction, or other structural causes of cardiac arrest and no angina pectoris. Associations between silent myocardial ischemia due to coronary artery spasm and the occurrence and characteristics of life-threatening ventricular arrhythmias were studied by both invasive and noninvasive techniques. Silent ischemic events were associated with the initiation of life-threatening ventricular arrhythmias in 5 patients with induced or spontaneous focal coronary artery spasm (or both). These patients were identified among a group of 356 survivors of out-of-hospital cardiac arrest who were evaluated between 1980 and 1991. In 2 of the 5 patients reperfusion, rather than ischemia itself, correlated with the onset of the ventricular arrhythmia. Only 1 of the 5 had an inducible arrhythmia during electrophysiologic testing. Titration of the dose of a calcium antagonist against the ability of ergonovine to provoke spasm was successful in preventing both the provocation of spasm and arrhythmias in all 4 patients who were tested. Silent myocardial ischemia due to coronary artery spasm can initiate potentially fatal arrhythmias in patients without flow-limiting structural coronary artery lesions.

Ozaki and associates[74] from Anjo and Nagoya, Japan, studied chronologic changes of coronary spasm by repeated *ergonovine provocation* tests during angiography. A total of 322 patients who had variant angina without severe atherosclerosis demonstrated a positive response to the first test. Ninety patients had recurrent variant anginal symptoms after an angina-free period of 38 ± 12 months. Of these 90 patients, 76 (84%) had symptoms or electrocardiographic findings similar to those of the first test. The initial 9 of these 76 patients underwent a second provocation test and showed coronary responses analogous to those on the first test. Of the 90 patients, 14 (16%) had different symptoms or electrocardiographic findings from those elicited at the first episode. All 14 patients again had a positive response to a second ergonovine test and the following angiographic changes were observed in the 3 major vessels between the 2 tests. Of the 21 vessels that had spasm on the first test, 8 vessels (19%) did not have spasm on the second test. Of the 21 vessels that did not demonstrate spasm on the first test, 10 (24%) demonstrated spasm on the second test. In the present study it is concluded that most patients with recurrent angina seemed to have consistency in the location of coronary spasm, while in some patients the fluctuation of coronary spasm was confirmed by 2 ergonovine provocation tests.

Harding and associates[75] in Durham, North Carolina, evaluated the utility of *ergonovine testing* for coronary artery spasm in 3,447 patients with angiographically insignificant or no CAD. No patients clinically had Prinzmetal's variant angina. Overall, 4% of patients had a positive ergonovine test result defined as coronary artery spasm causing ≥75% focal stenosis. Complications related to ergonovine use occurred in 11 patients. In a training sample of 1,136 patients studied between 1980 and 1984, two independent predictors of spasm were found using multivariate analysis: 1) the amount of visible CAD on the coronary angiogram and 2) a smoking history. A model to predict spasm based on these variables was validated in a test group 2,311 patients who received ergonovine from 1985 to 1989. The model allowed the identification of a subset of 400 patients in the validation sample who had a 10% positive test rate compared with a 2% positive test rate in the remaining patients. These data should permit clinicians who use provocative testing in the cardiac catheterization laboratory to reserve such testing for the subset of patients most likely to have abnormal findings.

To elucidate the *circadian variation of fibrinolytic components* in vasospastic angina, plasma levels of tissue plasminogen activator antigen, free plasminogen activator inhibitor antigen complex, and total free plasminogen activator inhibitor antigen were measured in venous plasma samples by Sakata and associates[76] from Shizuoka, Japan. Samples were taken every 6 hours (6AM, noon, 6PM, and midnight) for 24 hours in 14 patients with vasospastic angina, in 9 patients with exertional angina, and in 19 normal individuals. Twenty-four-hour Holter monitoring was also carried out in all subjects. All of the fibrinolytic components showed circadian variation, with a peak level at 6AM in every study group except for the tissue plasminogen activator antigen/free plasminogen activator inhibitor antigen complex in the group of patients with exertional angina. The values for all of the fibrinolytic components at each sampling time were higher in patients with CAD than in normal individuals. In particular, the mean value of free plasminogen activator antigen at 6AM in patients with vasospastic angina was significantly higher than that in normal individuals and that in patients with exertional angina. This value of free plasminogen activator antigen in patients with vasospastic angina was closely associated with the duration of ischemic attacks. These results suggested that the circadian fluctuation of fibrinolytic components may be an important factor that leads to coronary thrombosis at the time of coronary spasm, especially in the early morning.

MICROVASCULAR ANGINA

Vrints and colleagues[77] in Antwerp, Belgium, evaluated the coronary vasomotor responses to selected infusion of graded concentrations of acetylcholine (10^{-6} to 10^{-4} M) into the LAD using quantitative coronary arteriography in 24 patients with normal coronary arteriograms (12 patients with atypical symptoms and 12 patients with typical angina) as well as in 36 patients with CAD with varying degrees of atherosclerosis involving the LAD. In the patients with normal coronary arteries and atypical chest pain, acetylcholine induced primarily a vasodilator response, maximal during a 10^{-5} M acetylcholine infusion. However, patients with CAD demonstrated acetylcholine caused dose-dependent vasoconstriction, even if the LAD itself was smooth. Marked vasoconstriction was also induced in the patients with typical anginal and angiographically normal coronary arteries. In nine of the patients, the constrictor response was associated with anginal pain and electrocardiographic evidence of myocardial ischemia. Isosorbide dinitrate (1 mg) relieved the anginal pain and dilated all vessels when given by the intracoronary route. These data suggest that patients with normal coronary arteriograms and angina pectoris have impaired endothelium-dependent vasodilation similar to that observed in patients with overt coronary atherosclerosis. Abnormal coronary vasoconstrictor responses resulting from this impairment may contribute to the pathogenesis of myocardial ischemia and angina in these patients.

Sütsch and associates[78] in Zurich, Switzerland, measured coronary flow reserve by the coronary sinus thermodilution technique in 6 control subjects (group 1) and 12 patients with microvascular angina (group 2). Microvascular angina is characterized by exercise-induced angina in patients with normal coronary arteries and reduced coronary flow reserve. Coronary flow reserve was calculated from maximal coronary flow after 0.5 mg/kg of dipyridamole divided by flow at rest. Cutaneous flow ratio was estimated by laser Doppler fluxmetry (right forearm) before and after 4 minutes of suprasystolic blood pressure occlusion. Coronary flow at rest was identical in the 2 groups, but after coronary vasodilation with dipyridamole, coronary flow was higher in group 1 than in group 2. Coronary flow reserve differed significantly between the 2 groups. Coronary Doppler flux at rest was higher in group 1 than in group 2. The hyperemic response was identical in both groups. Thus, cutaneous flux ratio in patients with microvascular angina is not impaired. Local peripheral vasomotor tone appears to be increased in patients with microvascular angina because cutaneous flow at rest is reduced. These data suggest that a generalized disorder of vascular reactivity is not present in patients with microvascular angina.

DIET AND DRUGS FOR MYOCARDIAL ISCHEMIA

Diet ± cholestyramine

To assess the effect of dietary reduction of plasma cholesterol concentrations on coronary arterial atherosclerosis, Watts and associates[79] from London and Manchester, UK, and Dunedin, New Zealand, performed a randomized, controlled, end-point-blinded trial based on quantitative image analysis of coronary angiograms in patients with angina or past AMI. Another intervention group received diet and cholestyramine, to determine the effect of a greater reduction in circulating cholesterol concentrations. Ninety men with CAD, who had a mean (SD) plasma cholesterol of 7.23 (0.77) mmol/l were randomized to receive usual care (U, controls), dietary intervention (D), or diet plus cholestyramine (DC), with angiography at baseline and at 39 (SD 3.5) months. Mean plasma cholesterol during the trial period was 6.93 (U), 6.17 (D), and 5.56 (DC) mmol/l. The proportion of patients who showed overall progression of coronary narrowing was significantly reduced by both interventions (U 46%, D 15%, DC 12%), whereas the proportion who showed an increase in luminal diameter rose significantly (U 4%, D 38%, DC 33%). The mean absolute width of the coronary segments studied decreased by 0.201 mm in controls, increased by 0.003 mm in group D, and increased by 0.103 mm in group DC, with improvement also seen in the minimum width of segments, percentage diameter stenosis, and edge-irregularity index in intervention groups. The change in mean absolute width of the coronary segments was independently and significantly correlated with LDL cholesterol concentration and LDL/HDL cholesterol ratio during the trial period. Both interventions significantly reduced the frequency of total cardiovascular events. Dietary change alone retarded overall progression and increased overall regression of CAD, and diet plus cholestyramine was additionally associated with a net increase in coronary lumen diameter. These findings support the use of a lipid-lowering diet, and if necessary of appropriate drug treatment, in men with CAD who have even mildly raised serum cholesterol concentrations.

Low-fat diet + exercise

Schuler and associates[80] in Heidelberg, Germany, tested the effects of intensive physical exercise and a low fat diet on progression of coronary atherosclerotic lesions and stress-induced myocardial ischemia in patients with stable angina pectoris. Eighteen patients participated in the program for 1 year. They consumed a low fat, low cholesterol diet and exercise for >3 hours every week. Changes in coronary morphology were assessed by angiography and digital image processing. Stress-induced myocardial ischemia was measured by thallium-201 scintigraphy. Results were compared with those in patients receiving "usual care." In the intervention group, significant regression of coronary atherosclerotic lesions was found in 7 of the 18 patients and no change or progression was present in 11. In patients receiving "usual care," regression was found in only 1 patient with no change or progression in 11. There was a significant reduction in stress-induced myocardial ischemia not limited to patients with regression of coronary atherosclerotic lesions. Therefore, regular physical exercise and a low fat diet may retard progression of CAD. However, improvement of myocardial perfusion may be achieved independently from regression of stenotic lesions in some patients.

Significant regression of coronary and femoral atherosclerotic lesions has been documented by angiographic studies using aggressive lipid-lowering treatment. Schuler and coworkers[81] in Heidelberg, Germany, tested the applicability and effects of intensive physical exercise and low-fat diet on coronary morphology and myocardial perfusion in nonselected patients with stable angina pectoris. Patients were recruited after routine coronary angiography for stable angina pectoris; they were randomized to an intervention group (n = 56) and a control group on "usual care" (n = 57). Treatment comprised intensive physical exercise in group training sessions (minimum 2 hours per week), daily home exercise periods (20 minutes per day), and low-fat, low-cholesterol diet (American Heart Association recommendation, phase 3). No lipid-lowering agents were prescribed. After 12 months of participation, repeat coronary angiography was performed; relative and minimal diameter reductions of coronary lesions were measured by digital image processing. Change in myocardial perfusion was assessed by Thalium scintigraphy. In patients participating in the intervention group, body-weight decreased by 5%, total cholesterol by 10% and triglycerides by 24%: HDL increased by 3%. Physical work capacity improved by 23%, and myocardial oxygen consumption, as estimated from maximal rate-pressure product, by 10%. Stress-induced myocardial ischemia decreased concurrently, indicating improvement of myocardial perfusion. Based on minimal lesion diameter, progression of coronary lesions was noted in nine patients (23%), no change in 18 patients (45%), and regression in 13 patients (32%). In the control group, metabolic and hemodynamic variables remained essentially unchanged, whereas progression of coronary lesions was noted in 25 patients (48%), no change in 18 patients (35%), and regression in 9 patients (17%). These changes were significantly different from the intervention group. In patients participating in regular physical exercise and low-fat diet, CAD progresses at a slower pace compared with a control group on usual care.

Gould and associates[82] from Houston, Texas, and San Francisco, California, in a randomized, controlled, blinded, arteriographic trial to determine the effects of a low-cholesterol, low-fat, vegetarian diet, stress management and moderate aerobic exercise examined geometric dimensions, shape and fluid dynamic characteristics of coronary artery stenoses in humans. Complex changes of different primary stenosis dimensions in opposite directions or to different degrees caused stenosis shape change with profound effects on fluid dynamic severity, not accounted for by simple percent narrowing. Accordingly, all stenosis dimensions were analyzed, including proximal, minimal, distal diameter, integrated length, exit angles and exit effects, determining stenosis shape and a single integrated measure of stenosis severity, stenosis flow reserve reflecting functional severity. In the control group, complex shape change and a stenosis—molding characteristic of statistically significant progressing severity occurred with worsening of stenosis flow reserve. In the treated group, complex shape change and stenosis molding characteristic of significant regressing severity was observed with improved stenosis flow reserve, thereby documenting the multidimensional characteristics of regressing CAD in humans (Figure 2-8).

Cholesterol-lowering goals

LaRosa and experts[83] in cardiology, lipidology, epidemiology, and health economics in Washington, D.C., met to suggest approaches to cholesterol intervention in patients with established CAD. Based on current knowledge and reports, the conference participants suggested the following guidelines for the treatment of established CAD. LDL cholesterol should be the primary target of therapy. Patients with LDL cholesterol levels equal to or greater than 100 mg/dl should be considered candidates for both diet and if necessary drug therapy to lower such levels to less than a 100 mg/dl. In addition, drug therapy may be considered in patients with HDL cholesterol <35 mg/dl or triglyceride levels >250 mg/dl to raise HDL cholesterol >35 mg/dl and to lower triglyceride levels <250 mg/dl. Special attention should be given to simultaneous intervention on other CAD risk factors such as diabetes mellitus and hypertension. Once CAD is clinically manifest, gender and age should not substantially affect the intensity of intervention except in those whose myocardial damage has resulted in various significant clinical manifestation. Invasive interventions including PTCA and CABG are and will remain important in the acute management of CAD. Long-term reduction of recurrent events however is more dependent on medical intervention, including aspirin, B-

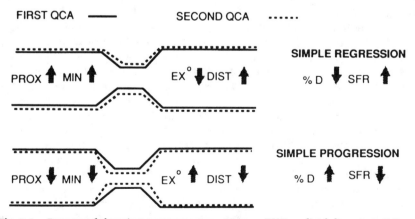

Fig. 2-8. Patterns of changing coronary artery stenoses. DIST = distal diameters; % D = percent diameter stenosis; EX° = exit angle; MIN = minimum; PROX = proximal; QCA = quantitative coronary arteriography showing simple progression and regression; SFR = stenosis flow reserve accounting for all stenosis dimensions. Reproduced with permission from Gould, et al.[82]

blockers and cholesterol lowering. Of these only cholesterol lowering has been shown to arrest the progression and induce regression of atherosclerosis. A cause-and-effect relation between circulating cholesterol and CAD has been established, and the benefit of cholesterol lowering in established CAD is very large—much larger even than the benefit in primary prevention.

Aspirin

Willard and associates[84] from Dallas, Texas, provided a superb review on the uses of aspirin in CAD. They concluded that low-dose aspirin (225 mg daily or every other day) is recommended for patients with stable angina, unstable angina, and evolving AMI. In addition, it is beneficial in patients undergoing coronary angioplasty or bypass grafting. The authors believe the data supporting its use in survivors of AMI was less compelling. The authors were also cautious in recommending the use of aspirin among patients without clinically apparent CAD because of the possible hemorrhagic complications which may outweigh its benefit unless the subjects had risk factors of considerable significance for atherosclerotic cardiovascular disease.

Nitrates

Knuuti and associates[85] from Turku, Finland, Basel, Switzerland, Goteborg, Sweden, Helsinki, Finland, and Jerusalem, Israel, compared the efficacy and safety of continuous and intermittent transdermal nitrate therapy using ambulatory electrocardiographic (Holter) monitoring. Eighty-five patients with stable angina pectoris and positive exercise test results participated during their concomitant antiischemic medication in a randomized open trial lasting 12 weeks. After a 3-week run-in period with continuous therapy (10 mg/24 hours), patients were randomized to either continuous- or intermittent-therapy groups. In the intermittent-therapy group the patients removed their patch at night (the mean patch-off period was 10 hours). Forty-eight-hour Holter monitoring was performed in each patient after randomization, and again after 2 and 12 weeks. Eighteen patients withdrew, 9 in each group. A total of 11,194 hours of electrocardiography were recorded and 607 ischemic episodes were detected, of which 79% were asymptomatic and 95% appeared during daytime. The number of ischemic episodes per 48 hours with intermittent therapy was 3.1 ± 0.7 (mean $\pm$ SEM) after randomization, 1.8 ± 0.4 at 2 weeks and 2.0 ± 0.6 at 12 weeks. With continuous therapy the respective numbers were 3.8 ± 1.1, 3.5 ± 0.9 and 4.2 ± 1.2. The differences were not statistically significant because a large number of patients (30%) had no ischemic episodes on Holter recording. However, when examining 47 patients with episodes during the study, the number of episodes was significantly reduced in the intermittent-therapy group. The changes in asymptomatic and symptomatic episodes were concordant. No changes and differences between the treatment groups were seen in nighttime episodes. Results suggest that intermittent transdermal nitrate therapy is superior to continuous therapy in reducing ischemic episodes. The nighttime nitrate-free interval does not lead to increased ischemia in patients with concomitant antiischemic medication.

Dubiel and associates[86] from Krakow, Poland, performed a double-blind study in 32 patients with stable angina pectoris to assess the effects of slow release *isosorbide dinitrate* (ISDN) (a single dose of 120 mg/day) on the frequency and duration of painless and painful ischemic episodes, and on electrocardiographic changes and exercise tolerance. Forty-eight-hour electrocardiographic monitoring and treadmill exercise tests were performed before, and at 20 and 21 days of therapy. Holter monitoring showed a significant decrease in the frequency of pain and silent episodes, and in the duration of painful (1,623 ± 664 seconds vs 323 ± 161 seconds); and silent episodes (2,818 ± 1,496 seconds vs 223 ± 102 seconds). The magnitude of painful and silent ST-segment depression was significantly reduced (2.7 ± 0.9 mm to 0.7 ± 0.7 mm and 2.0 ± 1.1 mm to 0.7 ± 0.5 mm, respectively). Time of exercise testing to the onset of ST-segment depression (442 ± 137 seconds vs 858 ± 110 seconds) or anginal pain was doubled (461 ± 128 seconds vs 830 ± 130 seconds). The work load increased from 6 to 10 METs. ISDN in a single dose of 120 mg/day is a valuable drug for stable angina pectoris, decreasing the frequency of silent and painful ischemic episodes and the magnitude of ST-segment depressions, and increasing exercise tolerance. It particularly shortened the duration of silent episodes. For patients' compliance, a once-daily dose of ISDN could be advantageous.

Isosorbide dinitrate + captopril

Metelitsa and associates[87] from Moscow, Russia, designed a study to assess whether the angiotensin-converting enzyme inhibitor captopril could potentiate the efficacy of a single dose of oral isosorbide dinitrate (ISDN) in patients with CAD. Fourteen men (mean age 53 years) with stable angina pectoris were studied. In each patient the efficacy of placebo, captopril (50 to 100 mg), ISDN (10 mg), and a combination of captopril (50 to 100 mg) and ISDN (10 mg) was assessed by repeated exercise treadmill tests performed before and 1, 2, 3 and 6 hours after administration of a single dose. A single-blind, randomized technique was applied. According to the mean data in the whole group of 14 patients, captopril alone produced no improvement in exercise duration to the onset of angina and to angina of moderate severity compared with placebo. The magnitude of ST-segment depression did not significantly change after captopril administration. ISDN alone significantly increased exercise duration to onset of angina and to angina of moderate severity (antianginal effect) and decreased the magnitude of ST-segment depression (antiischemic effect) 1 to 3 hours after administration. Combined administration of ISDN and captopril resulted in more expressed antianginal and antiischemic effects; at 2, 3 and 6 hours these effects with ISDN plus captopril were significantly more pronounced than those with ISDN alone. According to individual data, the most marked potentiation of ISDN efficacy was observed in patients who had poor response to ISDN alone. In all 6 patients in whom ISDN alone was ineffective, after the addition of captopril the desired antianginal effect was obtained. It is concluded that captopril can potentiate the efficacy of nitrates, especially in patients who do not respond to conventional doses.

Enalapril

An association between raised renin levels and AMI has been reported. Yusuf and associates[88] of the Studies of Left Ventricular Dysfunction (SOLVD) Trials studied the effects of enalapril on the development of AMI in unstable angina in 6,797 patients with an ejection fraction ≤35%. Patients were randomly assigned to placebo (n = 3,401) or enalapril (n = 3,396) at doses of 2.5–20 mg per day in 2 concurrent double-blind trials with the same protocol. Patients with CHF entered the treatment trial (n = 2,569) and those without CHF entered the prevention trial (n = 4,228). Follow-up averaged 40 months. In each trial there were significant reductions in the number of patients developing AMI (treatment trial: 158 placebo vs 127 enalapril, prevention trial: 204 vs 161) or unstable angina (240 vs 187; 355 vs 312). Combined, there were 362 placebo group patients with AMI compared with 288 in the enalapril group (risk reduction 23%). Five hundred and ninety-five placebo group patients developed unstable angina compared with 499 in the enalapril group (risk reduction 20%) (Figure 2-9). There was also a reduction in cardiac deaths (711 placebo, 615 enalapril), so that the reduction in the combined endpoint of deaths, AMI, and unstable angina was highly significant (20% risk reduction) (Figure 2-10). Enalapril treatment significantly reduced AMI, unstable angina, and cardiac mortality in patients with low EF.

Intravenous diltiazem + metoprolol

The anti-ischemic efficacy of diltiazem may improve with increments in dosage and with additional B-blocking therapy. The combined administration, however, could lead to adverse effects through amplification of negative inotropic and chronotropic properties. To evaluate hemodynamic tolerability and safety of high-dose intravenous diltiazem in patients with CAD receiving long-term metoprolol treatment, Wiesfeld and associates[89] from Rotterdam, The Netherlands, studied 9 such patients for 30 minutes after onset of intravenous diltiazem administration (0.5 mg/kg for 5 minutes, followed by 15 mg/hour). Diltiazem plasma levels peaked at 5 minutes (641 ± 74 µg/liter), decreasing to 177 µg/liter at 30 minutes. Average metoprolol levels 943 ± 12 µg/liter) did not change.

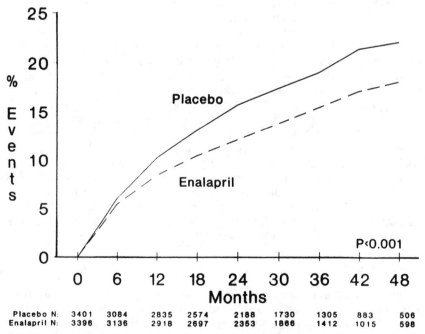

| Placebo N: | 3401 | 3084 | 2835 | 2574 | 2188 | 1730 | 1305 | 883 | 506 |
| Enalapril N: | 3396 | 3136 | 2918 | 2697 | 2353 | 1866 | 1412 | 1015 | 598 |

Fig. 2-9. Cumulative incidence of unstable angina, combined trials. Reproduced with permission from Yusuf, et al.[88]

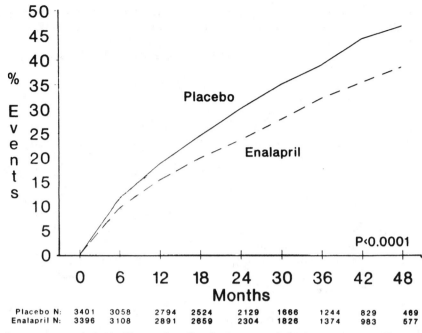

Placebo N:	3401	3058	2794	2524	2129	1666	1244	829	469
Enalapril N:	3396	3108	2891	2659	2304	1826	1374	983	677

Fig. 2-10. Cumulative incidence of cardiac death, myocardial infarction, or unstable angina, combined trials. Reproduced with permission from Yusuf, et al.[88]

Diltiazem immediately decreased systemic vascular resistance, LV systolic and mean aortic pressures (29, 21 and 20%, respectively, at 5 minutes), and they remained significantly reduced at 30 minutes. Heart rate initially increased by 11% during the bolus infusion. Concomitantly, contractility indexes V_{max} and Vce_{40}, measured at fixed heart rates, also increased significantly by 11%. Both heart rate and contractility indexes returned to baseline levels thereafter. Cardiac output increased by 10%, stroke index remained unchanged, but stroke work decreased significantly by 20%. Also, the tension-time index was significantly reduced (23%). Diltiazem induced moderate negative lusitropic effects, the first derivative of negative LV pressure decline decreased by 12% and Tau_2 lengthened by 13%. Concomitantly, LV filling pressure increased from 19 ± 2 to 23 ± 3 mm Hg, but only at 5 and 15 minutes. PQ, QRS and QTc intervals were not affected. Thus, high dosages of intravenous diltiazem are hemodynamically well tolerated and preserve cardiac pump function in patients taking chronic B blockade. The predominant systemic vasodilating effects and subsequent reduction in myocardial oxygen demand and cardiac work are likely to magnify the anti-ischemic potential of diltiazem, already afforded by coronary flow improvement after high-dose administration.

PERCUTANEOUS TRANSLUMINAL CORONARY ANGIOPLASTY

In New York State

Hannan and associates[90] from Albany, Buffalo, Syracuse, and New York, New York, sought to identify significant independent risk factors for major PTCA outcomes by doing a retrospective analysis using univariate and logistic regression analysis to identify the significant independent risk factors for adverse outcomes. The data was collected from all 31 hospitals performing PTCA in New York State in 1991. All 5,827 patients undergoing PTCA between January 1, 1991, and June 30, 1991, in New York State were analyzed. The main outcome measures were in-hospital mortality, major complications (in-hospital mortality, AMI, and/or emergency CABG), and absence of angiographic success (stenosis reduction of less than 20% on any attempted narrowing or residual stenosis of at least 50% on any attempted narrowing). Before discharge from the hospital, a total of 37 patients (9.63%) died; 67 patients (1.1%) suffered an AMI, with a mortality rate of 4.5%; and 97 patients (1.7%) underwent emergency CABG, with a mortality rate of 2.1% (no deaths in 85 patients who were hemodynamically stable and 2 deaths among 12 patients who were hemodynamically unstable). A total of 187 patients (3.2%) experienced a major complication. Angiographic success was achieved for 88% of all patients. Multivariate analysis found 4 independent preprocedural variables related to death: female gender, hemodynamic instability, shock, and EF. PTCA outcomes in New York compare favorably with other recent results reported in the literature. Several preprocedural variables markedly increase the incidence of adverse events.

For single-vessel disease

Despite the widespread use of PTCA, only a few prospective trials have assessed its efficacy. Parisi[91] of the Veterans Affairs ACME (Angioplasty Compared to Medicine) Study investigators compared the effects of PTCA with those of medical therapy on angina and exercise tolerance in patients with stable single-vessel CAD. Patients with 70 to 99% stenosis of 1 epicardial coronary artery and with exercise-induced myocardial ischemia were randomly assigned either to undergo PTCA or to receive medical therapy and were evaluated monthly. The patients assigned to PTCA were urged to have repeat angioplasty if their symptoms suggested restenosis. After 6 months, all the patients had repeat exercise testing and coronary angiography. A total of 107 patients were randomly assigned to medical therapy and 105 to PTCA. PTCA was clinically successful in 80 of the 100 patients who actually had the procedure, with an initial reduction in mean percent stenosis from 76 to 36%. Two patients in the PTCA group required emergency CABG. By 6 months after the procedure, 16 patients had had repeat PTCA. Myocardial infarction occurred in 5 patients assigned to PTCA and in 3 patients assigned to medical therapy. At 6 months 64% of the patients in the PTCA group (61 of 96) were free of angina, as compared with 46% of the medically treated patients (47 of 102) (Figure 2-11). The patients in the PTCA group were able to increase their total duration of exercise more than the medical patients (2.1 vs 0.5 minutes) and were able to exercise longer without angina on treadmill testing. For patients with single-vessel CAD, PTCA offers earlier and more complete relief of angina than medical therapy and is associated with better performance on the exercise test. However, PTCA initially costs more than medical treatment and is associated with a higher frequency of complications.

In an investigation by Kadel and associates[92] from Frankfurt/Main, Germany, 798 patients with symptomatic single-vessel disease who underwent PTCA between 1977 and 1985 were reevaluated by questionnaire 78 ± 23 months after dilatation. Indication for PTCA was stenosis of ≥70%, anginal symptoms, and objective signs of myocardial ischemia. The immediate success rate was 82%, and severe complications occurred in 7.1%,

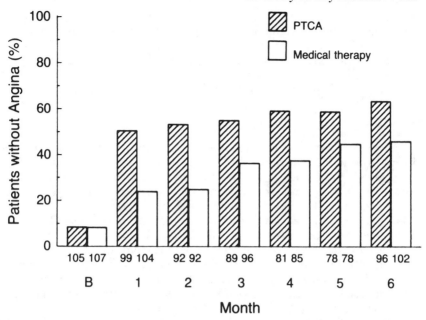

Fig. 2-11. Percent of Patients Who Were Free of Angina Each Month after Randomization. The horizontal axis shows the month before randomization (base line [B]) and clinic visits at months 1 through 6 for each treatment group. The numbers below the bars indicate the numbers of patients who were evaluated. Reproduced with permission from Parisi, et al.[91]

which included 2 fatal complications (0.3%). Repeat angiograms were performed in 582 of 648 patients who underwent successful dilatation and showed restenosis in 143 cases (25%). Within 1 year after the first dilatation, 586 patients had been successfully revascularized by PTCA (there was no evidence of restenosis or redilatation was successful), and 113 patients had undergone CABG. The remaining 99 patients were treated medically if PTCA was unsuccessful or if restenosis (≥70%) that was not amenable to redilatation was present. The 8-year overall survival probability was 92%, and cardiac survival was 96%. The 8-year event-free survival probability was 53% for all patients: 63% in patients who had successful PTCA and 15% in patients who had unsuccessful PTCA. The cardiac survival probabilities of patients with lasting PTCA success at 1 year and of surgically treated patients were significantly better than those of patients who did not have successful revascularization (at 8 years 97% and 98% vs 89%). Late events (≥1 year) occurred more often in patients who did not have successful revascularization compared with patients who had successful PTCA (at 8 years 58% were event-free vs 74%); even fewer late events were observed in surgically treated patients (at 8 years 88% were event-free). Cox's proportional hazards regression analysis revealed LVEF and revascularization status at 1 year as determinants of overall, cardiac, infarct-free, and event-free survival probabilities. At the time of reevaluation significantly more patients in the successful PTCA subgroup were still free of symptoms or had experienced improvement than patients in the CABG or medical subgroups (87% vs 69% and 60%, respectively), and more patients in the successful PTCA subgroup were still working (75% vs 53% and 57%, respectively). It was concluded that patients with single-vessel CAD who have undergone successful dilatation have an excellent long-term prognosis with regard to survival, cardiac symptoms, and vocational status. The long-term prognosis of patients who received medical therapy after failed PTCA was less favorable than that of patients who had undergone successful PTCA or that of patients who had undergone CABG after unsuccessful PTCA. If PTCA (or repeat PTCA because of restenosis) was unsuccessful, CABG improved long-term outcomes in these patients with symptomatic single-vessel CAD.

For multi-vessel disease

Incomplete revascularization is a common occurrence following PTCA in patients with multivessel disease. In an investigation by Faxon and associates[93] from Boston, Massachusetts, to determine the short-term and long-term consequences of incomplete revascularization and the influence of the functional nature of the incomplete revascularization, 139 consecutive patients with multivessel disease were analyzed: 72 were completely revascularized and 67 had incomplete revascularization. The former patients had a lower incidence of prior myocardial infarction and prior CABG. All patients had ≥1 lesion successfully dilated. In-hospital complications were insignificantly greater in incompletely revascularized patients compared with completely vascularized patients (mortality 3% vs 1%, myocardial infarction 11% vs 4%, and emergency CABG 5% vs 0%). After 1 year of follow-up, incompletely revascularized patients had similar outcomes (mortality 6% vs 3%, myocardial infarction 13% vs 7%, CABG 18% vs 15%, and repeat PTCA 19% vs 31%). The degree of incomplete revascularization was categorized as functionally adequate if all stenoses in bypassable vessels supporting viable myocardium were successfully dilated. Significantly fewer adverse events (death, myocardial infarction, or CABG) occurred in the functionally adequate group than in the functionally inadequate group (27% vs 6%). This study demonstrates that incompletely revascularized patients have a favorable 1-year outcome and that patients with incomplete but functionally adequate revascularization have long-term results comparable with those of patients with complete revascularization. This study also emphasizes the need to assess the functional significance of a stenosis when considering incomplete revascularization in a patient with multivessel CAD.

To determine the efficacy of multivessel PTCA, 569 consecutive patients undergoing multivessel PTCA were compared with 569 age- and sex-matched control patients undergoing single-vessel PTCA in an investigation carried out by Hollman and associates[94] from Cleveland, Ohio. Baseline variables were similar except for number of diseased vessels and greater LV dysfunction in the multivessel group. Major in-hospital complication rates (death 0% vs 0.5%; Q wave myocardial infarction 0.5% vs 0.9%; emergency CABG 2.5% vs 3.2%) were similar for multivessel and single-vessel PTCA. The 5-year actuarial survival rate was 93% for multivessel PTCA and 92% for single-vessel PTCA. Event-free survival was similar except that patients undergoing multivessel PTCA had an 8% higher incidence of repeat PTCA in the first year of follow-up. Multivessel PTCA can be performed with results comparable to those of single-vessel angioplasty with the exception of a higher incidence of repeat PTCA.

PTCA is increasingly performed in patients with multivessel CAD despite reports showing relatively low rates of complete revascularization and poorer long-term prognosis for patients with significant residual narrowings. Reasons for incomplete revascularization were assessed by Bourassa and coinvestigators[95] of the National Heart, Lung, and Blood Institute Percutaneous Transluminal Coronary Angioplasty Registry in

618 patients with multivessel CAD in the 1985–1986 NHLBI PTCA Registry. The PTCA operator was asked to describe the treatment plan and outcome for each of the 1,942 significant lesions (50% luminal diameter stenosis) in the Registry patients. Although all significant narrowings were considered amenable to balloon angioplasty in 77% of patients, complete correction was intended only for 34% of them. It was attempted in 28% and successful in 19%. Only 63% of total occlusions were considered amenable to PTCA and only 54% of those attempted were successfully dilated. PTCA was intended for 38% with 50 to 69% stenoses versus 80% with 70 to 89% stenoses and for 85% with narrowings >90%. Dilatation in narrowings of the LC and LAD arteries was intended less frequently than in narrowings of the right coronary artery. Finally, there was wide variability in operator strategy among the different Registry sites. It is concluded that (1) complete revascularization is infrequent after PTCA in patients with multivessel CAD, (2) major reasons for incomplete correction include total occlusions that are not PTCA amenable or are unsuccessfully attempted, and less than severe (50 to 69%) coronary narrowings by visual estimation for vascularization is often part of the PTCA strategy, and can usually be predicted before PTCA.

In an investigation by Warner and associates[96] from Richmond, Virginia, between May 1982 and December 1988, a total of 103 patients underwent PTCA of all 3 major coronary arteries at a single institution. Angiographic success was achieved in 334 of 352 vessels (95%) and in 441 of 460 lesions (96%). No patients required urgent CABG, and none died during the procedure; 6 had non-Q wave AMI. The mean length of follow-up time was 49 ± 15 months (range 28 to 107 months). There were 11 deaths, and 2 patients underwent cardiac transplantation. Thirty-six patients had a clinical recurrence; 30 had repeat PTCA and 5 had CABG. Another 9 patients eventually had CABG after the clinical recurrence. At 48 months actuarial event-free rates were AMI 98%%; CABG 88%; and death 89%. Of 86 current survivors, 58 are in functional class 0 to 1, 21 are in class II, and 7 are in class III.

Effectiveness ≥70 years of age

To study the immediate and long-term clinical success of PTCA in patients over 70 years of age, de Jaegere and associates[97] from Rotterdam-Dijkzigt, The Netherlands, prospectively entered in a specially designed database patients undergoing PTCA who were over 70 years of age. A total of 166 patients over 70 (median 73, range 70–84) underwent PTCA because of unstable angina (81 patients), stable angina (76 patients), or AMI (9 patients). The initial clinical success rate was 86% (142 of 166 patients). A major procedural complication occurred in 10 patients (6%): 4 patients (2%) died, 6 patients (4%) underwent emergency bypass surgery, and 5 patients (3%) sustained an AMI. In 14 patients (8%) coronary angioplasty did not significantly reduce the diameter stenosis but there were no associated complications. A total of 226 lesions were attempted. The initial angiographic success rate was 192 out of 226 lesions (85%). The median follow up was 21 (range 0.5–66) months. Sixteen patients (10%) died during follow up, 8 patients (5%) sustained a non-fatal AMI, 21 patients (13%) underwent a second or third balloon dilatation, and 17 patients (10%) underwent elective bypass surgery. Of the 146 survivors, 99 patients (68%) had sustained clinical improvement. The estimated survival at 4 years (Kaplan-Meier method) was 89 (SD4)%. The event free survival at 4 years for the total study population was 61 (8%). Multivariate logistic regression analysis showed that the extent of vessel disease was the only independent predictive factor for event free survival: the event free survival rate was 81 (10)% at 4 years for patients with single vessel CAD, compared with 45 (12)% for patients with multivessel CAD. Coronary angioplasty in patients over 70 was a safe and effective treatment for obstructive CAD. The extent of CAD, and not the completeness of revascularization, was the only independent predictive factor for event free survival.

PTCA was performed on 58 lesions in 53 patients ≥80 years of age with unstable angina in a study carried out by Santana and associates[98] from Newark, New Jersey. Most patients had previous myocardial infarction, abnormal LV contraction patterns, and multivessel coronary disease. In most (48) patients only 1 vessel was dilated. PTCA was successful in 48 (83%) lesions, but complications were frequent. Eight patients died, 6 after anatomically successful PTCA (3 with cardiac complications, 2 with noncardiac complications, and 1 with both cardiac and noncardiac complications). Two patients died after unsuccessful PTCA (1 of cardiac complications and 1 of noncardiac complications), and 11 patients with PTCA were alive with significant complications (all noncardiac). Twenty-nine patients had successful PTCA with no complications; 40 (75%) patients were discharged with clinically successful PTCA. It was concluded that PTCA is feasible in patients ≥80 years of age but that both cardiac and noncardiac complications are common in this group of very fragile patients.

For total occlusions

There has been increasing application of coronary angioplasty to patients with chronic total occlusions. Ruocco and co-investigators of the National Heat, Lung, and Blood Institute Percutaneous Transluminal Coronary Angioplasty Registry[99] compared the acute and long-term outcome in 271 patients after coronary angioplasty (142 single and 129 multiple stenoses of a total occlusion with 1,429 patients undergoing angioplasty of subtotal (≤99% stenosis) occlusions (885 single and 544 multiple) participating in the 1985–1986 National Heart, Lung, and Blood Institute Percutaneous Transluminal Coronary Angioplasty Registry. Baseline characteristics were similar for each lesion group except for a higher incidence of prior AMI and LV dysfunction (EF <50%) in patients with total occlusion. Major complications (death, AMI or emergency bypass surgery) were similar between patients with total and subtotal occlusions for single (6 vs 7%) and multilesion angioplasty (9 vs 6%). At 2 years, after making adjustments for baseline variables, patients with a total occlusion had a significantly increased risk of death compared with those with subtotal occlusion. There were no significant differences in cumulative event rates for AMI or CABG. Approximately three-fourths of patients in each group were free of angina at 2 years. In conclusion, angioplasty of chronic total occlusions is associated with a similar acute complication rate. Despite similar relief of anginal symptoms, patients in the total occlusion group have a higher 2-year mortality.

PTCA of chronically totally occluded vessels has been associated with a success rate well below the restenosis rate well above that for PTCA of stenosed segments. However, long-term clinical outcome after successful revascularization of a chronically totally occluded vessel has not been reported in detail. Accordingly, Ivanhoe and colleagues[100] in Atlanta, Georgia, analyzed data for 480 patients undergoing PTCA for chronic total occlusion at Emory University Hospital, in Atlanta, Georgia, from 1980 to 1988 for predictors of in-hospital procedural and clinical success, restenosis, and 4-year clinical follow-up. The study population was grouped by procedural and clinical success and failure. The groups were then compared for outcome, both in hospital and long term. The initial clinical success rate was 66*5. Independent correlates of failure were the number of vessels diseased, vessel location of the lesion, and absence of any distal antegrade filling. Follow-up data revealed 98% cardiac survival and 96% overall survival at 4 years for the group as a whole. Freedom from AMI or cardiac death was significantly greater in patients with clinical success than with clinical failure. In the successful group, 87% were free from coronary surgery after 4 years compared with 65% in the failure group. Two thirds of the patients were free of angina at last follow-up. The presence of angina at follow-up was the same for patients successfully treated and for those with failed PTCA, which may be related to the frequent use of coronary surgery in the failure group. In well-selected cases, the success rate for PTCA of chronic total occlusion is.acceptable. Furthermore, long-term clinical benefit is suggested by the high freedom from CABG, AMI, and death in the patients who underwent successful revascularization.

PTCA of chronic total occlusions is associated with relatively low success rates and a high incidence of restenosis. Whether there is long-term benefit in performing PTCA of these lesions is unknown. Bell and colleagues[101] in Rochester, Minnesota, analyzed the long-term outcome of a large series of patients undergoing this PTCA for chronic total occlusion. A computerized database of 354 consecutive patients (from 1979 to 1990) who underwent coronary PTCA of a chronic total coronary occlusion was performed. Initial success was achieved in 69%; in 66%, success was achieved without procedural death or need for CABG. During hospitalization, 6 patients suffered AMI, 9 required emergency CABG and 9 patients expired. During a mean follow-up period of 2.7 years, no difference was found in survival or freedom from AMI among 234 successfully dilated patients compared with 120 patients with a failed attempt. However, the use of CABG was significantly less after successful dilation. No significant difference in the cumulative incidence of severe angina was observed between these two patient populations, with the majority remaining asymptomatic. Restenosis occurred in 59% of 69 patients who returned for follow-up angiography. Successful recanalization is achieved in the majority of patients undergoing PTCA of chronic total occlusions and reduces the need CABG. However, no major impact on either survival or incidence of AMI was noted after successful recanalization when patients with surgery were included.

In a retrospective study by Maiello and associates[102] from Milano, Italy, of 365 chronic total occlusions that were submitted for PTCA, the influence of 27 clinical, morphologic, and procedural variables were analyzed as possible predictors of successful outcomes. Success rate was shown to be significantly influenced by the following variables: operator experience (41% in early patients, first 6 months; 73% in late patients, last 6 months of entire series), duration of occlusion (≤1 month 89%; 1 to 3 months 87%; ≥3 months 45%; unknown 60%), morphology of occlusion (tapered 83%; abrupt 51%), length of occlusion (≤15 mm 71%; >15 mm 60%), and bridging collaterals (present 29%; absent 67%). None of the other clinical, angiographic, or procedural variables correlated with the success rate of PTCA. The calculated probability for an experienced operator (>100 occlusions attempted) to successfully open an occlusion with favorable morphology (≤1 month old, short, tapered, without bridging collaterals) was 99%. An attempt by the same operator to open an occlusion with unfavorable structure (≥3 months old, long, untapered) has only 47% probability of success. The probability increases to 84% when the occlusion is tapered. It was concluded that in addition to the duration and the length of occlusion, tapered morphology, bridging collaterals, and operator experience can predict successful PTCA in chronic total coronary occlusion.

Prolonged inflations

Prolonged balloon inflation with or without autoperfusion techniques is a common initial approach to major dissection or abrupt occlusion after PTCA. To assess such a strategy in the setting of unsuccessful PTCA, Jackman and associates[103] from Durham, North Carolina, studied 40 patients who underwent prolonged balloon inflations of >20 minutes between January and July of 1991 after initially unsuccessful PTCA. These patients (median age 59 years) underwent PTCA for progressive or unstable angina (16 [40%]), symptomatic or asymptomatic residual stenosis after AMI (10 [25%]), AMI (3 [8%]), stable angina (3 [8%]), reinfarction ([5%]), and other indications ([15%]). The significant stenoses were primarily in the proximal and midportions of the right coronary (53%), left anterior descending (30%) and left circumflex (17%) coronary arteries. Before prolonged balloon inflation, the longest single inflation was 11 ± 6 minutes and the total time of all inflations was 17 ± 8 minutes (mean ± standard deviation). Stenosis was reduced from 91 ± 9 to 68 ± 16% before prolonged inflation. After prolonged balloon inflation of 30 ± 9 minutes, the residual stenosis was 47 ± 21%. Furthermore, improvements in the appearance of filling defects or dissections, or both, occurred in 19 patients (48%). Procedural success was obtained in 32 of 40 patients (80%). Coronary bypass grafting was performed in 8 patients (20%): 4 after unsuccessful PTCA (3 emergently) and 4 electively after initially successful PTCA. Although 5 patients had creatine kinase-MB elevations >20 IU/liter after the procedure, only 1 sustained a Q-wave myocardial infarction. There were no deaths in the hospital. In summary, prolonged balloon inflations of >20 minutes are successful in 80% of patients in whom initial extensive PTCA attempts were not. Prolonged inflations may thus be desirable before consideration of CABG or stenting.

Before non-cardiac operations

Huber and associates[104] from Rochester, Minnesota, evaluated the risk of perioperative AMI and death in 50 patients (mean age, 68 years) with severe CAD who underwent a noncardiac operation after revascularization had been achieved by successful PTCA. Before angioplasty, all patients were thought to be at high risk for perioperative complications on the basis of assessment of clinical variables and findings on specialized diagnostic tests. Of the 50 patients, 31 had Canadian Heart Association class III or IV angina or unstable angina. All patients who underwent functional testing had positive results. At catheterization, 38 patients (76%) had multivessel disease. The 50 patients underwent 54 noncardiac operations at a median of 9 days after angioplasty. The overall frequency of perioperative AMI was 5.6%, and the mortality was 1.9%. Two nonfatal non-Q-wave infarctions and 1 fatal Q-wave infarction occurred. In patients who have undergone successful angioplasty for severe CAD, the risk of major cardiac complications associated with a noncardiac surgical procedure is low.

Intravascular ultrasound assessment

Histological examination of the effects of balloon PTCA have been described from in vitro experiments and a limited number of pathologic specimens. Intravascular ultrasound imaging permits real time-cross-sectional observation of the effect of balloon dilation on the atherosclerotic plaque in vivo. Honye and co-investigators[105] in Orange, California, visualized morphological effects of PTCA in 47 patients immediately after balloon dilatation with an intravascular ultrasound imaging catheter. Cross-sectional images were obtained at 30 frames per second as the catheter passed along the length of the artery. Quantitative and qualitative assessments of the dilated atherosclerotic plaque were made from the angiograms and the ultrasound images. Six morphological patterns after PTCA were appreciated by ultrasound imaging. Type A consists of a linear, partial tear of the plaque from the lumen toward the media (7 lesions); Type B is defined by a split in the plaque that extends to the media (12 lesions); (Figure 2-12) Type C demonstrates a dissection behind the plaque that subtends an arc of up to 180° (4 lesions); and Type D was a more extensive dissection that encompasses an arc of more than 180° (4 lesions); and Type E may be present in either concentric (Type E_1, 14 lesions) or eccentric (Type$_2$, 11 lesions) plaque is defined as an ultrasound study without any evidence of a fracture or a dissection in the plaque. There was a large amount of residual atheroma in each type of morphology; there was no difference, however, in lumen or atheroma cross-sectional area among these six patterns. There was a good correlation between ultrasound and angiography for the recognition of a dissection. Calcification was seen in only 14% of lesions on angiography, whereas 83% of lesions revealed calcification on ultrasound imaging. As determined by intravascular ultrasound, calcified plaque was more likely to fracture in response to balloon dilatation than noncalcified plaque. Thirteen of 66 lesions developed clinical and angiographic restenosis. Restenosis was more likely to occur when the original dilation left a concentric plaque without a fracture or dissection (50% incidence) compared with a mean restenosis rate of 12% in the remaining morphological patterns. Intravascular ultrasound provides a more complete quantitative and qualitative description of plaque geometry and composition than angiography after PTCA. In addition, intravascular ultrasound identifies a subset of atherosclerotic plaque that has a higher incidence of restenosis. This information could be used prospectively to consider other therapeutic options in this subset.

Gerber and associates[106] from Mainz, Germany, performed a study to assess and classify the morphologic effects of PTCA by intravascular ultrasound (IU). Fifty-eight patients were examined immediately after PTCA with a 4.8Fr, 20 MHz rotational tip IU system. In 10 patients (17%), IU images could not be analyzed due to failure of the imaging system or poor image quality. In 48 patients (83%; 40 men and 8 women, aged 55 ± 9 years), IU images of 48 PTCA segments, as well as 41 distal and 44 proximal sites, were analyzed. The LAD artery was studied in 30 patients, the right coronary artery in 17 and the LM coronary artery in 1. Calcium was present in 32 of 48 PTCA segments (67%). Plaque morphology was concentric in 18 patients (38%) and eccentric in 30 (62%). Seven distinct morphologic patterns were observed. In concentric plaques, plaque com-

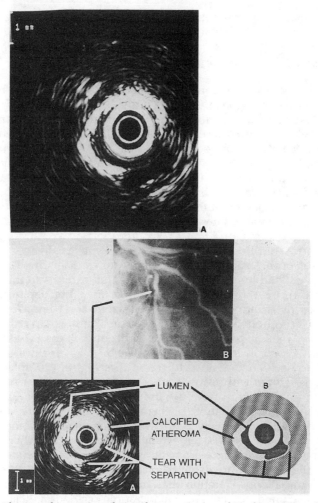

Fig. 2-12. Ultrasound image (panel A) and composite (panel B) of Type B morphology. In this pattern, the tear extends through the depth of the plaque to the media, but there is no evidence of a dissection behind the plaque, even though the two ends of the atheroma are separated and were observed in real time to move apart with each heartbeat. Calcified plaque is seen around the lumen. Reproduced with permission from Honye, et al.[105]

pression without significant wall alterations (type 1) was found in 2 patients (4%), superficial tears within the plaque (type 2) in 1 (2%) and deep tears (type 3) in 8 (17%). Deep tearing associated with submedial or subintimal dissection (type 4) was found in 2 patients (4%). Dissection between plaque and vessel wall without noticeable intimal tearing (type 5) was the most common morphology (n = 15; 31%) and in concentric and eccentric plaques. In eccentric plaques, no significant tearing of the plaque (type 6) was found in 6 patients (13%), and tearing of the plaque close to its base with dissection (type 7) in 14 (29%). In the PTCA segment, minimal luminal diameter was 3.5 ± 0.7 mm, maximal luminal diameter 4.3 ± 0.8 mm, luminal area 12 ± 4 mm², plaque area 10 ± 5 mm² and vessel area 23 ± 7 mm². Mean residual stenosis was 40%, mean recoil was =13%, and the correlation between luminal diameter and balloon size was low.

Intracoronary electrocardiogram

This prospective study by Pande and associates[107] from Geneva, Switzerland, examined data derived from the intracoronary electrocardiogram (derived from the coronary guide wire) compared with that from 4 standard surface leads (I, II, III, and V_2) in documenting myocardial ischemia during PTCA. Intracoronary and surface electrocardiograms were simultaneously recorded in 300 consecutive patients (mean age 59 ± 10; range 33 to 80 years) during PTCA in 368 lesions (167 LAD [46%], 85 LC [23%], 107 right coronary arteries [29%], and 9 bypass grafts [2%]), before balloon inflation, at 1 minute of inflation, and at the end of the procedure. ST segment changes (>0.1 mV) were observed in the intracoronary electrocardiogram in 306 lesions (83%) (151 LAD [88%], 75 LC [89%], and 80 right coronary arteries [73%]) vs in 245 lesions (67%) in the surface electrocardiogram (126 LAD [73%], 43 LC [47%], and 76 right coronary arteries [70%]). The mean ST segment shift was 0.5 ± 0.4 mV in intracoronary and 0.1 ± 0.2 mV in standard leads. ST elevation was seen in 97% of cases with intracoronary electrocardiographic changes versus in 83% with surface electrocardiographic changes. The remainder had ST depression. A total of 48 lesions (13%) did not produce electrocardiographic changes and 62 (16%) had silent ischemia. In 75 lesions (21%), electrocardiographic changes were seen only in the intracoronary electrocardiogram, compared with 14 lesions (4%) with changes only in the surface electrocardiogram. The intracoronary electrocardiogram more readily detects acute ischemia and is a valuable adjunct to surface leads during PTCA, particularly in the LC.

Coronary hemoperfusion

DiSciascio[108] for the Coronary Hemoperfusion Ischemia Prevention Study Investigators evaluated a new flow adjustable pump for coronary hemoperfusion to prevent ischemia during routine PTCA in 110 patients. The protocol included patients who had angina or ST segment elevation during a control balloon inflation of ≤3 minutes. Hemoperfusion was performed by means of a new large lumen angioplasty catheter utilizing the patient's renal vein or femoral artery blood. Arteries perfused were the LAD (n = 74), right coronary artery (n = 39), LC artery (n = 9) and coronary vein grafts (n = 15). Mean perfusion rate was 41 ± 9 ml/min and mean perfusion time was 9 ± 4 minutes. Chest pain score decreased from 2.9 ± 1 to 1.4 ± 1 during hemoperfusion, ST segment elevation score decreased from 2.6 to 0.7 and inflation time increased from 1.3 to 7 minutes. At least a 50% increase in tolerated inflation time was obtained in 104 patients (95%). PTCA was successful in 107 patients (97%) with mean stenosis reduced from 87 ± 11 to 20 ± 17%. Three patients required urgent CABG, 2 had an AMI, and 2 died later in the hospital of probable noncoronary causes. Complications related to hemoperfusion were transient heart block during dilation of the right coronary artery in 2 patients and hematoma requiring transfusion in 5. Therefore, this study indicates that a new hemoperfusion system is safe and effective in reducing ischemia and allowing longer balloon inflations during PTCA.

Exercise testing afterwards

To evaluate both the safety and clinical use of predischarge symptom-limited exercise testing after successful uncomplicated PTCA, Balady and associates[109] from Boston, Massachusetts, randomized 100 patients to undergo exercise testing (n = 50) or no exercise testing (n = 50). There was no differences in clinical or angiographic characteristics between the groups. Exercise testing was performed 38 ± 14 hours after PTCA. Patients who exercised achieved 71 ± 12% of predicted maximal heart rate, with 38% reaching stage III of the Bruce protocol. No patient in either group developed cardiac complications during 48-hour follow-up. Of the 11 patients with a positive test result, 92% had angiographically incomplete revascularization. Attending physicians (n = 16) were questioned both before and after exercise testing about when, after discharge, they would allow their patient to perform each of 11 specific activities of daily living. Questionnaires were administered to physicians at similar time frames for patients in the no-exercise group. Comparison of the responses between initial and repeat questionnaires showed that patients in the exercise group (with a test result negative for ischemia) were allowed to perform 7 of 11 activities, including return to work, earlier than the no-exercise patients. These data indicate that in this well-defined group of patients, symptom-limited exercise testing early after PTCA appears to be safe, and alters physician management in allowing patients with a negative test result to return to various activities at an earlier date. Such testing may be useful in counseling patients after PTCA.

Restenosis

To assess whether complicated pre-PTCA coronary stenosis morphology is associated with restenosis, 41 patients (47 stenoses) who underwent repeat PTCA 6 to 8 months after PTCA were studied by Tousoulis and associates[110] from London, England. Stenosis diameter and morphology were assessed by computerized quantitative coronary angiography before and immediately after PTCA and at follow-up angiography. Before PTCA 18 stenoses were concentric (symmetric narrowings with smooth borders), 12 were eccentric (asymmetric narrowings with smooth borders), and 17 were complicated (asymmetric with rough borders and overhanging edges). Restenosis occurred in 18 lesions: 2 (11%) concentric, 4 (33%) eccentric, and 12 (70%) complicated, whereas 29 lesions remained unchanged. Stenosis diameter before and immediately after PTCA was not significantly different in the 18 patients with and the 23 patients without restenosis. Follow-up angiograms showed that 11 (61%) stenoses in the group with stenosis and 18 (63%) in the group without restenosis had morphology similar to that before PTCA. Restenosis occurred in 7 (30%) patients who initially had chronic stable angina and in 11 (61%) who were first seen with unstable angina. In patients with stable angina 1 of 13 concentric stenoses, 2 of 8 eccentric stenoses, and 4 of 5 complicated lesions restenosed. In patients with unstable angina 1 of 5 concentric, 2 of 5 eccentric, and 8 of 12 complicated lesions had restenosis. Stenoses that were complicated before PTCA tended to adopt an irregular morphology if they recurred, whereas concentric stenoses rarely recurred. These findings indicate that complicated coronary stenoses are associated with a higher risk of restenosis than concentric stenoses. In most instances, the morphology of a restenosed lesions is similar to that observed before PTCA. It appears that coronary stenosis morphology rather than clinical presentation determines the possibility of restenosis.

Beatt and associates[111] in Rotterdam, The Netherlands, studied 490 coronary artery lesions using quantitative angiographic measurements in an attempt to predict mechanisms responsible for restenosis after

PTCA. Restenosis was defined as an absolute deterioration in the minimal luminal diameter by ≥ 0.72 mm. The principal determinants of restenosis were a large improvement in the minimal lumen diameter at the time of dilation (1.13 mm for the restenosis group compared with 0.86 for the no restenosis group) and an optimal post PTCA result (minimal lumen diameter 2.28 mm in the restenosis group compared with 2.05 mm in the no restenosis group corresponding to a 25% and 30% diameter stenosis, respectively). These observations suggest that a distinction needs to be made between a "clinical restenosis" of $\geq 50\%$ diameter stenosis and the "restenosis process" as measured by absolute changes occurring during and after PTCA. These data lend support to the hypothesis that the degree of mechanical stretch produced by the dilating balloon on the vessel wall may be important in stimulating the restenosis process.

Serum lipoprotein (a) (Lp[a]) has been associated with CAD. Its association with restenosis after PTCA has not been previously studied. Hearn and associates[112] from Atlanta, Georgia, and Birmingham, Alabama, examined serum levels of Lp(a) in addition to other lipoproteins and their components using standard assays, in subjects undergoing cardiac catheterization within 10 months after PTCA. Clinical (e.g., sex, diabetes, angina class) and angiographic (e.g., PTCA percent diameter reduction) factors were not different between the group without (diameter reduction <50%; group A) and the group with (diameter reduction $\geq 50\%$; group B) restenosis. Total cholesterol, triglycerides, high- and LDL cholesterol, apolipoprotein A-1, apolipoprotein B and Lp(a) were compared (Table 2-3). Univariate predictors of restenosis were serum triglycerides (2.50 $\pm$ 1.07 mmol/L for group A vs 1.72 $\pm$ 0.79 $\pm$ mmol/L for group B), and Lp(a)

TABLE 2-3. *Serum Lipids, Lipoproteins and Apolipoproteins. Reproduced with permission from Hearn, et al.[112]*

No. of patients	20	49
Cholesterol (mmol/liter)		
Total	5.70 ± 1.02	5.16 ± 1.12
VLDL	1.12 ± 0.49	0.79 ± 0.42*
LDL	3.47 ± 1.05	3.32 ± 0.96
HDL	1.06 ± 0.26	1.06 ± 0.24
Total: HDL ratio	5.59 ± 1.33	5.04 ± 1.42
Triglycerides (mmol/liter)	2.50 ± 1.07	1.72 ± 0.91*
Apo A-I (mg/dl)	99 ± 15.6	99 ± 17.7
Apo B (mg/dl)	135 ± 26.8	119 ± 30.8
Apo B: A-I ratio	1.38 ± 0.30	1.22 ± 0.34
Lp(a) (mg/dl)	7.0 (0.5–44.0)	18.8 (1–120)*

*Significantly different (p < 0.01).
All values are mean ± SD, except for Lp(a), which is the median (range in parentheses).
Apo = apolipoprotein; HDL = high-density lipoprotein; LDL = low-density lipoprotein; Lp(a) = lipoprotein (a); VLDL = very low density lipoprotein; + = present; 0 = absent.

(median: 7.0 mg/dl [range 0 to 44] for group A vs 19 mg/dl [range 1 to 120] for group B). Stepwise logistic regression revealed the only significant independent predictor of restenosis to be serum Lp(a). Each quintile of Lp(a) was associated with a progressively higher risk of restenosis, with the highest quintile (40 to 120 mg/dl) having an odds ratio of 11 compared with the lowest quintile (0 to 3.9 mg/dl). A serum Lp(a) of >19 mg/dl was associated with an odds ratio of 5.9 (restenosis rates of 58% in the group with 0 to 19 mg/dl and 89% in the group with 19 to 120 mg/dl). Hence, serum Lp(a) appears to be a potent predictor of restenosis in subjects returning for coronary arteriography after PTCA.

To determine the relation of post-PTCA restenosis to serum lipid fractions and to circulating levels of endogenous tissue plasminogen activator and its rapid inhibitor, 68 patients with CAD who underwent a successful PTCA were studied by Shah and Amin[113] in Los Angeles, California. During a mean follow-up of 9 months, 28 (41%) patients developed restenosis. A low HDL cholesterol level was independently and strongly related to both the risk of restenosis and to the time of restenosis. The mean HDL cholesterol level was 32 mg/dl in the restenosis group and 45 mg/dl in the nonrestenosis group (Figure 2-13). Restenosis developed in 22 of 34 (64%) patients with an HDL cholesterol ≤40 mg% compared with 6 of 34 (17%) patients with an HDL cholesterol >40 mg%. The only other variable that was significantly related to restenosis was a low rapid inhibitor level. The strong relation between a low HDL cholesterol level and the risk of restenosis suggests that lipid fractions could be important in the pathogenesis and prevention of restenosis.

Dimas and associates[114] in Cleveland, Ohio, evaluated 465 patients with multivessel CAD who underwent a second angioplasty procedure at the same site as the original procedure. The procedure was successful

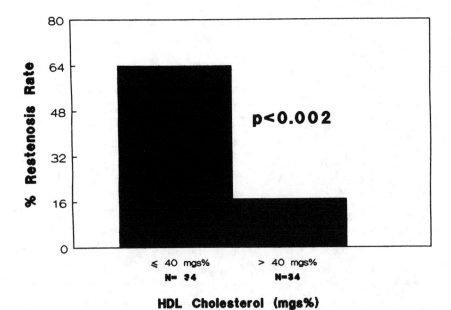

Fig. 2-13. Bar graph shows restenosis rate after percutaneous transluminal coronary angioplasty in 68 patients. Note the nearly fourfold higher restenosis rate in patients with a high density lipoprotein (HDL) cholesterol level ≤40 mg% compared with those whose level is >40 mg%. Reproduced with permission from Shah P and Amin J.[113]

in 97% of patients with a 1.5% rate of in-hospital CABG, a 0.9% incidence of AMI, and no procedural deaths (Figure 2-14). Four hundred sixty-three patients (99.6%) were followed for a mean of 41 months. Forty-nine patients (11%) underwent a third PTCA at the same site, 55 (12%) had CABG and 33 (7%) underwent PTCA at a different site. During follow-up, 12 patients (3%) sustained an AMI and 21 (5%) died, including 13 (3%) with cardiac death. Of the 442 surviving patients, 88% had functional improvement and 78% were free of angina. The actuarial 5 year cardiac survival rate was 96% and the rate of freedom from cardiac death and AMI was 92%. For the 49 patients who had a third PTCA procedure at the same site, the success rate was 94% with a 2% incidence of AMI. There were no in-hospital deaths or CABG. The mean follow-up interval for this subgroup was 31 months with a 22% cross-over rate to CABG, a 4% incidence rate of AMI, and a 2% cardiac mortality rate. At last follow-up, 89% of patients had sustained functional improvement and 76% were free of angina. The combined angiographic and clinical restenosis rate was 48%. Repeat PTCA as treatment for restenosis is an effective approach with a high success rate, low risk of complications, and sustained functional improvement. However, there is a trend toward diminished PTCA efficacy after a second restenosis.

Hernández and associates[115] in Madrid, Spain, evaluated the clinical implications of asymptomatic coronary restenosis in 277 consecutive patients with restenosis after PTCA. One hundred thirty three (48%) of these patients were asymptomatic (group I) and 144 (52%) were symptomatic (group II). Restenosis was documented 6 to 9 months after the procedure or earlier if angina recurred and was defined as a >50% luminal narrowing. Group I asymptomatic patients included fewer females and hypertensive patients and more patients with a previous AMI and single-

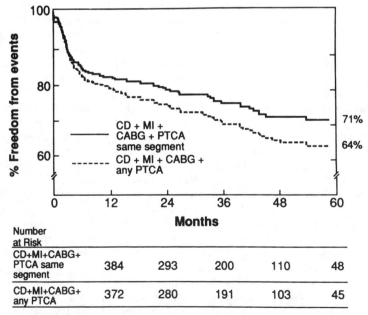

Number at Risk

CD+MI+CABG+ PTCA same segment	384	293	200	110	48
CD+MI+CABG+ any PTCA	372	280	191	103	45

Fig. 2-14. Five-year Kaplan-Meier actuarial freedom from cardiac death (CD), myocardial infarction (MI), coronary artery bypass surgery (CABG), third angioplasty (PTCA) for a second restenosis and any coronary angioplasty (PTCA) in 465 patients undergoing repeat angioplasty for restenosis. Reproduced with permission from Dimas, et al.[114]

vessel CAD. Before PTCA, symptoms had lasted for a shorter period, ischemia after recent AMI was a more frequent indication, and total revascularization more frequently obtained in group I than in group II patients. Only a normal BP, previous AMI, single-vessel CAD and shorter duration of symptoms were independent correlates of asymptomatic restenosis. No differences were found in stenosis severity before PTCA or after PTCA in the two groups. By follow-up angiography, group I had exercised more and had achieved a faster heart rate and more of them had a negative exercise test result. After 17 ± 13 months, 15 asymptomatic patients had recurrence of angina and recurrence was considered related to restenosis in 6 (21%) of 29 patients with exercise-induced ST changes, in 4 (9.5%) of 42 without ST changes, in none of the 15 with ST changes and elective PTCA. No group I patient died or was operated on and only six underwent another PTCA procedure for angina. By contrast, 6 patients (4%) in group II died, 11 (8%) required CABG, and 81 (56%) underwent repeat PTCA. Thus, asymptomatic coronary restenosis after PTCA is a frequent phenomenon with a good prognosis mainly in patients with a negative exercise test.

Trapidil (triazolopyrimidine), a platelet-derived growth factor antagonist, is a potential inhibitor of intimal proliferation after PTCA. In an investigation by Okamoto and associates[116] from Tsu, Japan, to study its efficacy, 72 patients were randomized to receive trapidil (600 mg/day orally for 1 week before PTCA and for 4 to 6 months after PTCA: n = 36) or aspirin and dipyridamole (aspirin, 300 mg/day, and dipyridamole, 150 mg/day; n = 36). At entry, both groups were comparable with regard to age, sex, dilated vessels, severity of pre-PTCA stenosis, residual stenosis after PTCA, and prevalence of coronary risk factors. Repeat coronary angiography was performed 6 months after PTCA. Restenosis, defined as the loss of at least 50% of the gain in luminal diameter accomplished by dilation, was present in 7 patients (19%) in the trapidil group and 15 patients (42%) in the aspirin-dipyridamole group. The progression of stenosis in patients with <30% residual stenosis was significant in both groups. Furthermore, in the patients with residual stenosis >30%, progression of stenosis was less in a trapidil group than in the aspirin-dipyridamole group. Thus trapidil was useful in preventing intimal proliferation after PTCA, especially in patients with >30% residual stenosis after PTCA.

Restenosis remains a critical limitation of PTCA. Weintraub and associates[117] from Atlanta, Georgia, reviewed the experience with restenosis in 1,490 patients who had restenosis of at least 1 site within 1 year of their PTCA. The source of data was the clinical database at Emory University. Patients who had previous coronary bypass surgery or PTCA and patients who underwent PTCA in the setting of AMI were excluded. When restenosis was angiographically documented, 363 were treated medically, 1,051 with repeat PTCA, and 76 with coronary bypass surgery. In the repeat PTCA group there were 778 patients who originally had 1-vessel disease and 273 with multiple vessel disease. Re-dilatation of restenotic sites was performed in 95%. Angiographic success of all lesions dilated was achieved in 99%. CABG was required in 2.5% of patients with restenosis first treated with repeat PTCA. One patient with multiple vessel CAD died. Two (1.6%) of the CABG patients had Q-wave AMI and there were no deaths. In the PTCA group, 5-year actuarial survival was 95%, and cardiac survival 96%. Freedom from cardiac events or further revascularization procedures was 51% at 5 years. Patients treated with PTCA and medically treated patients had similar cardiac survival rates. The most important correlates of cardiac survival were age and the presence of diabetes mellitus. At 5 years, cardiac survival without diabetes was 97 and 83% with diabetes. Selection of the appropriate form of therapy for restenosis cannot be easily determined from grouped data, but rather requires patient by patient selection. In patients with restenosis, with careful selection of therapy, excellent results may be obtained with low initial morbidity and mortality and high long-term survival.

The results of routine PTCA using gradual and prolonged balloon inflation with a perfusion balloon catheter were evaluated by Tenaglia and colleagues[118] from Durham, North Carolina, and Cincinnati, Ohio. Treated were 140 patients with inflation of the balloon to 6 atmospheres over 3 minutes, with a median inflation time of 15 minutes. The procedural success rate (residual stenosis ≤50%) was 99%. In-hospital major complications occurred in 5 patients (3.6%), with 1 patient experiencing a periprocedural AMI, 3 patients requiring CABG for abrupt closure, and 1 patient dying after elective CABG following previous successful PTCA of a culprit lesion. The restenosis rate in the 117 patients with angiographic follow-up (87% of those eligible) was 42%. Thus gradual and prolonged inflation using a perfusion balloon catheter resulted in a high procedural success rate and a restenosis rate similar to that reported in large studies of patients treated with standard PTCA.

Bauters and colleagues[119] in Lille, France, analyzed the angiographic rate of recurrent restenosis in patients who underwent repeat PTCA for a first restenosis within 3 months or >3 months after the first procedure. Between January 1981 and December 1990, 423 patients underwent a repeat PTCA procedure because restenosis had occurred at the site of a successful first PTCA procedure. The clinical characteristics, immediate outcome, and angiographic rate of recurrent restenosis were compared in patients who underwent repeat dilation within 3 months (early redilation group, n = 77) or >3 months (late redilation group, n = 346) after the first procedure. The incidence of unstable angina at the time of the repeat procedure was significantly higher in the patients who underwent early redilation (42% vs 8%). The procedural success (95%) and complication rates were similar in both groups. Follow-up angiography was performed in 86% of patients with an initially successful procedure. The incidence of restenosis was significantly higher in the group that underwent early redilation (56% vs 37%) and was similar in patients in this group who presented with stable (55%) or unstable (57%) angina. Therefore, rapidly recurring coronary stenoses have an extremely high rate of restenosis when treated by PTCA the second time and this is independent of the clinical presentation at the time of repeat dilation.

In an investigation by Foley and colleagues[120] from Toronto, Canada, the frequency, clinical pattern, and timing of recurrent angina following successful single-lesion PTCA was assessed in a consecutive group of 104 patients with stable angina and in 85 with unstable angina. In addition, the relationship between lesion morphology and angiographic features and the pattern of recurrent angina was determined. Restenosis, defined as recurrence of symptoms with >50% stenosis at the site of PTCA, similarly occurred in 25 (24%) of the stable group and in 23 (27%) of the unstable group. However, the pattern of angina at repeat presentation was aggressive in nature in only 8% of the stable group compared to 48% in the unstable group. The time interval between the recurrence of symptoms and repeat coronary angiogram or PTCA was longer in the nonaggressive group than in the aggressive group (16 ± 12 and 5 ± 6.8 weeks, respectively). The key factors predicting the recurrent angina pattern identified by multiple logistic regression analysis were the angina status pre-PTCA and the presence of double-vessel disease. An aggressive pattern of angina at the time of restenosis is frequent in patients with unstable angina at the time of PTCA, and close post-PTCA surveillance is necessary in these patients.

Complications

To determine whether complex cardiovascular interventional procedures (including coronary stent implantation, directional atherectomy, aortic valvuloplasty, and the use of an intraaortic balloon pump or cardiopulmonary bypass support) are associated with an increased likelihood of vascular access site complications, Muller and associates[121] from Ann Arbor, Michigan, prospectively screened 2,400 consecutive cardiac catheterization procedures over a 12-month study period. Complications occurred in 35 patients after 39 procedures (1.6%) and included the need for vascular surgical repair (17 patients), blood transfusion (28 patients) and systemic antibiotic therapy (7 patients). The incidence of complications after 1,519 diagnostic studies was 0.6%, after 698 conventional coronary balloon angioplasties 2.6%, and after 183 complex interventions 6.0% (Figure 2-15); 43% of the complications occurred after procedures of >2 hours' duration and 14% occurred in patients in whom arterial sheaths remained in situ for >24 hours. Detailed demographic and procedural characteristics were compared between the 35 patients with vascular complications and 150 patients randomly drawn from a computerized database of the uncomplicated procedures performed during the screening period. By univariate analysis with correction for multiple comparisons, variables predicting the likelihood of vascular complications included: periprocedural use of heparin or fibrinolytic therapy, arterial sheath size ≥8Fr, patient age ≥65 years, and the presence of peripheral vascular disease. The results of this study suggest that the overall inci-

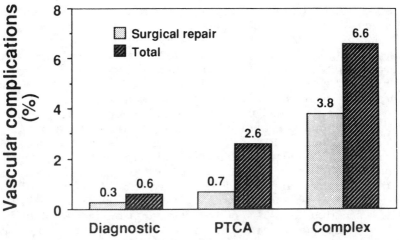

Fig. 2-15. Comparison of the incidence of access site complications and need for surgical intervention in patients undergoing diagnostic cardiac catheterization, conventional percutaneous transluminal coronary angioplasty (PTCA), and complex cardiovascular interventional procedures. Differences between the groups were highly statistically significant (p <0.0001). Reproduced with permission from Muller, et al.[121]

dence of access site complications is low but increases with the use of complex cardiovascular interventional procedures. Further refinements in the caliber of the new devices, vigilant monitoring of adjunctive anticoagulant therapy, and careful patient selection may reduce the morbidity and increase the safety of these procedures.

Lincoff and associates[122] in Ann Arbor, Michigan, and Cleveland, Ohio, assessed the clinical, angiographic, and procedural correlates of outcome after abrupt vessel closure during PTCA in 109 patients who had abrupt vessel closure during 1,319 consecutive PTCA procedures between July, 1989 and June, 1990. The 109 patients had a mean age of 59 ± 11 years; 63% were males, 57% had a prior AMI, and 61% had multivessel disease. PTCA was performed during AMI in 14%, after recent AMI in 36%, in patients with unstable angir.a in 34%, and those with stable coronary heart disease in 29% of patients. Abrupt vessel closure occurred at a median of 27 minutes (range 0 minutes to 5 days) from the first balloon inflation. By angiographic criteria, thrombus or coronary dissection was found in 20% and 28% of cases, respectively and both thrombus and dissection were present in 7% of closures and 45% were due to indeterminate mechanisms. Successful reversal of abrupt vessel closure, defined as restoration of normal coronary flow without resultant Q wave AMI, emergent CABG or death was achieved in 47 patients (43%). The incidence of death, need for emergent CABG, Q wave and non-Q wave AMI were 8%, 20%, 9%, and 11%, respectively (Figure 2-16). Univariate analysis using 23 clinical, morphologic and procedural variables demonstrated that successful outcome after abrupt closure was associated with prolonged balloon inflations (>120 seconds), unstable angina, and placement of an intracoronary stent. By multivariate analysis, independent correlates of

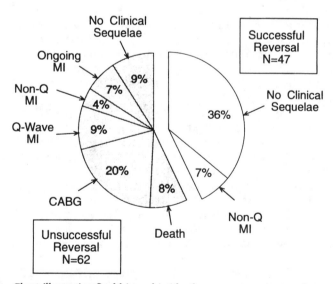

Fig. 2-16. Chart illustrating final hierarchic (death, emergency coronary bypass surgery, Q wave myocardial infarction, non-Q wave myocardial infarction) outcome for all 109 patients after abrupt vessel closure. The shaded pie slices represent unsuccessful outcome among 57% of patients; the white slices successful resolution in 43% of patients. MI = myocardial infarction; ongoing MI = patients undergoing rescue angioplasty for acute myocardial infarction, in whom development of Q waves or serum creatine kinase elevations could not be attributed to abrupt closure; other abbreviations as in Figure 1. Reproduced with permission from Lincoff, et al.[122]

successful outcome were prolonged balloon inflations and intracoronary stenting. Therefore, whereas prolonged balloon inflations and intracoronary stents may improve outcome after abrupt vessel closure, the cumulative mortality and morbidity risk remain significant.

Myler and associates[123] in Daly City, California, studied 533 consecutive patients with 764 target vessel and 1,000 lesions undergoing PTCA in the period July 1, 1990 to February 28, 1991. Procedural success was achieved in 92%, major cardiac events occurred in 3% with 0.8% AMI. An unsuccessful uncomplicated outcome occurred in 5% of patients. Lesion analysis using a modified American College of Cardiology/American Heart Association classification system showed that 8% were type A, 48% were type B, and 44% were type C. PTCA success was achieved in 99% of type A, 92% of type B and 90% of type C lesions. Major cardiac events occurred in 1% of type A, 2% of type B and 2% of type C lesions. An unsuccessful uncomplicated outcome occurred in no patients in type A, 6% in type B, and 7% in type C. Among the unsuccessful uncomplicated outcome group, occlusion occurred in 49%: 38% of type B and 59% of type C lesions. Statistical analysis of morphologic factors associated with PTCA success included absence of old occlusions and unprotected bifurcation lesions, decreasing lesion length, and no thrombus. The only significant factor associated with major cardiac events was the presence of thrombus. Predictors of an unsuccessful uncomplicated outcome included old occlusion and increasing length >20 mm, unprotected bifurcation lesion, and thrombus.

The degree of coagulation and its effect on the frequency of abrupt coronary artery closure, coronary ischemia, bleeding complications requiring transfusion, and death were examined in 336 patients after elective PTCA in a study carried out by McGarry and associates[124] from Philadelphia, Pennsylvania. All patients received a bolus of 10,000 U of heparin at the beginning of the procedure followed by a continuous infusion of 2000 U/hr. At the conclusion of the procedure the infusion was reduced to 1000 U/hr and continued for 18 to 24 hours at which time the heparin infusion was suspended to allow removal of arterial and venous access sheaths. Partial thromboplastin time was examined while patients continued to receive the heparin infusion. There was a variable degree of partial thromboplastin time prolongation in response to a standard dose of heparin with a range of 34 seconds to >150 seconds. Patients were divided into 2 groups according to the degree of heparin-induced partial thromboplastin time prolongation: group A included 271 patients with partial thromboplastin time ≥3 times the control value, and group B comprised 65 patients with partial thromboplastin time <3 times the control value. Ischemic complications were analyzed on day 1 after PTCA and at hospital discharge. Bleeding complications and mortality were examined only at hospital discharge. There was a significant reduction in the incidence of abrupt coronary artery closure in group A on day 1 (1.5% vs 11%), and at hospital discharge (2.6% vs 11%). There was also a statistically significant reduction in the frequency of coronary ischemic events in group A on day 1 (0.4% vs 9.2%) and at hospital discharge (1.5% vs 9.2%). There was no statistical difference in the incidence of bleeding complications requiring transfusion (2.9% vs 4.6%) or mortality (0.4% vs 3%) between the 2 groups. Of the 11 ischemic complications in group A, 6 occurred after suspension of the heparin infusion and therefore at a time of diminished anticoagulation. All ischemic complications observed in group B occurred during continuous infusion of heparin. Thus heparin therapy for 18 to 24 hours with resultant partial thromboplastin time ≥3 times the control value is effective in preventing ischemic complications after elective PTCA without an increase in bleeding complications. It may be necessary to monitor the anticoagulation level after elective PTCA to avoid the risk of inadequate anticoagulation.

A retrospective analysis of experience with intraprocedural thrombus complicating PTCA was undertaken in a study by Vaitkus and associates[125] from Philadelphia, Pennsylvania. Of 983 PTCA procedures reviewed, 62 (6.3%) were complicated by thrombus. Patients were managed conservatively (group I, n = 18), with redilation (group II, n = 17), or with intracoronary urokinase and redilation (group III, n = 27). The 3 groups did not differ with respect to demographic or baseline angiographic variables, but complications, defined as death, AMI, CABG, or threatened occlusion requiring emergency stenting, occurred in 11% of patients in group I, 24% in group II, and 48% in group III. Occlusive thrombus behavior was observed in 80% of these 62 patients. Patients with complications were less likely to have received antecedent antiplatelet therapy (79% vs 95% of patients without complications), had more complex baseline lesion morphology, more often had thrombus present at baseline (42% vs 19%), and more often had a low activated clotting time at the start of PTCA (53% vs 8%). Thrombi that led to complications more frequently exhibited occlusive behavior before therapy was begun (95% vs 71%) and more often occurred in the setting of intimal dissection (42% vs 14%). Patients undergoing PTCA at the time of diagnostic catheterization were more likely to have complications than those in whom PTCA was delayed. A successful outcome was more likely (83% vs 27%) in group III if at least 140,000 U of urokinase were administered within 50 minutes of the appearance of thrombus. Thus intracoronary thrombus formation during PTCA remains a significant source of morbidity. Antecedent antiplatelet therapy and intensive anticoagulation at the start of PTCA are important in avoiding complications resulting from thrombus formation. Intracoronary infusion of urokinase when initiated promptly appeared to minimize the frequency of complications and improve the angiographic results.

Agrawal and associates[126] in Birmingham, Alabama, performed a study to describe the initial experience and follow-up of ultrasound-guided compression of pseudoaneurysms in patients receiving systemic anticoagulants; antiplatelet therapy, or both, after recent cardiac catheterization or PTCA. Femoral artery pseudoaneurysm formation after an interventional procedure is becoming more common as larger caliber catheters and prolonged anticoagulant and antiplatelet therapy are used. Traditional therapy of this complications has been surgical repair. This study describes a new method of closing femoral pseudoaneurysms by using external compression guided by Doppler color flow imaging. Fifteen patients, 3 undergoing cardiac catheterization and 12 undergoing PTCA, developed an expansible growing mass at the vascular access site diagnosed as a femoral artery pseudoaneurysms by Doppler ultrasound. Seven of the patients had undergone coronary stenting and were receiving postprocedural anticoagulant therapy. These patients underwent progressive graded mechanical (C-clamp) external compression guided by ultrasound. Mechanical compression was continued to obliterate the vascular tracts to these aneurysms and maintain adequate flow in the femoral artery. After an average compression time of 30 minutes (range 10 to 120 minutes), these tracts remained closed. Follow-up ultrasound examination at 24 hours or later confirmed continued closure in all. Thus, these data suggest that nonsurgical closure of femoral pseudoaneurysms is feasible and effective.

Hermans and colleagues[127] in Rotterdam, The Netherlands, examined the relation between an angiographically visible coronary artery dissection immediately after successful coronary balloon angioplasty and a subsequent restenosis and long-term clinical outcome. The study population comprised all 693 patients who participated in the MERCATOR trial which was a randomized, double-blind, placebo-controlled restenosis prevention trial with an angiotensin converting enzyme inhibitor, cilazapril. Cineangiographic films were processed and analyzed at a central angiographic core facility without knowledge of clinical data and with the use of an automated interpolated edge detection technique. Angiographic follow-up was obtained in 94% of patients with 778 lesions. Two approaches were used to assess the restenosis phenomenon: 1) categoric, using the traditional cutoff criterion of >50% diameter stenosis at follow-up, and 2) continuous, defined as absolute change in minimal lumen diameter between the postcoronary angioplasty and follow-up, adjusted for the vessel size. Clinical outcome was ranked according to the most serious adverse clinical event for each patient during the 6-month follow-up, ranging from death, nonfatal AMI, CABG, and recurrent angina following medical therapy to none of these. Dissection occurred in 247 (32%) of the 778 dilated lesions. The restenosis rate was 29% in lesions with and 30% in lesions without dissection. The relative decrease in lumen diameter in both groups was 0.10 (mean difference). Clinical outcome included death in 4 patients (0.9%) without dissection and in 1 patient (0.4%) with dissection; nonfatal AMI in 4 (0.9%) without and 8 (3.2%) with dissection; CABG in 73 (17%) without and 32 (13%) with dissection; and recurrent angina requiring medical therapy in 88 (20%) without and 47 (19%) with dissection. There were no serious adverse events in 272 (62%) without and 114 patients (65%) with dissections. These data indicate that a successfully dilated coronary artery with angiographically visible dissection is no more likely to develop restenosis than one without dissection. Furthermore, dissection occurring in an otherwise successfully dilated coronary artery is not associated with a worse clinical outcome at 6-month follow-up than is a dilated lesion without visible dissection.

The availability of circulatory support devices has increased the importance of accurately identifying patients at risk for hemodynamic compromise during PTCA. Bergelson and associates[128] from Boston, Massachusetts, performed prospective evaluation of 3 criteria to predict hemodynamic compromise (defined as a decrease in systolic BP ≥20 to <90 mm Hg during balloon inflation) in 157 patients (group A) undergoing PTCA. LVEF <35% had a sensitivity of 13% and a specificity of 95%. Greater than 50% of the myocardium at risk was associated with a sensitivity of 31% and a specificity of 85%. The angiographer's assessment of high risk for hemodynamic compromise had the highest sensitivity of 56% and a specificity of 86%. The clinical and angiographic characteristics of these patients were reviewed to identify risk factors retrospectively. Multivariate analysis of 28 variables identified multivessel CAD, diffuse CAD, myocardium at risk, and stenosis before PTCA as independent predictors of hemodynamic compromise. With use of this analysis, a 13-point weighted scoring system was created based on the regression of coefficients of the variables. Defining high risk for hemodynamic compromise as a risk score ≥4, the sensitivity of this criterion in group A patients was 81% and the specificity was 74%. The scoring system was then prospectively applied to 61 consecutive patients (group B) undergoing PTCA. In using a risk score ≥4 to define high risk, this scoring system had a sensitivity of 92% and a specificity of 92%. In the same population, EF <35% had a sensitivity of 6% and >50% of myocardium at risk had a 13% sensitivity. Therefore, it is concluded that this scoring system substantially improves the ability to predict hemodynamic compromise during PTCA with a high sensitivity and specificity.

CORONARY ATHRECTOMY

Directional coronary atherectomy can cause ectasia, presumably due to an excision deeper than the angiographically "normal" arterial lumen. In a multicenter series in which quantitative coronary angiography was performed after directional atherectomy in 382 narrowings in 372 patients, De Cesare and associates[129] from several centers identified ectasia after atherectomy in 50 (13%) narrowings. By univariate analysis, ectasia was seen more often within the circumflex coronary artery, in complex, probably thrombus-containing lesions, and with higher device:artery ratios. Ectasia occurred less often in lesions within the right coronary artery. Histologic analysis demonstrated adventitia or media, or both, in all patients with angiographic ectasia. Repeat angiography was performed in 188 of 271 eligible patients (69%) 6.1 ± 2.4 months after atherectomy. Restenosis, defined as a follow-up area stenosis ≥75%, was present in 50% of patients without procedural ectasia and in 70% of patients with marked ectasia (residual area stenosis < −20%). It is concluded that excision beyond the normal arterial lumen may occur after directional coronary atherectomy, related, in part, to angiographic and procedural features noted at the time of atherectomy. Restenosis tends to occur more often in patients with marked ectasia after coronary atherectomy.

Identification of genes that are specifically activated in restenosis lesions after PTCA represents a necessary step toward molecular manipulation designed to inhibit cellular proliferation responsible for such lesions. Whereas quiescent smooth muscle cells preferentially express smooth muscle myosin, proliferating smooth muscle cells have been shown to preferentially express nonmuscle myosin in vitro. Accordingly, Leclerc and co-investigators[130] in Boston, Massachusetts, analyzed the expression of a recently cloned isoform of human nonmuscle myosin heavy chain in fresh human restenotic lesions. A total of 10 lesions, including 4 restenosis and 6 primary obtained percutaneously by directional atherectomy, were processed for examination by in situ hybridization. In total, 150 tissue sections of restenotic lesions, primary lesions, and normal internal mammary artery were hybridized with nonmuscle heavy chain probe. Restenotic lesions showed intense hybridization to the nonmuscle RNA probe, as demonstrated by a clustering of >20 grains per cell nucleus in 80% of the cells examined within a high-power field; in contrast, an equivalent degree of hybridization was observed in only 7% of cells within primary lesions. Results of immunocyto-chemistry using monoclonal antibody to smooth muscle actin indicated that cells demonstrating strong hybridization were smooth muscle in origin. These findings demonstrate that (1) human vascular tissue obtained by percutaneous directional atherectomy constitutes appropriate biopsy material for gene expression studies at the RNA level, and (2) nonmuscle myosin heavy chain RNA is present in greater abundance among restenotic versus primary vascular stenoses.

Bertrand and associates[131] from Lille, France, Rotterdam, the Netherlands, and Mainz, Germany, reported the results from 3 European centers using rotary ablation with rotablator, a device that is inserted into the coronary artery and removes atheroma by grinding it into millions of tiny fragments. Rotary ablation was performed in 129 patients. Primary success (reduction in percent luminal narrowing >20%, residual stenosis <50%, without complications) was achieved by rotary angioplasty alone in 73 patients (57%). An additional 38 patients (29%) had successful adjunctive balloon angioplasty. Thus primary success was achieved in 111 patients (86%) at the end of the procedure. Acute occlusion occurred in 10 patients (7.7%). Recanalization was achieved by balloon angioplasty in 7: urgent bypass grafting was undertaken in 2. Q-wave and on-Q-wave AMI occurred in 3 and 7 patients, respectively. No deaths occurred. Follow-up angiography was performed in 74 patients (60%). Restenosis, defined as the recurrence of significant luminal narrowing (>50%) occurred in 17 of 37 patients (46%) who underwent rotary ablation alone, and 11 of 37 patients (30%) who had adjunctive balloon angioplasty. The overall angiographic restenosis rate was 37.8%. In conclusion, rotary ablation is technically feasible, and relatively safe in the coronary circulation. The low primary success rate reflects the limited size of the device, which can be introduced through available guiding catheters, and limits the use of rotary ablation as a stand-alone procedure to lesions in small arteries or in distal locations.

Popma and the U.S. Directional Atherectomy Investigator Group[132] used directional coronary atherectomy in the period October 1, 1986, to December 31, 1989, during 1,020 procedures in 1,140 lesions at 14 clinical centers. Abrupt vessel closure, defined as a total coronary occlusion or subtotal occlusion associated with clinical evidence of ischemia, occurred in 43 procedures (4%). It developed in the catheterization laboratory in 34 patients, but it was delayed 1 to 96 hours in 9 patients. By univariate analysis, the incidence of abrupt closure was higher in directional atherectomy of de novo lesions, lesions in the right coronary artery and diffuse lesions. The incidence of abrupt closure tended to be lower in directional atherectomy of saphenous vein grafts as compared to native coronary arteries (1.6% vs 4%). Clinical findings during abrupt closure included severe angina in 26 patients, AMI in 17 patients, hypotension in 5 patients, and death in 2 patients. PTCA was attempted in 32 patients after abrupt vessel closure. In 16 patients, PTCA resulted in initial resolution of the closure episode, although 1 patient died 96 hours after the procedure. Fifteen of 16 patients without initial improvement after PTCA underwent CABG; 9 additional patients without abrupt closure were referred directly for CABG. Thus, abrupt vessel closure develops relatively infrequently after directional coronary artherectomy. In the absence of severe coronary dissection, abrupt closure after directional atherectomy may be managed by PTCA, although CABG is often required.

Between June 1988 and July 1991 Mansour and associates[133] from Boston, Massachusetts, performed 464 new device interventions (Palmaz–Schatz stent or Simpson directional atherectomy) in 410 patients. Chest pain occurred within 72 hours after the procedure in 94 patients (23%). All patients were evaluated with electrocardiograms and cardiac isoenzymes on the day after the procedure, and urgent repeat coronary angiography was performed in 29 chest pain patients (31%). Whereas all 14 patients with abnormal findings on repeat angiography had electrocardiographic changes, 6 of the 20 restudied patients (30%) with electrocardiographic changes had no angiographic explanation for chest pain. Non-Q-wave myocardial infarction occurred in 22 patients (5%) (10 of 35 [29%] with chest pain and electrocardiographic changes, 3 of 44 [7%] with chest pain and no electrocardiographic change, and 9 of 316 [3%] without chest pain). Factors associated with chest pain after new device intervention included a decreased residual percent stenosis, incomplete revascularization and the presence of multivessel disease. Vessel dissection after stenting but not atherectomy was associated with postprocedure chest pain. Chest pain is common (23%) after new device intervention. Electrocardiographic changes are a sensitive marker of angiographic abnormality and confer a higher risk of non-Q-wave AMI, but no increase of in-hospital mortality. Determinants of postprocedure chest pain are lower residual percent stenosis, incomplete revascularization and the presence of multivessel disease. Patients with chest pain but no electrocardiographic changes early after successful stent placement or atherectomy need not routinely undergo urgent recatheterization.

Over a 37-month period, Pomerantz and associates[134] from Boston, Massachusetts, used either directional coronary atherectomy (n = 35) or Palmaz–Schatz intracoronary stents (n = 84) in 119 of 176 interventions (68%) on saphenous vein grafts (average age 8.5 years from CABG to graft intervention), representing 37% of all stents and 15% of all atherectomies during the study period, respectively. Of the 57 saphenous vein graft lesions treated with conventional balloon angioplasty during this period, 49 (86%) had 1 or more contraindications to stenting or directional atherectomy (thrombus, total occlusion, reference vessel <3 mm in diameter). The acute success rate was 99% for stents (1 failure to dilate) and 94% for directional atherectomy (2 failures to cross the lesion with the atherectomy device). Lumen diameter increased from 0.9 to 3.6 mm (reference vessel 3.6) for stents, and from 0.9 to 3.5 mm (reference 3.8) for atherectomy (for all comparisons), with no major complications (abrupt or subabrupt closure, emergent CABG, death, or Q-wave AMI). During the same time period 50 of 57 vein grafts (88%) rejected for stenting or atherectomy were dilated successfully by conventional balloon angioplasty, with 3 patients (5%) requiring emergent coronary bypass surgery. Angiographic follow-up was available for 50 of 64 eligible patients (78%). Restenosis (defined as ≥50% stenosis at 6-month angiographic follow-up) was present in 13 of 50 lesions (26%), including 8 of 32 stented lesions (25%) and 5 of 18 atherectomy lesions (28%). These data suggest that saphenous vein bypass graft stenoses may be treated safely and effectively using Palmaz-Schatz stenting or directional atherectomy, with short- and long-term results that may be better than those traditionally expected with conventional balloon angioplasty.

Garratt and associates[135] from Rochester, Minnesota, performed directional coronary atherectomy (DCA) in 158 patients over a 2-year period at the Mayo Clinic. Primary atheromatous lesions were treated in 92 patients (group 1) and restenosis lesions were treated in 66 (group 2). Technical success (recovery of tissue and ≥40% luminal enlargement with a residual stenosis of <50%) was achieved in 152 lesions (92%); clinical success (technical success and no in-hospital death, Q-wave AMI or CABG) was achieved in 143 patients (91%). Adjunctive balloon angioplasty was used in 41 patients. DCA was successful less often in group 1 than in group 2 (86 vs 97%). A major complication occurred in 7% of patients; in-hospital death, Q-wave AMI and emergency CABG occurred in 3, 1 and 4% of patients, respectively. Major complications were more frequent in group 1 than in group 2 (10 vs 1). During a follow-up period of 14 ± 8 months, no difference between the groups was found in the incidence of late (4%), Q-wave AMI (1%), recurrent severe angina (29%), CABG surgery (15%) or repeat interventional procedure of the same vascular segment (24%). Vein graft and restenosis lesions tended to have greater success and fewer complications. Angiographic restenosis (increase of ≥30% in stenosis severity by visual assessment) occurred in 62% of patients and 58% of lesions with successful DCA, and was similar in the 2 groups; a tendency toward higher restenosis rates was seen in patients with vein graft DCA. Late clinical events appeared to occur at rates similar to those reported for patients after balloon angioplasty. These findings support the need for a randomized, prospective trial to compare DCA with balloon angioplasty.

The periprocedural events and myocardial function during nonocclusive coronary atherectomy by Rotablator or transluminal extraction catheter (TEC) may differ from events during balloon angioplasty. This difference may have important clinical consequences. Pavlides and associates[136] from Royal Oak, Michigan, assessed 17 patients undergoing Rotablator and 18 patients undergoing TEC atherectomy by clinical, hemodynamic, and electrocardiographic monitoring and simultaneous transesophageal echocardiography. The findings were compared with similar parameters during subsequent balloon angioplasty performed in 16 of 17 patients undergoing Rotablator and 14 of 18 undergoing TEC atherectomy. Chest pain occurred more frequently during balloon inflation than during either atherectomy, whereas ST-segment and T-wave electrocardiographic changes were equally frequent. Transient second- or third-degree atrioventricular block occurred in 6 patients during Rotablator but in none during TEC atherectomy or balloon inflation. Hemodynamic parameters and global LV function remained unchanged during atherectomy. Regional myocardial function in the distribution of the target coronary artery, assessed by a wall motion score, was not affected during Rotablator, but deteriorated slightly during TEC atherectomy and more significantly during balloon inflation (score from 0.3 ± 0.5 to 1.0 ± 0.7 during TEC and 2.0 ± 0.6 during balloon inflation). Thus, chest pain is infrequent, whereas hemodynamics and global LV function are preserved during Rotablator and TEC atherectomy. Transient AV block during Rotablator and regional myocardial dysfunction during TEC atherectomy may occur without significant consequences.

High-speed rotational atherectomy uses a diamond-coated, elliptical burr to abrade occlusive atherosclerosis, especially noncompliant calcified plaque. Mintz and colleagues[137] in Washington, DC, used intravascular ultrasound to analyze 28 patients after atherectomy. Arteries treated and imaged were LM, LAD, LC, right coronary artery and saphenous vein. Twenty patients had adjunct balloon angioplasty. Twenty-two target lesions were calcified; the intimal arc of calcium was 160°. After atherectomy, the intima-lumen interface was unusually distinct and circular. The lumen was larger than the largest burr used for both stand-alone and adjunct balloon procedures. Three-dimensional reconstruction of the ultrasound images showed a smooth lumen, especially in calcified plaque. Deviations from cylindrical geometry occurred only in areas of soft plaque or superficial tissue disruption of calcified plaque. Five patients were studied before and after rotational atherectomy. Intravascular ultrasound showed an increase in lumen size, a decrease in plaque-plus-media area and in arc of target lesion calcification, and no change in target lesion external elastic membrane cross-sectional area. Rotational atherectomy causes atheroablation with only moderate evidence of barotrauma in heavily calcified arteries, even after adjunct balloon angioplasty. The lumen is cylindrical, especially in areas of calcified plaque, and somewhat larger than the largest burr tip used.

Fishman and associates[138] in Boston, Massachusetts, studied the long-term clinical efficacy of directional coronary atherectomy. A total of 225 atherectomies performed in 190 patients between August, 1988 and July, 1991 were examined. Minimal lumen diameter of the treated segments was measured on angiograms obtained before, after, and 6 months after intervention. Although most lesions (97%) had one or more characteristics predictive of unfavorable short- or long-term results after conventional PTCA, atherectomy was successful in 205 lesions (91%) with a mean residual stenosis of 7 ± 16%. After subsequent PTCA in 16 unsuccessful atherectomy attempts, procedural success was 98%. There were no deaths or Q wave AMIs, and one patient underwent emergency CABG. Six-month angiographic follow-up was obtained in 77% of the eligible patients. The overall angiographic restenosis rate was 32%. Predictors of a lower restenosis rate included a postprocedural lumen diameter >3 mm, serum cholesterol ≤200 mg/dl, and recent AMI. Life-table analysis showed a 2% mortality rate and a 26% incidence of other events, including AMI, and repeat revascularization during the first year. The annual 5% mortality rate and 7% incidence of other events during years 2 and 3 were related in large part to the progression of CAD at other locations. Therefore, six-month angiographic follow-up of patients who underwent directional coronary atherectomy during the first 3 years of this group's experience showed an overall restenosis rate of 32%, with lower rates in patients with a postatherectomy lumen diameter ≥3 mm, cholesterol ≤200 mg/dl or a recent AMI.

In comparing the restenosis rates among different interventions, 1 potential confounder might be the differences in the arteries treated, as dictated by the technical limitations of particular devices. Kuntz and associates[139] from Boston, Massachusetts, and Edward City, California, utilized acute gain-late loss analysis to determine what influence coronary artery selection had on the restenosis rate after coronary stenting or directional atherectomy. The minimal luminal diameter of native coronary lesions was measured before and immediately after intervention in 102 single Palmaz-Schatz stents and 347 atherectomies, 367 (82%) of which had repeat angiographic measurement 6 months after intervention. Atherectomy-treated lesions had a higher proportion of LAD to right coronary arteries (68 vs 24%) compared with stents (31 vs 54%). Although subsequent restenosis rates were similar for stenting (25%) and atherectomy (30%), LAD versus right coronary lesions had a significantly higher restenosis rate for the overall group (35 vs 18%), for stents (44 vs 13%) and for atherectomy (35 vs 22%), respectively. Multivariable analysis demonstrated that post-procedure luminal diameter and coronary location (the proportion of LAD vessels treated, but not device type (stent vs atherectomy), were strong independent determinants of restenosis according to both binary (50% diameter stenosis) and continuous (late percent stenosis) definitions. The higher restenosis rate seen for left anterior descending as compared with right coronary lesions was associated with a larger "loss index" (late loss in luminal diameter divided by acute gain: 0.52 vs 0.35), which would suggest intrinsically greater intimal hyperplastic responsiveness. This study shows that LAD lesion location carries an independent increased risk of restenosis after either Palmaz-Schatz stenting or directional atherectomy, apparently because of a larger potential for luminal renarrowing of the LAD compared with the right or LC arteries.

Strauss and colleagues[140] in Rotterdam, The Netherlands; Toulouse, France; Redwood City, California; Brussels and Aalst, Belgium determined the safety and long-term results of directional coronary atherectomy in stented coronary arteries in 9 patients (10 procedures) 82 to 1,179 days after stenting. The tissue was assessed for histologic features of restenosis, smooth muscle cell phenotype, markers of cell proliferation and cell density. A control (no stenting) group consisted of 13 patients treated with directional coronary atherectomy for restenosis 14 to 597 days after coronary PTCA, directional coronary atherectomy or laser intervention. Directional coronary atherectomy procedures within the stent were successful with results similar to those of the initial stenting procedure. Of 5 patients with angiographic follow-up, three had restenosis requiring reintervention, including surgery in 2 and repeat atherectomy followed by laser angioplasty in one. Intimal hyperplasia was identified in 80% of specimens after stenting and in 77% after PTCA or atherectomy. In 3 patients with stenting, 70% to 76% of the intimal cells showed morphologic features of contractile phenotype by electron microscopy 47 to 185 days after coronary intervention. Evidence of ongoing proliferation was absent in all specimens studied. Although wide individual variability was present in the maximal cell density of the intimal hyperplasia, there was a trend toward a reduction in cell density over time. Although atherectomy is feasible for the treatment of restenosis in stented coronary arteries and initial results are encouraging, recurrence of restenosis is common. Intimal hyperplasia is a ubiquitous response to injury regardless of the device used and smooth muscle cell proliferation and phenotypic modulation toward a contractile phenotype are early events and largely completed by the time of clinical presentation with restenosis.

Bell and associates[141] in Rochester, Minnesota, studied the relation between deep arterial injury with directional coronary atherectomy and the subsequent development of coronary artery aneurysms in a consecutive series of 64 successfully treated patients in a total of 69 lesions with a mean angiographic follow-up of five months. Quantitative coronary arteriographic data were used for evaluation. Coronary artery aneurysms occurred in 7 patients (10%). The only significant clinical correlate of aneurysm formation was a relatively shorter duration of angina. There were no significant preprocedural angiographic predictors of aneurysms, although 6 (86%) of the 7 aneurysmal lesions arose from restenosis lesions compared with 30 (48%) of 62 lesions with no subsequent aneurysm development. Histopathologic examination of 414 specimens from 68 treated lesions showed no significant difference in the occurrence of subintimal resection between those with and those without subsequent aneurysm formation (29% vs 22%). Media alone was found in 14% of specimens from lesions that later became aneurysmal versus 15% of those that did not and adventitial resection was found in 14% and 7% of specimens, respectively. Aneurysms occur relatively frequently after directional coronary atherectomy. There were no statistically significant correlation with the depth of arterial resection, but the data from this study suggest that the role of adventitial resection in the occurrence of late aneurysm development should be explored further.

To assess the procedural results after coronary angioplasty using the transluminal extraction catheter (TEC) in patients with complex narrowings, Popma and associates[142] from Washington, D.C., reviewed their experience with 51 patients undergoing this procedure. One or more adverse lesion morphologic features were present in 45 patients (88%) and ≥2 adverse features were present in 38 (74%). Procedural success (<50% final diameter stenosis and the absence of major complications) was obtained in 42 patients (82%); major complications occurred in 7 patients (death, 3; Q-wave AMI, 4; emergency bypass operation, 2). Distal embolization was noted in 5 patients with thrombus-containing sapheous vein graft stenoses. Only lesion thrombus correlated with an unsuccessful outcome. After TEC use, diameter stenosis was reduced from 76 ± 13 to 50 ± 22%. Adjunct balloon angioplasty was used in 44 procedures (86%), further reducing the diameter stenosis to 32 ± 22%. High-frequency intracoronary ultrasound was performed in 11 patients after TEC use. Plaque fissuring was present in all lesions and intraluminal dissection was noted in 4 (36%). Residual plaque after TEC use was found in virtually all lesions. During the 5.2 ± 2.8-month follow-up period, 17 patients (40%) developed recurrent symptoms. Coronary bypass surgery was performed in 4 patients and repeat coronary angioplasty was required in 3. In addition, 3 patients died from cardiac causes.

CORONARY STENTING

The coronary stent has been investigated as an adjunct to PTCA to obviate the problems of early occlusion and late restenosis. From March 1986 to March 1990, Strauss and associates[143] from multiple European medical centers implanted in 265 patients and in 308 narrowings the coronary wall stent in 6 European centers. For this study, the patients were analyzed according to date of implantation (group 1, March 1986 to January 1988; group 2, February 1988 to March 1990) and vessel type (native arteries versus bypass grafts). Quantitative angiographic follow-up was performed in 82% of the study patients. The early in-hospital occlusion rate in the overall group was 15%. Group 1 patients had a 20% rate in contrast to 12% rate in group 2. The early occlusion rate in the overall group was 15%. Group 1 patients had a 20% rate in contrast to 12% rate in group 2. The early occlusion rate in native vessels and bypass grafts was 19 and 8%, respectively. Restenosis was determined by 2 criteria (criterion 1, ≥0.72 mm loss in minimal luminal diameter from poststent to follow-up; criterion 2, ≥50% diameter stenosis at follow-up) within the stent and in the segments immediately proximal and distal to the stent. The restenosis rate with criterion 1 was 43% in the overall group of patients, 35% in group 1 versus 49% in group 2, and 34% in native vessels versus 54% in bypass grafts. The second criterion was met by 27% of patients in the overall group, 21% in group 1 versus 32% in group 2, and 18% in native vessel versus 39% in bypass grafts. The overall mortality during the study period was 6.6% in native arteries and 9% in bypass grafts (6 and 7.9% at 1 year, respectively). The actuarial event-free survival (freedom from death, AMI, bypass surgery or angioplasty) for native artery patients was 46% at 40 months and for bypass graft patients 37% at 20 months. It is concluded that early in-hospital occlusions remain a major problem with this device despite improvement in the later experience. Although patients with bypass grafts had a significantly lower early occlusion rate than those with implantation of native arteries, a significantly higher rate of late restenosis limited the early benefits of stenting. The indications for stenting remain unknown and require results of randomized clinical studies.

Intracoronary stenting has been introduced as an adjunct to PTCA aimed at overcoming its limitations, namely acute arterial closure and late restenosis. de Jaegere and associates[144] from multiple international medical centers reported the first experience with Wiktor stent implanted in the first 50 consecutive patients. All patients had restenosis of a native coronary artery lesion after prior balloon angioplasty. The target coronary artery was the left anterior descending artery in 26 patients, the circumflex artery in 7 patients and the right coronary artery in 17 patients. The implantation success rate was 98% (49 of 50 patients). There were no procedural deaths. Acute or subacute thrombotic stent occlusion occurred in 5 patients (10%). All 5 patients sustained a nonfatal AMI. Four of these patients underwent recanalization by means of balloon angioplasty; the remaining patient was referred for bypass surgery. A major bleeding complication occurred in 11 patients (22%): groin bleeding necessitating blood transfusion in 6, gastrointestinal bleeding in 3 and hematuria in 2. Repeat angiography was performed at a mean of 5.6 ± 1.1 months in all but 1 patient undergoing implantation. Restenosis, defined by a reduction of ≥0.72 mm in the minimal luminal diameter or a change in diameter stenosis from < to ≥50%, occurred in 20 (45%) and 13 (29%) patients, respectively. In this first experience, the easiness and high technical success rate of Wiktor stent implantation are overshadowed by a high incidence of subacute stent occlusion and bleeding complications.

In an investigation by de Scheerder and associates[145] from Rotterdam and Leiden, The Netherlands, and Brussels and Aalst, Belgium, during a 2-year period, 136 self-expanding Wall-stents were implanted in sapheous vein bypass grafts in 69 patients with end-stage CAD. All patients had severe symptoms and the majority were poor candidates for either repeat surgery or conventional bypass CABG because of unfavorable native anatomy, impaired LV function, or a high-risk bypass lesion anatomy for PTCA. All procedures were technically successful without major complications and without need for emergency CABG. However, during the hospital stay acute thrombotic complications occurred in 7 patients (10%) resulting in 1 death and AMI in 5 patients and necessitating emergency repeat PTCA in 2 patients and repeat CABG in 4. Twenty-three patients had serious hemorrhagic complications directly related to the rigorous anticoagulation schedule. Two patients died of fatal cerebral bleeding. During follow-up, another 5 patients died accounting for a total mortality rate of 12%. At late angiographic follow-up (4.9 ± 3.4 months, n = 53), 25 patients (47%) had a restenosis (≥50%) within or immediately adjacent to the stent, necessitating reintervention in 19 patients (PTCA, n = 12; repeat CABG, n = 7). In the group without stent-related stenosis (n = 28), 15 patients had progression of disease in either the native or bypass vessels leading to recurrence of major anginal symptoms within 1 to 24 months. Ten of these patients required further intervention (stent, n = 6; PTCA, n = 3; repeat CABG, n = 1). Stenting in saphenous CABG grafts can be performed safely with excellent immediate angiographic and clinical results. Early occlusion, late restenosis, and bleeding complications associated with the aggressive anticoagulant treatment remain significant limitations. Reintervention as a result of restenosis or progression of disease in other lesions is common. Stenting of diseased bypass grafts in symptomatic patients with end-stage CAD (who are at high risk for conventional PTCA or CABG reintervention) is useful as palliative therapy.

Balloon-expandable stents may reduce the restenosis rate following PTCA. To evaluate this potential in saphenous vein grafts, 26 patients with 30 discrete stenoses underwent conventional balloon dilatation and successful Palmaz-Schatz stent implantation as part of a multicenter trial carried out by Strumpf and associates[146] from Phoenix, Arizona. All patients had resolution of their angina following the procedure. In a mean 5-month follow-up period, 14 patients (54%, 16 lesions) had repeat arteriography; 2 patients (14%) developed recurrent ischemia ascribed to their venous grafts from in-stent restenosis (2 of 16 lesions, 13%). Two asymptomatic patients (8%) died: 1 from cardiac arrest (stent patient) and 1 from stroke. The clinical recurrent rate (cardiac death, AMI, CABG, repeat PTCA, or symptom recurrence) was 15%. These results show trends toward an improved primary success rate with combined vein graft angioplasty/stenting and a lower restenosis rate in stented saphenous vein grafts.

Carrozza and associates[147] in Boston, Massachusetts, studied 220 patients who had 250 endovascular procedures between June, 1988 and July, 1991. Minimal lumen diameter of the treated segments was measured on angiograms obtained before, after and 6 months after intervention. Stent placement was successful in 246 (98%) of 250 lesions, reducing diameter stenosis from 77% to −2.5%. There were no deaths or Q wave AMI. One patient required emergency CABG and one developed subacute thrombosis. Femoral vascular complications occurred in 36 patients (16%). Six-month angiographic follow-up was obtained in 91% of eligible patients. The overall angiographic restenosis rate was 25%. The rate of restenosis was higher for stents in the left anterior descending than in the right coronary artery, in diabetic patients, and in vessels with post-stent lumen diameters <3.3 mm. Stenting of the left anterior descending coronary artery was the strongest predictor of restenosis. Total survival was 97% and event-free survival from death, AMI, or revascularization was 70% at 36 months. Thus, intracoronary stents can be placed successfully with a low incidence of major complications. The angiographic restenosis rate was 25% and 70% of patients remained free of cardiovascular events at 3 years. Diabetes, small postprocedure lumen diameter and stenting of the left anterior descending coronary artery are associated with the highest rates of restenosis.

In an investigation carried out by Lau and associates[148] from London, United Kingdom, follow-up angiographic study was performed in 86 patients after initially successful Wallstent stent (Medinvent, Lausanne, Switzerland) implantation between April 1986 and October 1990. The stent angiographic restenosis rate was 16% at a mean of 8 months after stenting despite the inclusion of a substantial number of patients at high risk of restenosis after PTCA. Of a total 15 variables analyzed, only suboptimal stent placement was found to be a significant predictor of stent restenosis. Age; gender; baseline New York Heart Association functional class; previous PTCA; indication for stenting; LVEF; preangioplasty and immediate postangioplasty diameter stenosis severity; stented vessel site; lesional morphology; number, diameter, and length of stents implanted; and the interval between stenting and follow-up angiographic restudy were not significant risk factors of stent restenosis. This study suggests that intracoronary stent implantation with the Wallstent may be a useful and promising adjunctive option after PTCA, particularly in patients at high risk of restenosis after PTCA. However, because of the significantly enhanced risk of restenosis after suboptimal stent implantation, it is strongly recommended in the selection and placement of Wallstent stents that they adequately cover the entire length of the dilated coronary segment.

LASER ANGIOPLASTY

The role of excimer laser angioplasty in treating CAD remains uncertain. In a cohort of 764 patients who had 858 coronary stenoses treated with excimer laser-facilitated angioplasty, Bittl and associates[149] for the Percutaneous Excimer Laser Coronary Angioplasty Registry from several USA medical centers used relative risk analysis to examine acute success, complications and restenosis rates, and the results were compared with those of balloon angioplasty to identify the lesion types that show the greatest benefit with the new treatment. Clinical success was achieved in 657 patients (86%), as indicated by ≤50% residual stenosis and no in-hospital complications. A major in-hospital complication (death, CABG, or Q-wave or non-Q-wave AMI) occurred in 58 patients (7.6%). Follow-up angiography was obtained in 70% of eligible patients. Combining angiographic and noninvasive restenosis rates yielded an overall restenosis rate of 46%. Relative risk analysis showed that major complications occurred frequently in lesions at an arterial bifurcation. However, certain complex lesions that are difficult to treat with balloon angioplasty (saphenous vein graft lesions, lesions >10 mm, ostial lesions, calcified stenoses, total occlusions and unsuccessful balloon dilatations), analyzed together as a group, had lower complication rates by univariate (OR 0.59) and multivariate logistic regression analyses. Restenosis rates were higher for lesions >10 mm in length (OR 1.28) and for those treated with laser alone (OR 1.69). In conclusion, the use of excimer laser-facilitated angioplasty to treat many lesion types will be limited by significant restenosis, despite acceptable initial clinical results. Favorable success rates with this new technology were found for a group of 6 lesions that comprise the "alpha class" (saphenous vein graft lesions, long lesions, ostial lesions, calcified stenoses, total occlusions and unsuccessful balloon dilatations). Direct, controlled comparison with other interventional technologies will define the ultimate role of the excimer laser angioplasty procedure.

CORONARY ARTERY BYPASS GRAFTING

Factors influencing operative rates

Goldberg and associates[150] from Milwaukee, Wisconsin, Rochester, Minnesota, and Baltimore, Maryland, examined the differences in the rates of CABG between white and black Medicare patients in a cross-sectional study with data from the 1986 Health Care Financing Administration hospital claims records on all Medicare patients in the USA in 1986. Sex and age-adjusted CABG rates for whites and blacks over the age of 65 years were computed for each of 50 states and 305 Standard Metropolitan Statistical Areas (Figure 2-17). Nationally, the CABG rate was 27.1/10,000 for whites (40.4 for white men and 16.2 for white women), and 7.6 for blacks (9.3 for black men and 6.4 for black women). Racial differences were greater in the southeast, particularly in nonmetropolitan areas, than in other regions. Neither white nor black Standard Metropolitan Statistical Area rates were associated with the rate of admission for AMI (an indication of the amount of CAD). White rates, but not black rates, were associated with the number of thoracic surgeons per 100,000 people. For patients insured by Medicare, race is strongly associated with CABG rates, and this association is greater for men than for women and greater in the Southeast than in other parts of the country. Physician supply may relate to the CABG rates for whites.

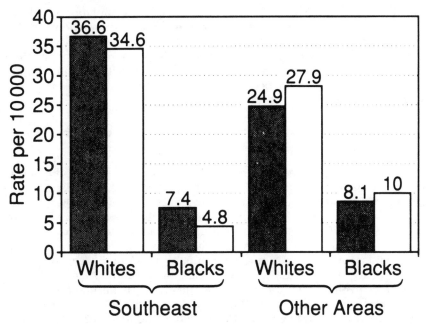

Fig. 2-17. National coronary artery bypass graft rates by race, community size, and region. Shaded bars indicate Standard Metropolitan Statistical Areas; and unshaded bars, non-Standard Metropolitan Statistical Areas. Reproduced with permission from Goldberg, et al.[150]

Versus angioplasty

Little data directly compare the outcomes of patients treated with PTCA and CABG. Vacek and associates[151] from Kansas City, Missouri, examined the characteristics and outcomes of 152 patients who underwent multivessel PTCA and 134 patients who had multivessel CABG. Patients who had prior PTCA or CABG were excluded. Baseline characteristics such as age, sex, and prior AMI were similar in the 2 groups. EF was significantly lower in the CABG group (48 ± 14%) versus the PTCA patients (53 ± 15%). Narrowing distribution when analyzed by major vascular beds (left anterior descending, circumflex and right coronary arteries) as well as by individual arteries was not significantly different between the groups when left main stenosis was excluded. The surgical group received a larger number of bypasses per patient (3.9) when compared with narrowings dilated in the angioplasty group (3.7). The left internal mammary artery was used in 75% of patients as one of the grafts. Angioplasty success was 95% by standard criteria. Over a mean follow-up of 110 weeks for PTCA patients and 134 weeks for CABG patients the occurrence of death was similar (10 and 14%, respectively) as was AMI (4 and 2%, respectively). However, all other cardiac events including subsequent cardiac catheterization (49 vs 10%), PTCA (30 vs 2%) and CABG (23 vs 2%) occurred significantly more often in the PTCA group. Of the 152 PTCA patients, 74 (49%) underwent repeat catheterization once, 26 (17%) twice, 8 (5%) 3 times, and 4 (3%) 4 times. At the time of final follow-up, 87% of surviving patients in the CABG group were angina-free and 84% had negative treadmill test results, whereas these findings were seen in 78 and 73% of PTCA patients, respectively, despite the greater number of intervening procedures in the PTCA group. It is concluded that although both PTCA and CABG can provide good symptomatic relief for patients with multivessel CAD, with comparable midterm survival rates, a need for repeat interventions occurs significantly more often in patients of this type undergoing angioplasty as opposed to those undergoing surgery, with greater evidence of residual or recurrent ischemia in those who received PTCA.

Effects of age

Carey and associates[152] from Torrance, California, studied the effect of increasing age on quality of life, survival, and risk of reoperation in 2,479 patients followed up prospectively 2 to 20 years after CABG. Quality of life was determined from annual questionnaires, which were used to calculate a health status index from the patient's symptomatic status and subjective response to the operation, which was graded between zero and 1.00 (asymptomatic). Four age groups were studied: age ≤49 years (AG40), 50 to 59 years (AG50), 60 to 69 years (AG60), and ≥70 years (AG70). Associated problems (LV aneurysm, valve disease, AMI) necessitating treatment were present in 17% (61/361) of AG40 patients, 19% (165 of 859) of AG50 patients, 23% (213/927) of AG60 patients, and 31% (102/332) of AG70 patients. The hospital mortality rate was higher in older patients undergoing combined procedures but not in patients undergoing coronary bypass grafts only. Probability of survival and health status indexes were calculated excluding patients with valve disease and cardiogenic shock. Probability of survival was significantly better in patients less than age 60 than in those 60 years or older, but in patients with an EF ≥0.40, probability of survival at 12 years was 0.64 (age <60) versus 0.62 (age ≥60). The actuarial risk of reoperation, calculated as the difference between probability of survival and probability of survival without reoperation, progressively increased in younger patients but not in patients aged ≥60 years. At 15 years, the reoperation rates were 26% (AG40), 14% (AG50), 5% (AG60), and 7% (AG70). Mean health status index for years 1 to 5 was 0.85 in AG40 patients, 0.84 in AG50 patients, 0.89 in AG60 patients, and 0.90 in AG70 patients; for years 6 to 10, 0.81, 0.89, 0.86, and 0.89; and for years 11 to 15, 0.77, 0.78, 0.84, and 0.84, respectively. Thus, quality of life after myocardial revascularization is better, improvement lasts longer, and reoperation rate is less in patients aged ≥60 years.

Older patients represent a growing proportion of patients undergoing CABG. Although functional benefits after CABG have been demonstrated, most assessments of outcomes have involved patients aged <65 years. Therefore, little is known concerning the impact of CABG on older patients, compared with that on younger ones. Guadagnoli and associates[153] from Boston, Massachusetts, compared a number of postsurgical (6 months) health-related quality-of-life outcomes (e.g., symptoms, cardiac functional status, instrumental activities of daily living, and emotional and social functioning) reported by patients aged <65 (n = 169) and ≥65 (n = 99) years who underwent elective CABG at 4 major teaching hospitals in Massachusetts and California. The proportion of patients reporting cardiac-related symptoms after surgery did not vary by age, and quality-of-life outcome scores of younger and older patients did not differ even after adjustment for clinical and demographic characteristics. The exception to this was mental health status, an outcome for which older patients reported better functioning than did younger ones. On average, patients in the 2 age groups reported equivalent improvement over preadmission status in instrumental activities of daily living, and emotional and social functioning. The independent relation of clinical and sociodemographic factors to quality-of-life outcomes was also investigated. Patients who functioned better before admission, those with less severe co-morbid disease, and married patients reported better functioning after discharge. In general, older patients who underwent elective CABG reported functional benefits similar to those reported by younger ones, and the factors associated with better functioning did not vary by age group.

Although CABG effectively eliminates or diminishes symptoms of myocardial ischemia, the overall performance status and functional outcome in elderly patients undergoing CABG is poorly documented. Glower and associates[154] from Durham, North Carolina, reviewed 86 consecutive patients aged 80 to 93 years undergoing isolated CABG. Preoperative, intraoperative, and postoperative characteristics and pre- and postoperative performance status (Karnofsky score) were examined. Forty patients (47%) were women, and most patients had highly symptomatic CAD with class III or IV angina in 94% and unstable angina in 90%. Significant co-morbid disease was present in 49% of patients, and cardiac catheterization revealed left main or 3-vessel disease in 74% of patients. The rate of significant in-hospital complications was 29%, with infection in 14%, stroke in 9%, and respiratory failure in 8% being most frequent. Median performance status (Karnofsky score) improved from 20 to 70% with 89% of hospital survivors being discharged home. Factors associated with failure to achieve a successful functional outcome at discharge were presence of 1 or more preoperative co-morbid conditions, preoperative AMI within 7 days of operation, and postoperative low cardiac output. Survival at 30 days, 6 months, and 3 years were 90, 78, and 64%, respectively. These data demonstrate that CABG can be offered to selected elderly patients with acceptable morbidity and mortality, marked improvement in performance status, and an acceptable quality of life.

Tuman and associates[155] from Chicago, Illinois, prospectively studied 2,000 patients undergoing CABG to compare the influence of age on the incidence of neurologic, cardiac, and other complications. Postoperative neurologic events were found in 56 (2.8%) of patients, with an incidence in patients ≥75 years (8.9%) more than twice that of patients 65 to 74 (3.6%) and 9 times larger than in patients <65 (0.9%). Cardiac complications did not differ between age groups except for low cardiac output state, which occurred 1.7 times more frequently in patients ≥75 years compared with those <65. Patients with postoperative neurologic events had a ninefold increase in mortality—35.7% versus 4.0%. Logistic regression analysis demonstrated the most important predictors of a postoperative neurologic event to be age, preoperative neurologic abnormality, recent AMI, and duration of cardiopulmonary bypass. The risk of neurologic complications increases disproportionately to the risk of cardiac complications in the elderly undergoing CABG with cardiopulmonary bypass. Despite neurologic improvement (32 of 56 patients), a postoperative neurologic event was second only to low cardiac output state as the postoperative complication most highly associated with in-hospital death.

Twenty-year follow-up

Ulicny and associates[156] from Cincinnati, Ohio, reviewed the clinical records of their first 100 patients to undergo saphenous vein aortocoronary artery bypass grafting at their hospital. The procedures were performed between March 19, 1970, and March 30, 1972. The patient population included 84 men, and the mean age was 51.4 years. There were 12 patients with single-vessel, 36 with 2-vessel, and 52 with 3-vessel CAD, an average of 2.4 involved arteries per patient. Forty-eight patients were judged to have diffuse atherosclerotic disease. Twelve patients had LM CAD. Each patient received an average of 1.8 sapheous vein grafts. Thirty-six patients underwent repeat CABG after an average of 133 months resulted in cumulative reoperative rates of 5%, 14%, 27%, and 36% at 5, 10, 15, and 20 years, respectively. The 5-, 10-, 15-, and 20-year survival rates were 90%, 68%, 53%, and 41%, respectively (Figure 2-18). Survival was not significantly related to the cause of death, cardiac-related causes being predominant. There were no significant relations between the length of survival and sex, the number of grafts received, or the presence of LM CAD. Survival was inversely related to age at initial operation as well as initial LV end-diastolic pressure. Survival positively correlated with the occurrence of triple-vessel disease and the presence of diffuse disease. Survival correlated with the occurrence of repeat grafting, the interval to repeat grafting, and survival after repeat grafting, but again did not correlate with the operation received. The 5- and 10-year survival rates for repeat operation were 77% and 71%, respectively. Saphenous vein CABG in this era yielded a 41% 20-year survival. Cardiac-related events continued to account for most late deaths. Thirty-six percent of all patients and 53% of all long-term survivors underwent repeat operation. Repeat operation significantly influenced long-term survival.

In 3-vessel disease

Complete revascularization after CABG is a logical goal and improves symptomatic outcome and survival. However, the impact of complete revascularization in patients with 3-vessel CAD with varying severities of angina and LV dysfunction has not been clearly defined. Bell and colleagues[157] in Rochester, Minnesota performed a retrospective analysis of 3,372 nonrandomized surgical patients from the Coronary Artery Sur-

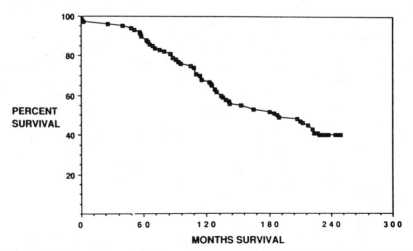

Fig. 2-18. Kaplan-Meier survival curve for the 100 patients undergoing primary coronary artery bypass grafting. Reproduced with permission from Ulicny, et al.[156]

gery Study (CASS) Registry who had 3-vessel CAD. Group 1 (894 patients) had class I or II angina and group 2 (2,478 patients) had class III or IV angina. In group 1, adjusted cumulative 4-year survivals according to the number of arteries bypassed were 85% for 1 artery, 94% for 2, 96% for 3, and 96% for >3 arteries. Adjusted event-free survival (death, AMI, definite angina or reoperation) was not influenced by the number of arteries bypassed, nor was the anginal status among patients remaining alive after 5 years. In group 2, adjusted cumulative 5-year survivals were 78% for 1 artery, 85% for 2, 90% for 3 and 87% for >3 arteries. Adjusted event-free survivals after 6 years were 23% for 1, 23% for 2, 29% for 3, and 31% for >3 arteries; at 5 years, those with more complete revascularization were more likely to be asymptomatic or free of severe angina. Among group 2 patients with EF <0.35, 6-year survival was 69% for those with grafts to ≥3 arteries versus 45% for those with grafts to 2 arteries (Figure 2-19).

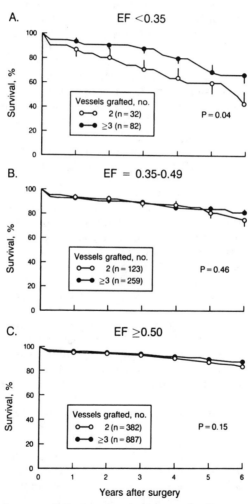

Fig. 2-19. Graphs show cumulative 6-year survival in group 2 patients, comparing complete revascularization (three or more bypassed vessels) and incomplete revascularization (two bypassed vessels) and stratified according to preoperative left ventricular ejection fraction (EF). Survival is shown for those with ejection fractions of <0.35 in panel A, ejection fractions between 0.35 and 0.49 in panel B, and ejection fractions ≥0.50 in panel C. Reproduced with permission from Bell, et al.[157]

Placing grafts to 3 or more vessels was independently associated with improved survival and event-free survival in group 2 but not group 1 patients. The case-fatality rates among 529 patients experiencing a myo-cardial infarction during follow-up was significantly higher for patients with less complete revascularization. Complete revascularization (grafts to 3 or more vessels) in patients with 3-vessel CAD appears to most benefit those with severe angina and LV dysfunction.

Risk factors for perioperative morbidity and mortality

King and associates[158] from Rochester, New York, performed a study to compare women and men undergoing CABG. Factors before and after CABG were examined to identify variables related to mortality and morbid-ity. The study population included 465 women and 465 men watched for age (mean age 64.2 years) who underwent first time isolated CABG between 1983 and 1988. There were higher incidences of systemic hyper-tension, diabetes mellitus, postmyocardial infarction angina, thyroid gland disease, arthritis, AMI, CHF, and emergency surgery in women, whereas more men had peptic ulcer disease. The in-hospital death rate was not significantly different (women 4.3% vs men 3.7%). For all subjects, emergency surgery, significant LM narrowing and renal disease were related to death only in men. Age and body surface area were not related to death. After surgery men had a higher incidence of atrial arrhythmia, and women had a higher incidence of CHF. Although women did not have a higher mortality rate, the data suggest that women and men do not share all the same predictors of mortality after surgery.

This study by Hannan and associates[159] from Albany, New York, utilized a state-wide data base containing clinical risk factors for cardiac surgery to investigate differences in in-hospital mortality rates for men and women undergoing CABG. The crude mortality rates for CABG for men and women were 3.08% and 5.43%, respectively, in New York State in 1989. When logistic regression analysis was used to control for preoperative risk, gender remained a significant predictor of mortality. Risk-adjusted mortality rates were 3.33% and 4.45% for men and women, respectively. The risk-adjusted odds ratio of women to men experiencing in-hospital death was 1.52.

To relate morbidity and mortality risk to preoperative severity of illness in patients undergoing CABG, Higgins and associates[160] from Cleveland, Ohio, in a retrospective analysis of 5,051 patients used univariate and logistic regression to identify risk factors associated with perioperative morbidity and mortality (Table 2-4). Prospective application of models was applied to a subsequent 2-year validation cohort numbering 4,069 persons. Included in the study were all adult patients undergoing CABG between July 1, 1986, and June 30, 1988 (reference group), and July 1, 1988, and June 30, 1990 (validation group). The main outcome measures were mortality and morbidity (AMI and use of intra-aortic balloon pump, mechanical ventilation for 3 or more days, neurological deficit, oliguric or anuric renal failure, or serious infection). Emergency procedure, preop-erative serum creatinine levels of >168 μmol/L, severe LV dysfunction, preoperative hematocrit of 0.34, increasing age, chronic pulmonary dis-ease, prior vascular surgery, reoperation, and mitral valve insufficiency were found to be predictive of mortality. In addition to these factors, diabetes mellitus, body weight of 65 kg or more, aortic stenosis, and cerebrovascular disease were predictive of morbidity. Logistic regression

TABLE 2-4. *Potential Factors Considered and Univariate Analysis Results (N = 5051).* Reproduced with permission from Higgins, et al.[160]*

Factor	Occurrence, %	Morbidity P	Morbidity OR	Mortality P	Mortality OR
Emergency case	3.1	<.001	7.01	<.001	6.25
Serum creatinine ≥168 μmol/L	3.5	<.001	4.27	<.001	7.39
Reoperation	18.5	<.001	1.94	<.001	2.10
Severe LV dysfunction	11.3	<.001	2.35	<.001	4.33
Mitral valve insufficiency	3.3	<.001	2.93	.002	2.96
Age ≥70 y	22.9	<.001	1.81	<.001	2.43
Diabetes, on medication	17.2	<.001	1.54	<.02	1.66
Weight ≤65 kg	15.1	<.001	1.89	<.001	2.22
Anemia (HCT ≤0.34)	8.7	<.001	2.60	<.001	4.66
COPD, on medication	7.5	<.001	1.71	<.001	2.70
Cerebrovascular disease	6.6	<.001	1.78	.09	1.65
Aortic stenosis, operated	4.0	<.001	2.20	<.001	3.42
Prior vascular surgery	5.6	<.001	1.98	<.001	3.59
Female gender	20.6	<.001	1.66	<.001	1.97
Aortic insufficiency, operated	1.9	<.001	2.34	.009	3.23
Left main trunk ≥70%	9.5	<.001	1.57	<.02	1.82
Congestive heart failure	9.0	<.001	2.30	<.001	3.65
Kidney disease by history	5.8	<.001	2.82	<.001	4.27
Kidney transplant or dialysis	0.2	.003	8.07	.02	11.33
History of angina†	65.9	<.02	0.75	<.02	0.61
Mitral valve stenosis	1.0	<.04	1.99	.1	2.49
History of cigarette smoking‡	41.6	.08	1.18	.6	1.10
Prior myocardial infarction	41.9	.1	1.14	.9	1.01
Prior lung surgery	0.4	.1	2.01	.09	4.16
Hypertension, treated	43.8	.3	1.09	.6	1.09
Liver disease	3.0	.7	1.08	1.0	0.77
Coronary artery stenosis >50%	99.6	1.0	0.97	.4	0.50
Total serum cholesterol ≥7.37 mmol/L§	12.7	.4	1.10	.4	1.23
Triglycerides ≥3.17 mmol/L§	12.4	.1	0.80	.9	0.98

*OR indicates odds ratio; LV, left ventricular; HCT, hematocrit; and COPD, chronic obstructive pulmonary disease.
†Sample size equals 3529.
‡Sample size equals 3804.
§Sample size equals 3782.

equations were developed, and a simple additive score for clinical use was designed by allocating each of these risk-factor values of 1 to 6 points. Both methods predict mortality. Increased morbidity was demonstrated with increases in score. The logistic or clinical models developed are superior to the currently available methods for comparing mortality outcome and provide previously unavailable information on morbidity based on preoperative status. The clinical scoring system is useful for preoperative estimates of morbidity and mortality risks.

Mortality: Medicare experience

Hartz and associates[161] from multiple USA medical centers compared mortality rates for Medicare patients who underwent CABG with those who had PTCA or both PTCA and CABG. Two data sets were used for the study: The first contained information on demographic factors, comorbidities and subsequent mortality on all 96,666 Medicare patients who had bypass surgery or angioplasty in 1985; the second contained additional detailed clinical data collected using the MedisGroups method on a random sample of 2,931 revascularization patients from 6 states.

From the national data set 30-day and 1-year mortality rates were 3.8 and 8.2% for 25,423 angioplasty patients and 6.4 and 11.8% for 71,243 bypass surgery patients. Mortality rates for the MedisGroups data were 4.4 and 8.5% for the angioplasty patients and 6.5 and 11.9% for the bypass surgery patients. After eliminating patients admitted with an AMI, mortality rates were 1.9 and 6.0% for 632 angioplasty patients and 5.1 and 10.8% for 1,730 bypass surgery patients. The risk-adjusted relative risk of mortality for bypass surgery versus angioplasty was 1.72 for all patients, 2.15 for low-risk patients and 0.90 for high-risk patients. Results suggest that low-risk patients have better survival with angioplasty because of lower short-term mortality.

Vein-graft stenosis

The influence of coronary artery stenoses on patient survival and event-free survival is known, but no studies have reported the long-term outcome of patients with stenoses in saphenous vein bypass grafts. Lytle and associates[162] from Cleveland, Ohio, retrospectively studied 723 patients who underwent a postoperative angiographic study that documented a stenosis of 20–99% in at least 1 saphenous vein graft and who did not undergo reoperation or PTCA within 1 year after that catheterization (Table 2-5). The mean follow-up interval was 83 months (range 1 to 237 months). For comparison, a group of 573 patients who underwent a postoperative catheterization that did not show any vein graft stenosis were also followed up. Cox regression analyses were used to identify

TABLE 2-5. *Characteristics at catheterization of patients with and without stenotic vein grafts. Reproduced with permission from Lytle, et al.*[162]

Variable	Patients with stenotic vein grafts (N = 723)		Patients with no stenotic vein grafts (N = 573)		p Value
	n	%	n	%	
Men	664	91.8	522	91.1	0.64
Age (mean)	57.4 years		57.2 years		0.70
Functional class at cath					
NYHA					
I	310	42.9	328	57.2	
II	294	40.7	186	32.5	<0.001
III	75	10.4	41	7.2	
IV	44	6.1	18	3.1	
CHF	49	6.8	17	3.0	0.002
Indication for cath					
Angina	368	50.9	199	34.7	
Myocardial infarction	67	9.3	69	12.0	<0.001
Routine	180	24.9	172	30.0	
Other	108	14.9	133	23.2	
LVF					
Normal-mild	553	76.5	437	76.3	
Moderate-severe	170	23.5	136	23.7	0.93
Extent of native vessel disease (≥50% stenosis)					
LMT	118	16.3	83	14.5	
1VD	49	6.7	75	13.1	<0.001
2VD	149	20.6	153	26.7	
3VD	407	56.3	262	45.7	
No. of stenotic vein grafts					
1	617	85.3	None		
2	98	13.6			
3	8	1.1			
No. of patent ITA grafts	195		138		
No. of patent vein grafts					
0	372		106		
1	269		288		
2	73		136		
≥3	9		43		

NYHA, New York Heart Association; *CHF*, congestive heart failure; for other abbreviations see Tables I to V.

predictors of late survival, reoperation-free survival, and event-free survival. For the entire group of patients with stenotic vein grafts, moderate or severe impairment of LV function, interval between operation and catheterization, older age, triple-vessel or LM CAD, and stenosis of the vein graft to the LAD coronary artery were associated with decreased late survival. Patients with an operation-to-catheterization interval ≥5 years were at particularly high risk, and multivariate analyses of that subgroup confirmed that a stenotic graft to the LAD artery was a strong predictor of decreased survival, decreased reoperation-free survival, and decreased event-free survival. Patients ≥5 years postoperatively with ≥50% stenosis of vein grafts to the LAD had survival of 70% and 50% at 2 and 5 years after catheterization, compared with 97% and 80% for those with ≥50% stenosis of the native LAD artery. Late vein graft stenoses are more dangerous than native coronary stenoses. Late stenoses in saphenous vein grafts to the LAD coronary artery predict a high rate of death and cardiac events and are an indication for reoperation.

Ventricular arrhythmias

To determine the incidence and characteristics of ventricular dysrhythmias (VPCs >30/min, VT ≥4 beats, and VF) and whether a relationship exists between VT and myocardial ischemia in patients undergoing CABG, Smith and associates[163] from San Francisco, California, continuously monitored 50 patients for 10 perioperative days using 2-lead electrocardiography. Electrocardiographic changes consistent with ischemia were defined as a reversible ST depression ≥1.0 mm, or ST elevation ≥2.0 mm from baseline, lasting at least 1 minute. Ventricular dysrhythmias developed in 10% of patients preoperatively and in 16% intraoperatively before CABG. The highest incidence occurred postoperatively, with ventricular dysrhythmias developing in 66% of patients (22% to 44% of patients on any postoperative day 0 to 7). VPCs were >30/hr in 6% of patients preoperatively, in 8% intraoperatively before bypass, and in 34% postoperatively (6% to 23% of patients on any postoperative day). Twenty-nine patients (58%) developed 76 verified episodes of ≥3 beats of VT. VT occurred in 6% of patients preoperatively (4 episodes), in 8% of patients intraoperatively prior to CABG (4 episodes), and 54% of patients postoperatively (5% to 21% on any postoperative day). No patient developed VF. All postoperative VT episodes (after tracheal intubation) were asymptomatic. Postoperatively, 48% of patients developed ischemia, compared with 12% preoperatively and 10% intraoperatively before CABG. Only 5 of 68 (7%) postoperative VT episodes occurred within 3 hours of an ischemic episode. None of the 5 adverse cardiac outcomes were preceded by VT. It was concluded that perioperative ventricular dysrhythmias are common and silent, and are most prevalent in the postoperative period; however, postoperative VT usually is not associated with myocardial ischemia or with an adverse cardiac outcome.

Atheroembolism from ascending aorta

As the ages of patients undergoing cardiac operations have increased, noncardiac causes of death have increased. To identify these causes of death, Blauth and associates[164] from Cleveland, Ohio, analyzed necropsy findings in 229 patients having CABG or cardiac valve operations between

1982 and 1989. The mean age was 66 ± 10 years and the range 32–94 years; 130 patients (59%) were male. Autopsies were complete in 129 patients (58%) and limited to the chest and abdomen in the remainder. Embolic disease was identified in 69 patients (31%). Atheroemboli or abnormalities consistent with atheroemboli were identified in 48 patients (22%). Fourteen patients had thromboembolism and 7 had disseminated intravascular coagulation. The prevalence of athereoembolic disease increased dramatically from 4.5% in 1982 to 48% in 1989 (Figure 2-20). Atheroembolic disease was found in the brain in 16% of patients, spleen in 11%, kidney in 10%, and pancreas in 7%. Thirty (62.5%) of the 48 patients had multiple athereoembolic sites. Atheroemboli were more common in patients undergoing coronary artery procedures (43/165; 26%) than in those undergoing valve procedures (5/56; 9%). There was a high correlation of atheroemboli with severe atherosclerosis of the ascending aorta. Atheroembolic events occurred in 46 of 123 patients (37%) with severe disease of the ascending aorta but in only 2 of 98 patients (2%) without significant ascending aorta disease. Forty-six of 48 patients (96%) who had evidence of atheroemboli had severe atherosclerosis of the ascending aorta. There was a direct correlation between age, severe atherosclerosis of the ascending aorta, and atheroemboli. Incremental risk factors for atheroemboli are peripheral vascular disease and severe atherosclerosis of the ascending aorta.

Cigarette smoking afterwards

Cavender and associates[165] in Birmingham, Alabama, ascertained how continued cigarette smoking or smoking cessation related to long-term survival and morbidity in patients with established CAD managed with medical therapy or CABG. Seven hundred eight patients were randomized to medical therapy or CABG surgery in the Coronary Artery Surgery Study (CASS) and were subgrouped according to smoking behavior during a

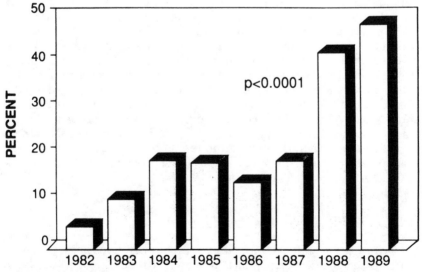

Fig. 2-20. Annual incidence of atheroembolic disease, 1982 to 1989. Reproduced with permission from Blauth, et al.[164]

mean 11-year follow-up interval. Survival at 10 years after entry into the study was 82% among 468 patients who reported no smoking during follow-up compared with 77% among the 312 patients who continued to smoke. Survival was 80% among those who smoked at entry but stopped versus 69% among those who continued smoking (Figure 2-21). Among those who smoked at baseline, continued smoking increased the relative risk of death by 1.73. After 10 years, those who smoked, in comparison with nonsmokers, were less likely to be angina free and more likely to be unemployed. They also had more activity limitation and hospital admissions, especially for chest pain, AMI, cardiac catheterization, peripheral vascular surgery, and stroke. Thus, among patients with documented CAD, continued cigarette smoking may result in decreased survival, especially among those who undergo CABG. Smokers have more angina, greater physical activity limitation, and more hospital admissions.

Exercise testing afterwards

The predictive value of a postoperative exercise test in terms of cardiac events after CABG was prospectively studied by Yli-Mayry and associates[166] from Oulu, Finland, in 231 consecutive patients. During a 5-year follow-up there were 28 cardiac events (12%), of which 15 were cardiac deaths (13 sudden), and 13 were nonfatal AMIs. There was no difference in the rate of graft patency between groups with and without cardiac events, but EF was lower in patients with than without events (51 ± 16% vs 58 ± 10%). Duration of the exercise test was shorter, and maximal work load was lower in patients with cardiac events. The prevalence of ≥1 mm ST-segment depression was 22% (symptomatic in 25%, and silent in 75%) and did not differ between groups with and without cardiac events. After adjustment for prognostic variables using the proportional hazards method, diuretic treatment and a low postoperative EF remained signifi-

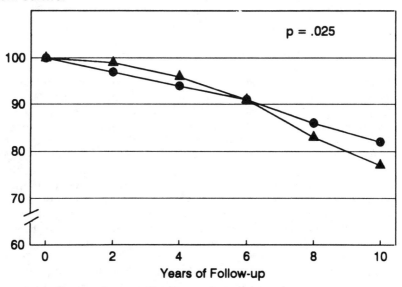

Fig. 2-21. Ten-year survival among all randomized patients. Survival among nonsmokers (circles, n = 468) was greater than among smokers (triangles, n = 312) at 10-year follow-up (82% vs. 77%). Reproduced with permission from Cavender, et al.[165]

cant for predicting the risk of cardiac events within 5 years of CABG, but exercise duration and work load did not have any significant predictive value. Thus, the predictive value of a postoperative exercise test is limited, and signs of impaired LV function are of greater significance for the 5-year prognosis after CABG than are those of AMI.

Exercise echocardiography afterwards

Exercise echocardiography was used by Crouse and associates[167] from Kansas City, Missouri, to assess the adequacy of regional myocardial perfusion in 125 patients who had undergone CABG. There were 108 men and 17 women (mean age 65 years) evaluated from 6 weeks to 16 years (mean 7 years) after surgery. Resting parasternal long- and short-axis and apical 4- and 2-chamber echocardiograms were recorded, digitized and stored. Maximal, symptom-limited upright treadmill exercise was then performed with continuous electrocardiographic monitoring. Repeat echocardiographic imaging and digitization were repeated within 1 minute of exercise termination. Resting and postexercise digitized echocardiograms were compared. A normal regional wall motion response to exercise consisted of improved segmental contraction and was used to predict uncompromised regional vascular supply. Unimproved or worsened segmental contraction after exercise was abnormal and was used as a predictor of regional vascular insufficiency. All patients underwent cardiac catheterization within 1 month after exercise testing. Regional coronary insufficiency was considered to exist when a segment's major vascular conduit exhibited ≥50% luminal diameter reduction. Compared with the simultaneously acquired stress electrocardiogram, exercise echocardiography had superior sensitivity (98 vs 41%), specificity (92 vs 67%), positive predictive value (99 vs 91%), and negative predictive value (86 vs 12%). In addition, exercise echocardiography correlated closely with the extent and regional distribution of compromised vascular supply. Exercise echocardiography is a highly sensitive, specific and accurate screening test for abnormal global and regional myocardial vascular supply in patients who have undergone CABG.

Ultrasound of internal mammary artery

De Bono and associates[168] from Leicester, UK, used transcutaneous Doppler ultrasound to examine internal-mammary-artery (IMA) blood-flow in 26 patients with IMA coronary bypass grafts. The ungrafted right IMA could be seen in all of 19 patients, the grafted left IMA in 16 of 26, and the grafted right IMA in 3 of 7. The velocity profile recorded from the proximal part of the grafted IMA is distinct from that of an ungrafted artery, with a systolic peak which reflects graft capacitance in the face of high intramyocardial resistance, and a diastolic peak which represents graft conductance when intramyocardial resistance is low. Total graft blood-flow can be estimated from the mean velocity and the measured vessel diameter; resting flows ranged from 22 to 79 ml/min. In recently grafted patients, resting graft blood-flow correlated with myocardial "run-off" estimated from preoperative arteriograms; graft blood-flow increased appropriately with exercise. This simple, noninvasive technique to measure IMA graft blood-flow may find applications for routine postoperative follow-up of patients with IMA grafts and for studies on the physiology and pharmacology of coronary artery blood-flow.

In chronic renal failure

Insulin-dependent diabetic patients found to have substantial CAD at the time of assessment for renal transplantation have 2-year survival of <50%. Because most of these patients have no angina, their management is controversial. Manske and associates[169] from Minneapolis, Minnesota, tried to find out whether coronary artery revascularization in such patients might decrease the combined incidence of unstable angina, AMI, and cardiac death. One hundred and fifty-one consecutive insulin-dependent diabetic candidates for renal transplantation underwent coronary angiography. Thirty-one had stenoses >75% in ≥1 coronary arteries, atypical chest pain or no chest pain, and a LVEF >0.35. Of these, 26 agreed to be randomly assigned medical treatment (a calcium-channel-blocking drug plus aspirin) or revascularization (angioplasty or CABG). Ten of 13 medically managed and 2 of 13 revascularized patients had a cardiovascular endpoint within a median of 8.4 months of coronary angiography. Four medically managed patients died of AMI during follow-up. Thus, revascularization decreased the frequency of cardiac events in insulin-dependent diabetic patients with chronic renal failure and symptomless CAD (Figure 2-22).

In radiation-induced atherosclerosis

Radiation-associated coronary atherosclerosis is a potential problem for patients who have had mediastinal irradiation for malignant tumors. Hicks[170] from Rochester, New York, reviewed 14 patients with radiation-associated coronary atherosclerosis and analyzed post-surgical problems and long-term outcome. Fourteen patients with radiation-associated coronary atherosclerosis and class III and IV New York Heart Association

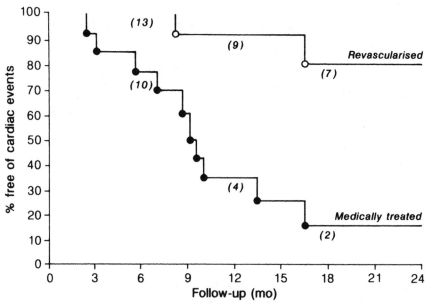

Fig. 2-22. Cardiovascular events in medically treated and revascularised patients. Nos in parentheses = patients available for follow-up. Reproduced with permission from Manske, et al.[169]

symptoms were identified because of mediastinal or chest wall irradiation (30 Gy) associated with anterior epicardial discoloration or fibrosis, aortitis with adventitial thickening, and inflammatory process over a proximal coronary artery. Two distinct treatment groups were analyzed. Coronary artery operation resulted in one hospital death, with vein grafts being used predominantly. The internal mammary artery could only be used in 3 patients because of vessel friability and mediastinal fibrosis. Postoperative RV dysfunction and pulmonary problems were frequent. Severe pericardial inflammatory complications (fibrosis with graft closure, and constrictive pericarditis) present in 2 early patients resulted in routine anterior pericardiectomy after coronary artery operation without further problems. Long-term follow-up (100%) (range, 11 to 74 months) revealed that 1 patient died late and of the remainder (12 patients), 11 were in New York Heart Association class I and 1 in class II, experiencing 3 myocardial events. Thus, patients with radiation-associated coronary atherosclerosis have a low operative mortality but have risk of early RV and pulmonary dysfunction. The routine use of internal mammary artery may not be possible and anterior pericardiectomy is recommended. Long-term results are excellent and no evidence of accelerated disease has been noted.

Heart size as prognostic sign

Goor and associates[171] from Tel Aviv, Israel, investigated the effect of cardiomegaly by chest x-ray (cardiothoracic ratio >0.5) on operative and late mortality in patients with LV dysfunction undergoing CABG. The study group consisted of 178 patients with an LVEF <45% and the patients were operated on from 1978–1985: 45 patients had an LVEF <30% and 133 patients had LVEF from 31% to 45%. Twenty-four of the 45 patients (53%) and 54 of the 133 patients (41%) had cardiomegaly (Figure 2-23).

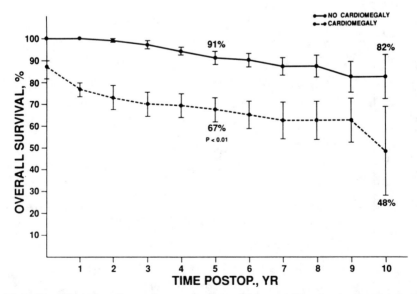

Fig. 2-23. Effect of cardiomegaly on operative and late mortality of patients with infarct-borne left ventricular dysfunction undergoing coronary bypass operations. Reproduced with permission from Gour, et al.[171]

All 4 deaths in the group of 45 patients with LVEF <30% and all 6 deaths in the group with LVEF from 31% to 45% had cardiomegaly. Regardless of the severity of the LV dysfunction, there were no operative deaths among the patients with normal heart size. Cardiomegaly appears to be a poor prognostic sign in patients undergoing CABG.

Aspirin afterwards

In an investigation by Johnson and colleagues[172] from Milwaukee, Wisconsin, for the years 1968 through 1981, 5618 patients in a single cardiovascular surgery practice underwent CABG. Detailed clinical information was obtained during hospitalization and entered into a data base. All surviving patients were surveyed for aspirin use on 4 occasions: in 1984, 1985, 1986 and 1987. A subgroup of 2395 patients gave consistent answers on every returned survey. The group that answered consistently positive, had a 5-year survival rate of 79%; those who answered consistently negative had a 5-year survival rate of 67%. Stepwise logistic regression showed that, after adjusting for patient characteristics, the relative risk of death was 58% for consistent aspirin users compared with consistent non-aspirin users. This study provides evidence that regular aspirin use after CABG may enhance survival.

Re-operation

Between January 1980 and May 1988, Dougenis and associates[173] from New Castle-Upon-Tyne, UK, performed CABG for the first time in 1,363 patients and 49 had a second CABG for recurrent angina by the same surgeon. There were 42 males and 5 females with a mean age of 53.6 years. Mean time since first operation was 68.9 (37 SD) months. Prior to surgery only 8 (16.3%) were still working. There were 3 hospital deaths and 2 late deaths at 2.5 and 3.5 years after surgery and 1 patient underwent cardiac transplantation at 1.5 years. Follow-up has been completed up to March 1989, mean 3.7 years, range 10–108 months. Questionnaires were sent to all patients concerning the financial and functional situation. Hospital expenses were calculated (a) prospectively for 15 consecutive first time CABGs and for 5 second time CABGs, (b) retrospectively from patients' records with the help of a simple computer program. The final figures were corrected for inflation rates. The 1- and 5-year actuarial probability of angina-free interval was 87.5% and 40% respectively. Eight patients (12.2%) had no benefit, 6 (13.6%) had benefit but were not able to work, 16 (36.4%) were able to work but unemployed and 14 (13.8%) were fully employed producing a total salary of 69,072 pounds per annum. Hospital expenses were: first time CABG 3645–4049 pounds, second time CABG 6290–7235 pounds. The total for the entire group was 308,166 pounds. Repeated CABG can be accomplished with reasonable mortality and has good late results. However, financially, in this region it is not as cost effective, being 1.8 times more expensive and half as good as a first operation at restoring patients to work.

To define the incidence, possible causes, operative procedure, and early and medium term results of patients undergoing the reoperation of CAD, Akl and associates[174] from Harefield, UK, performed a retrospective analysis of 115 patients who had reoperation for recurrent angina 1–17 years (mean 7.4) after primary CABG (Figure 2-24). They received 279 grafts

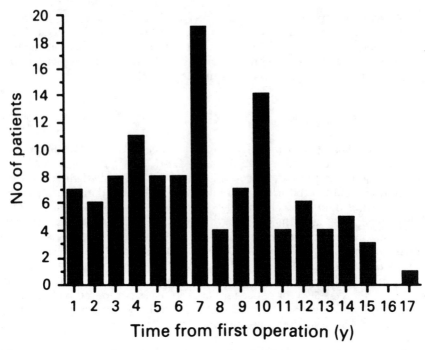

Fig. 2-24. Time interval to repeat CABG. Reproduced with permission from AKI, et. al.[174]

(2.4 grafts per patient); 58% of the grafts were anasatomosed to previously grafted vessels. The internal mammary artery was used in 87% of patients who required grafts to the LAD coronary artery. Reoperation accounted for 8.3% of the total number of patients who underwent CABG. Graft failure alone or in combination with other factors was judged to be the cause of recurrence of symptoms in 87%. Forty-two percent of patients had ≥2 coronary risk factors. The early mortality was 5.2% and the actuarial survival at 5 and 10 years was 90% and 88% respectively. Eighty-five percent of the survivors had initial complete relief of angina and 14% had partial involvement. Freedom from recurrent symptoms at 5 and 10 years was 67% and 35%, respectively (Figure 2-25). Vein graft failure either alone or in combination with progression of native CAD was the main cause for symptomatic deterioration after CABG.

Cosgrove and associates[175] from Cleveland, Ohio, tested the efficacy and safety of *aprotinin* in 169 patients undergoing isolated CABG. Patients were randomly assigned to high-dose aprotinin, low-dose aprotinin, or placebo treatment groups in a double-blind, placebo-controlled study. Treatment groups did not differ significantly with respect to age, sex, red cell mass, number of grafts, use of internal thoracic artery, or incidence of preoperative aspirin therapy. Patients treated with aprotinin had a significant reduction in postoperative chest tube drainage (720 ± 753, 866 ± 1,636, and 1,121 ± 683 mL, respectively), for high-dose aprotinin, low-dose aprotinin, and placebo. Transfusion requirements were reduced in aprotinin-treated patients (2.1 ± 4.2, 4.8 ± 11.8, and 4.1 ± 6.2 units for high-dose, low-dose, and placebo, respectively). A similar reduction

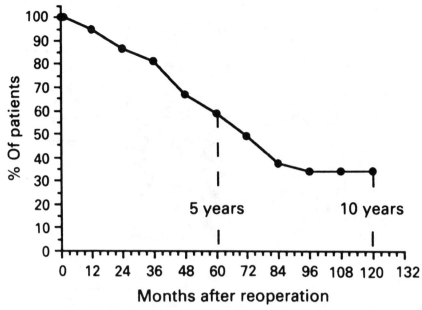

Fig. 2-25. Freedom from recurrence of symptoms after reoperation (n = 115). Reproduced with permission from AKI, et. al.[174]

in chest tube drainage and transfusion requirements was seen in patients using aspirin preoperatively. Q-wave AMIs were increased in the aprotinin subgroups (17.5%, 14.3%, and 8.9% for high-dose, low-dose, and placebo groups; not significant). Acute vein graft thrombosis was found in 6 of 12 vein grafts studied at postmortem examination in patients receiving aprotinin but not in any of 5 grafts in patients receiving placebo. The authors concluded that aprotinin is extremely effective in reducing bleeding and transfusion requirements and may increase the risk of graft thrombosis.

Composition of plaques in saphenous vein conduits

Mautner and associates[176] from Bethesda, Maryland, described quantitatively the composition of atherosclerotic plaques in saphenous vein grafts used for aortocoronary bypass and compared the findings to those in the native coronary arteries in the same men. A total of 607 five-mm segments of saphenous veins and 797 five-mm segments of native coronary arteries were examined by computerized planimetric technique in 19 men, aged 39 to 82 years (mean 61), who had survived bypass operation for >1 year. Comparison of the mean percentages of the plaque components in saphenous vein grafts in place for 14 to 26 months with those of the native coronary arteries revealed significant differences: cellular fibrous tissue, 86 vs 7%; dense fibrous tissue, 13 vs 82%. As survival time after the bypass operation increased, composition of the plaques in the saphenous veins changed so that by approximately 80 months the amounts of cellular and dense fibrous tissue in both saphenous vein grafts and native coronary arteries were similar: 10 vs 16%, and 75 vs 71%

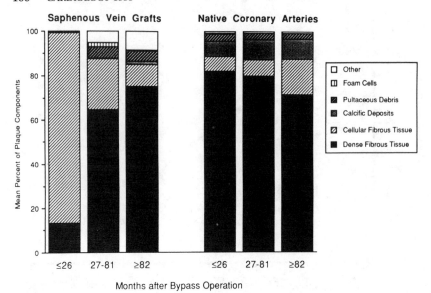

Fig. 2-26. Graph showing the relation of plaque composition in saphenous vein grafts and in the native epicardial coronary arteries according to the time interval from bypass operation to death. In patients surviving ≤26 months cellular fibrous tissue was the dominant component in the plaques of the saphenous vein grafts. After ≥82 months the plaques of the saphenous vein grafts consisted predominantly of dense fibrous tissue, similar to the plaque composition in the native coronary arteries. The composition of the plaques in the native coronary arteries remained constant after bypass operation. The category "Other" includes foam cells plus lymphocytes and pure inflammatory infiltration. Reproduced with permission from Mautner, et al.[176]

(Figure 2-26). Thus, by about 7 years after a coronary bypass operation the composition of plaques in saphenous vein grafts is similar to that in the native coronary arteries of the same patients.

References

1. Coronary heart disease incidence, by Sex—United States, 1971–1987. MMWR 1992 (July 24);41:526–529.

2. Trends in Coronary Artery Disease Mortality USA 1980–1988. Morbidity and Mortality Weekly Report 1992(July 31);41(no. 30):548.

3. Bickell NA, Pieper KS, Lee KL, Mark DB, Glower DD, Pryor DB, Califf RM: Referral patterns for coronary artery disease treatment: Gender bias or good clinical judgment? An Intern Med 1992 (May 15);116:791–797.

4. Eysmann SB, Douglas PS: Reperfusion and revascularization strategies for coronary artery disease in women. JAMA 1992 (Oct 14);268:1903–1907.

5. Graboys TB, Biegelsen B, Lampert S, Blatt CM, Lown B: Results of a second-opinion trial among patients recommended for coronary angiography. JAMA 1992 (Nov 11);268:2537–2540.

6. Sheldahl LM, Wilke NA, Dougherty SM, Levandoski SG, Hoffman MD, Tristani FE: Effect of age and coronary artery disease on response to snow shoveling. J Am Coll Cardiol 1992 (November);20:1111–7.

7. Mautner SL, Lin F, Roberts WC: Composition of atherosclerotic plaques in the epicardial coronary arteries in juvenile (type I) diabetes mellitus. Am J Cardiol 1992 (Nov 15);70:1264–1268.

8. Om A, Warner M, Sabri N, Cecich L, Vetrovec G: Frequency of coronary artery disease and left ventricular dysfunction in cocaine users. Am J Cardiol 1992 (June 15);69:1549–1552.

9. Akagi T, Rose V, Benson LN, Newman A, Freedom RM: Outcome of coronary artery aneurysms after Kawasaki disease. J Pediatr (November) 1992;121:689–694.

10. Hubbard BL, Gibbons RJ, Lapeyre AC III, Zinsmeister AR, Clements IP: Identification of severe coronary artery disease using simple clinical parameters. Arch Intern Med 1992 (Feb);152:309–312.

11. Tranchesi B Jr, Barbosa V, Piva DE, Albuquerque C, Caramelli B, Gebara O, Filho RDD, Nakano O, Bellotti G, Pileggi F: Diagonal earlobe crease as a marker of the presence and extent of coronary atherosclerosis. Am J Cardiol 1992 (Dec 1);70:1417–1420.

12. Loecker TH, Schwartz RS, Cotta CW, Hickman JR Jr: Fluoroscopic coronary artery calcification and associated coronary disease in asymptomatic young men. J Am Coll Cardiol 1992 (May);19:1167–72.

13. Bobbio M, Detrano R, Schmid J-J, Janosi A, Righetti A, Pfisterer M, Steinbrunn W, Guppy KH, Abi-Mansour P, Deckers JW, Colombo A, Lehmann KG, Olson HG: Exercise-induced ST depression and ST/heart rate index to predict triple-vessel or left main coronary disease: a multicenter analysis. J Am Coll Cardiol 1992 (January);19:11–18.

14. Miranda CP, Liu J, Kadar A, Janosi A, Froning J, Lehmann KG, Froelicher FV: Usefulness of exercise-induced ST-segment depression in the inferior leads during exercise testing as a marker for coronary artery disease. Am J Cardiol 1992 (Feb 1);69:303–307.

15. Watson G, Mechling E, Ewy GA: Clinical significance of early vs late hypotensive blood pressure response to treadmill exercise. Arch Intern Med 1992 (May);152:1005–1008.

16. Iskandrian AS, Kegel JG, Lemlek J, Heo J, Cave V, Iskandrian B: Mechanism of exercise-induced hypotension in coronary artery disease. Am J Cardiol 1992 (June 15);69:1517–1520.

17. Hambrecht RP, Schuler GC, Muth T, Grunze MF, Marburger CT, Niebauer J, Methfessel SM, Kubler W: Greater diagnostic sensitivity of treadmill versus cycle exercise testing of asymptomatic men with coronary artery disease. Am J Cardiol 1992 (July 15);70:141–146.

18. Ribisl PM, Morris CK, Kawaguchi T, Ueshima K, Froelicher VF: Angiographic patterns and severe coronary artery disease: Exercise test correlates. Arch Intern Med 1992 (Aug);152:1618–1624.

19. Quinones MA, Vernai MS, Haichin RM, Mahmarian JJ, Suarez J, Zoghbi WA: Exercise Echocardiography Versus [201]TI Single-Photon Emission Computed Tomography in Evaluation of Coronary Artery Disease Analysis of 292 Patients. Circulation 1992 (March);85:1026–1031.

20. Marwick TH, Nemec JJ, Pashkow FJ, Stewart WJ, Salcedo EE: Accuracy and limitations of exercise echocardiography in a routine clinical setting. J Am Coll Cardiol 1992 (January);19:74–81.

21. Sawada SG, Ryan T, Segar D, Atherton L, Fineberg N, Davis C, Feigenbaum H: Distinguishing ischemic cardiomyopathy from nonischemic dilated cardiomyopathy with coronary echocardiography. J Am Coll Cardiol 1992 (May);19:1223–8.

22. Christian TF, Miller TD, Bailey KR, Gibbons RJ: Noninvasive identification of severe coronary artery disease using exercise tomographic thallium-201 imaging. Am J Cardiol 1992 (Jul 1);70:14–20.

23. Dilsizian V, Freedman NMT, Bacharach SL, Perrone-Filardi P, Bonow RO: Regional Thallium Uptake in Irreversible Activity After Reinjection Distinguishes Viable From Nonviable Myocardium. Circulation 1992 (February);85:627–634.

24. Delonca J, Camenziend E, Meier B, Righetti A: Limits of thallium-201 exercise scintigraphy to detect coronary disease in patients with complete and permanent bundle branch block: A review of 134 cases. Am Heart J 1992 (May);123;1201–1207.

25. O'Keefe JH Jr, Bateman TM, Silvestri R, Barnhart C: Safety and diagnostic accuracy of adenosine thallium-201 scintigraphy in patients unable to exercise and those with left bundle branch block. Am Heart J 1992 (September);124;614–621.

26. Gupta NC, Esterbrooks DJ, Hilleman DE, Mohiuddin SM, for the GE SPECT Multicenter Adenosine Study Group: Comparison of adenosine and exercise thallium-201 single-photon emission computed tomography (SPECT) myocardial perfusion imaging. J Am Coll Cardiol 1992 (February);19:248–57.

27. Nishimura S, Mahmarian JJ, Boyce TM, Verani MS: Equivalence between adenosine

and exercise thallium-201 myocardial tomography: a multicenter, prospective, cross-over trial. J Am Coll Cardiol 1992;20:265–75.

28. Lette J, Waters D, Bernier H, Champagne P, Lassonde J, Picard M, Cerino M, Nattel S, Boucher Y, Heyen F, Dube S: Preoperative and long-term cardiac risk assessment: Predictive value of 23 clinical descriptors, 7 multivariate scoring systems, and quantitative dipyridamole imaging in 360 patients. An of Surg 1992 (Aug);216:192–204.

29. Simons DB, Schwartz RS, Edwards WD, Sheedy PF, Breen JF, Rumberger JA: Noninvasive definition of anatomic coronary artery disease by ultrafast computed tomographic scanning: A quantitative pathologic comparison study. J Am Coll Cardiol 1992 (November);20:1118–26.

30. St. Goar F, Pinto F, Alderman E, Fitzgerald P, Stinson E, Billingham M, Popp R: Detection of Coronary Atherosclerosis in Young Adult Hearts Using Intravascular Ultrasound. Circulation 1992 (September);86:756–763.

31. Goel M, Wong ND, Eisenberg H, Hagar J, Kelly K, Tobis JM: Risk factor correlates of coronary calcium as evaluated by ultrafast computed tomography. Am J Cardiol 1992 (Oct 22);70:977–980.

32. Lichtlen P, Nikutta P, Jost S, Deckers J, Wiese B, Rafflenbeul W, and the INTACT Study Group: Anatomical Progression of Coronary Artery Disease in Humans as Seen by Prospective, Repeated, Quantitated Coronary Angiography, Relation to Clinical Events and Risk Factors. Circulation 1992 (September);86:828–838.

33. Raby KE, Barry J, Creager MA, Cook EF, Weisberg MC, Goldman L: Detection and significance of intraoperative and postoperative myocardial ischemia in peripheral vascular surgery. JAMA 1992 (July 8);268:222–227.

34. Lee TH, Ting HH, Shammash JB, Soukup JR, Goldman L: Long-term survival of emergency department patients with acute chest pain. Am J Cardiol 1992 (Jan 15);69:145–151.

35. Liao Y, Cooper RS, Ghali JK, Szocka A: Survival rates with coronary artery disease for black women compared with black men. JAMA 1992 (Oct 14);268:1867–1871.

36. Boehrer JD, Lange RA, Willard JE, Hillis LD: Markedly increased periprocedure mortality of cardiac catheterization in patients with severe narrowing of the left main coronary artery. Am J Cardiol 1992 (Dec 1);70:1388–1390.

37. Lim R, Dyke L, Dymond DS: Effect on prognosis of abolition of exercise-induced painless myocardial ischemia by medical therapy. Am J Cardiol 1992 (Mar 15);69:733–735.

38. Mark DB, Lam LC, Lee KL, Clapp-Channing NE, Williams RB, Pryor DB, Califf RM, Hlatky MA: Identification of Patients with Coronary Disease at High Risk for Loss of Employment, A Prospective Validation Study. Circulation 1992 (November);86:1485–1494.

39. Galderisi M, Lauer MS, Levy D: Echocardiographic determinants of clinical outcome in subjects with coronary artery disease (the Framingham Heart Study). Am J Cardiol 1992 (Oct 15) 70:971–976.

40. Hilton TC, Shaw LJ, Chaitman BR, Stocke KS, Goodgold HM, Miller DD: Prognostic significance of exercise thallium-201 testing in patients aged 70 years with known or suspected coronary artery disease. Am J Cardiol 1992 (Jan 1);69:45–50.

41. Shaw L, Chaitman BR, Hilton TC, Stocke K, Younis LT, Caralis DG, Kong BA, Miller D: Prognostic value of dipyridamole thallium-201 imaging in elderly patients. J Am Coll Cardiol 1992 (June);19:1390–8.

42. Eitzman D, Al-Aouar Z, Kanter HL, vom Dahl J, Kirsh M, Deeb GM, Schwaiger M: Clinical outcome of patients with advanced coronary artery disease after viability studies with positron emission tomography. J Am Coll Cardiol 1992 (September);20:559–65.

43. Mangano DT, Browner WS, Hollenberg M, Li J, Tateo IM: Long-term cardiac prognosis following noncardiac surgery. JAMA 1992 (July 8);268:233–239.

44. Hollenberg M, Mangano DT, Browner WS, London MJ, Tubau JF, Tateo IM: Predictors of postoperative myocardial ischemia in patients undergoing noncardiac surgery. JAMA 1992 (July 8);268:205–209.

45. Romeo F, Rosano GM, Martuscelli E, Valente A, Reale A: Unstable angina: Role of silent ischemia and total ischemia time (silent plus painful ischemia), a 6-year follow-up. J Am Coll Cardiol 1992 (May);19:1173–9.

46. Warner M, Disciascio G, Kohli R, Sabri N, Goudreau E, Cowley MJ, Vetrovec GW: Frequency

and predictors of left ventricular segmental dysfunction in patients with recent rest angina. Am J Cardiol 1992 (June 15);69:1521–1524.

47. Neri Seneri G, Abbate R, Gori A, Attanasio M, Martini F, Giusti B, Dabizzi P, Poggesi L, Modesti P, Trotta F, Rostagno C, Boddi M, Gensini G: Transient Intermittent Lymphocyte Activation Is Responsible for the Instability of Angina. Circulation 1992 (September);86:790–797.

48. Hamm CW, Ravkilde J, Gerhardt W, Jorgensen P, Peheim E, Ljungdahl L, Goldmann B, Katus HA: The prognostic value of serum troponin T in unstable angina. N Engl J Med 1992 (July 16);327:146–150.

49. Mizuno K, Satomura K, Miyamoto A, Arakawa K, Shibuya T, Arai T, Kurita A, Nakamura H, Ambrose JA: Angioscopic evaluation of coronary-artery thrombi in acute coronary syndromes: Angioscopic evaluation of coronary-artery thrombi in acute coronary syndromes. N Engl J Med 1992 (Jan 30);326:287–291.

50. Freeman MR, Langer A, Wilson RF, Morgan CD, Armstrong PW: Thrombolysis in Unstable Angina Randomized Double-Blind Trial of t-PA and Placebo. Circulation 1992 (January);85:150–157.

51. Chaudhary H, Crozier I, Hamer A, Foy S, Shirlaw T, Ikram H: Tissue plasminogen activator using a rapid-infusion low-dose regimen for unstable angina. Am J Cardiol 1992 (Jan 15);69:173–175.

52. Bar FW, Verheugt FW, Col J, Materne P, Monassier JP, Geslin PG, Metzger J, Raynaud P, Foucault J, de Zwaan C, Vermeer F: Thrombolysis in Patients With Unstable Angina Improves the Angiographic but Not in Clinical Outcome, Results of UNASEM, A Multicenter, Randomized, Placebo-Controlled, Clinical Trial with Anistreplase. Circulation 1992 (July);86:131–137.

53. Hegele R, Freeman M, Langer A, Connelly P, Armstrong P: Acute Reduction of Lipoprotein(a) by Tissue-Type Plasminogen Activator. Circulation 1992 (June);85:2034–2038.

54. Schreiber TL, Rizik D, White C, Sharma GVRK, Cowley M, Macina G, Reddy PS, Kantounis L, Timis GC, Margulis A, Bunnell P, Barker W, Sasahara A: Randomized Trial of Thrombolysis Versus Heparin in Unstable Angina. Circulation 1992 (November);86:1407–1414.

55. Theroux P, Waters D, Lam J, Juneau M, McCans J: Reactivation of unstable angina after the discontinuation of heparin. N Engl J Med 1992 (July 16);327:141–145.

56. Grambow DW, Topol EJ: Effect of maximal medical therapy on refractoriness of unstable angina pectoris. Am J Cardiol 1992 (Sept 1);70:577–581.

57. Stammen F, De Scheerder I, Glazier JJ, Van Lierde J, Vrolix M, Willems JL, De Geest H, Piessens, J: Immediate and follow-up results of the conservative coronary angioplasty strategy for unstable angina pectoris. Am J Cardiol 1992 (June 15);69:1533–1537.

58. Taki J, Yasuda T, Flamm SD, Hutter A, Gold HK, Leinbach R, Strauss HW: Comparison of painful and painless left ventricular dysfunction recorded during ambulatory ventricular function monitoring in angina pectoris secondary to coronary artery disease. Am J Cardiol 1992 (Dec 15);70:1555–1558.

59. Panza JA, Diodati JG, Callahan TS, Epstein SE, Quyyumi AA: Role of increases in heart rate in determining the occurrence and frequency of myocardial ischemia during daily life in patients with stable coronary artery disease. J Am Coll Cardiol 1992 (November);20:1092–8.

60. Diodati JG, Cannon RO III, Epstein SE, Quyyumi AA: Platelet Hyperaggregability Across the Coronary Bed in Response to Rapid Atrial Pacing in Patients With Stable Coronary Artery Disease. Circulation 1992 (October);86:1186–1193.

61. Juul-Moller S, Edvardsson N, Jahnmatz B, Rosen A, Sorensen S, Omblus R: Double-blind trial of aspirin in primary prevention of myocardial infarction in patients with stable chronic angina pectoris. Lancet 1992 (Dec 12);340:1421–1425.

62. Parmley WW, Nesto RW, Singh BN, Deanfield J, Gottlieb SO, and the N-CAP Study Group: Attenuation of the circadian patterns of myocardial ischemia with nifedipine GITS in patients with chronic stable angina. J Am Coll Cardiol 1992 (June);19:1380–9.

63. Mulcahy D, Keegan J, Phadke K, Wright C, Sparrow J, Purcell H, Fox K: Effects of coronary artery bypass surgery and angioplasty on the total ischemic burden: A study of exercise testing and ambulatory ST segment monitoring. Am Heart J 1992 (March);123:597–603.

64. The VA Coronary Artery Bypass Surgery Cooperative Study Group: Eighteen-Year Fol-

low-up in the Veterans Affairs Cooperative Study of Coronary Artery Bypass Surgery for Stable Angina. Circulation 1992 (July);86:121–130.

65. Naka M, Hiramatsu K, Aizawa T, Momose A, Yoshizawa K, Shigematsu S, Ishihara F, Niwa A, Yamada T: Silent myocardial ischemia in patients with non-insulin-dependent diabetes mellitus as judged by treadmill exercise testing and coronary arteriography. Am Heart J 1992 (January);123:46–53.

66. Nyman I, Larsson H, Areskog M, Areskog N-H, Walletin L, and the RISC study group: The predictive value of silent ischemia at an exercise test before discharge after an episode of unstable coronary artery disease. Am Heart J 1992 (February);123:324–331.

67. Kurita A, Takase B, Uehata A, Sugahara H, Nishioka T, Maruyama T, Satomura K, Mizuno K, Nakamura H: Differences in plasma β-endorphin and bradykinin levels between patients with painless or with painful myocardial ischemia. Am Heart J 1992 (February);123:304–309.

68. Quyyumi AA, Panza JA, Diodati JG, Dilsizian V, Callahan TS, Bonow RO: Relation between left ventricular function at rest and with exercise and silent myocardial ischemia. J Am Coll Cardiol 1992 (April);19:962–967.

69. Nyman I, Larsson H, Wallentin L, The Research Group on Instability in Coronary Artery Disease in Southeast Sweden: Lancet 1992 (Aug 29);340:497–501.

70. Kaski JC, Tousoulis D, McFadden E, Crea F, Pereira WI, Maseri A: Variant Angina Pectoris Role of Coronary Spasm in the Development of Fixed Coronary Obstructions. Circulation 1992 (February);85:619–626.

71. Caralis DG, Deligonul U, Kern MJ, and Cohen JD: Smoking Is a Risk Factor for Coronary Spasm In Young Women. Circulation 1992 (March);85:905–909.

72. Nobuyoshi M, Abe M, Nosaka H, Kimura T, Yokoi H, Hamasaki N, Shindo T, Kimura K, Nakamura T, Nakagawa Y, Shiode N, Sakamoto A, Kakura H, Iwasaki Y, Kim K, Kitaguchi S: Statistical analysis of clinical risk factors for coronary artery spasm: Identification of the most important determinant. Am Heart J 1992 (July); 124:32–38.

73. Myerburg RJ, Kessler KM, Mallon SM, Cox MM, Demarchena E, Interian A Jr, Castellanos A: Life-threatening ventricular arrhythmias in patients with silent myocardial ischemia due to coronary artery spasm. N Engl J Med 1992 (May 28);326:1451–1455.

74. Ozaki Y, Takatsu F, Osugi J, Sugiishi M, Watarai M, Anno T, Tyama J: Long-term study of recurrent vasospastic angina using coronary angiograms during ergonovine provocation tests. Am Heart J 1992 (May);123:1191–1198.

75. Harding MB, Leithe ME, Mark DB, Nelson CL, Harrison JK, Hermiller JB, Davidson CJ, Pryor DB, Bashore TM: Ergonovine maleate testing during cardiac catheterization: A 10-year perspective in 3,447 patients without significant coronary artery disease or Prinzmetal's variant angina. J Am Coll Cardiol 1992 (July);20:107–11.

76. Sakata K, Hoshino T, Yoshida H, Ono N, Ohtani S, Yokoyama S, Mori N, Kaburagi T, Kurata C, Urano T, Takada Y, Takada A: Circadian fluctuations of tissue plasminogen activator antigen and plasminogen activator inhibitor-1 antigens in vasospastic angina. Am Heart J 1992 (October);124:854–860.

77. Vrints CJM, Bult H, Hitter E, Herman AG, Snoeck JP: Impaired endothelium-dependent cholinergic coronary vasodilation in patients with angina and normal coronary arteriograms. J Am Coll Cardiol 1992 (January);19:21–31.

78. Sütsch G, Hess OM, Franzeck UK, Dörffler T, Bollinger A, Krayenbühl HP: Cutaneous and coronary flow reserve in patients with microvascular angina. J Am Coll Cardiol 1992 (July);20:78–84.

79. Watts GF, Lewis B, Brunt JNH, Lewis ES, Coltart DJ, Smith LDR, Mann JI, Swan AV: Effects of coronary artery disease of lipid-lowering diet, or diet plus cholestyramine, in the St. Thomas' Atherosclerosis Regression Study (STARS). Lancet 1992 (Mar 7);339:563–569.

80. Schuler G, Hambrecht R, Schlierf G, Grunze M, Methfessel S, Hauer K, Kubler W: Myocardial perfusion and regression of coronary artery disease in patients on a regimen of intensive physical exercise and low fat diet. J Am Coll Cardiol 1992 (January);19:34–42.

81. Schuler G, Hambrecht R, Schlierf G, Niebauer J, Hauer K, Neumann J, Hobert E, Drinkmann A, Bacher F, Grunze M, Kubler W: Regular Physical Exercise and Low-

Fat Diet, Effects on Progression of Coronary Artery Disease. Circulation 1992 (July);86:1–11.

82. Gould KL, Ornish D, Kirkeeide R, Brown S, Stuart Y, Buchi M, Billings J, Armstrong W, Ports T, Scherwitz L: Improved stenosis geometry by quantitative coronary arteriography after vigorous risk factor modification. Am J Cardiol 1992 (Apr 1);69:845–853.

83. LaRosa JC, Cleeman JI: Cholesterol Lowering as a Treatment for Established Coronary Heart Disease. Circulation 1992 (March);85:1229–1235.

84. Willard JE, Lange RA, Hillis LD: The use of aspirin in ischemic heart disease. N Engl J Med 1992 (July 16);327:175–181.

85. Knuuti MJ, Wahl M, Wiklund I, Smith P, Alhainen Harkonen R, Puska P, Tzivoni D: Acute and long-term effects on myocardial ischemia of intermittent and continuous transdermal nitrate therapy in stable angina. Am J Cardiol 1992 (June 15);69:1525–1532.

86. Dubiel JP, Moczurad KW, Bryniarski L: Efficacy of a single dose of slow-release isosorbide dinitrate in the treatment of silent or painful myocardial ischemia in stable angina pectoris. Am J Cardiol 1992 (May 1);69:1156–1160.

87. Metelitsa VI, Martsevich SY, Kozyreva MP, Slastnikova ID: Enhancement of the efficacy of isosorbide dinitrate by captopril in stable angina pectoris. Am J Cardiol 1992 (Feb 1);69:291–296.

88. Yusuf S, Pepine CJ, Garces C, Pouleur H, Salem D, Kostis J, Benedict C, Rousseau M, Bourassa M, Pitt B: Effect of enalapril on myocardial infarction and unstable angina in patients with low ejection fractions. Lancet 1992 (Nov 14);340:1173–1178.

89. Wiesfeld ACP, Remme WJ, Look MP, Kruijssen DACM, Van Hoogenhuyze CA: Acute hemodynamic and electrophysiologic effects and safety of high-dose intravenous diltiazem in patients receiving metoprolol. Am J Cardiol 1992 (Oct 22);70:997–1003.

90. Hannan EL, Arani DT, Johnson LW, Kemp HG Jr, Lukacik G: Percutaneous transluminal coronary angioplasty in New York state: Risk factors and outcomes. JAMA 1992 (Dec 2);268:3092–3097.

91. Parisi AF, Folland ED, Hartigan P: A comparison of angioplasty with medical therapy in the treatment of single-vessel coronary artery disease. N Engl J Med 1992 (Jan 2);326:10–16.

92. Kadel C, Vallbracht C, Buss F, Kober G, Kaltenbach M: Long-term follow-up after percutaneous transluminal coronary angioplasty in patients with single-vessel disease. Am Heart J 1992 (November);124:1159–1169.

93. Faxon DP, Ghalilli K, Jacobs AK, Ruocco NA, Christellis EM, Kellett MA, Jr, Varrichione TR, Ryan TJ: The degree of revascularization and outcome after multivessel coronary angioplasty. Am Heart J 1992 (April) 123:854–859.

94. Hollman J, Simpfendorfer C, Franco I, Whitlow P, Goormastic M: Multivessel and single-vessel coronary angioplasty: A comparative study. Am Heart J 1992 (July);124:9–12.

95. Bourassa MG, Holubkov R, Yeh W, Detre KM, Co-Investigators of the National Heart, Lung, and Blood Institute Percutaneous Transluminal Coronary Angioplasty Registry: Strategy of complete revascularization in patients with multivessel coronary artery disease (A report from the 1985–1986 NHLBI PTCA Registry). Am J Cardiol 1992 (July 15);70:174–178.

96. Warner MF, DiSciascio G, Kohli RS, Vetrovec GW, Sabri MN, Goudreau E, Kelly KM, Cowley MJ: Long-term efficacy of triple-vessel angioplasty in patients with severe three-vessel coronary artery disease. Am Heart J 1992 (November);124:1169–1174.

97. De Jaegere P, De Feyter P, Van Domburg R, Suryapranata H, Van Den Brand M, Serruys PW: Immediate and long term results of percutaneous coronary angioplasty in patients aged 70 and over. Br Heart J 1992 (Feb);67:138–143.

98. Santana JO, Haft JI, LaMarche NS, Goldstein JE: Coronary angioplasty in patients eighty years of age or older. Am Heart J 1992 (July);124:13–18.

99. Ruocco NA Jr, Ring ME, Holubkov R, Jacobs AK, Detre KM, Faxon DP, Co-Investigators of the National Heart, Lung, and Blood Institute Percutaneous Transluminal Coronary Angioplasty Registry: Am J Cardiol 1992 (Jan 1);69:69–76.

100. Ivanhoe RJ, Weintraub, Douglas JS, Lembo NJ, Furman M, Gershony G, Cohen CL, King SB: Percutaneous Transluminal Coronary Angioplasty of Chronic Total Occlusions

Primary Success, Restenosis, and Long-term Clinical Follow-up. Circulation 1992 (January);85:106–115.

101. Bell MR, Berger PB, Bresnahan JF, Reeder GS, Bailey KR, Holmes DR: Initial and Long-term Outcome of 354 Patients After Coronary Balloon Angioplasty of Total Coronary Artery Occlusions. Circulation 1992 (March);85:1003–1011.

102. Maiello L, Colombo A, Gianrossi R, Mutinelli M-R, Bouzon R, Thomas J, Finci L: Coronary angioplasty of chronic occlusion: Factors predictive of procedural success. Am Heart J 1992 (September);124:565–570.

103. Jackman JD Jr, Zidar JP, Tcheng JE, Overman AB, Phillips HR, Stack RS: Outcome after prolonged balloon inflations of >20 minutes for initially unsuccessful percutaneous transluminal coronary angioplasty. Am J Cardiol 1992 (June 1);69:1417–1421.

104. Huber RC, Evans MA, Breshahan JF, Gibbons RJ, Holmes DR Jr: Outcome of noncardiac operations in patients with severe coronary artery disease successfully treated preoperatively with coronary angioplasty. Mayo Clin Proc 1992 (Jan);67:15–21.

105. Honye J, Mahon DJ, Jain A, White CJ, Ramee SR, Wallis JB, Al-Zarka A, Tobis JM: Morphological Effects of Coronary Balloon Angioplasty in Vivo Assessed by Intravascular Ultrasound Imaging. Circulation 1992 (March);85:1012–1025.

106. Gerber TC, Erbel R, Gorge G, Ge J, Rupprecht HJ, Meyer J: Classification of morphologic effects of percutaneous transluminal coronary angioplasty assessed by intravascular ultrasound. Am J Cardiol 1992 (Dec 15);70:1546–1554.

107. Pande AK, Meier B, Urban P, Moles V, Dorsaz P-A, Favre J: Intracoronary electrocardiogram during coronary angioplasty. Am Heart J 1992 (August);124:337–341.

108. DiSciascio G, Angelini P, Vandormael MG, Brinker JA, Cowley MJ, Dean LS, Douglas JS Jr, and the Coronary Hemoperfusion Ischemia Prevention Study (CHIPS) Investigators: Reduction of ischemia with a new flow-adjustable hemoperfusion pump during coronary angioplasty. J Am Coll Cardiol 1992 (March);19:657–62.

109. Balady GJ, Leitschuh ML, Jacobs AK, Merrell D, Weiner DA, Ryan TJ: Safety and clinical use of exercise testing one to three days after percutaneous transluminal coronary angioplasty. Am J Cardiol 1991 (May 15);69:1259–1264.

110. Tousoulis D, Kaski JC, Davies G, Pereira W, El Tamimi H, McFadden E, Maseri A: Preangioplasty complicated coronary stenosis morphology as a predictor of restenosis. Am Heart J 1992 (January);123:15–20.

111. Beatt KJ, Serruys PW, Luijten HE, Rensing BJ, Suryapranata H, de Feyter P, van den Brand M, Laarman GJ, Roelandt J, van Es GA: Restenosis after coronary angioplasty: The paradox of increased lumen diameter and restenosis. J Am Coll Cardiol 1992 (February);19:258–66.

112. Hearn JA, Donohue BC, Baalbaki H, Douglas JS, King SB III, Lembo NJ, Roubin GS, Sgoutas DS: Usefulness of serum lipoprotein (a) as a predictor of restenosis after percutaneous transluminal coronary angioplasty. Am J Cardiol 1992 (Mar 15);69:736–739.

113. Shah P, Amin J: Low High Density Lipoprotein Level Is Associated With Increased Restenosis Rate After Coronary Angioplasty. Circulation 1992 (April);85:1279–1285.

114. Dimas AP, Grigera F, Arora RR, Simpfendorfer CC, Hollman JL, Frierson JH, Franco I, Whitlow PL: Repeat coronary angioplasty as treatment for restenosis. J Am Coll Cardiol 1992 (May);19:1310–4.

115. Hernández RA, Macaya C, Iñiguez A, Alfonso F, Goicolea J, Fernandez-Ortiz A, Zarco P: Midterm outcome of patients with asymptomatic restenosis after coronary balloon angioplasty. J Am Coll Cardiol 1992 (June);19:1402–9.

116. Okamoto S, Inden M, Setsuda M, Konishi T, Nakano T: Effects of trapidil (triazolopyrimidine), a platelet-derived growth factor antagonist, in preventing restenosis after percutaneous transluminal coronary angioplasty. Am Heart J (June);123:1439–1444.

117. Weintraub WS, Ghazzal ZMB, Douglas JS Jr, Liberman H, Morris DC, Cohen CL, King SB III: Initial management and long-term clinical outcome of restenosis after initially successful percutaneous transluminal coronary angioplasty. Am J Cardiol 1992 (Jul 1);70:47–55.

118. Tenaglia AN, Quigley PJ, Kereiakes DJ, Abbottsmith CW, Phillips HR, Tcheng JE, Rendall D, Ohman EM: Coronary angioplasty performed with gradual and prolonged inflation using a perfusion balloon catheter: Procedural success and restenosis rate. Am Heart J 1992 (September);124:585–589.

119. Bauters C, Lablanche J-M, McFadden EP, Leroy F, Bertrand ME: Clinical characteristics and angiographic follow-up of patients undergoing early or late repeat dilation for a first restenosis. J Am Coll Cardiol 1992 (October);845–8.

120. Foley JB, Chisholm RJ, Common AA, Langer A, Armstrong PW: Aggressive clinical pattern of angina at restenosis following coronary angioplasty in unstable angina. Am Heart J (November);124:1174–1180.

121. Muller DWM, Shamir KJ, Ellis SG, Topol EJ: Peripheral vascular complications after conventional and complex percutaneous coronary interventional procedures. Am J Cardiol 1992 (Jan 1);69:63–68.

122. Lincoff AM, Popma JJ, Ellis SG, Hacker JA, Topol EJ: Abrupt vessel closure complicating coronary angioplasty: Clinical, angiographic and therapeutic profile. J Am Coll Cardiol 1992 (April);19:926–35.

123. Myler RK, Shaw RE, Stertzer SH, Hecht SH, Ryan C, Rosenblum J, Cumberland DC, Murphy MC, Hansell HN, Hidalgo B: Lesion morphology and coronary angioplasty: Current experience and analysis. J Am Coll Cardiol 1992 (June);19:1641–52.

124. McGarry TF, Jr, Gottlieb RS, Morganroth J, Zelenkofske SL, Kasparian H, Duca PR, Lester RM, Kreulen TH: The relationship of anticoagulation level and complications after successful percutaneous transluminal coronary angioplasty. Am Heart J 1992 (June);123:1445–1451.

125. Vaitkus PT, Herrmann HC, Laskey WK: Management and immediate outcome of patients with intracoronary thrombus during percutaneous transluminal coronary angioplasty. Am Heart J 1992 (July);124:1–8.

126. Agrawal SK, Pinheiro L, Roubin GS, Hearn JA, Cannon AD, Macander PJ, Barnes JL, Dean LS, Nanda NC: Nonsurgical closure of femoral pseudoaneurysms complicating cardiac catheterization and percutaneous transluminal coronary angioplasty. J Am Coll Cardiol 1992 (September);20:610–5.

127. Hermans WRM, Rensing BJ, Foley DP, Deckers JW, Rutsch W, Emanuelsson H, Danchin N, Wijns W, Chappuis F, Serruys PW, on behalf of the MERCATOR Study Group: Therapeutic dissection after successful coronary balloon angioplasty: no influence on restenosis or on clinical outcome in 693 patients. J Am Coll Cardiol 1992 (October);20:767–80.

128. Bergelson BA, Jacobs AK, Cupples A, Ruocco NA Jr, Kyller MG, Ryan TJ, Faxon DP: Prediction of risk for hemodynamic compromise during percutaneous transluminal coronary angioplasty. Am J Cardiol 1992 (Dec 15);70:1540–1545.

129. Decesare NB, Popma JJ, Holmes DR Jr, Dick RJ, Whitlow PL, King SB, Pinkerton CA, Kereiakes DJ, Topol EJ, Haudenschild CC, Ellis SG: Clinical angiographic and histologic correlates of ectasia after directional coronary atherectomy. Am J Cardiol 1992 (Feb 1);69:314–319.

130. Leclerc G, Isner JM, Kearney M, Simons M, Safian RD, Baim DS, Weir L: Evidence Implicating Nonmuscle Myosin in Restenosis Use of In Situ Hybridization to Analyze Human Vascular Lesions Obtained by Directional Atherectomy. Circulation 1992 (February);85:543–553.

131. Bertrand ME, Lablanche JM, Leroy F, Bauters C, De Jaegere P, Serruys PW, Meyer J, Dietz U, Erbel R: Percutaneous transluminal coronary rotary ablation with rotablator (European experience). Am J Cardiol 1992 (Feb 15);69:470–474.

132. Popma JJ, Topol EJ, Hinohara T, Pinkerton CA, Baim DS, King SB III, Holmes DR Jr, Whitlow PL, Kereiakes DJ, Hartzler GO, Kent KM, Ellis SG, Simpson JB, for the U.S. Directional Atherectomy Investigator Group: Abrupt vessel closure after directional coronary atherectomy. J Am Coll Cardiol 1992 (June);19:1372–9.

133. Mansour M, Carrozza JP Jr, Kuntz RE, Fishman RF, Pomerantz RM, Senerchia CC, Safian RD, Diver DJ, Baim DS: Frequency and outcome of chest pain after two new coronary interventions (Atherectomy and stenting). Am J Cardiol 1992 (June 1);69:1379–1382.

134. Pomerantz RM, Kuntz RE, Carrozza JP, Fishman RF, Mansour M, Schnitt SJ, Safian RD, Baim DS: Acute and long-term outcome of narrowed saphenous venous grafts treated by endoluminal stenting and directional atherectomy. Am J Cardiol 1992 (July 15);70:161–167.

135. Garratt KN, Holmes DR Jr, Bell MR, Berger PB, Kaufmann UP, Bresnahan JF, Vlietstra RE: Results of directional atherectomy of primary atheromatous and restenosis

lesions in coronary arteries and saphenous vein grafts. Am J Cardiol 1992 (Aug 15);70:449–454.

136. Pavlides GS, Hauser AM, Grines CL, Dudlets PI, O'Neill WW: Clinical, hemodynamic, electrocardiographic and mechanical events during nonocclusive, coronary atherectomy and comparison with balloon angioplasty. Am J Cardiol 1992 (Oct 1);70:841–845.

137. Mintz GS, Potkin BN, Keren G, Satler LF, Pichard AD, Kent KM, Popma JJ, Leon MB: Intravascular Ultrasound Evaluation of the Effect of Rotational Atherectomy in Obstructive Atherosclerotic Coronary Artery Disease. Circulation 1992 (November);86:1383–1393.

138. Fishman RF, Kuntz RE, Carrozza JP Jr, Miller MJ, Senerchia CC, Schnitt SJ, Diver DJ, Safian RD, Baim DS: Long-term results of directional coronary atherectomy: Predictors of restenosis. J Am Coll Cardiol 1992 (November);20:1101–10.

139. Kuntz RE, Hinohara T, Robertson GC, Safian RD, Simpson JB, Baim DS: Influence of vessel selection on the observed restenosis rate after endoluminal stenting or directional atherectomy. Am J Cardiol 1992 (Nov 1);70:1101–1108.

140. Strauss BH, Umans VA, van Suylen R-J, de Feyter PJ, Marco J, Robertson GC, Renkin J, Heyndrickx G, Vuzevski VD, Bosman FT, Serruys PW: Directional atherectomy for treatment of restenosis within coronary stents: Clinical, angiographic and histologic results. J Am Coll Cardiol 1992 (December);20:1465–73.

141. Bell MR, Garratt KN, Bresnahan JF, Edwards WD, Holmes DR Jr: Relation of deep arterial resection and coronary artery aneurysms after directional coronary atherectomy. J Am Coll Cardiol 1992 (December);20:1474–81.

142. Popma JJ, Leon MB, Mintz GS, Kent KM, Satler LF, Garrand TJ, Pichard AD: Results of coronary angioplasty using the transluminal extraction catheter. Am J Cardiol 1992 (Dec 15);70:1526–1532.

143. Strauss BH, Serruys PW, Bertrans ME, Puel J, Meier B, Goy JJ, Kappenberger L, Rickards AF, Sigwart U, Morel MA, Van Swijndregt EM: Quantitative angiographic follow-up of the coronary wallstent in native vessels and bypass grafts (European experience—March 1986 to March 1990). Am J Cardiol 1992 (Feb 15);69:475–481.

144. De Jaegere PP, Serruys PW, Bertrand M, Wiegand V, Kober G, Marquis JF, Valeix B, Uebis R, Piessens J: Wiktor stent implantation in patients with restenosis following balloon angioplasty of a native coronary artery. Am J Cardiol 1992 (Mar 1);69:598–602.

145. de Scheerder IK, Strauss BH, de Feyter PJ, Beatt KJ, Bauer LHB, Wijns W, Heyndrix GR, Suryapanata H, van den Brand M, Buis B, Serruys PW: Stenting of venous bypass grafts: A new treatment modality for patients who are poor candidates for reintervention. Am Heart J 1992 (April);123:1046–1054.

146. Strumpf RK, Mehta SS, Ponder R, Heuser RR: Palmaz-Schatz stent implantation in stenosed saphenous vein grafts: Clinical and angiographic follow-up. Am Heart J 1992 (May);123:1329–1336.

147. Carrozza JP Jr, Kuntz RE, Levine MJ, Pomerantz RM, Fishman RF, Mansour M, Gibson CM, Senerchia CC, Diver DJ, Safian RD, Baim DS: Angiographic and clinical outcome of intracoronary stenting: immediate and long-term results from a large single-center experience. J Am Coll Cardiol 1992;20:328–37.

148. Lau KW, Gunnes P, Williams M, Rickards A, Sigwart U: Angiographic restenosis after successful Wallstent stent implantation: An analysis of risk predictors. Am Heart J 1992 (December);124:1473–1477.

149. Bittl JA, Sanborn TA, Tcheng JE, Siegel RM, Ellis SG: Clinical success, complications and restenosis rates with excimer laser coronary angioplasty. Am J Cardiol 1992 (Dec 15);70:1533–1539.

150. Goldberg KC, Hartz AJ, Jacobsen SJ, Krakauer H, Rimm AA: Racial and community factors influencing coronary artery bypass graft surgery rates for all 1986 Medicare patients. JAMA 1992 (Mar 18);267:1473–1477.

151. Vacek JL, Rosamond TL, Stites HW, Rowe SK, Robuck W, Dittmeier G, Beauchamp GD: Comparison of percutaneous transluminal coronary angioplasty versus coronary artery bypass grafting for multivessel coronary artery disease. Am J Cardiol 1992 (Mar 1);69:592–597.

152. Carey JS, Cukingnan RA, Singer LKM: Quality of life after myocardial revascularization: Effect of increasing age. J Thorac Cardiovasc Surg 1992 (Jan);103:108–115.

153. Guadagnoli E, Ayanian JZ, Cleary PD: Comparison of patient-reported outcomes after

elective coronary artery bypass grafting in patients aged ≥ and <65 years. Am J Cardiol 1992 (Jul 1);70:60–64.

154. Glower DD, Christopher TD, Milano CA, White WD, Smith LR, Jones RH, Sabiston DC Jr: Performance status and outcome after coronary artery bypass grafting in persons aged 80 to 93 years. Am J Cardiol 1992 (Sept 1);70:567–571.

155. Tuman KJ, McCarthy RJ, Najafi PH, Ivankovich AD: Differential effects of advanced age on neurologic and cardiac risks of coronary artery operations. J Thorac Cardiovasc Surg 1992 (Dec);104:1510–1517.

156. Ulicny KS Jr, Flege JB Jr, Callard GM, Todd JC: Twenty-year follow-up of saphenous vein aortocoronary artery bypass grafting. Ann Thorac Surg 1992 (Feb);53:258–262.

157. Bell M, Gersh B, Schaff H, Holmes D, Fisher L, Alderman E, Myers W, Parsons L, Reeder G, and the Investigators of the Coronary Artery Surgery Study: Effect of Completeness of Revascularization on Long-term Outcome of Patients With Three-Vessel Disease Undergoing Coronary Artery Bypass Surgery, A Report From the Coronary Artery Surgery Study Registry. Circulation 1992 (August);86:446–457.

158. King KB, Clark PC, Hicks GL Jr: Patterns of referral and recovery in women and men undergoing coronary artery bypass grafting. Am J Cardiol 1992 (Jan 15);69:179–182.

159. Hannan EL, Bernard HR, Kilburn HC, Jr, O'Donnell JF: Gender differences in mortality rates for coronary artery bypass surgery. Am Heart J 1992 (April);123:866–872.

160. Higgins TL, Estafanous FG, Loop FD, Beck GJ, Blum JM, Paranandi L: Stratification of morbidity and mortality outcome by preoperative risk factors in coronary artery bypass patients; A clinical severity score. JAMA 1992 (May 6);267:2344–2348.

161. Hartz AJ, Kuhn EM, Pryor DB, Krakauer H, Young M, Heudebert G, Rimm AA: Mortality after coronary angioplasty and coronary artery bypass surgery (The National Medicare Experience). Am J Cardiol 1992 (July 15);70:179–185.

162. Lytle BW, Loop FD, Taylor PC, Simpfendorfer C, Kramer JR, Ratliff NB, Goormastic M, Cosgrove DM, Schnauffer MJ: Vein graft disease: The clinical impact of stenoses in saphenous vein bypass grafts to coronary arteries. J Thorac Cardiovasc Surg 1992 (May);103:831–840.

163. Smith RC, Leung JM, Keith FM, Merrick S, Mangano DT, and the Study of Perioperative Ischemia (SPI) Research Group: Ventricular dysrhythmias in patients undergoing coronary artery bypass graft surgery: Incidence, characteristics, and prognostic importance. Am Heart J 1992 (January);123:73–81.

164. Blauth CI, Cosgrove DM, Webb BW, Ratliff NB, Boylan M, Piedmonte MR, Lytle BW, Loop FD: Atheroembolism from the ascending aorta: An emerging problem in cardiac surgery. J Thorac Cardiovasc Surg 1992 (June);103:1104–1012.

165. Cavender JB, Rogers WJ, Fisher LD, Gersh BJ, Coggin CJ, Myers WO, for the CASS Investigators: Effects of smoking on survival and morbidity in patients randomized to medical or surgical therapy in the Coronary Artery Surgery Study (CASS): 10-year follow-up. J Am Coll Cardiol 1992;20:287–94.

166. Yli-Mayry S, Huikuri HV, Airaksinen KEJ, Ikaheimo MJ, Linnaluoto MK, Takkunen JT: Usefulness of a postoperative exercise test for predicting cardiac events after coronary artery bypass grafting. Am J Cardiol 1992 (Jul 1);70:56–59.

167. Crouse LJ, Vacek JL, Beauchamp GD, Porter CB, Rosamond TL, Kramer PH: Exercise echocardiography after coronary artery bypass grafting. Am J Cardiol 1992 (Sept 1);70:572–576.

168. De Bono DP, Samani NJ, Spyt TJ, Hartshorne T, Thrush AJ, Evans DH: Transcutaneous ultrasound measurement of blood-flow in internal mammary artery to coronary artery grafts. Lancet 1992 (Feb 15);339:379–381.

169. Manske CL, Wang Y, Rector T, Wilson RF, White CW: Coronary revascularization in insulin-dependent diabetic patients with chronic renal failure. Lancet 1992 (Oct 24);340:998–1002.

170. Hicks GL Jr: Coronary artery operation in radiation-associated atherosclerosis: Long-term follow-up. Ann Thorac Surg 1992 (Apr);53:670–674.

171. Goor DA, Golan M, Bar El Y, Modan M, Lusky A, Rozenman J, Mohr R: Synergism between infarct-borne left ventricular dysfunction and cardiomegaly in increasing the risk of coronary bypass surgery. J Thorac Cardiovasc Surg 1992 (Oct);104:983–989.

172. Johnson WD, Kayser KL, Hartz AJ, Saedi SF: Aspirin use and survival after coronary bypass surgery. Am Heart J 1992 (March);123:603–608.

173. Dougenis D, Naik S, Brown AH: Is repeated coronary surgery for recurrent angina cost effective? Euro Heart J (Jan);13:9–14.

174. Akl ES, Ozdogan E, Ohri SK, Barbir M, Chei K, Gaer JAR, Mitchell AG, Yacoub MH: Early and long term results of re-operation for coronary artery disease. Br Heart J 1992 (Aug);68:176–180.

175. Cosgrove DM III, Heric B, Lytle BW, Taylor PC, Novoa R, Golding LAR, Stewart RW, McCarthy PM, Loop FD: Aprotinin therapy for reoperative myocardial revascularization: A placebo-controlled study. Ann Thorac Surg 1992 (Dec);54:1031–1038.

176. Mautner SL, Mautner GC, Hunsberger SA, Roberts WC: Comparison of composition of atherosclerotic plaques in saphenous veins used as aortocoronary bypass conduits with plaques in native coronary arteries in the same men. Am J Cardiol 1992 (Dec 1);70:1380–1387.

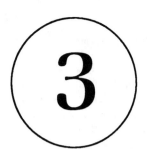

Acute Myocardial Infarction and Its Consequences

Circadian symptom onset

A circadian variation of symptom onset in AMI with an increased frequency in the late morning and possibly also in the evening has been found in several studies. It has been suggested that different circadian rhythms may exist in various subgroups of patients. Hansen and associates[1] from Malmo, Sweden, examined the possibility in a population of 10,791 patients collected between 1973 and 1987 in a continuously operating register of patients with AMI in Malmo, Sweden. In 6,763 patients (63%) in whom a distinct symptom onset could be established, symptom onset occurred with an increased frequency between 6:01 A.M. and 12:00 Noon (30.6%) and between 6:01 P.M. and 12:00 midnight (26.9%). Similar bimodal circadian rhythms were seen in patients aged > 70 years (n = 2,923), ≤70 years (n = 3,840), men (n = 4,528), women (n = 2,235), smokers (n = 653), patients with (n = 1,872) and without (n = 4,891) a history of previous AMI, and in patients with recent non-Q-wave AMI (n = 333). In 455 patients receiving cardioselective B blockers the circadian distribution did not differ from a random, whereas in patients taking non-selective B blockers or calcium antagonists significant bimodal rhythms were found. Statistically significant interactions were found between symptom onset and age dichotomized at 70 years, and between patients with and without a history of previous AMI. In a multivariate analysis only these variables (age ≤/>70 years; ± history of a previous AMI) were found to modify the circadian rhythm of symptom onset in the population.

To investigate the circadian pattern of AMI in a large international patient population, the collaborative group of the Second International

Study of Infarct Survival (ISIS-2)[2] prospectively determined the time of day of the onset of symptoms in 12,163 consecutive patients randomized in the ISIS-2 Trial. Overall there was a marked circadian variation in the incidence of AMI characterized by a sharp increase from 0600 h to 0800 h, with a peak period from 0800 h to 1100 h followed by a gradual decline from 1100 h to 1800 h (Figure 3-1). During the evening and night there was a steady trough, with no evidence of a second peak. Although there was some scatter, this circadian pattern was similar among patients of 5 different geographic regions on 3 continents and in various subcategories of patients defined with respect to age, gender, previous AMI, and aspirin intake prior to AMI. The circadian pattern of diabetics, however, was different compared with non-diabetics, and it demonstrated no significant variation. This increased morning incidence of AMI indicates specific triggering mechanisms that are particularly likely to occur during, or just before, that time of day.

Circadian variation of arrhythmias

Circadian variation in the onset of cardiovascular events including sudden coronary death, AMI, and ventricular arrhythmias has been described. Gillis and associates[3] from Calgary, Canada, and Baltimore, Maryland, evaluated in 132 patients with frequent VPCs and reduced LV function after AMI the effect of LV dysfunction on the circadian variation of VPC frequency. Patients were prospectively divided into 20 groups based on LVEF (those with LVEF ≤0.30, and those with LVEF between 0.30 and 0.45). Median hourly VPC frequencies and heart rates were compared between the 2 groups. Subgroup analyses based on treatment with B-adrenoceptor blocking agents and on New York Heart Association functional class were also performed. In patients with LVEF ≤0.30, a distinct circadian variation of VPCs, and the expected morning increase in VPC frequency were present. In contrast, a distinct circadian variation of VPCs was absent in patients with LVEF 0.30. A circadian variation of VPC fre-

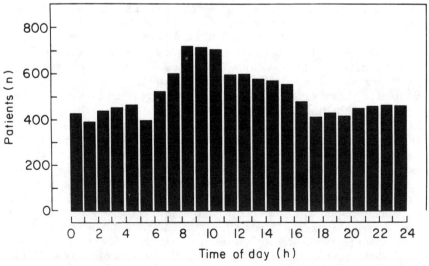

Fig. 3-1. Time of onset of symptoms of suspected acute myocardial infarction in the total study population (n = 12163). Reproduced with permission from Second International Study of Infarct Survival Collaborative Group.[2]

quency was also absent in patients with severe symptomatic CHF (New York Heart Association class III-IV). Treatment with B-adrenoceptor blocking agents was associated with a loss of the circadian variation of VPC frequency. The circadian variation of heart rate was also blunted in the group treated with B-adrenoceptor blocking agents. The proportion of subjects manifesting a positive correlation between heart rate and VPC frequency was lower in subjects with LVEF >0.30 (26%) than in those with LVEF ≤0.30 (46%). Thus, circadian variation of VPC frequency is absent in patients with severe LV dysfunction.

Heart period variability

To determine the reproducibility of frequency domain measures of heart period variability in patients with previous AMI, Bigger and associates[4] for the CAPS and ESVEM Investigators, studied 2 random samples of 40 patients each (1 from the Cardiac Arrhythmia Pilot Study [CAPS] [unsustained ventricular arrhythmias], and 1 from the Electrophysiologic Studies Versus Electrocardiographic Monitoring [ESVEM] [sustained ventricular arrhythmias] trial). For each patient, 2 24-hour continuous electrocardiographic recordings were analyzed, and the average normal RR interval, total power and 4 components of total power were calculated. Group means and standard deviations for each sample were virtually identical for the pairs of 24-hour recordings. Furthermore, measurements for individual patients were stable from day to day, as measured by the intraclass correlation coefficients and the standard errors of measurement. Reproducibility of heart period variability measurements is excellent in patients with previous AMI and ventricular arrhythmias, and is comparable to the high stability previously found in a small group of normal subjects. The stability of measures of heart period variability facilitates distinguishing real changes due to progression or regression of cardiac disease or to drug effects from apparent changes due to random variation.

In an investigation by Lombardi and associates[5] from Milano and Pavia, Italy, the circadian variations of spectral indices of heart rate variability were analyzed in 20 patients 4 weeks after a first and uncomplicated AMI and in 20 control individuals. R-R interval and variance showed a characteristic day-night pattern with a significant reduction of the latter parameter in patients after myocardial infarction (10967 ± 1109 msec^2 vs 16860 ± 2132 msec^2). Control individuals were characterized by a predominance of low-frequency component during the day and of high-frequency component during the night, which reflected the expected 24-hour pattern of variation of sympathovagal balance. A 24-hour elevation of the low-frequency component and a smaller high-frequency component during the night differentiated patients after myocardial infarction from control individuals. The difference between the 2 groups was even more evident when the 24-hour sympathovagal balance was assessed with the low frequency/high frequency ratio. Thus spectral analysis of heart rate variability indicates that in patients after myocardial infarction there is an alteration of neural control mechanisms as indicated by the presence of signs of sympathetic activation and by the attenuation of the nocturnal increase in vagal tone.

Pre-infarction angina

In an investigation by Hirai and associates[6] from Toyama, Japan, the effect of preinfarction angina on the preservation of LV function was evaluated with the use of cineventriculography in 37 patients who had either total or subtotal occlusion of the proximal LAD during the convalescent period of myocardial infarction. In 15 patients who had preinfarction angina >1 week before the onset of AMI (group A), the global LVEF was 54 ± 3% and regional wall motion in the infarct area was 10 ± 3%. In 10 patients who had preinfarction angina within 1 week before the onset of AMI (group B), the LVEF and regional wall motion in the infarct area were 42 ± 3% and 1 ± 2%, respectively. In 12 patients without preinfarction angina (group C), the LVEF and regional wall motion in the infarct area were 38 ± 3% and −1 ± 2%, respectively. In groups B and C, both the LVEF and regional wall motion in the infarct area were lower than those in group A. The collateral circulation at the onset of AMI was better in group A compared with groups B and C. Thus the collateral circulation, promoted by repetitive anginal episodes indicative of myocardial ischemia, causes the preservation of myocardial function.

Tobacco consumption

To estimate the risk of AMI in snuff users, cigarette smokers, and non-tobacco users in northern Sweden, where using snuff is traditional, Huhtasaari and associates[7] from Lulea, Umea, and Kalix, Sweden, performed a case-controlled study involving men aged 35-64 years old who had had a first AMI and also a population-based sample of men aged 35-64 years who had not had an AMI and both lived in the same geographic area. The main outcome measure was tobacco consumption (regular snuff dipping, regular cigarette smoking, and non-tobacco use) and risk of AMI. Fifty-nine of 585 (10%) patients who had a first AMI and 87 of 589 (15%) randomly selected men without AMI were non-smokers who used snuff daily. The age adjusted odds ratio for AMI was 0.89 for exposure to snuff and 1.87 for cigarette smoking compared with non-tobacco users, showing an increased risk in smokers but not in snuff dippers. Regular cigarette smokers had a significantly higher risk of AMI than regular snuff dippers. Smoking, but not snuff dipping, predicted AMI in a multiple logistic regression model that included age and level of education. In middle aged men snuff dipping is associated with a lower risk of AMI than cigarette smoking.

Serum ferritin

Iron can induce lipid peroxidation in vitro and in vivo in humans and has promoted ischemic myocardial injury in experimented animals. Salonen and co-investigators[8] in Kuopio, Finland, tested the hypothesis that high serum ferritin concentration and high dietary iron intake are associated with an excess risk of AMI. Randomly selected men (n = 1,931), aged 42, 48, 54, or 60 years, who had no symptomatic CAD at entry, were examined in the Kuopio Ischaemic Heart Disease Risk Factor Study (KIHD) in Eastern Finland between 1984 and 1989. Fifty-one of these men experienced an AMI during an average follow-up of 3 years. On the basis of a Cox proportional hazards model adjusting for age, examination year, cigarette pack-years, ischemic electrocardiogram in exercise test, maximal oxygen uptake, systolic BP, blood glucose, serum copper, blood leukocyte count, and serum HDL cholesterol, apolipoprotein B, and triglyceride concentrations, men with serum ferritin ≥200 μg/1 had a 2.2-fold risk factor-adjusted risk of AMI compared with men with a lower serum ferritin. An elevated serum ferritin was a strong risk factor for AMI in all multivariate models. This association was stronger in men with serum LDL cholesterol concentration of 5.0 mmol/1 (193 mg/dl) or more than in others (Figure 3-2). Also, dietary iron intake had a significant association with the disease risk in a Cox model with the same covariates. These data suggest that a high stored iron level, as assessed by elevated serum ferritin concentration, is a risk factor for CAD.

Occupation

While some analytical studies have suggested that individuals in occupations representing higher compared with lower socioeconomic status have a decreased risk of CAD, it is unclear whether occupation itself has an etiologic role in the development of CAD or whether differences in as yet uncontrolled coronary risk factors may account for these differences in risk. Hebert and associates[9] from Boston, Massachusetts, and Hanover, New Hampshire, evaluated white-collar versus blue-collar occupation and risk of CAD among 230 men hospitalized for a first AMI and 222 control subjects of the same age, sex, and neighborhood of residence. Information on coronary risk factors was obtained from home interviews, and blood specimens were drawn to test lipid and lipoprotein levels. Usual occupation was dichotomized into white-collar and blue-collar occupation according to the Edwards' classification. The relative risk of AMI of white-collar compared with blue-collar workers was 0.74 after controlling for age, cigarette smoking, family history of premature AMI, history of treatment for high BP, body mass index, history of diabetes, alcohol consumption, type A personality, leisure-time physical activity, total calories, and percentage of calories consumed as saturated fat. However, there was no residual association after control for HDL cholesterol yielding a relative

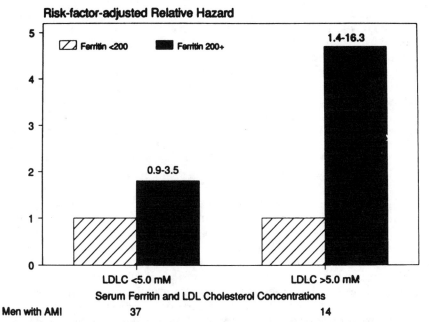

Fig. 3-2. Bar graph of risk factor-adjusted relative hazard of acute myocardial infarction (AMI) associated with serum ferritin concentration ≥200 μg/l (with 95% CI) in men with serum low density lipoprotein cholesterol (LDLC)≥5 mmol/l and those with serum LDLC <5 mmol/l. Reproduced with permission from Salonen, et al.[8]

risk of 0.98. These results suggest that white-collar occupation per se does not appear to protect from CAD. Any apparent protective effect on AMI that has been previously observed in white-collar compared with blue-collar workers may be attributable to differences in HDL cholesterol levels.

Relation to lipids

A large and consistent body of evidence supports the judgment that elevation of total plasma blood cholesterol is a cause of AMI and that high levels of LDL cholesterol have a positive relation and high levels of high HDL cholesterol an inverse relation with AMI. At present, however, the roles, if any, of the major subfractions of HDL, namely, HDL_2 and HDL_3, have not been clarified. In addition, the relation of plasma apolipoprotein concentrations to AMI and whether they provide predictive information over and above their lipoprotein cholesterol associations is unknown. Buring and co-workers[10] in Brookline, Massachusetts, evaluated these questions in a case-control study of patients hospitalized with a first AMI and neighborhood controls of the same age and sex. Cases had significantly lower levels of total HDL as well as HDL_2 and HDL_3 cholesterol. These differences persisted after controlling for a large number of demographic, medical history, and behavioral risk factors and levels of other lipids. There were significant inverse dose-response relations with odds ratios for those in the highest quartile relative to those in the lowest of 0.15 for total HDL, 0.17 for HDL_2, and 0.29 for HDL_3 cholesterol levels. Levels of LDL and VLDL cholesterol and triglycerides were also higher among cases than controls, but only for triglycerides was the difference statistically significant after adjustment for coronary risk factors and other lipids. Apolipoproteins A-I and A-II were both significantly lower in cases, and difference remained even after adjustment for coronary risk factors and lipids. There were significant dose-response relations for both apolipoprotein A-I and A-II. Neither apolipoprotein B nor E was significantly related to AMI after adjustment for lipids and other coronary risk factors. When all 4 apolipoproteins were taken together, there was an increased level of prediction of AMI over the information provided by the lipids and other coronary risk factors, but this appeared present only for the individual apolipoproteins A-I and A-II. These data indicated that both HDL_2 and HDL_3 cholesterol levels are significantly associated with AMI. They also raise the possibility that apolipoprotein levels, especially A-I and A-II, may add relevant information to determination of risk of AMI.

Plasma homocystine

To assess prospectively the risk of CAD associated with elevated plasma levels of homocyst(e)ine, Stampfer and associates[11] from Boston, Massachusetts, and Beaverton and Portland, Oregon, performed a nested case-controlled study using prospectively collected blood samples. A total of 14,916 male physicians, aged 40 to 84 years, with no prior AMI or stroke provided plasma samples at baseline and were followed up for 5 years. Samples from 271 men who subsequently developed AMI were analyzed for homocyst(e)ine levels together with paired controls, matched by age and smoking. AMI or death due to CAD was the main outcome measure. Levels of homocyst(e)ine were higher in cases than in controls (11.1 ± 4.0 [SD] vs 10.5 ± 2.8 nmol/mL). The difference was attributable to an excess of high values among men who later had AMIs. The relative risk for the highest 5% vs the bottom 90% of homocyst(e)ine levels was 3.1. After additional adjustment for diabetes, hypertension, aspirin assignment, Quetelet's Index, and total/HDL cholesterol, this relative risk was 3.4. Thirteen controls and 31 cases (11%) had values above the 95th percentile of the controls. Moderately high levels of plasma homocyst(e)ine are associated with subsequent risk of AMI independent of other coronary risk factors. Because high levels can often be easily treated with vitamin supplements, homocyst(e)ine may be an independent, modifiable risk factor.

Prehospital delay times

Substantial time delays from symptom onset to diagnosis and treatment of patients with AMI have been demonstrated. In an investigation by Kereiakes and colleagues[12] from Cincinnati, Ohio, and Durham, North Carolina, to determine the relative importance of prehospital mode of patient transport and the relative impact of emergency medical system transport with or without a prehospital cellular electrocardiogram on hospital time delays to initiation of thrombolytic therapy, 4 prospective parallel groups of patients with AMI were evaluated. The median hospital time delay to treatment was 64 minutes for patients transported by private automobile (walk-in); 55 minutes for patients transported by local ambulance; 50 minutes for patients transported by the emergency medical system without a prehospital electrocardiogram; and 30 minutes for patients transported by the emergency medical system who had a 12-lead electrocardiogram transmitted from the field. Patients transported by the emergency medical system were randomized to receive cellular telephone transmission of a prehospital 12-lead electrocardiogram. Specialized emergency medical system transport alone did not facilitate in-hospital initiation of thrombolytic therapy in patients with AMI when compared with those brought by local ambulance or by private automobile. A significant reduction in hospital time delay to treatment was observed only in patients transported by the emergency medical system who had cellular transmission of a prehospital 12-lead electrocardiogram from the field.

To evaluate whether patients who recognize the symptoms of myocardial ischemia and have easy access to medical care have shortened time delays between onset of symptoms and hospital presentation, Ridker and associates[13] from Boston, Massachusetts, compared the total time interval between symptom onset and hospital arrival for 258 U.S. male physicians experiencing a first AMI in the Physicians' Health Study (PHS) with that of a comparable group of 240 men enrolled in the U.S. component of the Second International Study of Infarct Survival (ISIS-2), as well as those of previously published series of patients with AMI. For patients presenting for medical care within 24 hours of symptom onset, the median time delay from onset of symptoms to presentation for medical care was 1.8 hours in the PHS (Figure 3-3) and 4.9 hours in the U.S. component of ISIS-2 (Figure 3-4). Furthermore, 56% of participants in the PHS presented for medical care within 2 hours and 72% within 4 hours of symptom onset compared with 20% and 44%, respectively, for ISIS-2 participants. In previously published series, the average time to presentation was comparable to that in the ISIS-2 trial, with variation depending on country of origin and on local population density. The median time to medical presentation in any previous series was not shorter than that in the PHS. Thus, physicians in the PHS had significantly shorter time delays between onset of symptoms and presentation for medical care. This difference

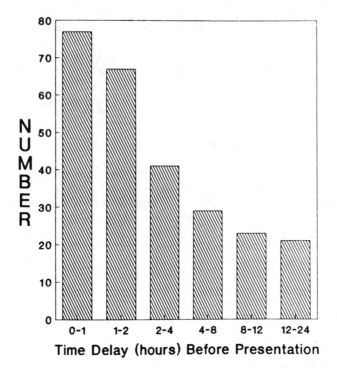

Fig. 3-3. Distribution of time delay between onset of symptoms and treatment for 258 subjects with first myocardial infarction in Physicians' Health Study. Reproduced with permission from Ridker, et al.[13]

may help explain the far lower than expected cardiovascular mortality rates among physician participants in the PHS. Furthermore, the data provide encouraging evidence that shorter delay times from onset of symptoms to hospital presentation can be achieved.

Goldberg and associates[14] from Worcester and Boston, Massachusetts, examined the duration of patient delay from the time of onset of symptoms of AMI to hospital presentation and the relation of delay time and various patient characteristics to receipt of thrombolytic therapy as part of a community-based study of patients hospitalized with AMI in the Worcester, Massachusetts, metropolitan area. In all, 800 patients with validated AMI hospitalized at 16 hospitals in the Worcester metropolitan area in 1986 and 1988 constituted the study sample. Patients delayed on average 4 hours between noting symptoms suggestive of AMI and presenting to area-wide emergency departments with no significant change observed between 1986 and 1988. The shorter the time interval of delay, the greater the likelihood of receiving thrombolytic therapy; patients arriving at the emergency department within 1 hour of the onset of acute symptoms were approximately 2.5 and 6.5 times more likely to receive thrombolytic agents than were those presenting to the hospital between 4 and 6, and > 6 hours, respectively, after the onset of symptoms. Results of a multivariate analysis showed increasing length of delay, older age, history of hypertension or AMI and non-Q-wave AMI to be significantly associated with failure to receive thrombolytic therapy.

To measure the delays between onset of symptoms and admission

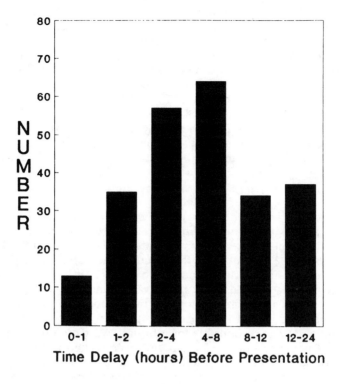

Fig. 3-4. Distribution of time delay between onset of symptoms and treatment for 240 subjects with first myocardial infarction in U.S. component of Second International Study of Infarct Survival. Reproduced with permission from Ridker, et al.[13]

to hospital and provision of thrombolysis in patients with possible AMI, Birkhead[15] on behalf of the Joint Audit Committee of the British Cardiac Society and a Cardiology Committee of the Royal College of Physicians of London performed an observational study involving 1,934 patients admitted with suspected AMI. Patients who made emergency calls did so sooner after onset of symptoms than those who called their doctor (median time 40) minutes v 70 (70 to 90) minutes. General practitioners took a median of 20 (20 to 25) minutes to visit patients, rising to 30 (20 to 30) minutes during 0800-1200. The median time from call to arrival in hospital was 41 (38 to 47) minutes for patients who called an ambulance from home and 90 (90 to 94) minutes for those who contacted their doctor. The median time from arrival at hospital to thrombolysis was 80 (75 to 85) minutes for patients who were treated in the cardiac care unit and 31 (25 to 35) minutes for those treated in the accident and emergency department.

Electrocardiographic criteria in children

Myocardial infarction, a common occurrence in adults, is generally considered to be rare in children. Electrocardiographic criteria for diagnosis of AMI in adults are well known and accepted, but no general criteria exist for children. Towbin and associates[16] from Houston, Texas, reported 37 autopsy proven cases of transmural AMI and electrocardiographic evidence of AMI in 30 of these cases. A variety of conditions previously reported to produce "pseudo-infarction" are included in these cases of AMI, including myocarditis, HC, and the cardiomyopathy of Duchenne's muscular dystrophy (Figure 3-5). Compilation of the electrocardiographic data in all patients allowed for the development of criteria for this diagnosis of AMI in childhood, and include wide Q waves (>35 ms) with or without Q-wave notching, ST-segment elevation (>2 mm), and prolonged QT interval corrected for heart rate (QTc >440 ms) with accompanying Q-wave abnormalities. With use of these electrocardiographic criteria, an additional 3 patients were subsequently diagnosed prospectively with AMI and confirmed on autopsy. Pathologic evaluation confirmed the location of infarct predicted by the electrocardiograms in all 3 cases.

Infarct location to coronary narrowing

To determine whether the site of AMI can be predicted on the basis of a previous arteriogram, Giroud and associates[17] from Geneva, Switzerland, evaluated 184 consecutive angiograms obtained between March 1972 and August 1990 in 92 patients who had undergone coronary angiography both before and after AMI without intervening CABG or PTCA. Median time between the first coronary angiography and AMI was 26 months (range 1 to 144). On the first angiogram, most patients (89%) had 1- or 2-vessel disease, and 56 (61%) had an abnormal ventriculography. Seventy-two segments (78%) responsible for a future AMI were not significantly stenosed. On the second angiogram, AMI was related to the previously most stenotic segments in only 29 patients (32%). For these patients, median time between first coronary angiography and AMI was slightly shorter (22 vs 28 months). The severity of the narrowing on the first angiogram was a poor predictor of subsequent AMI. It is concluded that in a selected, medically treated cohort, AMI is frequently related to a segment that was not the most stenotic one or was not even significantly

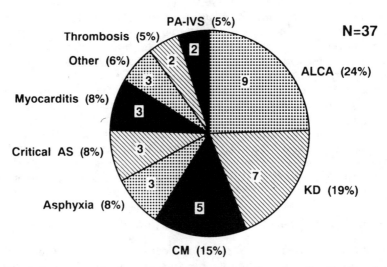

Fig. 3-5. Myocardial infarction in childhood. The distribution of cardiac disorders in 37 patients in which myocardial infarction occurred as seen at autopsy. ALCA = anomalous left coronary artery from the pulmonary artery; AS = aortic stenosis; CM = cardiomyopathy; KD = Kawasaki disease; PA-IVS = pulmonary atresia with intact ventricular septum. Reproduced with permission from Towbin, et al.[16]

stenosed at previous angiography, particularly with a long interval between the first angiogram and AMI.

Ultrafast magnetic resonance imaging

Van Rugge and associates[18] from Leiden and Utrecht, The Netherlands, assessed the value of ultrafast magnetic resonance imaging (MRI) for dynamic contrast enhancement and myocardial perfusion abnormalities in 20 patients with healed myocardial infarction. At baseline and after bolus injection of the paramagnetic contrast agent gadolinium-diethylenetriaminepentaacetic acid (0.04 mmol/kg body weight), single-level short-axis MRI was performed every third RR interval with an acquisition time of 500 ms. Myocardial signal intensities were measured in transmural myocardial regions of interest. After gadolinium-diethylenetriaminepentaacetic injection, infarcted and normal myocardium demonstrated a signal intensity enhancement of 50 and 134%, respectively. A signal intensity of normal relative to infarcted myocardium increased from 1.25 ± 0.22 (SD) before to 1.91 ± 0.41 after gadolinium-diethylenetriaminepentaacetic acid. The rate of signal increase in the infarcted and normal myocardium was 5.17 ± 2.22 and 18.99 ± 9.96 s^{-1}, respectively. Ultrafast MRI using gadolinium diethylenetriaminepentaacetic acid bolus administration clearly identifies myocardial perfusion abnormalities in patients with healed myocardial infarction. The infarct site on MRI corresponded with the location of wall motion asynergy determined by echocardiography.

Persons excluded from clinical trials

To determine the extent to which the elderly have been excluded from trials of drug therapies used in the treatment of AMI, to identify factors associated with such exclusions, and to explore the relation between the exclusion of the elderly and the representation of women, Gurwitz and associates[19] from Boston and Worcester, Massachusetts, conducted a systematic search of English language publications from January, 1960 through September, 1991, to identify all relevant studies of specific pharmocotherapies employed in the treatment of AMI. Only trials in which patients were randomly allocated to receive a specific therapeutic regimen or a placebo or nonplacebo control regimen were included for review. A total of 214 trials met inclusion criteria, involving 150,920 study subjects. Over 60% of trials excluded persons over the age of 75 years. Studies published after 1980 were more likely to have age-based exclusions compared with studies published before 1980. Trials of thrombolytic therapy involving an invasive procedure were more likely to exclude elderly patients compared with other studies. Studies with age-based exclusions had a smaller percentage of women compared with those without such exclusions (18% vs 23%), with the mean age of the study population significantly associated with the proportion of women participants. Age-based exclusions are frequently used in clinical trials of medications used in the treatment of AMI. Such exclusions limit the ability to generalize study findings to the patient population that experiences the most morbidity and mortality from AMI.

An excellent editorial on this topic was prepared by Nanette K. Wenger[20] from Atlanta, Georgia, who concluded with the following statement: "When the police queried the notorious criminal Willie Sutton as to why he robbed banks, he replied, 'because that's where the money is.'

Similarly, data applicable to elderly patients and to women must be derived from the relevant research source: studies conducted in these specific populations."

Diagnostic and therapeutic gender bias

Maynard and associates[21] from Seattle, Washington, designed a study to compare treatment and outcome of AMI in women and men. Patient hospital records were reviewed, and information about patient characteristics, treatments, and hospital events was entered in the Myocardial Infarction Triage and Intervention Registry. Between January 1988 and June 1990, a total of 4,891 consecutive patients, including 1,659 women, were hospitalized for AMI in 19 hospitals in the Seattle, Washington, metropolitan area (Figure 3-6). In-hospital thrombolytic therapy, coronary angiography, angioplasty, and CABG were examined, as were in-hospital complications and death. Women were older and more often had histories of previous hypertension and previous CHF. Thrombolytic therapy was used less often in women, although information about eligibility for treatment was not available to determine if this difference was due to treatment bias or differences in eligibility. Both coronary angiography and PTCA were used less frequently in women (Figure 3-7). Of patients who had coronary angiography, equal proportions of women and men received angioplasty and/or CABG. Hospital mortality was 16% for women and 11% for men, although this difference was diminished by age adjustment (Figure 3-8). Mortality was higher in women undergoing CABG, but this difference, too, was less apparent after age adjustment. Despite high levels of risk factors and mortality, coronary angiography and angioplasty were used less often in women, although among those who underwent coronary angiography, there were no gender differences in the use of angioplasty or bypass surgery.

To determine whether a gender bias exists in the selection of patients for diagnostic and therapeutic cardiovascular procedures early after AMI, Krumholz and associates[22] from Boston, Massachusetts, performed a retrospective cohort study involving 2,473 consecutive patients with a princi-

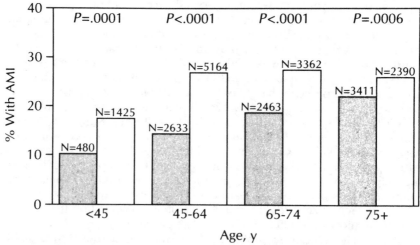

Fig. 3-6. Proportion of women (shaded bars) and men (open bars) admitted to coronary care units with a discharge diagnosis of acute myocardial infarction (AMI) according to age. Reproduced with permission from Maynard, et al.[21]

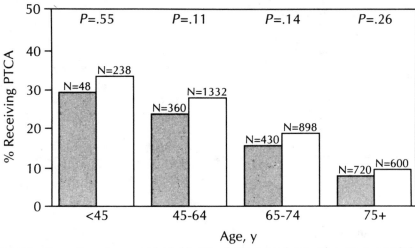

Fig. 3-7. Proportion of women (shaded bars) and men (open bars) with acute myocardial infarction who underwent percutaneous transluminal coronary angioplasty (PTCA), according to age. Reproduced with permission from Maynard, et al.[21]

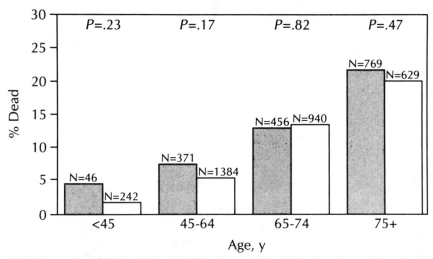

Fig. 3-8. Age-related hospital mortality in women (shaded bars) and men (open bars). Reproduced with permission from Maynard, et al.[21]

pal discharge diagnosis of AMI and a peak creatine kinase MB fraction of at least 4%. The study compared men and women regarding frequency with which they underwent various cardiac procedures (Figure 3-9). Women had coronary angiography during hospitalization for AMI much less frequently than men, but the age-adjusted rates were similar in women and men. An abnormal EF (< 50%) was equally frequent in women and men who underwent left ventriculography. Among patients who had coronary angiography, women had a significantly lower rate of severe CAD, defined as either a LM stenosis of >50%, 3-vessel, or 2-vessel CAD with a proximal LAD stenosis of >70%. When adjustments were made for age, women had PTCA as often as men but had CABG significantly less frequently. When adjustments were made for age and the severity of CAD, the difference in rates was of borderline significance. No evidence

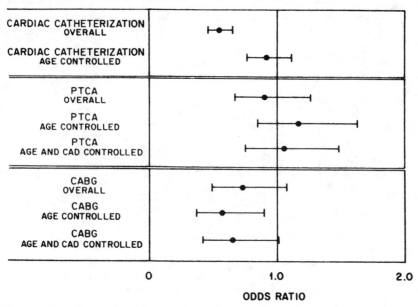

Fig. 3-9. Female-to-male odds ratios for cardiac procedures. Overall and age-controlled odds ratios are shown for cardiac catheterization. For both percutaneous transluminal coronary angioplasty (*PTCA*) and coronary artery bypass graft (*CABG*), overall odds ratios are shown, along with odds ratios adjusted for age and severity of coronary artery disease (*CAD*). Bars represent 95% CIs. Reproduced with permission from Krumholz, et al.[22]

of a difference in the rate of coronary angiography early after AMI between women and men was found after age adjustment. Among patients who have cardiac catheterization early after AMI, women and men are equally likely to have angioplasty, but women are less likely than men to have CABG.

Return to work and emotional distress

Rost and Smith[23] from Little Rock, Arkansas, examined how return to work predicted subsequent change in emotional distress in 143 patients who had been employed at the time of initial AMI. Ninety patients (63%) returned to work by 4 months and remained employed at 12 months. There were no differences in mental health at baseline between those who returned to work and those who did not, but emotional distress decreased significantly between 4 and 12 months only in the group who returned to work. Emotional distress declined after resuming work even when employees returned to jobs with which they reported dissatisfaction at the time of the AMI. The relationship between return to work and decreasing emotional distress remained after controlling for initial physical and psychological adjustment as well as sociodemographic and social support characteristics. The improvements in mental health associated with return to work should reassure clinicians who emphasize the emotional as well as economic value of work after an initial AMI.

Silent myocardial ischemia afterwards

Petretta and associates[24] from Naples, Italy, evaluated characteristics and prognostic significance of ischemic ST changes at predischarge Holter monitoring in 270 consecutive post AMI patients. The 64 patients with ST changes had a greater incidence of non-Q-wave AMI and VPCs; they were more frequently in Moss class >2 and they had a lower wall motion score. At 2-year follow-up, patients with ST changes had a higher incidence of cardiac death and reinfarction. At multivariate analysis, Killip class and ST changes were the most predictive variables; when multivariate analysis was repeated including an additional variable—the inability to perform a stress test—Killip class was the most significant variable, and the presence of ST changes showed only borderline statistical significance. In the subset of patients who did not perform the stress test, ST change was the most important variable, followed by Killip class. Thus, after AMI, ST changes during Holter monitoring are associated with a poor prognosis and appear useful for stratifying patients who do not perform exercise stress tests.

PROGNOSTIC INDICES

Age

To determine whether advancing age is an independent predictor of increased mortality following AMI or simply a marker for more extensive cardiac disease, a higher prevalence of comorbid conditions, and/or differences in therapeutic approach, Rich and associates[25] from St. Louis, Missouri, studied 261 consecutive patients with AMI admitted to a university teaching hospital during a 1-year interval. Seventy-four variables were analyzed to determine univariant predictors of in-hospital and 1-year post-discharge mortality. Multiple linear regression models were constructed to determine independent predictors of early and late mortality after adjusting for baseline and therapeutic differences between younger and older patients. Compared with patients <70 years (n = 124), patients ≥70 years (n = 137) were more likely to be female and have a prior history of ischemic heart disease. New York Heart Association functional class and Killip class on admission were higher in older patients, as were the admission serum creatinine and blood urea nitrogen levels. Serum albumin and peak creatine kinase levels were lower in older patients, but older patients were more likely to exhibit LV hypertrophy or atrioventricular block on the initial electrocardiogram. Finally, younger patients were 3 times as likely to receive a thrombolytic agent and 66% more likely to receive intravenous B-blockade than older patients, and younger patients were also more likely to receive heparin and intravenous nitroglycerin. Hospital mortality was 5.6% in patients <70 years versus 16.1% in patients ≥70 years. After adjusting for baseline and therapeutic differences, independent predictors of hospital mortality were systolic BP on admission (inverse correlation), B-blocker therapy (inverse correlation), age, peak creatine kinase level, and Killip class. Among hospital survivors, 1-year post discharge mortality was 6.8% in patients <70 years versus 19.1% in those ≥70 years. Independent predictors of post-discharge mortality after adjusting for age-related baseline and therapeutic differences were admission heart rate, age, LVEF (inverse correlation), initial non-Q-wave AMI and the blood urea nitrogen level. After adjusting for multiple baseline and therapeutic differences between older and younger patients, age per se remained a strong independent predictor of both inhospital and 1-year post-discharge mortality rates in patients with AMI.

Ventricular arrhythmias

To determine of the signal-averaged (SA) electrocardiogram (ECG) predicts the occurrence of sustained ventricular arrhythmia and sudden death after AMI, Steinberg and associates[26] from New York, New York, performed SAECG in 82 consecutive patients. Seventy-one patients (39%) had an abnormal SAECG. The presence of an abnormal SAECG was not related to underlying LV dysfunction or any other clinical or measured variable. There were 16 end points (sustained ventricular arrhythmia or sudden cardiac death) during 14-month follow-up. The SAECG was a significant predictor of these events, and an abnormal SAECG conferred a 2.7-fold increase in risk. The risk associated with an abnormal SAECG was independent of both LV function and ventricular arrhythmia on Holter ECG. The SAECG had excellent negative predictive accuracy (95%), but the positive predictive accuracy was low (15%). When the results of the SAECG were combined with the results of the Holter ECG, a group of very high-risk patients was identified; at 18 months, the presence of abnormal SAECG and Holter ECG was associated with a risk of 26% compared with only 4% if both tests were normal. Furthermore, all published studies with a similar design were pooled for meta-analysis. The meta-analysis revealed a 6-fold increase in risk, independent of LV function, and an 8-fold increase in risk, independent of Holter results when the SAECG was abnormal. The SAECG is a noninvasive test that can rapidly and easily provide potent prognostic information regarding the risk of sustained ventricular arrhythmias for patients after AMI.

To compare 1-, 6- and 24-hour ambulatory electrocardiograms for prediction of mortality after AMI, Connolly and associates[27] on behalf of the CAMIAT Pilot Study Group identified all patients with AMI hospitalized in Hamilton, Canada, during a one-year period. There were 683 patients discharged alive after AMI. One-, 6- and 24-hour ambulatory electrocardiographic results were available in 565 patients, and follow-up mortality data at 1 year was available in 560. Mean age of the patients was 64 years; 160 (29%) had previous AMI and 105 (19%) had had CHF. One hundred and fifty-two patients (27%) were receiving B blockers, and 31 (6%) were receiving antiarrhythmic drugs. Regression modeling of survival times up to 1 year showed that all 3 durations of recording were univariate predictors of mortality. Using 10 ventricular premature complexes/hour as the criterion of a positive test, neither the 6- nor 24-hour data contained statistically significant residual explanatory power after the 1-hour data were accounted for by the model. The longer durations of recording increased sensitivity at a cost of decreased specificity. The positive and negative predictive values of the 3 durations of recording were virtually identical. The presence of VT was not a significant predictor of mortality in this population. There appears to be no benefit to ambulatory electrocardiographic recordings > 1 hour when they are to be used for prediction of 1-year mortality after AMI.

Rodriguez and associates[28] from Maastricht, the Netherlands, Heidelberg, Germany, and Liege, Belgium, developed a prognostic index for nonfatal recurrences of VT using a retrospective analysis of a group of 206 patients with sustained monomorphic VT or VF after healing of the AMI. Seventy-four patients (36%) (64 with VT and 10 with VF) had recurrences of sustained monomorphic VT during 3.4 ± 9 years of follow-up. Three clinical variables were selected and weighted by stepwise logistic discriminant analysis of the study group. They were coded as follows: interval of AMI to arrhythmia (<2 months = 1; 2 to 6 months = 2; >6 months = 3), drug therapy with or without sotalol (with = 1, without = 2), and VT or VF as the presenting arrhythmia (VT − 1, VF − 2). The prognostic index was: 3.41 − (0.56 × interval) − (1.94 × therapy) + (0.86 × arrhythmia). This index was validated prospectively in a test group of 158 consecutive patients with VT or VF after healing of AMI. Patients were allocated into different classes with decreasing prognostic index values associated with increasing risk for recurrences of VT. In the test group, 27 of 158 (17%) patients (22 with VT and 5 with VF) had recurrences of VT (follow-up of 2 ± 2 years). Two risk classes of patients were identified: high risk for recurrences of VT (61%) corresponding to patients with a negative index; and low risk (4%) consisting of those with a positive index. Thus, using 0 as the cutoff point, the sensitivity, specificity, and positive and negative predictive values were 81, 89, 62 and 96%, respectively. This prognostic index may be used in selecting treatment for patients with severe ventricular arrhythmias after healing of AMI.

In survivors of complicated AMI, the inducibility of sustained VT may help identify a subset that is at increased risk for subsequent sudden cardiac death or spontaneous sustained VT. Bhandari and associates[29] from Los Angeles, California, performed prehospital discharge programmed ventricular stimulation in 86 survivors of AMI complicated by CHF, angina pectoris, or nonsustained VT. These patients also underwent cardiac catheterization with coronary angiography and 24-hour ambulatory electrocardiographic recording. Programmed ventricular stimulation induced sustained VT in 19 patients (22%) and VF in 6 (7%) and did not induce these arrhythmias in 61 patients (71%). During an average follow-up of 18 ± 13 months, 11 patients had arrhythmic events (7 sudden death and 4 nonfatal spontaneous sustained VT) and 10 patients had nonsudden cardiac death. The total cardiac mortality rate was 20%. Arrhythmic events occurred in 32% of the 19 patients with inducible sustained VT compared with 7% of the remaining 67 patients. By multivariate analysis the occurrence of arrhythmic events was independently predicted by both inducible sustained VT and Killip class III or IV heart failure. The risk of arrhythmic events was 4.4% in the absence of both variables versus 38% when both variables were present. The total cardiac mortality rate was best predicted by low LVEF (<30%). Thus programmed ventricular stimulation is useful in risk stratification of survivors of complicated AMI. The prognostic utility appears to be particularly high in patients with infarction complicated by Killip class III or IV heart failure.

Wilson and Kostis[30] for the Beta-Blocker Heart Attack Trial followed survivors of AMI with <2 VPCs per hour on 24-hour ambulatory echocardiogram for an average of 25 months (11-40 months) while receiving a placebo (1,222 patients) or propranolol, 180-240 mg/day (1,234 patients). Three quarters of the participants with VPCs had an average of <2 VPCs per hour (Figure 3-10). Only 16% did not have any ventricular ectopic activity during the 24 hours. Analysis of total mortality according to the number of VPCs per hour showed that patients who had VPCs with a very low frequency (<0.5 per hour) had 49% higher mortality than patients who did not have any VPC (Figure 3-11). Patients who had >0.5 VPC per hour but <1 VPC per hour had a statistically significant higher mortality rate, 11.7 versus 4.1% than patients who had no VPC. These data indicate that low ventricular ectopic activity frequency is associated with increased mortality in survivors of AMI.

% OF POPULATION

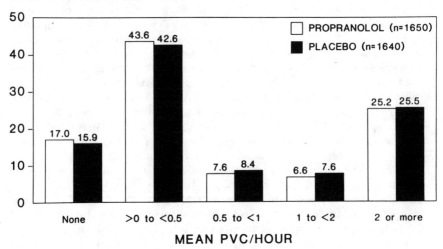

Fig. 3-10. Prevalence of ventricular ectopic activity in survivors of acute myocardial infarction. The population is the 3,290 BHAT trial participants who were being monitored by 24-h ambulatory electrocardiography at baseline. Reproduced with permission from Wilson AC and Kostis JB.[30]

DEATHS PER 100 PATIENTS

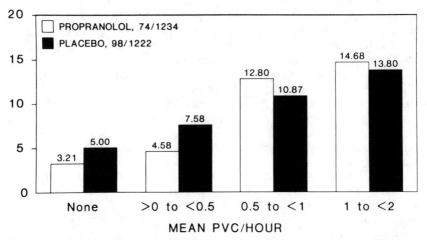

Fig. 3-11. Relationship between mortality rate and increasing mean number of PVC per hour in the BHAT trial patients at baseline over an average followup period of 25 months. The population is the 2,456 BHAT trial participants who had an average of <2 PVC/h. Reproduced with permission from Wilson AC and Kostis JB.[30]

Non-Q wave infarction

In a study by Schechtman and associates[31] from St. Louis, Missouri, Boston, Massachusetts, Providence, Rhode Island, Cheyenne, Wyoming, Houston, Texas, and Charlottesville, Virginia, the association between 1-year mortality and infarct location was evaluated in 544 patients with non-Q wave AMI. Infarcts were anterior (alone or including other locations) in 51% (n = 278) of cases, localizable but not anterior 30% (n = 161) of the time, and nonlocalizable in 19% (n = 105) of patients. One-year actuarial mortality (73 deaths) was 17% in the anterior group, 13% in the nonanterior group, and 6.8% in nonlocalizable patients. Anterior and localizable nonanterior mortality were similar. However, there were differences when mixed location infarcts were excluded. Mortality in the inferior infarction only group (2.8%, n = 36) was less than in the lateral infarction only group (17%, n = 79) and almost significantly less than in the anterior only group (15%, n = 62). The positive prognosis in the inferior infarction only group may be associated with the low rate of ST depression among these patients compared with those with other infarct locations. Mortality among localizable infarcts (16%) was greater than among those that were nonlocalizable (6.8%). Despite the low overall risk of the nonlocalizable infarcts, 42% (n = 44) of these patients developed ≥1 important risk factor while in hospital. It was concluded that among patients with relatively small non-Q wave myocardial infarction: 1) anterior mortality is similar to localizable nonanterior mortality; 2) inferior only infarcts have a better prognosis than infarcts with other non-mixed locations; 3) infarct localizability implies increased risk; and 4) nonlocalizable infarcts define a heterogeneous group among which a substantial proportion will develop in-hospital risk factors that are associated with decreased survival.

To compare the short and long-term prognosis after a first Q-wave or non-Q-wave AMI, Berger and associates[32] from Framingham and Boston, Massachusetts, and Bethesda, Maryland, followed 227 men and 136 women, mean age 67 years, for a mean of 5.1 ± 4.9 years, 77% of whom had a first Q-wave AMI and 23% of whom had a non-Q-wave first AMI. Reinfarction and death from CAD were the mean outcome measures. During the follow-up period, subjects with non-Q-wave infarction had a significantly higher rate of reinfarction than subjects in the Q-wave group (Figure 3-12). The 10-year reinfarction rates were 44.8% vs. 27.4%. When analyzed separately by age and sex, differences in reinfarction rates were only noted in men and in those under the age of 65 years. There were no differences in CAD death rates based on Q-wave status, even when

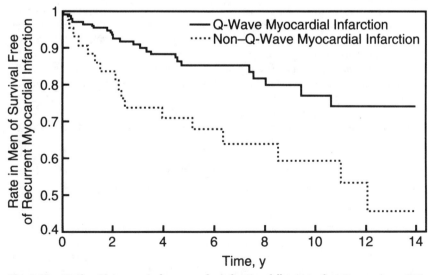

Fig. 3-12. Kaplan-Meier survival curves of reinfarction following a first Q-wave (n = 172) and non–Q-wave (n = 52) myocardial infarction in male subjects. There were 23 reinfarctions in the Q-wave group and 17 reinfarctions in the non–Q-wave group (*P* = .005). Reproduced with permission from Berger, et al.[32]

examined separately by age and sex. Multivariate analysis revealed a 1.8-fold higher risk of reinfarction in the non-Q-wave group, and also demonstrated that baseline hypertension was an independent risk factor for predicting reinfarction. There were no differences in the rates of sudden death or all-cause mortality following the 2 types of AMI. Additionally, subjects with a first Q-wave infarction had a higher rate of subsequent CHF, while those with non-Q-wave infarctions had a significantly higher rate of coronary insufficiency (unstable angina with transient ST-T wave abnormalities). These results confirm and extend findings from prior studies that have identified patients with first non-Q-wave AMIs as potentially unstable, with greater subsequent morbidity and similar mortality to their counterparts with Q-wave infarctions.

The article was followed by an editorial entitled "Q-Wave Vs Non-Q-Wave Myocardial Infarction—An Oversimplified Dichotomy" by Arthur, J. Moss[33] from Rochester, New York. The final paragraph of his editorial was as follows: "Enormous progress has been made in the past decade in identifying patients at risk of a second myocardial infarction and cardiac death after a first coronary event. The risk is related largely to the magnitude of left ventricular dysfunction and to the amount of residual jeopardized ischemic myocardium, but not specifically to the electrocardiographic type of infarction. If a patient has recurrent angina or clinical evidence of left ventricular dysfunction after an initial coronary event, then coronary angiography is indicated. If a patient is asymptomatic after infarction, early exercise testing is the most cost-effective approach to stratify and identify high-risk patients with jeopardized ischemic myocardium, left ventricular dysfunction, or ventricular arrhythmias who may be amenable to treatment. These recommendations apply equally to patients with Q-wave and non-Q-wave infarctions, regardless of whether the patients received thrombolytic therapy."

Pulmonary congestion

The interrelation of different grades of pulmonary congestion evaluated by chest roentgenogram in the coronary care unit, predischarge LVEF and long-term prognosis was studied in 1,850 surviving patients of AMI by Gottlieb and associates[34] from Rochester, New York. Pulmonary congestion was categorized as: none, mild or moderate, or severe; LVEF was classified as: $\geq 40\%$, 25 to 39%, or $<25\%$. The majority of patients (1,060; 57%) had an LVEF $\geq 40\%$ and no signs of pulmonary congestion. Severe pulmonary congestion was noted in 63 patients (3.4%), 17 with LVEF $<25\%$ and 16 with LVEF $\geq 40\%$. One hundred twenty-five patients (6.8%) had an LVEF $<25\%$, 49 of whom had no signs of pulmonary congestion. During a mean 2-year follow-up, cardiac mortality occurred in 212 patients (11.5%). The cardiac mortality rate was related to both predischarge LVEF impairment and severity of pulmonary congestion. Cardiac mortality hazard ratios for LVEF $<25\%$, and 25 to 39% were 5.32 and 2.91, respectively, where a referent hazard ratio of 1 was assigned to patients with LVEF $\geq 40\%$ and to those with no pulmonary congestion. Development of pulmonary congestion during AMI significantly increased the cardiac mortality risk derived from LVEF, with a marked mortality effect in patients with severe pulmonary congestion. These findings emphasize the independent prognostic role of pulmonary congestion and highlight the interactive mechanisms (systolic and diastolic dysfunctions) responsible for unfavorable outcome in surviving AMI patients.

Living alone

To determine if the presence of a disrupted marriage or living alone would be an independent prognostic risk factor for a subsequent major cardiac event following an initial AMI, Case and associates[35] from New York, Rochester, and Manhasset, New York, performed a prospective evaluation in the placebo wing of a randomized, double-blind drug trial in patients with an enzyme-documented AMI who were admitted to a coronary care facility. Data for living alone and/or a marital disruption were entered into a Cox proportional hazards model constructed from important physiologic and nonphysiologic factors in the same database. All consenting patients who were 25 to 75 years of age and without other serious diseases were enrolled (placebo, N = 1234) within 3 to 15 days of the index infarction and followed for a period of 1 to 4 years (mean, 2.1 years). Nine hundred sixty-seven patients were followed for 1.1 years and 530 for 2.2 years. Recurrent major cardiac event (either recurrent nonfatal infarction or cardiac death) was the primary outcome measure. Living alone was an independent risk factor, with a hazard ratio of 1.54 (Figure 3-13). Using the Kaplan-Meier statistical method for calculation, the recurrent cardiac event rate at 6 months was 15.8% in the group living alone vs 8.8% in the group not living alone. Risk remained significant throughout the follow-up period. A disrupted marriage was not an independent risk factor. Living alone but not a disrupted marriage is an independent risk factor for prognosis after AMI when compared with all other known risk factors.

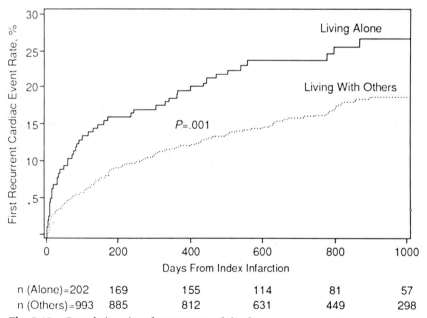

Fig. 3-13. Cumulative rate of occurrence of the first recurrent cardiac event (nonfatal myocardial infarction or cardiac death, whichever is first) over a 1-year to 4-year (mean, 2.7 years) follow-up period. At 6 months, the recurrent event rate in those patients living alone is 79% greater than in those living with others. Reproduced with permission from Case, et al.[35]

Emotional support

To compare the survival of elderly patients hospitalized for AMI who have emotional support with that of patients who lack such support, while controlling for severity of CAD, comorbidity, and functional status, Berkman and associates[36] from New Haven, Connecticut, performed a prospective, community-based cohort study involving 100 men and 94 women aged 65 years or more hospitalized for AMI between 1982 and 1988. Social support, age, gender, race, education, marital status, living arrangements, presence of depression, smoking history, weight, and physical function were assessed prospectively using questionnaires. The presence of CHF, pulmonary edema, and cardiogenic shock; the position of infarction; in-hospital complications; and history of AMI were assessed using medical records. Comorbidity was defined using an index based on the presence of 8 conditions. Of 194 patients, 76 (39%) died in the first 6 months after AMI. In multiple logistic regression analyses, lack of emotional support was significantly associated with 6-month mortality after controlling for severity of AMI, comorbidity, risk factors such as smoking and hypertension, and sociodemographic factors. When emotional support was assessed before AMI, it was independently related to risk for death in the subsequent 6 months.

Psychological stress

Because of their unstable pathophysiology, Frasure-Smith and associates[37] from Montreal, Canada, hypothesized that patients with non-Q-wave AMI would be more vulnerable to the negative effects of psychologic stress than patients with Q-wave AMI and thus would be more likely to benefit from programs aimed at relieving stress. This hypothesis was tested through secondary analysis of data from a 1-year randomized clinical trial of psychological stress monitoring and intervention after AMI. After discharge, treatment group patients were telephoned each month and asked to respond to an index of psychological stress symptoms (General Health Questionnaire GHQ-20). Those with high stress symptoms (GHQ ≥5) received home nursing visits. Control group patients received usual care. The sample consisted of 461 men, aged 31 to 86 years, who responded to the GHQ-20 before hospital discharge. Patients were followed for 5 years using record data. There were 321 Q-wave AMIs, 112 non-Q-wave AMIs and 28 indeterminate electrocardiograms. Life-table analyses showed that among patients with non-Q-wave AMIs receiving usual care, high stress in the hospital (GHQ ≥5) was associated with a 1-year relative risk of cardiac mortality of 5.49 ± 1.39. In comparison, control patients with Q-wave MIs had no stress-related increase in risk. In the treatment group, the patients with non-Q-wave AMIs did not experience an increase in risk associated with high stress. Further, this pattern of results was not altered by adjustment for covariates including previous history of AMI. In conclusion, the link between psychological stress and cardiac events is more apparent among patients with non-Q-wave than Q-wave AMI, and therefore stress-relieving interventions may be of particular value after non-Q-wave AMI.

In Medicare population

Udvarhelyi and associates[38] from Boston, Massachusetts, described the process of care and clinical outcomes associated with AMI in the

Medicare population. They examined differences in process of care and outcome of care as a function of patient age, gender, and race. They used a longitudinal data base created from Medicare utilization and administrative files. They studied a cohort of AMI patients covered by Medicare in 1987 and a random sample of Medicare patients without AMI. The main outcome measurements were the following: (1) The use of coronary angiography, CABG, and PTCA during the first 90 days after a new AMI; (2) mortality at 30 days, 1 year, and 2 years; (3) reinfarction rates; and (4) reoperation rates for CABG and PTCA. The mortality rates were high: 26% at 1 month, 40% at 12 months, and 47% at 24 months (Figure 3-14). They varied greatly by age, less so by gender and race, and were high even among patients who survived the first 1 month. Compared with mortality, reinfarction was uncommon, occurring in 7.3% of patients. During the first 90 days, 23% of all patients underwent angiography and

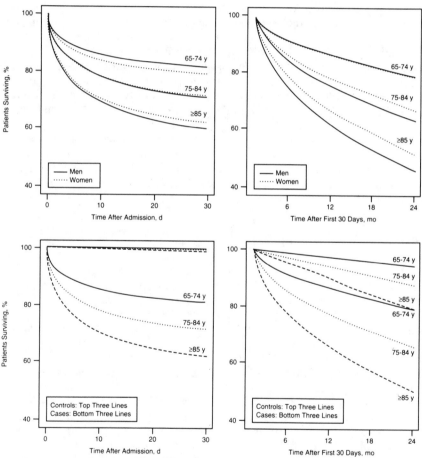

Fig. 3-14. Gender- and age-specific survival during the 2 years following an acute myocardial infarction (AMI) for the 1987 AMI cohort and the Medicare control population. The ordinate represents the cumulative proportion of patients surviving over time. Top left, Differences in survival between men and women during the first 30 days after their index AMI. Top right. Differences in survival between men and women for those surviving the first 30 days. Bottom left, Survival of the AMI cohort by age compared with the control population for the first 30 days. Bottom right, Survival of the AMI cohort by age groups compared with the control population for those surviving the first 30 days. Reproduced with permission from Udvarhelyi, et al.[38]

13% underwent coronary revascularization (CABG, 8%; PTCA, 5%). The use of all 3 procedures decreased with age and was less common among women and blacks than among men and whites. Differential use by age and race was greater for angiography than for revascularization procedures. The prognosis following AMI in patients aged 65 years and above is much worse than is commonly realized. Procedure use in these patients varies as a function of gender and race, even though mortality does not.

Preceding angina pectoris

Behar and associates[39] from Tel Hashomer, Israel, examined the role of chronic (> 1 month) angina before AMI in predicting hospital and long-term mortality rates among 4166 patients with first AMI. The prevalence of angina in these patients was 43%. Chronic angina was more common in women (49%), patients with hypertension (49%), and diabetic patients (49%) than in men and counterparts free of the former conditions. In patients with angina the hospital course was more complicated and non-Q-wave AMI was more common than in counterparts without angina. In-hospital (16%), as well as 1- (8%) and 5-year postdischarge (26%), mortality rates in hospital survivors were higher among patients with previous angina than in patients without previous angina (12%, 6%, and 19%, respectively). After adjustment for age and all other predictors of increased mortality rates in this cohort of patients, angina preceding AMI emerged as an independent predictor of increased hospital mortality rates. For postdischarge mortality rates (mean follow-up 5.5 years), the covariate-adjusted relative risk of death in patients with angina was similar, according to estimation by Cox proportional hazards model. These data support the notion that preexisting angina identifies a group of patients at increased risk of death.

Collateral filling of the infarct artery

Reported studies have showed that long-term morbidity and mortality after AMI are influenced by the presence or absence of anterograde flow in the infarct artery. In comparison with patients with anterograde flow, those whose infarct artery remains occluded are more likely to have unstable angina, recurrent AMI, CHF, and sudden death. Boehrer and associates[40] from Dallas, Texas, performed a study to assess the influence of collateral filling of the infarct artery on long-term morbidity and mortality in surviving patients of initial AMI in whom the infarct artery was occluded. Over a 12.5 year period, 146 subjects (108 men and 38 women; aged 25 to 76 years) with AMI, no anterograde flow in the infarct artery, and no disease of other coronary arteries were medically treated and followed for 42 ± 28 months. Of these subjects, 120 had angiographic evidence of collateral filling of the infarct artery (group I), whereas the remaining 26 did not (group II). The groups were similar in age, sex, cardioactive medications, LV performance and infarct artery. They were also similar in incidence of unstable angina (19% of group I, 31% of group II), recurrent AMI (12% of group I, 8% of group II), congestive heart failure (16% of group I, 12% of group II) and cardiac death (16% of group I, 19% of group II). Thus, angiographic evidence of collateral filling of the infarct artery in surviving patients of AMI exerts no demonstrable influence (beneficial or detrimental) on long-term morbidity or mortality.

Electrocardiographic left ventricular hypertrophy

Behar and associates[41] of the SPRINT Study Group involving 13 coronary care units between July 1981 and August 1983 found the electrocardiographic evidence of LV hypertrophy to be 6.1% among the 4,720 consecutive hospital survivors of AMI. The prevalence of electrocardiographic LV hypertrophy increased with age and was higher in patients with previous AMI, angina, and systemic hypertension. Mean age of patients with electrocardiographic LV hypertrophy was 67.2 vs 61.4 years in counterparts free of electrocardiographic LV hypertrophy. Patients with electrocardiographic LV hypertrophy had a higher rate of CHF on admission, or developing during their stay in coronary care units. The 1- and 5-year mortality rates were 19.7 and 46.6% among patients with electrocardiographic LV hypertrophy versus 8.7 and 26.2%, respectively in patients without this finding. The covariate-adjusted odds ratio of 1-year mortality was 1.88 for the presence of electrocardiographic LV hypertrophy when age alone was adjusted for, and 1.51 when multiple covariate adjustment was undertaken. After multiple covariate adjustment for 5-year mortality after discharge, the relative risk associated with electrocardiographic LV hypertrophy was 1.51. The results of the present study showed that the presence of electrocardiographic LV hypertrophy on the discharge electrocardiogram of survivors from AMI is associated with a 1.5-fold increase of short- and long-term mortality. Patients with electrocardiographic LV hypertrophy, potentially at an increased post-discharge risk, may be candidates for early noninvasive testing and more intensive follow-up after recovering from AMI.

Intermittent ST depression

Ruberman and colleagues[42] in Edmonton, Canada, conducted a case-control analysis to determine the contribution made to mortality by intermittent ST depression among patients enrolled in the already completed Beta Blocker Heart Attack Trial. ST-depression was determined by computer analysis of 24-hour electrocardiographic tapes as a change in ST level by ±0.1 mV or more from the median value of ST-segments of all normally conducted complexes for ≥1 minute. All computer-detected ST events were verified by trained readers. To estimate risk of dying associated with ST-depression, 261 deaths were compared with controls matched for age, sex, drug status, and time elapsed since AMI. In a model including relevant covariates, ST-segment depression had a relative risk of 1.73. The relative risk was 2.56 in untreated patients and 0.98 in propranolol-treated patients. A history of angina, although not independently significant, was found to enhance these relative risks. A gradient of risk was shown in the placebo group by a relative risk of 1.91 in those with 1-30 minutes of ST-segments depression and 4.33 in those with >30 of ST-segment depression. The findings in this large study show a significant contribution to mortality among untreated early post-AMI survivors from transient ST-segment depression on 24-hour monitoring. The absence or reduction of effect in the treated group also suggest an anti-ischemic mechanism by which propranolol exerts a protective effect on mortality.

Early resting echocardiogram

To develop improved prognostic algorithms for routine bedside use in AMI, Berning and associates[43] from Copenhagen, Denmark, defined in

201 consecutive patients the prognostic value concerning 2- and 12-month mortality of an early (within 72 hours after AMI) resting echocardiogram. The relation between (1) the clinical variables (age, sex, prior and repeat AMI, arrhythmias, cardiac arrest, early [<72 hours after AMI] and late CHF, early and maximal in-hospital Killip class, and maximal creatine kinase-MB (isoenzyme), (2) early myocardial performance by echocardiography, and (3) mortality was characterized by Kaplan-Meier survival curves and receiver-operating characteristic curves based on Cox regression model. Only age and clinical CNF in terms of the maximal in-hospital Killip class had independent predictive value of death when an early echocardiographic estimate of LVEF was included in the multivariate statistical models (Table 3-1).

In a prospective clinical trial of 195 consecutive unselected patients with AMI, systematic blinded clinical and echocardiographic examinations were performed by 2 observers on day 5 in a study carried out by Launbjerg and colleagues[44] from Hillerød, Denmark. The purpose was to define low-risk patients with regard to in-hospital and 2-month mortality and predict the potential costs (lost patient lives) and benefits (saved in-patient days) if as a routine procedure these low-risk patients were discharged earlier. By design, low-risk patients as defined by clinical criteria were allocated to discharge on days 7 to 10 and by echocardiographic criteria on days 5 to 7 after AMI. The sensitivity of the echocardiographic low-risk identification procedure was more than twofold higher than the sensitivity of clinical low-risk identification (49% vs 24%). Both procedures were safe with a specificity of 100% for cardiac mortality. Optimal identification of low-risk patients was provided by combining data from echocardiographic and clinical evaluations (sensitivity 59%). Results of the study suggest that a bedside echocardiographic approach to estimation of global LV function is more sensitive and equally specific and therefore more efficient for risk stratification on post-AMI day 5 than clinical examination alone. Thus, echocardiographic examination allows identification of a larger subset of patients with AMI (>40% of the population alive on day 5) who can be discharged earlier and safely, with a

TABLE 3-1. *Clinical Variables According to Survival Status One Year After Acute Myocardial Infarction. Reproduced with permission from Berning, et al.[43]*

Clinical Variables	Survivors (n = 149)	Nonsurvivors (n = 52)	p Value*
Sex (women/men)	36/113	20/32	<0.05
Age (yr) (median [range])	61.2 (35–83)	66.3 (43–90)	<0.005
AMI number (1/2/3/4)	109/31/8/1	40/7/2/3	NS
Reinfarction†	7	1	NS
Asystole†	1	2	NS
Atrial fibrillation†	12	8	NS
Supraventricular tachycardia†	1	0	NS
Ventricular premature complexes†	6	3	NS
Ventricular fibrillation†	11	6	NS
Early heart failure	39	33	<0.0001
Late heart failure	58	43	<0.0001
Early Killip class (1/2/3/4) (n)	110/32/3/4	19/22/3/8	<0.0001
Maximal Killip class (1/2/3/4) (n)	91/40/9/9	9/18/2/23	<0.0001
Maximal CKMB (median [range])	158 (10–1,492)	193 (19–1,524)	NS
Early echocardiographic LVEF (median [range])	41 (15–72)	28 (9–54)	<0.0001

*Kruskall Wallis test (univariate comparison).
†Present within the first 5 days after AMI.
AMI = acute myocardial infarction; CKMB = creatine kinase-MB; LVEF = left ventricular ejection fraction; NS = not significant.

potential saving of in-patient days of 436 days in 87 low-risk patients minus the cost of echocardiographic studies in 195 patients. However, the best prediction was obtained by combining clinical and echocardiographic examinations. This procedure identified 104 patients (53% of population) who were candidates for early discharge with even greater potential savings and no deaths within 2 months after AMI.

Dipyridamole-induced wall-motion abnormalities

Bolognese and associates[45] in Novara, Italy, determined the prevalence and prognostic significance of silent myocardial in 217 patients recovering from a first uncomplicated AMI and undergoing a dipyridamole echocardiography test before hospital discharge. Clinical, angiographic, exercise electrocardiographic and dipyridamole echocardiographic variables were examined. Among 217 patients, 89 had no echocardiographically proved dyssynergy after dipyridamole, whereas 128 had dipyridamole-induced wall motion abnormalities that were silent in 94 (Group I) and symptomatic in 34 (Group II). There were no intergroup differences with respect to dipyridamole time, prevalence of inferior AMI, ischemic electrocardiographic changes during the test, diabetes, ongoing medical therapy, multivessel disease, and baseline left ventricular ejection fraction. There was also no significant difference between Group I and Group II patients as regards wall motion score index at peak dipyridamole effect. Patients were followed for 24 ± 4 and 25 ± 5 months, respectively. Life table analysis revealed no difference in unstable angina, reinfarction and death between the 2 groups. A Cox survival analysis identified a positive echocardiogram after dipyridamole administration as the best predictor of cardiac events, whereas dipyridamole-induced chest pain showed no independent predictive value. Therefore, patients with silent and symptomatic ischemia had comparable (1) severity of dipyridamole-induced ischemia, (2) extent of angiographic CAD, and (3) frequency of important cardiac events subsequently.

COMPLICATIONS

Ventricular arrhythmia

Incidence and timing of recurrences of sustained VT or sudden death were studied by Rodriguez and associates[46] from Maastricht, the Netherlands, in 206 patients who survived their first episode of VF (n = 52) or sustained VT (n = 154) after AMI. All patients were treated with (empirically selected) antiarrhythmic drugs; 49% received amiodarone. After a mean follow-up of 36 months, 64 patients (41%) in the VT group and 10 (19%) in the VF group had nonfatal VT recurrences. Sudden death occurred in 22 (14%) and 9 (17%) patients in the VT and VF groups, respectively. Incidence of sudden death had 2 peaks at approximately 3 and 12 months. Nonfatal VT recurrences were more frequent (most often occurring in first 6 months) in the VT than in the VF group. Sudden death occurred during the following 3 years in only 10% of patients who survived 1 year. There was a much higher incidence of sudden death in patients with LVEF ≤40% than in those with LVEF >40% (28 of 65 vs 3 of 141), but no relation between LVEF and nonfatal VT recurrences.

To determine whether the beneficial effect of low-dose amiodarone on survival in patients with complex ventricular arrhythmias after AMI was dependent on LV function, Pfisterer and associates[47] of the Basel Antiarrhythmic Study of Infarct Survival were analyzed. Two hundred twelve patients after AMI with asymptomatic complex arrhythmias were randomly assigned to receive *amiodarone* 200 mg/day or to a control group and followed up for 1 year. Results of mortality and arrhythmic events were related to baseline radionuclide LVEF. With preserved (≥40%) LVEF, there was a significantly lower 1-year cardiac mortality in patients treated with amiodarone (1 of 68 or 1.5%) versus control subjects (5 of 56 or 8.9%). This was not the case for patients with LVEF <40%. Similarly, arrhythmic events were significantly reduced only in patients with preserved LV function. These results suggest an interaction between the effects of amiodarone on survival and LV dysfunction in patients after AMI.

To examine the immediate and long-term clinical and prognostic significance of primary VT, defined as tachycardia of ventricular origin occurring within the 48 hours of AMI in patients without hemodynamic compromise (Killip class I), Eldar and associates[48] for the SPRINT Study Group from Tel Hashomer, Israel, studied 162 patients with primary VT, both sustained and nonsustained (study group), and 2,578 counterparts without VT (reference group) in intensive coronary care units in 8 regional referral and university hospitals. The study and reference groups had similar mortality (in-hospital, 6.8% and 9.6% and at 1 year after discharge, 3.7% and 5.4%, respectively) and in-hospital complications rates (atrioventricular block, 12.0% and 9.7%; cardiogenic shock, 3.7% and 3.0%; cardiac arrest, 1.8% and 4.4%, respectively). Patients with sustained VT (18 patients) compared with those with nonsustained VT (134 patients) had higher rates of polymorphic tachycardia (50% compared with 6%), in-hospital total cardiac mortality (21% compared with 4%) and sudden-death mortality (14% compared with 2%); they also showed a trend toward a higher-in-hospital mortality than the reference group (21.4% compared with 9.6%) but had no increased mortality 1 year after discharge (4.6% compared with 5.4%). As a group, patients with primary VT do not differ from counterparts without primary VT in their in-hospital clinical course and 1-year prognosis. Primary sustained VT is often polymorphic and carries worse in-hospital prognosis than nonsustained tachycardia. However, it does not predict recurrent VT or increased sudden-death rates during the next year.

O'Hara and associates[49] from Maastricht, the Netherlands, studied 150 consecutive patients with sustained monomorphic VT (n = 116) or VF (n = 34) late after AMI, and found that 17 had reproduction of their sustained monomorphic VT during exercise testing. Data from these patients (group I) were compared with data from patients without exercise-induced VT (group II). No statistical difference was found between groups I and II with relation to age, sex, number of vessels with 70% stenosis, LVEF, number of previous myocardial infarctions, inducibility during programmed stimulation and total mortality during follow-up. In group I, only 1 patient (6%) developed ST depression during exercise compared with 47 patients (35%) in group II. After a 34-month mean follow-up, 6 patients in group I (35%) and 18 patients in group II (13%) died suddenly. It is concluded that sustained monomorphic VT is reproduced during exercise in only 11% of patients with spontaneous late sustained monomorphic VT or VF. Electrocardiographic findings do not support ischemia as a triggering mechanism of exercise-induced sustained monomorphic

VT. Patients with exercise-induced sustained monomorphic VT have a high incidence of sudden death.

Sudden death

Sudden arrhythmic cardiac death is a major unresolved health problem, yet there is no agreement on the chronologic definition of sudden death. Sweeney and associates[50] from Rochester, New York, in a retrospective study, investigated the frequency distribution of the chronology of the terminal cardiac event in a large post-AMI population and identified factors associated with instantaneous (<1 minute) cardiac death. The study involved 229 patients enrolled in the Multicenter Diltiazem Post-Infarction Trial who died during 2-year follow-up and had quantitative information on the chronology of the terminal event. Thirty-two percent of the cardiac deaths occurred instantaneously. Patients who died instantaneously were more likely to be men, to have a baseline EF <0.40, and to have a frequent (≥10/hour) and repetitive (≥3 in a row) VPC on an ambulatory electrocardiogram than those who did not die instantaneously. Patients who died instantaneously received more digitalis and class iA antiarrhythmic agents and less B blockers in the week before death than those dying noninstantaneously. Logistic regression analysis identified 3 independent factors that differentiated instantaneous from noninstantaneous death: frequent VPCs; digitalis and no B blocker medication. Instantaneous death (within 1 minute) was responsible for almost one third of the cardiac deaths that occurred in this postinfarction population. Frequent VPCs, digitalis, and absence of B-blocker therapy distinguished patients who died instantaneously from those who died noninstantaneously.

Heart block

As part of a community-based study of patients hospitalized with AMI in Worcester, Massachusetts, metropolitan area, Goldberg and associates[51] examined changes over time in the incidence rates of complete heart block (CHB) complicating AMI, and the prognostic impact of CHB on the in-hospital and long-term survival of these patients. In all, 4,762 patients with validated AMI hospitalized at 16 hospitals in the Worcester metropolitan area during 1975, 1978, 1981, 1984, 1986, and 1988 constituted the study sample. The incidence rates of CHB complicating AMI remained relatively stable at 5.8% over the 13-year (1975 to 1988) period studied. The incidence rates of CHB were approximately twice as high in patients with inferior/posterior wall AMI (7.7%) as in those with anterior wall AMI (3.9%). Use of a multivariate regression analysis to control for factors affecting the incidence rates of CHB revealed that patients were at highest risk for developing CHB during the latter 2 study years (1986 and 1988). Patients with AMI developing CHB had higher in-hospital case fatality rates than did those without CHB overall, as well as during each of the 6 periods studied. The in-hospital survival associated with CHB did not improve over time. After use of a multivariate regression analysis to control for additional prognostic factors, the independent effect of CHB on in-hospital prognosis remained. Patients with inferior wall AMI complicated by CHB were at significantly increased risk of dying during hospitalization compared with those without CHB. Long-term survival rates for up to a 14-year follow-up period for discharged surviving patients were not significantly different for AMI patients when compared with those without

CHB, with no significant differences in long-term survival observed concerning the location of the AMI. The results of this observational, population-based study suggest that the incidence rates of CHB resulting from AMI have not changed over time and that CHB is associated with an unfavorable short- but not long-term prognosis.

Berger and associates[52] and the TIMI Investigators determined the incidence and significance of second- or third-degree heart block among patients with inferior AMI treated with thrombolytic therapy. Data from the prethrombolytic era suggest that heart block occurs in approximately 20% of patients with acute inferior AMI and is associated with a marked increase in mortality. One thousand seven hundred and eighty-six patients with acute inferior AMI enrolled in the Thrombolysis in Myocardial Infarction (TIMI) II who received recombinant tissue-type plasminogen activator within 4 hours of symptom onset were evaluated. Heart block developed in 214 patients (12%). One hundred thirteen patients (6%) had heart block on presentation and 101 (6%) developed heart block in the 24 hours after treatment with tissue plasminogen activator. Patients with heart block at entry were slightly older and a greater proportion had cardiogenic shock. The 21-day mortality rate among patients with heart block at entry was 7% compared with 3% among patients without heart block at study entry. However, heart block was not independently associated with a 21-day mortality after adjustment for other variables, including shock. Mortality and other adverse cardiac events in the following year were similar among patients with and without heart block. Among patients without heart block at study entry, coronary arteriography among patients randomly assigned to coronary arteriography 18 to 48 hours after admission revealed that the infarct-related artery was occluded in 28% of patients who developed heart block versus 16% of patients without heart block. The 21-day mortality rate was increased among patients in whom heart block developed after thrombolytic therapy (10%) versus 2% in those patients without heart block. Analysis of the increased mortality among patients developing heart block suggested that mortality was due to severe cardiac dysfunction; no patient was thought to have died as a result of heart block or its treatment. These data demonstrate that heart block is common among patients with inferior AMI given thrombolytic therapy, and it is associated with increased mortality.

Cardiogenic shock

Gacioch and associates[53] in Ann Arbor, Michigan, and Cleveland, Ohio, evaluated 68 patients presenting to the University of Michigan with AMI and cardiogenic shock to determine whether hemodynamic support with new mechanical devices and emergency revascularization alter long-term prognosis in these patients. Interventions performed included thrombolytic therapy in 46%, intraaortic balloon counterpulsation in 70%, cardiac catheterization in 86%, PTCA in 73%, emergency CABG and VSD repair in 15%, hemopump insertion in 11%, percutaneous cardiopulmonary support in 4% and ventricular assist device usage in 3%. The 30-day survival rate was significantly better in patients who had successful PTCA of the infarct-related artery than in patients with failed angioplasty (61% vs. 7%) or no attempt at angioplasty (61% vs 14%) (Figure 3-15). This difference was maintained over a 1-year follow-up period. The only clinical variable that predicted survival was age <65 years. The early use of the new support devices in 10 patients was associated with death in 8, but this poor outcome may reflect a selection bias for an especially high risk population. These data suggest that emergency revascularization with PTCA may reduce the mortality rate in these patients.

Bengtson and colleagues[54] in Durham, North Carolina, evaluated a consecutive series of 200 patients admitted with AMI complicated by cardiogenic shock. The in-hospital mortality rate was 53%. Variables with significant univariate association with in-hospital death included patency of the infarct-related artery, patient age, lowest cardiac index, highest arteriovenous oxygen difference and left main CAD. The most important predictors of in-hospital death were patency of the infarct-related artery, cardiac index and peak creatine kinase, MB fraction. The mortality rate in patients with patent infarct-related arteries was 33% as compared to 75% in those with closed arteries and 84% in those in whom arterial patency was unknown. Patients who survived hospital discharge were followed for a median of 2 years with a mortality rate of 18% after 1 year. Thus, the best descriptor of the relation between the variables and postdischarge mortality included age, peak serum creatine kinase, LVEF, and patency of the infarct-related artery. Thus, in a large consecutive series of patients with cardiogenic shock with follow-up, patency of the infarct-related artery was most strongly associated with in-hospital and long-term mortality. These findings support an aggressive interventional strategy in patients with cardiogenic shock.

Mitral regurgitation

To investigate MR occurring early in the course of AMI, Lehmann and associates[55] of the TIMI Study Group performed a prospective observational study derived from patients entering phase I of the Thrombolysis in Myocardial Infarction (TIMI) trial involving 206 patients studied within 7 hours of symptom onset during their first AMI. Contrast left ventriculography was used to document MR. MR was present in 27 patients (13%). Although the presence of MR correlated with the site of the myocardial infarct (20 of the 27 had anterior wall infarcts) and the number of akinetic chords, it was not statistically related to the peak creatine kinase value

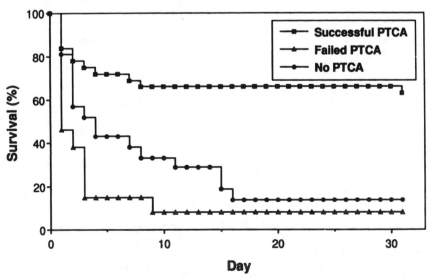

Fig. 3-15. The 30-day survival rate in 68 patients. PTCA = percutaneous transluminal coronary angioplasty. Reproduced with permission from Gacioch, et al.[53]

or to LV chamber size of LV filling pressure. A murmur of MR was heard in only 2 patients (1 incorrectly). The presence of early MR predicted cardiovascular mortality at 1 year. Thus, MR early during MI is generally clinically silent, is more common in anterior wall infarcts, is associated with regional dysfunction but not early LV dilation or peak enzyme release, and is an important predictor of cardiovascular mortality at 1 year.

To describe outcomes of patients sustaining an AMI complicated by MR managed with contemporary reperfusion therapies, Tcheng and associates[56] from Durham, North Carolina, studied 1,480 consecutive patients presenting between April, 1986 and March, 1989 who had emergency cardiac catheterization within 6 hours of the AMI. Fifty patients were found to have moderately severe or severe MR. Acute ischemic moderately severe to severe (3+ or 4+) MR was associated with a mortality of 24% at 30 days, 42% at 6 months, and 3+ or 4+ MR was an independent predictor of mortality (Figure 3-16). Patients with MR tended to be female, older, and to have cerebral vascular disease, diabetes mellitus, and pre-existing symptomatic CAD. Physical examination did not identify 50% of patients with moderately severe to severe MR. Acute reperfusion with thrombolysis or angioplasty did not reliably reverse the MR. In this obser-

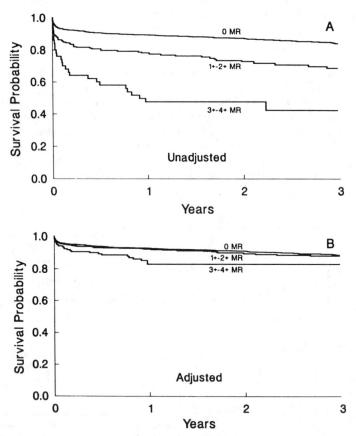

Fig. 3-16. Kaplan-Meier survival estimates grouped by degree of mitral regurgitation.The grade of mitral regurgitation was assessed by ventriculography at the time of emergency cardiac catheterization. Panel A. Unadjusted survival estimates. Panel B. Data adjusted to the overall mean for age, ejection fraction, New York Heart Association congestive heart failure score, and coronary artery disease severity score. MR = mitral regurgitation. Reproduced with permission from Tcheng, et al.[56]

vational study, the greatest in-hospital and 1-year mortalities were seen in patients reperfused with emergency PTCA, whereas patients managed medically or with CABG had lower mortalities. Moderately severe to severe (3+ or 4+) MR complicating AMI portends a grave prognosis. Acute reperfusion does not reduce mortality to levels experienced by patients with lesser degrees of MR nor does it reliably restore valvular competence.

Severe MR due to CAD unfavorably alters prognosis and is associated with increased mortality. Sharma and associates[57] from New York, New York, characterized clinical, angiographic and pathoanatomic findings in 50 consecutive patients with severe ischemic MR. Forty-two patients (84%) either presented with AMI or a well-documented prior AMI. Eleven patients (22%) were in cardiogenic shock at the time of catheterization. Forty patients (80%) had >70% stenosis of the right and LC coronary arteries with or without LAD CAD. Segmental asynergy of the LV wall was present in 48 patients (96%) and involved the inferior wall in 43 (86%). Mean EF for the group was $51 \pm 7\%$. A total of 15 patients had direct inspection of the mitral valve apparatus at surgery or autopsy. Posteromedial papillary muscle involvement was found in 14 patients, fibrosis or necrosis in 10 and rupture in 4, with anterolateral papillary muscle rupture in 1 patient. Thus, acute severe ischemic MR is usually associated with significant narrowing of both right and LC coronary arteries, and posteromedial papillary muscle involvement.

Rupture of the ventricular septum

Parry and associates[58] from New Castle upon Tyne, UK, from 1980-1989 observed 108 patients with rupture of the ventricular septum during AMI and 81 of them had operative repair: 43 (53%) survived the early postoperative period. Of 32 patients with cardiogenic shock who had surgery, early operative mortality in those operated on within 48 hours of rupture was 90% (18/20) compared with 33% (4/12) in those operated on later. All survivors with preoperative shock had intra-aortic balloon counterpulsation before operation. Concomitant CABG was not associated with improved survival. Three patients survived long-term without operation.

Since 1944, 91 patients (50 men and 41 women, mean age 68 years [range 39 to 86]) with ventricular septal rupture after AMI were seen at the Mayo Clinic and reviewed by Lemery and associates[59] from Rochester, Minnesota. Patients were divided into 4 groups according to therapy and timing of surgical intervention. Fourteen patients seen before 1965, when surgery was not performed for such a complication or not readily available, were excluded from the analysis. Group 1 (n = 22) had surgery within 48 hours of septal rupture, group 2 (n = 6) underwent operation between 2 and 14 days, group 3 (n = 24) had surgery after 14 days, and group 4 (n = 25) only received medical treatment (Figure 3-17). Short-term (30 days) survivors (45%, 35 of 77 patients) were compared with nonsurvivors. Using logistic regression, by univariate analysis, 3 variables were significantly associated with outcome: age, cardiogenic shock, and long delay between ventricular septal rupture and surgical intervention. By multivariate analysis, however, only cardiogenic shock and age correlated with an adverse outcome. In patients with cardiogenic shock after septal rupture, the prognosis was uniformly fatal unless patients undergo early surgery. None of the 23 patients in groups 2, 3 or 4 survived, whereas 5 of 13 patients (38%) who had surgery within 48 hours of septal rupture survived. In patients with CHF, the long-term outcome was similar among patients who underwent early surgery; 3 of 6 patients (50%) survived compared with 8 of 15 patients (53%) in whom surgery was delayed. In group 4 patients (no surgery), 12 of the 19 patients who were nonsurvivors were in cardiogenic shock and died within 48 hours of septal rupture, but in the remaining 7 patients, death occurred between 3 and 9 days in 5 patients, and at 20 and 30 days in 2 others. Thus, in patients with cardiogenic shock after septal rupture, only those who underwent operation within 48 hours survived; the potential for rapid and unpredictable deterioration in the nonsurgical group and the good surgical results warrant early repair for most patients with VSD after AMI.

Muehrcke and associates[60] from Boston, Massachusetts, described outcome in 75 patients who underwent repair of a postAMI VSD at the Massachusetts General Hospital between June, 1968, and April, 1991. Group I (n = 33) included patients who had 2 or 3-vessel CAD and had complete revascularization in addition to repair of the VSD. Group II (n = 19) patients also had 2 or 3-vessel CAD, but CABG was not performed; only the VSD was repaired. Group III (n = 23) patients had only 1-vessel CAD corresponded to the region of the AMI; they underwent VSD repair only. Follow-up of hospital survivors was 96% complete at a mean of 86 months (range, 1 to 288 months). Hospital mortality after VSD repair was 21% in the cohort with CABG (Group I), 26% in those without CABG (Group II), and 26% in those with only 1-vessel CAD (Group III). With follow-up after 5 and 10 years, the actuarial survival was 72% ± 8% and 48% ± 10% respectively in the bypass group, 29% ± 11% and 0% respectively in the unbypassed group, and 52% ± 10% and 36.5% ± 11%, respectively, in the cohort with single-vessel disease. Bypassing associated CAD significantly increased long-term survival when compared with patients with unbypassed CAD.

Westaby and associates[61] from Oxford, UK, studied all patients with post-AMI ventricular septal rupture referred to their hospital for operation

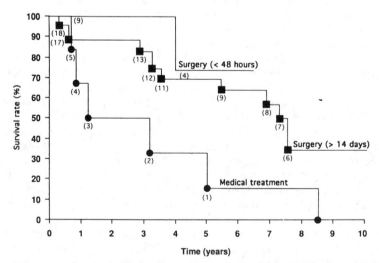

Fig. 3-17. Long-term survival in 30-day survivors after postmyocardial infarction-related ventricular septal defect with surgical intervention or medical therapy. Group 2 (not shown) includes only 1 patient (who survived >5 years). Numbers in *parentheses* indicate the number of patients at the beginning of each interval. Reproduced with permission from Lemery, et al.[59]

over a 4.5 year period. Twenty-one women and 8 men were admitted, 13 of whom had received streptokinase and 16 of whom had not. The median interval between symptomatic onset of AMI and the development of septal rupture was 24 hours for those treated with streptokinase and 6 days for those who were not. Of the 26 patients who underwent surgical repair, 3 were operated on less than 36 hours after streptokinase infusion, in 1 case within 12 hours. Macroscopic observation of the disintegrating myocardium showed muscle bundles dissected by blood rendered incoagulable by thrombolytic treatment, together with the histologic features of reperfusion injury. The overall surgical mortality rate for the streptokinase group was 33% and for the others 21%. The patient operated on within 12 hours of thrombolytic treatment recovered uneventfully. Six of the 7 surgical deaths were caused by LV or biventricular failure and 1 by gastrointestinal hemorrhage. All survivors were in New York Heart Association classes II or III between 2 weeks and 4.5 years after operation. The authors concluded that thrombolysis leads to early breakdown of the ventricular septum after AMI but does not preclude early repair.

Meuhrcke and associates[62] from Boston, Massachusetts, analyzed experiences with 86 patients who had an AMI and underwent surgical repair of an infarct related VSD between June 1968, and May 1991, at their hospital. Their Group I patients (n = 57) included those patients <70 years and Group II (n = 29) represented patients aged ≥70 years. Follow-up with hospital survivors ranged from 1 month to 24 years and was compiled in April and May, 1991. Three patients were lost to follow-up (4%), and these were younger than 70 years of age. There were no differences in the values of the preoperative variables for the younger and older groups with respect to sex, concomitant procedures performed (bypass vs no bypass), use of an intra-aortic balloon pump, location of VSD, presence of shock, total hospital days, or days between infarction and operation. There was, however, a difference between the 2 groups relative to the era when surgery was performed. More patients over the age of 70 underwent surgery after 1978 than before 1978. Most survivors are in New York Heart Association Class I or II, and there was no difference between the younger and older groups in functional class at the time of follow-up (83.3% vs 91.7% of survivors in Class I or II, respectively). Using the generalized Wilcoxon test to analyze these survival data, there was no apparent difference in long-term survival when comparing the 2 age groups. The mean follow-up period was 77.02 months for the younger group and 80.52 months for the older group. The fact that more older patients were repaired after the authors had significant experience in the surgical management of patients with VSDs probably accounted for the excellent results in the older age group. The data revealed that patients over the age of 70 can expect excellent long-term survival with >90% of these survivors remaining in New York Heart Association Functional Class I or II.

Rupture of the left ventricular free wall

López-Sendón and colleagues[63] in Madrid, Spain, have evaluated the sensitivity and specificity of clinical, hemodynamic and echocardiographic diagnostic variables obtained at the bedside in the identification of ventricular rupture following AMI in 1,247 consecutive patients, including 33 patients with subacute ventricular rupture diagnosed at operation (group A) and 1,214 patients without ventricular rupture (group B). The incidence of syncope, recurrent chest pain, hypotension, electromechanical dissociation, pericardial tamponade, pericardial effusion, high acoustic intrapericardial echoes, RA and RV wall compression identified from 2-dimensional echocardiograms and hemopericardium demonstrated during pericardiocentesis was greater in group A than in group B. The presence of cardiac tamponade, pericardial effusion >5 mm, high density intrapericardial echoes or RA or RV wall compression had a diagnostic sensitivity ≥70% and specificity >90%. The number of false positive diagnoses was always high for each diagnostic variable alone (>20%), but the combination of clinical (hypotension), hemodynamic (cardiac tamponade) and echocardiographic variables allowed a sensitivity of ≥ 65% with a small number of false positive diagnoses (<10%) and provided useful information for therapeutic decisions. The diagnosis of subacute ventricular rupture requires a surgical decision. Twenty-five (76%) of the 33 patients with subacute ventricular rupture survived the surgical procedure and 16 (48.5%) are long-term survivors. Subacute ventricular wall rupture is a relatively frequent complication after AMI that can be accurately diagnosed and successfully treated.

Left ventricular aneurysm

Komeda and associates[64] from Toronto, Canada, reviewed 336 consecutive patients who underwent repair of LV aneurysm from 1978 to 1989: 281 patients had partial resection of the aneurysm and conventional closure of the ventriculotomy; 17 patients had inverted T closure, and 38 had endocardial patch (Figure 3-18). These two latter techniques were developed in an attempt to restore normal LV geometry. The operative mortality was 6.8% (23 patients). A stepwise logistic regression analysis of various preoperative clinical, hemodynamic, and angiographic variables revealed that LVEF of ≤0.20, age >60 years, previous myocardial revascularization, lack of angina, and New York Heart Association functional class IV were independent predictors of operative mortality. The technique of repair was not a predictor of outcome, but when patients with poor LV

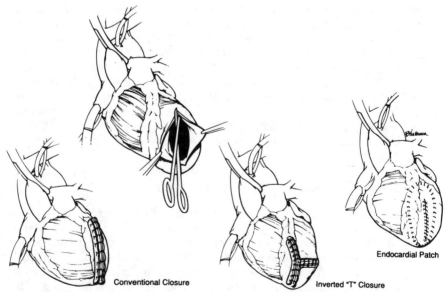

Conventional Closure   Inverted "T" Closure   Endocardial Patch

Fig. 3-18. Operative techniques. Reproduced with permission from Komeda, et al.[64]

function were analyzed separately, the operative mortality was reduced from 12.5% to 6.5% when newer techniques were employed. Patients were followed up during a mean of 6.3 years. There were 51 late deaths, 45 cardiac. Cox regression analysis indicated that poor LV function and LM CAD were the only 2 predictors of late mortality. The actuarial survival at 10 years was 63% ± 4% (Figure 3-19). Most patients (88%) were in New York Heart Association class I or II. These data indicate excellent long-term results after repair of LV aneurysm.

Silent myocardial ischemia

To determine the incidence of angina pectoris during induced myocardial ischemia in patients who have had thrombolytic therapy for AMI in comparison with patients with angina pectoris, Taylor and associates[65] from Springfield, Illinois, performed coronary artery occlusion by balloon dilatation catheter for 5 minutes in both groups. Twenty-five patients with angina pectoris who were undergoing PTCA were compared with 20 patients having PTCA 2 days after thrombolytic therapy for AMI. During balloon occlusion 16 (24%) of 25 patients in the angina pectoris group developed angina. In contrast, 9 (30%) of 30 patients in the thrombolysis group had angina pectoris during balloon occlusion of the infarct artery. The electrocardiographic response to ischemia and changes in PA wedge pressure were similar in the 2 study groups. After thrombolytic therapy for AMI, silent ischemia may be the rule rather than the exception.

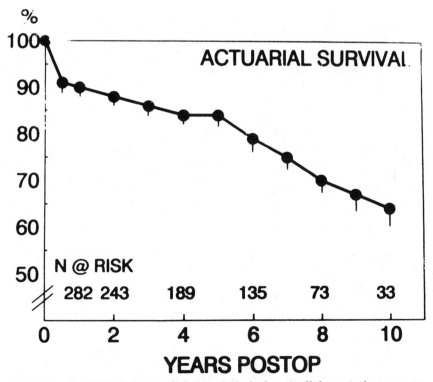

Fig. 3-19. Overall actuarial survival of patients who had repair of left ventricular aneurysm. Reproduced with permission from Komeda, et al.[64]

GENERAL TREATMENT

Diet change

To test whether a fat reduced diet rich in soluble dietary fiber, antioxidant vitamins, and minerals reduces complications and mortality after AMI, Singh and associates[66] from Moradabad, India, performed a randomized, single-blind, controlled trial involving 505 patients with suspected AMI. Those with definite or possible AMI and unstable angina were assigned to diet A (n = 204) or diet B (n = 202) within 24-48 hours of the AMI. Both groups were advised to follow a fat reduced diet. Group A was also advised to eat more fruit, vegetables, nuts, and grain products. The main outcome measures were mortality from cardiac disease and other causes. Blood lipoprotein concentrations and body weight fell significantly in patients in group A compared with those in group B (cholesterol fell by 0.74 mmol/l in group A vs. 0.32 mmol/l in group B, 95% confidence interval of difference 0.14 to 0.70, and weight by 7.1 vs 3.0 kg, 0.52 to 7.68). The incidence of cardiac events was significantly lower in group A than group B (50 vs 82 patients). Group A also had lower total mortality (21 vs 38 died) than group B. Comprehensive dietary changes in conjunction with weight loss immediately after AMI may modulate blood lipoproteins and significantly reduce complications and mortality after 1 year.

Home-based exercise program

A home-based exercise program has been found to be as useful as a hospital-based one in improving cardiovascular fitness after an AMI. To find out whether a comprehensive home-based program would reduce psychological distress, Lewin and associates[67] from Edinburgh and Livingston, UK, randomly allocated 176 patients with an AMI to a self-help rehabilitation program based on a heart manual or to receive standard care plus a placebo package of information and informal counseling. Psychological adjustment, as assessed by the Hospital Anxiety and Depression Scale, was better in the rehabilitation group at 1 year. They also had significantly less contact with their general practitioners during the following year and significantly fewer were readmitted to hospital in the first 6 months. The improvement was greatest among patients who were clinically anxious or depressed at discharge from hospital. The cost-effectiveness of the home-based program has yet to be compared with that of a hospital-based program, but the findings of this study indicate that it might be worth offering such a package to all patients with AMI.

Meta-analyses of trials

A splendid article[68] summarizing numerous randomized controlled trials of therapies for reducing the risk of total mortality in AMI was presented in the July 8, 1992, issue of the *Journal of the American Medical Association*. A sample of the multiple figures from this article is shown in Figure 3-20.

Metoprolol

Several postinfarction trials have evaluated the effect of secondary prophylaxis with different beta-blockers. Although so-called meta-analy-

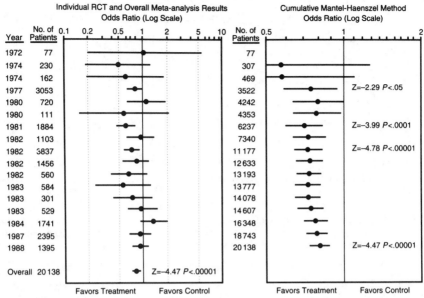

Fig. 3-20. Results of 17 randomized control trials (RCTs) of the effects of oral β-blockers for secondary prevention of mortality in patients surviving a myocardial infarction presented as two types of meta-analyses. On the left is the traditional one, revealing many trials with nonsignificant results but a highly significant estimate of the pooled results on the bottom of the panel. On the right, the same data are presented as cumulative meta-analyses, illustrating that the updated pooled estimate became statistically significant in 1977 and has remained so up to the present. Note that the scale is changed on the right graph to improve clarity of the confidence intervals. Reproduced with permission from Antman, et al.[68]

sis of the results from all the trials have shown a beneficial effect of postinfarction beta-blockade, many of the individual studies have shown inconclusive results, mainly due to low statistical power. To obtain an evaluation of the merits of postinfarction therapy with metoprolol, Olsson and associates[69] from multiple medical centers collected data from the 5 available studies with metoprolol and pooled them into 2 database. In the total material 5,474 patients (4,353 men, 1,121 women) have been studied during double-blind therapy with metoprolol 100 mg twice daily or matching placebo. The follow-up time ranged from 3 months to 3 years. In total 4,732 patient years of observation were obtained. In total there were 223 deaths in the placebo-treated patients and 188 deaths in the metoprolol-treated patients, which corresponds to mortality rates of 97.0 and 78.3 per 1,000 patient years, respectively. The mortality reduction was found both in men and women (Figure 3-21). As has been reported from individual postinfarction beta-blocker trials, the pooled results showed a marked reduction in sudden deaths (104 in the placebo group, 62 in the metoprolol group). In a Cox regression model the influence of sex, age and smoking habits on the effect of metoprolol was evaluated. None of these factors influenced the metoprolol effect significantly. It is concluded that metoprolol therapy after AMI infarction reduces the total number of deaths, and especially sudden cardiac deaths. The mortality reduction was independent of gender, age, and smoking habits. Available data support a continuous beneficial effect.

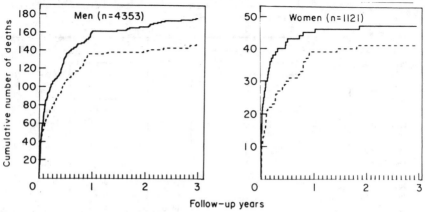

Fig. 3-21. Cumulative number of all deaths subdivided by gender from the five pooled postinfarction trials. Solid line = placebo; broken line = metoprolol. Reproduced with permission from Olsson, et al.[69]

Diltiazem

Wong and associates[70] in San Diego, California; New York, New York; and Farmingham, Connecticut, determined whether diltiazem reduced short and long-term in-hospital reinfarction in patients with non-Q wave AMI studied in the Multicenter Diltiazem Postinfarction Trial. There 514 patients with non-Q wave AMI; 279 patients were randomized to placebo and 235 to Diltiazem. The average follow-up period was 25 months. There were no differences in baseline clinical characteristics between the two groups. Early reinfarction (≤6 months) occurred in 17 patients in the placebo group and 2 patients in the diltiazem group. Late reinfarction (> 6 months) occurred in 13 patients in the placebo group and 14 patients in the diltiazem group. Initial and reinfarction electrocardiograms were analyzed by using a coding system that permitted identification of standard anatomic areas involved in the infarction process. Thirty-one of 46 patients had a localized AMI on index and reinfarction electrocardiograms. In the early reinfarction group, 10 (77%) of 13 AMIs occurred in the same electrocardiographic region in which the initial AMI had occurred; all 10 were in patients in the placebo group. Among the 18 patients with late reinfarction, the site of the second AMI was the same as for the first in 9 patients and differed in 9. There was no difference between the placebo and diltiazem treated groups with respect to location of the AMI. Thus, diltiazem reduces the early but not the late risk of reinfarction after non-Q wave AMI; early reinfarction tends to occur in the same electrocardiographic region as that of the index infarction; and diltiazem may reduce the early reinfarction rate by stabilizing the coronary lesion that caused the index.

Aspirin and diltiazem

Medical practice patterns change in response to a variety of stimuli, one of which may be the publication of the results of randomized clinical trials. Lamas and investigators for the Survival and Ventricular Enlargement (SAVE) Study[71] assessed the temporal association between the publication of clinical trials on AMI and changes in treatment practices for this disorder. The authors analyzed the use of aspirin before and after

AMI and that of calcium antagonist after AMI in 2,231 survivors of AMI enrolled in the SAVE study over a 3-year period (from January, 1987 through January, 1990). The proportion of patients using these treatments was analyzed before and after the publication dates of 3 clinical trials: the Physicians' Health Study, published in January, 1988, which supported the use of aspirin to prevent a first AMI; the Second International Study of Infarct Survival (ISIS-2), published in August, 1988, which supported the use of aspirin after AMI; and the Multicenter Diltiazem Postinfarction Trial, published in August, 1988, which reported a deleterious effect of diltiazem in some patients after AMI. The use of aspirin before AMI increased from 16.2% to 23.9% between January, 1987 and January, 1990. Enrollment in the study after the publication of the Physicians' Health Study independently predicted aspirin use before AMI. The use of aspirin after AMI increased from 38.8% to 71.9% during the 3-year study period. Enrollment in the study after the publication of ISIS-2 independently predicted the use of aspirin after AMI. The use of calcium antagonists after AMI decreased from 57.1% to 33.1% during the study period. Enrollment in the study after the publication of the Multicenter Diltiazem Postinfarction Trial independently predicted the use of calcium antagonists after AMI. These observations suggest that randomized clinical trials have a measurable influence on medical practice patterns.

Captopril

The left ventricle progressively dilates in some patients after AMI. Both systolic and diastolic LV dysfunction can be of significance in the development of CHF. Captopril has been shown to prevent the LV dilatation, but the effect on LV diastolic function is unknown. In a placebo-controlled, double-blind parallel study, Gotzsche and associates[72] from Aarhus, Denmark, randomized 58 consecutive AMI patients with CHF or low EF or both at day 7 to either placebo or captopril (25 mg twice daily). No differences were present between the groups at baseline. Fifty-three patients completed the 6-month study period. Both LV diastolic and systolic volume indexes increased significantly in the placebo group (17 and 14%, respectively); in the captopril group there was no change in LV diastolic volume index, but a 13% reduction in LV systolic volume index. EF increased significantly in the captopril group. The peak flow velocities of the early and atrial filling phases were measured, and the ratio between the velocities was calculated. A significant reduction was observed during the study period in early peak flow velocity (65 to 52) peak flow velocity (1.3 to 0.8) in the placebo group, but no significant changes occurred in the captopril group. No correlation was found between dilatation of the LV and reduction in early peak flow velocity or the ratio between early and atrial peak flow velocity. In conclusion, captopril prevented LV dilatation, improved EF and prevented LV diastolic dysfunction in AMI patients with early signs of LV systolic dysfunction.

LV dilatation and dysfunction after AMI are major predictors of death. In experimental and clinical studies, long-term therapy with the angiotensin-converting-enzyme inhibitor captopril attenuated LV dilatation and remodeling. Pfeffer and associates[73] on behalf of the SAVE Investigators investigated whether captopril could reduce morbidity and mortality in patients with LV dysfunction after an AMI. Within 3 to 16 days after AMI, 2,231 patients with an EF ≤40% but without overt CHF or symptoms of myocardial ischemia were randomly assigned to receive double-blind treatment with either placebo (1,116 patients) or captopril (1,115 patients) and were followed for an average of 42 months. Mortality from all causes was significantly reduced in the captopril group (228 deaths, or 20%) as compared with the placebo group (275 deaths, or 25%); the reduction in risk was 19% (Figure 3-22). In addition, the incidence of both fatal and non-fatal major cardiovascular events was consistently reduced in the captopril group (Figure 3-23). The reduction in risk was 21% for death from cardiovascular causes, 37% for the development of severe heart failure, 22% for CHF requiring hospitalization, and 25% for recurrent AMI. In patients with asymptomatic LV dysfunction after AMI, long-term administration of captopril was associated with an improvement in survival and reduced morbidity and mortality due to major cardiovascular events. These benefits were observed in patients who received thrombolytic therapy, aspirin, or beta-blockers, as well as those who did not, suggesting that treatment with captopril leads to additional improvement in outcome among selected survivors of AMI.

Enalapril

Long-term administration of angiotensin-converting-enzyme inhibitors has been shown to improve survival in patients with symptomatic LV failure and to attenuate LV dilatation in patients with AMI. Swedeberg and associates[74] on behalf of the CONSENSUS II Study Group studied whether mortality could be reduced during the 6 months after an AMI with use of enalapril. At 103 Scandinavian centers patients with AMI and BP above 100/60 mm Hg were randomly assigned to treatment with either enalapril or placebo, in addition to conventional therapy. Therapy was

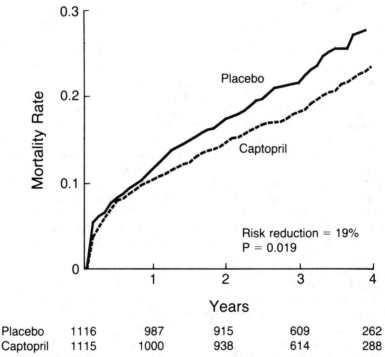

Placebo	1116	987	915	609	262
Captopril	1115	1000	938	614	288

Fig. 3-22. Cumulative Mortality from All Causes in the Study Groups. The number of patients at risk at the beginning of each year is shown at the bottom. Reproduced with permission from Pfeffer, et al.[73]

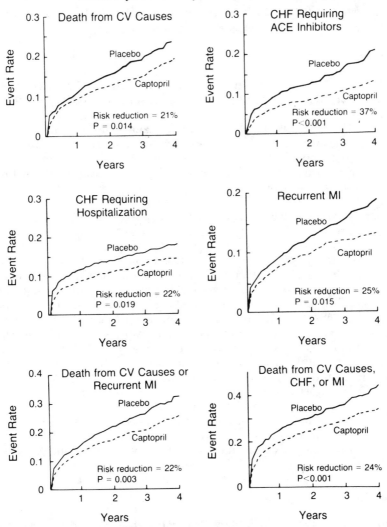

Fig. 3-23. Life Tables for Cumulative Fatal and Nonfatal Cardiovascular Events. CV denotes cardiovascular CHF congestive heart failure, and MI myocardial infarction. The bottom right panel shows the following events: death from cardiovascular causes, severe heart failure requiring angiotensin-converting–enzyme inhibitors or hospitalization, or recurrent myocardial infarction. For all the combined analyses, only the time to the first event was used. Reproduced with permission from Pfeffer, et al.[73]

initiated with an intravenous infusion of enalapril (enalaprilat) within 24 hours after the onset of chest pain, followed by administration of oral enalapril. Of the 6,090 patients enrolled, 3,046 were assigned to placebo and 3,044 to enalapril. The life-table mortality rates in the 2 groups at 1 and 6 months were not significantly different (6.3 and 10.2% in the placebo group vs. 7.2 and 11.0% in the enalapril group). The relative risk of death in the enalapril group was 1.10. Death due to progressive CHF occurred in 104 patients (3.4%) in the placebo group and 132 (4.3%) in the enalapril group. Therapy had to be changed because of worsening CHF in 30% of the placebo group and 27% of the enalapril group. Early hypotension (systolic pressure <90 mm Hg or diastolic pressure <50 mm Hg) occurred in 12% of the enalapril group and 3% of the placebo group. Enalapril therapy started within 24 hours of the onset of AMI does not improve survival during the 180 days after infarction.

Heparin

Kroon and co-workers[75] in Leiden, The Netherlands, investigated the anticoagulant response of 12,500 IU heparin subcutaneously in patients with AMI and healthy volunteers to determine variabilities in response and modifying factors. On the fourth day after thrombolytic therapy, blood samples were taken before and at frequent intervals until 10 hours after the injection of 12,500 IU heparin subcutaneously. Plasma anti-Xa activity, anti-IIa activity, and the activated partial thromboplastin time were measured in addition to body weight and thickness of the abdominal subcutaneous fat layer. Contrary to expectations, the increase of anti-Xa activity, anti-IIa activity, and activated partial thromboplastin time compared with baseline levels was very small, with an average maximal activated partial thromboplastin time of 43 seconds. Subsequently, the influence of the length of the injection needle on the anticoagulant effect of 12,500 IU heparin subcutaneously was studied in 10 healthy volunteers to find a factor that could be responsible for the poor response in the patients. The length of the injection needle did not influence the anticoagulant effect of heparin. Large interindividual and intraindividual variabilities were seen in the volunteers. Most volunteers had minimal prolongation of the activated partial thromboplastin time, but very strong prolongation was also seen. There was no correlation between the abdominal skinfold thickness and anti-Xa activity, anti-IIa activity, or activated partial thromboplastin time, but in the patient study, there was a correlation between weight and anti-Xa activity and activated partial thromboplastin time. Subcutaneous administration of heparin in a fixed dose for prophylactic and therapeutic purposes may be inadequate because of the large interindividual and intraindividual variations in anticoagulant effect.

Lidocaine

Antman and Berlin[76] in Philadelphia, Pennsylvania, reviewed the experience with the prophylactic use of lidocaine with the purposes of 1) to track the incidence of primary VF in the control and lidocaine-treated groups in the randomized control trials of lidocaine prophylaxis against primary VF in AMI, with particular emphasis on the time frame of the randomized trial, and 2) to estimate the number of patients who must receive lidocaine currently to prevent one episode of VF. The following variables from randomized control trials published between 1969 and 1988 were entered into logistical regression models to predict the percent of patients developing VF: year of publication of the randomized control trial, method of data analysis used in the trial, route and technique of lidocaine administration, duration of monitoring for VF, and exclusion criteria before randomization (CHF/cardiogenic shock, VT/VF, or bradycardia/AV block). Year of publication was a significant predictor of VF in both the control and lidocaine groups even after adjusting for other covariates. Based on a univariate logistic regression model with year as the predictor variable, it was estimated that the incidence of primary VF in the control group fell from 4.5% in 1970 to 0.4% in 1990 and from 4.3% down to 0.1% for the lidocaine group over the same time period. Thus, about 400 patients would currently need prophylaxis with lidocaine to prevent one episode of VF. Present estimates of the risk:benefit ratio of lidocaine prophylaxis should consider the low risk of VF in control patients and the large number who need lidocaine prophylaxis to prevent 1 episode of VF. When added to the previously reported trend toward excess mortality in lidocaine-treated patients, these data argue against the routine prophylactic use of lidocaine in patients with AMI.

Moricizine

The Cardiac Arrhythmia Suppression Trial (CAST) tested the hypothesis that the suppression of asymptomatic or mildly symptomatic VPCs in survivors of AMI would decrease the number of deaths from ventricular arrhythmias and improve overall survival. The second CAST study (CAST-II) tested this hypothesis with a comparison of moricizine and placebo. CAST-II was divided by the cardiac arrhythmia suppression trial II investigators into 2 blinded, randomized phases: an early 14-day exposure phase that evaluated the risk of starting treatment with moricizine after AMI (1,325 patients), and a long-term phase that evaluated the effect of moricizine on survival after AMI in patients whose VPCs were either adequately suppressed by moricizine (1,155 patients) or only partially suppressed (219 patients). CAST-II was stopped early because of the first 14-day period of treatment with moricizine after an AMI was associated with excess mortality (17 of 665 patients died or had cardiac arrests), as compared with no treatment or placebo (3 of 660 patients died or had cardiac arrests); and estimates of conditional power indicated that it was highly unlikely (8% chance) that a survival benefit from moricizine could be observed if the trial were completed. At the completion of the long-term phase, there were 49 deaths or cardiac arrests due to arrhythmias in patients assigned to moricizine, and 42 in patients assigned to placebo. As with the antiarrhythmic agents used in CAST-I (flecainide and encainide), the use of moricizine in CAST-II to suppress asymptomatic or mildly symptomatic VPCs to try to reduce mortality after AMI is not only ineffective but also harmful.

Amiodarone

Ceremuzynski and colleagues[78] in Warsaw, Lodz, Bydgoszcz and Krakow, Poland; and Bethesda, Maryland, evaluated the effect of amiodarone on mortality, ventricular arrhythmias, and clinical complications in high risk post-AMI patients. Patients who were not eligible to receive beta-blockers were randomized to receive amiodarone (n = 305) or placebo (n = 308) for 1 year. There were 21 deaths in the amiodarone group compared with 33 in the placebo group (Figure 3-24). There were two noncardiac deaths in the amiodarone group and none in the placebo group. There was a significant decrease in Lown class 4 ventricular arrhythmias in patients treated with amiodarone (8% vs 20%, respectively). Adverse effects developed in 30% of amiodarone-treated patients and 10% of placebo-treated patients. Pulmonary toxicity which was mild and reversible occurred in only one patient in the amiodarone group. This trial demonstrates a significant reduction in cardiac mortality and ventricular arrhythmias with amiodarone treatment. In this study, amiodarone or placebo were given at an initial dose of 800 mg/day for the first 7 days and 400 mg/day 6 days a week for the subsequent 12 months. The dose could be reduced to 200 mg/day and even to 100 mg/day if heart rate decreased to <55 beats/minute or if the QT interval was >0.48 seconds.

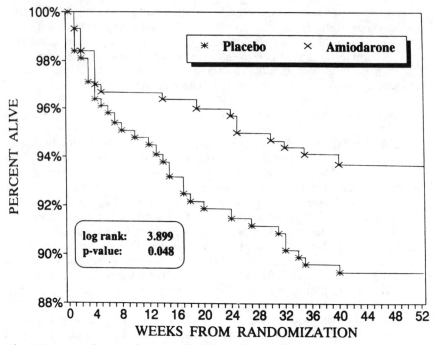

Fig. 3-24. Survival curves of patients who did not die of cardiac causes and were randomly allocated to treatment with amiodarone and placebo during the trial. Reproduced with permission from Ceremuzynski, et al.[78]

These data are provocative and indicate the need for a larger study of the potential influence of amiodarone in reducing cardiac mortality in patients after AMI.

Magnesium

To ascertain the effect of the intravenous administration of magnesium in AMI on the frequency of arrhythmias and mortality, Horner[79] in London, United Kingdom, performed a meta-analysis of randomized controlled trials. The study included 930 patients with AMI admitted to primary referral hospitals. Administration of magnesium in AMI was associated with a 49% reduction in VT and VF. The incidence of cardiac arrest was reduced by 58%. The frequency of supraventricular tachycardias was also lower. Overall, there was a 54% reduction in mortality. In conclusion, intravenous magnesium is a safe and effective method of reducing the frequency of arrhythmias and mortality in AMI.

THROMBOLYSIS

General recommendations

Doorey and associates[80] from Newark, Delaware, Philadelphia, Pennsylvania, and Cleveland, Ohio, prepared a review to assess the usefulness of thrombolytic therapy for AMI by evaluating whether inclusion and exclusion criteria should be altered as well as the public health implications of any such alterations. Data obtained were from English-language articles on the use of thrombolytic therapy in AMI. Articles that reported on inclusion and exclusion criteria as well as specific complications of this therapy were specifically sought. The review included articles under the terms thrombolytic therapy and AMI in the National Library of Medicine's MEDLINE database. Studies selected for detailed review were those reporting specifics about inclusion and exclusion criteria and efficacy. Data extraction guidelines for assessing data quality included study size, patient population, detail of patient information acquired, and consecutive patient enrollment. Thrombolytic therapy can provide substantial decrements of morbidity and mortality of AMI in the subset of patients who receive this therapy, but is underused in the United States. Advanced age per se should not be an exclusion criterion. Improvements can be made in electrocardiographic diagnosis of AMI. Many of the clinical conditions initially excluded from thrombolytic consideration, such as hypertension or having received cardiopulmonary resuscitation, are only relative contraindications. The benefit/risk ratio in treatment of these patients is often acceptable. Several well-documented points of delay from onset of symptoms to treatment can be minimized, and accelerated therapy can result in a reduction in mortality rates. Significant public health benefits will result from greater use of thrombolytic therapy in AMI.

Streptokinase

The large volume of published randomized, controlled trials has led to a need for meta-analyses to track therapeutic advances. Performing a new meta-analysis whenever the results of a new trial of a particular therapy are published permits the study of trends in efficacy and makes it possible to determine when a new treatment appears to be significantly effective or deleterious. Lau and associates[81] from Boston, Massachusetts, performed cumulative meta-analyses of clinical trials that evaluated 15 treatments and preventive measures for AMI. An example of this method is its application to the use of intravenous streptokinase as thrombolytic therapy for acute infarction. Thirty-three trials evaluating this therapy were performed between 1959 and 1988 (Figure 3-25). The authors found that a consistent, statistically significant reduction in total mortality was achieved in 1973, after only 8 trials involving 2,432 patients had been completed. The results of the 25 subsequent trials, which enrolled an additional 34,542 patients through 1988, had little or no effect on the odds ratio establishing efficacy, but simply narrowed the 95% confidence interval. In particular, 2 very large trials, the Gruppo Italiano per lo Studio della Streptochinasi nell' Infarto Miocardico trial in 1986 (11,712 patients) and the Second International Study of Infarct Survival trial in 1988 (17,187 patients) did not modify the already established evidence of efficacy. The authors used a similar approach to study the accumulating evidence of efficacy (or lack of efficacy) of 14 other therapies and preventive measures for AMI. Cumulative meta-analysis of therapeutic trials facilitates the determination of clinical efficacy and harm and may be helpful in tracking trials, planning future trials, and making clinical recommendations for therapy.

Cerqueira and colleagues[82] in Seattle, Washington, determined whether patients treated with streptokinase survived long-term after AMI. Thrombolytic therapy for AMI reduces early mortality and improves the

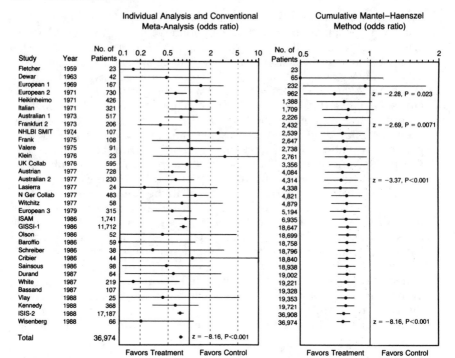

Fig. 3-25. Conventional and Cumulative Meta-Analyses of 33 Trials of Intravenous Streptokinase for Acute Myocardial Infarction. The odds ratios and 95 percent confidence intervals for an effect of treatment on mortality are shown on a logarithmic scale. A bibliography of the published trial reports is available from the authors. Reproduced with permission from Lau, et al.[81]

one year survival rate, but the long-term survival benefits of treatment and the relation between survival and baseline clinical characteristics, infarct size and ventricular function have not been established. In this study, survival status at a minimum of 3 and a mean of 5 ± 2.3 years in 618 patients randomized between 1981 and 1986 to receive conventional treatment (n = 298) or thrombolysis with streptokinase (n = 325) in the Western Washington Intracoronary (n = 250) and Intravenous (n = 368) Streptokinase in Myocardial Infarction trials was determined. The relation between long-term survival and thrombolytic therapy, admission baseline clinical characteristics and late radionuclide tomographic thallium-201 infarct sizes and LVEFs were assessed in subsets of patients. Survival at 6 weeks was 94% in patients who received streptokinase versus 88% in the control group. However, survival at 3 years was 84% in the streptokinase group and 82% in the control group and for the total period of follow-up, there was no significant benefit. Analysis by infarct location showed a higher survival rate at 3 years for patients treated with anterior AMI (76% vs 67%), but no overall survival benefit. Survival at 3 years for patients with an inferior AMI was 89% in the streptokinase-treated group and 91% in the control group. By stepwise Cox regression analysis, admission clinical variables associated with decreased long-term survival were anterior AMI, advanced age, history of prior AMI, and the presence of pulmonary edema or hypotension. Although streptokinase therapy was associated with improved survival, it was not an independent determinant of survival. LVEF and thallium-201 infarct size measured approximately eight weeks after enrollment had a strong association with long-term survival. Univariate analysis in a subgroup of 289 patients with complete data identified AMI size, LVEF, age and history of prior AMI as predictors of survival. In the multivariate model, only LVEF, age, and prior AMI were strong predictors. Thus, in the early trials of thrombolytic therapy for AMI, streptokinase improved early survival, but there was little long-term survival benefit. This failure to show improvement in the 3- to 8-year survival rate may reflect the need to study a larger group of patients or to initiate treatment earlier after symptom onset or deal with the consequences of progressive coronary heart disease in a more effective manner.

The value of thrombolytic therapy in myocardial infarction is well established, while any beneficial effect of adjunct therapy is more uncertain. In a double-blind, randomized, parallel-group study the effect of combined intravenous infusions of streptokinase and isosorbide dinitrate on enzyme-estimated infarct size was investigated by Hildebrandt and associates[83] from Hellerup, Denmark, and Monheim, Germany. One hundred consecutive patients with strong clinical and electrocardiographic suspicion of AMI, admitted to the coronary care unit within 8 hours after the onset of symptoms, were given a streptokinase infusion of 1.5 million units for 1 hour and a titrated dose of isosorbide dinitrate or placebo for 48 hours. From isoenzyme B of creatine kinase values measured every 4 hours, the infarct size was calculated and the possible presence of reperfusion was evaluated. The infarct size in patients receiving isosorbide dinitrate infusion was reduced compared with placebo. By subdividing the patients according to whether or not reperfusion had occurred, the infarct size appeared to be similar following isosorbide dinitrate and placebo in patients with reperfusion (419 vs 369 U/L), whereas the infarct size in patients not reperfused was markedly reduced after treatment with isosorbide dinitrate (223 vs 1320 U/L). In conclusion, the present study demonstrates that the infarct size may be reduced by other means than reperfusion and its supports the use of combined infusion of thrombolytic agents and nitrates in patients with suspected AMI.

Anistreplase

To assess the feasibility, safety, and efficacy of domiciliary thrombolysis by general practitioners, the Grampain Region Early Anistreplase Trial (GREAT) Group[84] performed a randomized, double-blind, parallel group trial of anistreplase 30 units intravenously and placebo given either at home or in hospitals in Aberdeen, UK. Anistreplase was administered at home 101 minutes after onset of symptoms, while anistreplase was given in hospital 240 minutes after onset of symptoms in 311 patients with suspected AMI and without contraindications to thrombolytic therapy and all were seen at home within 4 hours of onset of symptoms. Adverse events after thrombolysis were infrequent and, apart from cardiac arrest, not a serious problem when they occurred in the community: 7 of 13 patients were resuscitated after cardiac arrest out of hospital. By 3 months after trial entry the relative reduction of deaths from all causes in patients given thrombolytic therapy at home was 49% (13/163 [8.0%] v 23/148 [15.5%]; difference − 7.6%). Full thickness Q wave infarction was less common in patients with confirmed infarction receiving treatment at home (65/122 [53.3%] v 76/112 [67.9%]; difference 014.6%). General practitioners provided rapid pre-hospital coronary care of a high standard. Compared with later administration in hospital, giving anistreplase at home resulted in reduction in mortality, fewer cardiac arrests, fewer Q wave infarcts, and better LV function. Benefits were most marked where thrombolytic therapy was administered within 2 hours of the onset of symptoms.

Tissue-type plasminogen activator (t-PA)

Wall and the TAMI-7 Study Group[85] determined the clinical profile and efficacy of accelerated recombinant tissue-type plasminogen activator dose regimens in 232 patients systematically evaluated following AMI. Five different strategies of thrombolytic therapy were evaluated (Table 3-2). The fifth strategy involved a combination of accelerated tissue plasminogen activator and intravenous urokinase (regimen E). A weight-adjusted dose of 1.25 mg/kg body weight of tissue plasminogen activator over 90 minutes (regimen C) yielded the highest coronary patency rate (83%) at angiography. In-hospital reocclusion rates for this regimen were 4%. An exaggerated (60 minutes) dosage regimen yielded an inferior coronary patency rate (63%). Combination therapy (regimen E) was associated with a 72% patency rate and a 3% reocclusion rate. Marginal improvement in LVEF and regional wall function was demonstrated with all thrombolytic strategies. Bleeding complications were more common at the periaccess site and were not different from those reported with conventional 3 hour dosing regimens. Measurements at baseline, 30 minutes and 3 hours of levels of tissue plasminogen activator, fibrinogen and fibrinogen degradation products were obtained. Fibrinogen levels of <1 g/liter were demonstrated with combination therapy (regimen E) as well as with regimen C. Major clinical outcomes, including death, coronary artery reocclusion and reinfarction showed a tendency to be less common with regimen C. Thus, although accelerated dose regimens of tissue plasminogen activator do not reliably yield coronary patency rates >85%, an acute coronary patency rate of approximately 85% can be achieved. Exaggerated (60 minutes) accelerated therapy may be associated with inferior coronary patency rates compared with conventional regimens. The profile of improved rate of reperfusion, low reocclusion and a bleeding complication frequency comparable with that of conventional thrombolytic regimens

TABLE 3-2. *Dosing Regimens. Reproduced with permission from Wall, et al.*[85]

Regimen	rt-PA Dosage	Maximal rt-PA Dose (mg)
A	1 mg/kg over 30 min (10% bolus); 0.25 mg/kg over 30 min	120
B	1.25 mg/kg over 90 min (20-mg bolus)	120
C	0.75 mg/kg over 30 min (10% bolus); 0.50 mg/kg over 60 min	120
D	20-mg bolus; 30-min wait; 80 mg over 120 min	100
E	1 mg/kg over 30 min + urokinase (1.5 million U) over 1 h	90

rt-PA = recombinant tissue-type plasminogen activator.

suggests that an accelerated tissue plasminogen activator therapeutic regimen deserves more investigation.

The efficacy of multiple intravenous bolus injections of tissue-type plasminogen activator (t-PA) in inducing rapid coronary revascularization in patients with AMI was previously demonstrated. In a Bolus Dose-Escalation Study of Tissue-Type Plasminogen Activator (BEST), Hackett and associates[86] of the Bolus Dose-Escalation Study of Tissue-Type Plasminogen Activator (BEST) investigators investigated the efficacy of 3 different doses of a single rapid intravenous bolus injection of t-PA (duteplase, Wellcome Foundation, London) in inducing coronary patency (Thrombolysis in Myocardial Infarction perfusion grade 2 or 3) in 64 patients with AMI presenting <6 hours after onset of symptoms. At 60 minutes after administration of t-PA, the infarct-related coronary artery was patent in 9 of 17 patients (53%) after 0.3 MU/kg, in 14 of 23 (61%) after 0.45 MU/kg and in 10 of 14 (71%) after 0.6 MU/kg. At 90 minutes after t-PA, coronary patency was present in 9 of 17 cases (53%) after 0.3 MU/kg, in 12 of 24 (59%) after 0.45 MU/kg and in 10 of 13 (77%) after 0.6 MU/kg. One patient in each dose group had a silent reoccluded infarct-related artery by 24 hours, and there were 2 clinical reinfarctions before discharge. No major bleeding events were observed. There were 5 hospital deaths, all unrelated to t-PA. A single intravenous bolus injection of 0.7 MU/kg of t-PA appears to be effective in inducing rapid coronary patency and to be safe in patients with AMI.

Hsia and associates[87] in Washington, D.C.; Houston, Texas; and St. Louis, Missouri, have determined whether arterial patency after the administration of tissue plasminogen activator in patients with AMI may be sustained by effective anticoagulation. The Heparin Aspirin Reperfusion Trial (HART) included three clinical centers with eight hospitals and 24 investigators. In this study, patients presenting within 6 hours of onset of chest pain were eligible for entry if 0.1 mV ST elevation was identified in 2 contiguous electrocardiographic leads and if there were no contraindications to the administration of tissue plasminogen activator. Patients received 100 mg of tissue plasminogen activator, including a 6 mg bolus dose, 54 mg during the first hour, 20 mg during the second hour, and 5 mg per hour during each of the next 4 hours and were randomized to treatment with either oral aspirin (80 mg/day) or intravenous heparin (5,000 international units bolus followed an infusion at 1,000 units/hour) adjusted to maintain the activated partial thromboplastin time at 1.5 to two times control values. Mean activated partial thromboplastin times were higher among patients with an open infarct-related artery than in those with a closed artery (81 ± 4 vs 54 ± 9 s). Only 45% of patients with values <45 s at 8 and 12 hours after the administration of tissue plasminogen activator had Thrombolysis in Myocardial Infarction flow grades 2 or 3 in the infarct-related artery at 18 hours. However, 88% of patients with activated partial thromboplastin times >45 s and 95% of those with values >60 s had an open infarct-related artery at 18 hours. Among patients with initially patent infarct-related arteries who underwent repeat angiography at 7 days, activated partial thromboplastin times were similar in those with a persistently patent artery and those with late reocclusion. Excessive anticoagulation did not appear to increase hemorrhage risk except that access-site-related hemorrhage was more common in patients with activated partial thromboplastin times >100 s at 8 hours. These data indicate that effective heparanization maintains coronary artery patency after thrombolysis with tissue plasminogen activator.

Alteplase (rt-PA)

To determine whether concomitant treatment with intravenous heparin affects coronary artery patency and outcome in patients treated with alteplase thrombolysis for AMI, de Bono and associates[88] for the European Cooperative Study Group from multiple medical centers performed a double-blind, randomized trial using alteplase 100 mg plus aspirin (250 mg intravenously followed by 75-125 mg on alternate days) plus heparin (5000 units intravenously followed by 1000 units hourly without dose adjustment) compared with alteplase plus aspirin plus placebo for heparin. A total of 652 patients aged 21-70 years with clinical and electrocardiographic features of AMI were studied and all to be included had thrombolytic therapy started within 6 hours of the onset of major symptoms. The main outcome measure was angiographic coronary patency 48-120 hours after randomization. Coronary patency (TIMI grades 2 or 3) was 83% in the heparin group and 75% in the group given placebo for heparin. The relative risk of an occluded vessel in the heparin treated group was 0.66. Mortality was the same in both groups. There were nonsignificant trends towards a smaller enzymatic infarct size and a higher incidence of bleeding complications in the group treated with heparin. Concomitant intravenous heparin improves coronary patency in patients with alteplase. Whether this can be translated into improved clinical benefit needs to be tested in a larger trial.

Neuhaus and associates[89] in Munich, Germany, used a new front-loaded infusion regimen of 100 mg of tissue plasminogen activator with an initial bolus dose of 15 mg followed by an infusion of 50 mg over 30 minutes and 35 mg over 60 minutes in a randomized multicenter trial in 421 patients with AMI. The effects of this front-loaded administration of tissue plasminogen activator were compared with those with *anisoylated plasminogen streptokinase activator* (APSAC) on early patency and reocclusion of infarct-related coronary arteries. Coronary angiography 90 minutes after the start of treatment revealed a patent infarct-related artery in 84.4% of 199 patients given tissue plasminogen activator as compared with 70.3% of 202 patients given APSAC. Early reocclusion within 24 to 48 hours was documented in 10% of 174 patients given tissue plasminogen activator and 2.5% of 163 patients given APSAC. Late reocclusion within 21 days was observed in 2.6% of 152 patients given tissue plasminogen activator versus 6.3% of 159 patients given APSAC. There were 5 in-hospital deaths (2.4%) in the tissue plasminogen activator group and 17 deaths (8%) in the APSAC group. The reinfarction rates were 3.8% and 4.8%, respectively. Peak serum creatine kinase and LV ejection fraction were identical in both groups. There were more bleeding complications after APSAC (45% vs 31%). Two intracranial hemorrhages (0.9%) occurred in each group. Thus, front-loaded administration of 100 mg of tissue plasminogen activator yields a significantly higher early patency rate of the infarct-related artery in comparison with that occurring with APSAC. Although more early reocclusions occur after tissue plasminogen activator than after APSAC, hospital reinfarction rates are similar. In this small trial, there was a reduced mortality in the tissue plasminogen activator group as compared to patients treated with APSAC.

Carney and associates[90] for the RAAMI Study Investigators conducted a multicenter, randomized, open label trial in 281 patients with AMI receiving 100 mg of tissue plasminogen activator according to either the standard 3 hour infusion regimen with an initial 10 mg bolus followed by 50 mg for the first hour, then 20 mg for the second hour or an accelerated 90 minute regimen, including a 15 mg initial bolus followed by 50 mg over 30 minutes, then 35 mg over 60 minutes. All patients also received intravenous heparin and oral aspirin during and after the tissue plasminogen activator infusion. At 60 minutes after initiation of the tissue plasminogen activator infusion, the observed angiographic patency rates were 76% in the accelerated regimen and 63% in the control group. At 90 minutes, these rates were 81% and 77%, respectively. Both randomized groups experienced similar rates of recurrent ischemia, reinfarction, angiographic evidence of reocclusion, and other complications of AMI, including stroke and death as well as bleeding complications. Fifteen percent of the patients with a patent artery at 60 minutes had recurrent ischemia compared with 33% who had an occluded artery at 60 minutes and a patent artery at 90 minutes. These data demonstrate that an accelerated 100 mg dose of tissue plasminogen activator can produce more rapid reperfusion rates without an apparent change in safety.

Arnout and associates[91] in Leuven, Belgium, used the European Cooperative Study Group to determine whether the conjunctive use of intravenous heparin influences the efficacy of alteplase for coronary thrombolysis in patients with AMI. In this trial, patients with alteplase and aspirin were randomized to concomitant fixed doses of intravenous heparin of a bolus dose of 5,000 U followed by continuous infusion of 1,000 U/hour or placebo. The current study group comprised 149 of 324 patients allocated to heparin therapy and 132 of 320 patients allocated to placebo administration who had interpretable coronary arteriograms obtained within 6 days of treatment and sufficient plasma samples to assess the level of anticoagulation. Activated partial thromboplastin times, fibrinogen and D-dimer levels were determined on plasma samples at baseline and at 45 minutes and 3, 12, 24 and 36 hours after the start of alteplase administration. Coronary artery patency rate was higher in patients given heparin therapy than in those given placebo (80% and 71%, respectively). Patients given heparin were classified into 3 groups: 48 patients (32%) with all activated partial thromboplastin times at least twice their own baseline values were considered optimal anticoagulation; 40 patients (27%) with the lowest activated partial thromboplastin times at 3, 12, 24, or 36 hours between 130% and 200% of the baseline values (suboptimal anticoagulation); and 61 patients with at least one activated partial thromboplastin time less than 130% of baseline (inadequate anticoagulation). In the heparin group, coronary artery patency correlated with the level of anticoagulation: 90%, 80%, and 72%, respectively, in patients with optimal, suboptimal, and inadequate anticoagulation. Heparin administration was associated with a smaller reduction in fibrinogen and a smaller increase in D-dimer level during and after alteplase administration. There was no correlation identified between fibrinogen or D-dimer levels and coronary artery patency. There were no intracerebral hemorrhages in these patients. However, bleeding was more frequent in the subgroup with optimal anticoagulation with heparin. These data suggest that intense anticoagulation with intravenous heparin enhances coronary artery patency after alteplase treatment of patients with AMI.

Anderson and colleagues[92] in Salt Lake City, Utah, utilized a double-blind, randomized, multicenter trial to compare the effects of treatment with anistreplase (APSAC) and alteplase (rt-PA) on convalescent LV function, morbidity and coronary artery patency at day 1 in patients with AMI. Anistreplase is a new, easily administered thrombolytic agent approved for the treatment of AMI. Alteplase is a rapidly acting, relatively fibrin-specific thrombolytic agent widely used in the United States. Study entry requirements were age ≤75 years, symptoms duration ≤4 hours, ST segment elevation and no contraindications. The two study drugs, PSAC, 30 U/2 to 5 minutes, and rt-PA, 100 mg/3 hours were each given with aspirin (160 mg/day) and intravenous heparin. Prespecified end points were convalescent LV function (rest/exercise), clinical morbidity and coronary artery patency at 1 day. A total of 325 patients were entered, stratified into groups with anterior (37%) or inferior or other (63%) AMI, randomized to receive APSAC or rt-PA and followed up for 1 month. At entry, patient characteristics in the two groups were balanced. Convalescent LVEF at the predischarge study averaged 51% in the APSAC group and 54% in the rt-PA group. At 1 month, LVEF averaged 50% versus 55%, respectively. In contrast, LVEF showed similar augmentation with exercise at 1 month after APSAC and rt-PA and exercise times were comparable. Mortality and the incidence of serious clinical events, including stroke, VT, VF, CHF within 1 month, recurrent ischemia and reinfarction were comparable in the two groups. Mechanical interventions were applied with equal frequency. A combined clinical morbidity index was determined and showed a comparable overall outcome for the two treatments. Convalescent rest EF was high after both therapies but higher after rt-PA. Other clinical outcomes, including exercise function, morbidity index, and 1-day coronary artery patency were favorable and comparable after APSAC and rt-PA.

Duteplase (rt-PA)

Kalbfleisch and associates[93] from multiple medical centers evaluated in patients with AMI the hypothesis that an infusion of recombinant tissue-type plasminogen activator (rt-PA) maintained for up to 24 hours could prevent reocclusion after early patency had been established. The rt-PA studied was an investigational double chain rt-PA (Duteplase) administered according to body weight. Coronary patency was documented to 139 of 213 patients who had 90-minute angiograms recorded after an initial lytic dose of rt-PA. In these responders a further 90-minute infusion at one third the initial lytic dose was given before assignment to 1 of 4 maintenance dose rates (0.012, 0.024, 0.036, 0.048 MIU/kg/hour) which were continued for the subsequent 9 to 21 hours. The principal end point was the status of the infarct-related coronary artery 12 to 24 hours after the start of therapy, and before termination of rt-PA, in patients with initially patent vessels at 90 minutes. Of the 103 responders with repeat angiograms after a 9 to 21 hour maintenance infusion of rt-PA, a total of 17 (16.5%) patients reoccluded across all doses administered. There was no significant relationship between the maintenance dose rate and the incidence of reocclusion. However, there was strong association between total dose of rt-PA administered and the incidence (16%) of serious or life-threatening bleeding exclusive of surgery. Other factors associated with serious bleeding included low body weight, female gender, and total duration of rt-PA infusion. Reocclusion was independent of the 90-minute Thrombolysis in Myocardial Infarction trial perfusion grade and diameter of infarct vessel. Rethrombosis after establishment of early patency after rt-PA remains a significant problem that is unaffected by sustained rt-PA infusion in doses that can be tolerated.

Urokinase

To examine the fibrinolytic capacity in patients with AMI, Sakamoto and associates[94] from Kumamoto, Japan, measured baseline levels of plasma plasminogen activator inhibitor activity and tissue-type plasmino-gen activator (t-PA) antigen in 47 patients with Q-wave AMI who under-went emergent coronary angiography 3.0 ± 2.0 hours after symptom onset. They received intracoronary injection of urokinase if their infarct-related arteries were occluded. They were classified into 3 groups ac-cording to the patency of the infarct-related artery before and after throm-bolytic therapy: the patent group (13 patients), the recanalized group (23 patients) and the occluded group (11 patients). The mean level of plasma plasminogen activator inhibitor activity (IU/ml) was higher in patients with AMI as a whole than in the control group (12.8 ± 1.6 vs 5.4 ± 0.5). The level was lower in the patent group (3.0 ± 1.1) and higher in the recanalized (18.6 ± 2.2) and occluded (10.8 ± 2.5) groups than in the control group. The level was lower in the occluded than in the recanalized group and 62% of the patients in the occluded group had levels within range of the control group. The mean level of plasma t-PA antigen (ng/ml) was higher in patients with AMI as a whole than in the control group (10.3 ± 0.8 vs 5.8 ± 0.3). There was no difference in the level among the 3 groups with AMI. Thus, this study indicates that there is a significant relation between the baseline plasma fibrinolytic capacity and the patency of the infarct-related artery before and after thrombolytic therapy.

Ventricular arrhythmias during thrombolysis

Gressin and associates[95] from Corbeil-Essonnes, France, examined ventricular arrhythmias during thrombolysis for AMI in their relation to coronary artery patency. Twenty-four-hour Holter monitoring was begun 3.1 ± 20.2 hours after onset of pain in 40 patients (age 54 ± 2 years; anterior AMI 42.5%) treated with streptokinase (42.5%) or recombinant tissue-type plasminogen activator (57.5%) (delay from pain 3.3 ± 0.2 hours). A Marquette 8000 computer was used for Holter analysis. The infarct-related artery was considered as patent (72.5%) or non-patent (27.5%) according to coronary angiography (delay from pain 26.7 ± 2.5 hours; 60% <24 hours). Ventricular arrhythmias were present in all pa-tients. Tolerance was good (1 cardioversion for VF). The incidence of accelerated idioventricular rhythm was not different between patients with a patent and nonpatent artery (90 vs 82%), nor for VT (83 vs 73%). Coronary artery patency was associated with a 14-, 13- and 32-fold in-crease of VPC, VT and accelerated idioventricular rhythms, respectively. The increased incidence of sustained VT (patent 38%; nonpatent 0%) and early (before the first 6 hours) accelerated idioventricular rhythm (patent 76%; nonpatent 18%) associated with artery patency suggests that these arrhythmias may be noninvasive diagnostic criteria for reperfusion (sensi-tivity 38 vs 76%, and specificity 100 vs 82%). A positive correlation was found between the frequency of VPCs and VT, and peak creatine kinase.

In an investigation by Hohnloser and associates[96] from Freiburg, Ger-many, in 107 patients with AMI, the incidence of ventricular arrhythmias during the acute phase of thrombolysis was examined by means of Holter monitoring. In patients with a patent infarct-related artery as assessed angiographically at 90 minutes, the occurrence of accelerated idioventri-cular rhythms was noted significantly more frequently than in patients with a permanent occluded vessel. This arrhythmia peaked in the first 180 minutes after the start of thrombolysis. In addition, single VPC and runs of VT were also more common in patients with successful reperfu-sion. The effects of acute intravenous administration of beta-blockers were examined in 66 patients without contraindications to this therapeutic approach. There were no differences in the occurrence of any type of rhythm disorders in patients with (n = 43) or without beta-blockade (n = 23). Thus ventricular arrhythmias, particularly accelerated idioventricular rhythms and single VPC, occur more frequently in patients with a patent infarct artery within the first 24 hours after thrombolysis. Acute intravenous beta-blockade does not appear to exert significant antiarrhythmic effects during this period.

Additional ST segment elevation early

Shechter and colleagues[97] in Tel-Hashomer, Israel, evaluated the significance of further ST segment elevation that occurs during the first hour of thrombolytic therapy to evaluate whether further ST segment elevation developing during the first hour of therapy predicts thrombolysis. One hundred and seventy seven consecutive patients with a first AMI were divided into two groups: Group A, 98 patients with ST elevation ≥1 mm above the initial ST elevation during the first hour of thrombolytic therapy and Group B, 79 patients without this finding. The presence or absence of additional ST segment elevation was not associated with a clinical or prognostic difference in patients with first AMI or posterior acute AMI, but its presence indicated a more favorable clinical outcome in patients with anterior AMI. Among the patients with anterior AMI, the 65 patients in Group A had a higher LVEF (44 ± 9% vs 35 ± 11%, respectively), less heart failure (15% vs 35%), and a lower in-hospital mortality rate (0% vs 8%) than did the 37 patients in Group B. Therefore, additional ST segment elevation during early thrombolytic therapy in patients with anterior AMI suggests a more favorable clinical outcome and may be indicative of successful reperfusion.

Perfusion grades

The Thrombolysis in Myocardial Infarction (TIMI) study group designated patency grades 0 (occluded) or 1 (minimal perfusion) as thrombolysis failure and grade 2 (partial perfusion) or 3 (complete perfusion) as success. To evaluate their true functional significance, perfusion grades were compared with enzymatic and electrocardiographic indexes of myocardial infarction in 359 patients treated within 4 hours with anistreplase (APSAC) or streptokinase by Karagounis and associates[98] in Salt Lake City, Utah. Serum enzymes and electrocardiograms were assessed serially. Patency was determined at 90 to 240 minutes (median 2 hours) and graded by an observer without knowledge of patient data. Results for the two drug arms were similar and combined. Distribution of patency was grade 0 = 20%, n = 72; grade 1 = 8%, n = 27; grade 2 = 16%, n = 58 and grade 3 = 56%, n = 202. Interventions were performed after angiography but within 24 hours in 51% (n = 37), 70% (n = 19), 41% (n = 24) and 14% (n = 28) of patients with grades 0, 1, 2 and 3, respectively. Outcomes were compared among the four patency groups by the orthogonal contrast method. Patients with perfusion grade 2 did not differ significantly from those with grade 0 or 1 in enzymatic peaks, time to peak activity, and evolution of summed ST segments, Q and R waves. Conversely, comparisons of patients with grade 3 perfusion with those with grades 0 to 2 yielded significant differences for enzymatic peaks and time to peak activity for three of the four enzymes and electrocardiographic indexes of myocardial infarction. Thus, patients with grade 2 flow have indexes of myocardial infarction similar to those in patients with an occluded coronary artery. Only early grade 3 flow results in a significantly better outcome. Since early achievement of grade 2 flow does not appear to lead to optimal myocardial salvage, the frequency of achieving grade 3 perfusion alone may best measure the reperfusion success of thrombolytic therapy.

Predictors of early morbidity and mortality

Clinical variables collected prospectively for the 3,339 patients of the Thrombolysis in Myocardial Infarction II study were analyzed by Mueller and the TIMI Investigators[99] in Baltimore, Maryland retrospectively to identify predictors of clinical events of 42 days and earlier and to identify subgroups in which an invasive or conservative strategy might be superior. Pulmonary edema/cardiogenic shock presented as the strongest independent correlate with death. In two subgroups, mortality differed between the invasive and conservative strategies: 1) Patients with versus without prior AMI had a high mortality in the conservative strategy (12% vs 4%); in the invasive strategy, the mortality rates were similar (6% and 5%). 2) Patients with diabetes mellitus and no prior AMI had a higher mortality in the invasive than in the conservative strategy (15% vs 4%). Reinfarction was not independently correlated with baseline characteristics except with history of angina. Mortality was lower in current smokers and ex-smokers versus never-smokers. Current smokers had a lower risk profile, including age, pulmonary edema/cardiogenic shock, history of hypertension, and diabetes. The rate of reinfarction was lower in current smokers versus ex-smokers and never-smokers. "Not current smoker" was an independent correlate with reinfarction. The coronary anatomy did not differ among the current smokers, ex-smokers, and never-smokers. The strong independent correlation of pulmonary edema/cardiogenic shock with death suggests that thrombolysis is not sufficient to improve survival in these patients. The higher mortality in patients with versus without prior AMI in the conservative strategy suggest that early catheterization and revascularization of these patients might be beneficial. Conversely, the higher mortality in diabetics without prior AMI in the invasive than in the conservative strategy suggests that early aggressive management might not be suitable in this subgroup except for clinical indications. Reinfarction was not predictable by clinical variables except by history of angina. The finding that "not current smokers" was an independent correlate with reinfarction was unexpected.

Effect on morbidity and mortality

To evaluate the impact of introducing thrombolytic and aspirin therapy into the management policy of a coronary care unit, Ranjadayalan and associates[100] from London, UK, studied 336 patients with AMI comprising consecutive admissions to their coronary care unit over 2 separate 12-month periods: January-December, 1986 (n = 158) and September, 1989-August, 1990 (n = 178), before and after thrombolytic and aspirin therapy had been introduced into the management policy of the unit. Thrombolytic and aspirin therapy was given to 87% and 93%, respectively, of all patients in the 1989/1990 cohort. This high treatment rate led to substantial improvements in morbidity and mortality. Thus, comparison of the 1986 and 1989/1990 cohorts showed reductions in hospital mortality (24% to 11%), VF (22% to 13%), and cardiogenic shock (20% to 6%), particularly in patients aged over 60. Reductions in the incidence of lesser degrees of heart failure are reflected in the proportions of patients discharged with diuretic requirements, which declined from 43% in 1986 to 22% in 1989/1990. The duration of hospital stay for patients who survived showed no change between 1986 and 1989/1990, but time spent in the coronary care unit decreased from 3.1 ± 1.8 to 2.1 ± 1.4 days. Most nonselected patients with AMI are candidates for thrombolytic and aspirin therapy, which can be given safely, leading to profound reductions in mortality and the incidence of major complications, particularly in the older age group.

Mechanisms of death

Kleiman and associates[101] in Baltimore, Maryland, for the TIMI Investigators evaluated mechanisms of death among patients who died within 18 hours of enrollment in the Thrombolysis and Myocardial Infarction Phase II (TIMI II) study. Among 3,339 patients enrolled, 32 died within the first 4 hours and 31 died within the subsequent 14 hours. Thirteen of the 63 patients had shock at enrollment and 22 had advanced hemodynamic compromise without shock. Twenty-eight patients initially had minimal to no compromise hemodynamically. Prior AMI was present in 16 patients (25%). CHF resulting from extensive heart muscle damage was responsible for 39 early deaths (62%), ventricular rupture for 10 (16%), arrhythmia for 8 (13%) and complications of therapy in 6 (10%). Nine of 720 patients randomized to immediate intravenous beta-blocking therapy had an early death compared with 6 of 714 assigned to deferred beta-blocker therapy (Table 3-3). These data indicated that mortality is highest in the early hours after AMI, even in patients treated with thrombolytic therapy and is most frequently due to extensive heart muscle damage. Efforts to reduce mortality should be directed at prevention, limitation, or palliation of early pump failure and very early treatment with thrombolytic therapy.

Invasive vs non-invasive treatment afterwards

The thrombolysis in Myocardial Infarction (TIMI) Phase II Trial by Williams and colleagues[102] in Providence, Rhode Island, randomized 3,339 patients to either an invasive or a conservative strategy after intravenous recombinant tissue-type plasminogen activator for AMI. The patients assigned to the invasive strategy routinely underwent cardiac catheterization, and when anatomically appropriate, PTCA or CABG 18-48 hours after infarction. Conservative patients had these procedures only in response to the occurrence of spontaneous or provoked ischemia. One-year follow-up data were available in 3,316 patients (99%). The primary trial end point, death and nonfatal AMI, occurred in 15% of invasive patients and in 15% of conservative patients. When analyzed individually, there was no difference in death or recurrent AMI between the two groups. Anginal status at 1 year was also similar. Cardiac catheterization and PTCA were performed more often in invasive (98% and 61% respectively) compared with conservative (45% and 21%, respectively) patients. At 1 year, the cumulative number of patients who underwent CABG (17%) was similar in the two groups. The invasive and conservative strategies resulted in similar favorable outcomes at 1 year of follow-up. In particular, the rates of mortality and reinfarction were not different and were impressively low in both groups. One possible advantage of the invasive strategy was detected in subgroup analyses. In patients with a history of AMI, the data

TABLE 3-3. *Mechanism of Death According to Time to Death. Reproduced with permission from Kleiman, et al.*[101]

	Time to Death		
Cause of Death	≤4 h (N = 32)	>4 h–≤18 h (N = 31)	>18 h–≤42 days (N = 102)
Cardiovascular disease	30	27	68
Cardiac disease	30	27	64
Fatal MI	30	27	57
Qualifying MI	30	27	43
Recurrent	0	0	14
Cardiac death*			
Pump failure	22	17	35
Arrhythmia	4	4	19
Ventricular rupture	4	6	9
Other	0	0	1
Complications	2	4	34
Hemorrhage	2	3	13
Consequence of CABG	0	1	6
Consequence of PTCA	0	0	8
Other	0	0	7
Autopsy obtained	13	14	38

*Based on the Mortality and Morbidity Classification Committee classification of causes of death according to the following rule: all cardiac deaths with ventricular rupture present are attributed to rupture; in the absence of rupture, cardiac deaths with pump failure present are attributed to pump failure. CABG = coronary artery bypass graft surgery; MI = myocardial infarction; PTCA = percutaneous transluminal coronary angioplasty.

are suggestive that 1-year mortality was lower in invasive patients (10%) than in conservative patients (17%).

To test the hypothesis that delayed PTCA might provide clinical benefit compared with medical therapy alone, Ellis and co-investigators[103] in the treatment of post-thrombolytic stenosis study group in Cleveland, Ohio randomized 87 patients within 6 hours of chest pain onset with thrombolytic therapy and with negative functional tests between PTCA to be performed 4 to 14 days after AMI versus no PTCA. Both groups received medical therapy. Patients with postinfarct angina or prior Q wave infarction in the infarct distribution were excluded. The primary study end point was increase in LVEF with exercise measured by radionuclide studies 6 weeks after AMI, a parameter known from other studies to correlate inversely with future ischemic events. Clinical outcome was also monitored for 12 months. There were no differences between the study groups for any prerandomization variable recorded. Mean age was 57 years, 84% of patients were male, 21% had prior AMI, 36% had anterior AMI, 7% had multivessel disease, and the infarct stenosis measured 70% before randomization. PTCA was successful in 38 of 42 patients but resulted in non-Q wave MI due to acute closure of the treated site in 3 of 42 patients. There was no difference in 6-week resting EF or increase in EF with exercise between the 2 groups. There were no deaths in either group. Actuarial 12-month infarct-free survival was 98% in the no-PTCA group and 91% in the PTCA group. Thus there was no functional or clinical benefit from routine late PTCA after AMI treated with thrombolytic therapy in this relatively low-risk cohort of patients. These data strongly suggest that patients with an uncomplicated AMI after thrombolytic therapy, even if they have a "significant" residual stenosis of the infarct vessel, should be treated medically if they are without evidence of ischemia on stress testing before hospital discharge.

Ruocco and colleagues[104] in Boston, Massachusetts, and Baltimore, Maryland, for the Thrombolysis in Myocardial Infarction Investigators assessed the possibility that a subgroup of patients at high risk for recurrent ischemia and reinfarction after thrombolytic therapy might benefit from early intervention. The Thrombolysis in Myocardial Infarction Phase II study concluded that an obligatory invasive strategy after thrombolytic therapy offered no advantage over a more conservative therapy. Data from 3,534 patients enrolled in the Thrombolysis in Myocardial Infarction Phase II trial were analyzed to determine whether a history of antecedent angina before AMI identifies patients at high risk for subsequent ischemia and whether these patients benefit from an invasive strategy. Antecedent angina identified patients at increased risk for recurrent chest pain in the hospital (32% vs 21%, respectively) and recurrent AMI during the first year of follow-up compared with patients without antecedent angina. Among patients assigned to the invasive strategy, coronary arteriography revealed that those with antecedent angina had a more severe residual stenosis of the infarct-related artery after thrombolytic therapy and more multivessel disease. The clinical outcome of the patients with antecedent angina assigned randomly to either the invasive or the conservative strategy were compared. The invasive strategy patients had a slightly lesser incidence of recurrent chest pain in the hospital (30% vs 35%) and more negative findings on exercise tolerance tests (25% vs 19%), but there were no differences between the treatment strategies in the end point variables of recurrent AMI or death. These data demonstrate that antecedent angina identifies patients at increased risk for recurrent ischemic events after thrombolytic therapy. Similar to the results for the overall group, the invasive strategy does not alter the risk of repeat AMI or death compared with the conservative approach.

Effect on signal-averaged electrocardiogram

Pedretti and associates[105] from Tradate, Italy, evaluated the influence of intravenous thrombolysis on both prevalence of ventricular late potentials and incidence of late arrhythmic events in 174 consecutive patients surviving a first AMI; 106 patients (61%) received thrombolysis (group A) and 68 (34%) had conventional therapy (group B). In group A, 18 patients (17%) had late potentials compared with 23 (34%) in group B; mean LVEF was not different (0.50 ± 0.09 vs 0.50 ± 0.10 [NS]). Of 63 patients who underwent coronary arteriography because of post-infarction ischemia, 28 (44%) had a closed infarct-related artery; of these, 11 (39%) had late potentials compared with 3 of 35 (9%) with a patent artery. Mean LVEF was not significantly different between the 2 groups (0.49 ± 0.09 vs 0.53 ± 0.09). At a mean follow-up of 14 ± 9 months, 8 of 161 patients (5%)

had a late arrhythmic event; 6 of 8 (75%) with and 28 of 153 (18%) without events had late potentials. In group A, 4 of 99 patients (4%) had events compared with 4 of 62 (6%) in group B (p = NS, relative risk 1.6). Of 24 patients with anterior wall AMI and LV dyskinesia, 6 events occurred. In this group of patients, a higher rate of events was observed (25%); 3 of 16 (19%) treated with thrombolysis had an event compared with 3 of 8 (37%) treated conventionally. Thrombolysis and patency of the infarct-related artery significantly reduce the rate of late potentials independently of global LV function. ALthough no significant difference was found in the follow-up results, the reduced rate of late potentials suggests an improved ventricular electrical stability both in patients treated with thrombolysis and in those with a patent vessel.

Malik and associates[106] from London, UK, examined standard time domain variables from signal-averaged electrocardiograms in a population of 331 survivors of AMI. Of these subjects, 130 received early (<24 hours) thrombolytic therapy. During a follow-up of ≥10 months, there were 17 arrhythmic events (8.5%) (sudden death or sustained symptomatic VT) in the group without thrombolysis and 8 (6.2%) in those with thrombolysis. Statistically, highly significant differences between the signal-averaged electrocardiographic variables of patients with and without arrhythmic events were found in the group without thrombolysis, whereas only room-mean = square voltage of the terminal 40 ms of the signal-averaged QRS complex was statistically associated with outcome (the differences in the other 2 indexes being not significant) in patients with thrombolysis. When using 2 previously published categoric criteria for the diagnosis of abnormal signal-averaged electrocardiography, the performance of these criteria in predicting arrhythmic events was substantially better in the group without thrombolysis than in those with thrombolysis (positive predictive accuracy >3 times lower). Retrospectively adjusted receiver-operator characteristics showed that for a sensitivity of 30%, the maximum achievable positive predictive accuracy of signal-averaged electrocardiography for arrhythmic events was 100% in the group without thrombolysis, but only 27% in those with thrombolysis. It is concluded that standard signal-averaged electrocardiography after AMI is less informative in patients who receive thrombolytic treatment.

In an investigation by Moreno and associates[107] from Salt Lake City, Utah, to assess the effects of thrombolysis and reperfusion on late potentials after AMI, 101 patients (79 men, age 63 ± 11 years) underwent signal-averaged electrocardiographic studies at 11 ± 9.2 days, with the use of a 40 to 250 Hz band-pass filter. Patients were divided into 4 groups: 1) 54 patients treated with thrombolytic agents at 2.8 ± 1.1 hours, with 81% "early" patency/reperfusion; 2) 47 patients treated conventionally with 45% "late" patency/reperfusion; 3) 56 patients with patency; and 4) 26 patients without patency. A late potential was present when ≥2 of 3 defined criteria were present. There was a significant difference in the incidence of late potentials between groups 1 and 2 (22% vs 43%) and between groups 3 and 4 (18% vs 50%). Late potentials also tended to occur less often after "early" than after "late" patency/reperfusion (13% vs 25%). The odds ratio for developing a late potential was 0.39 for thrombolysis versus no thrombolysis and 0.22 for patency/reperfusion versus no patency/reperfusion. By analysis of covariance the effects of thrombolysis on late potentials were entirely explained by reperfusion. Thus the risk of late potentials after AMI is high but is reduced by thrombolysis and reperfusion. In addition, the effectiveness of "early" reperfusion appears to be greater than that of "late" but requires further clarification.

Effect of antecedent angina

Barbash and associates[108] in Tel Hashomer, Israel, have evaluated the importance of antecedent angina in predicting clinical outcome in 8,329 patients with AMI who received thrombolytic therapy with either recombinant tissue plasminogen activator or streptokinase. There were 2,370 patients with antecedent angina for >1 month, 1,512 patients with antecedent angina for ≤1 month and 4,447 patients with no antecedent angina. The longer the duration of angina, the worse the baseline characteristics in the three groups: the mean patient age was 65 versus 62 versus 61 years, respectively. The rate of previous AMI was 37% versus 18% versus 10% and the rate of hypertension was 40% versus 31% versus 27%, respectively, Antecedent angina was associated with a longer hospital stay (11.3 vs 11.7 vs 10.8 days), a higher incidence of CABG (2.2% vs 1.2% vs 0.7%), a worse Killip class at discharge, and a higher hospital and 6-month mortality (12% and 18% vs 8.9% and 11.6% vs 6.6% vs 9.2%, respectively) (Figure 3-26). A multivariate analysis taking into account all baseline characteristics confirmed the independent association of antecedent angina with mortality with a relative risk of 1.4 to 1.47. Therefore, antecedent angina predicts a worse clinical outcome and a more intensive use of medical resource in patients with AMI during thrombolytic therapy.

Left ventricular performance afterwards

Zaret and associates[109] for the TIMI investigators evaluated global and regional LV performance with equilibrium radionuclide angiography in patients in the Thrombolysis in Myocardial Infarction (TIMI) II trial at the time of hospital discharge. Studies at rest were available in 1,162 (69%) of the invasive and 1,150 (69%) of the conservative strategy patients, and exercise studies in 1,133 (67%) of the invasive and 1,145 (69%) of the conservative patients. Repeat studies were performed at the time of 6-week follow-up. Global and regional EF at rest were both comparable in

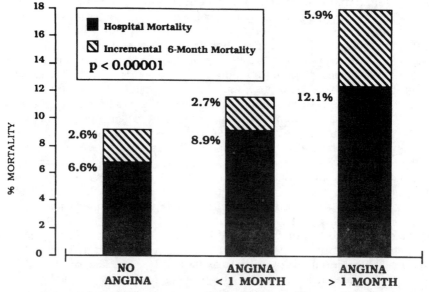

Fig. 3-26. Hospital and 6-month mortality by angina groups (by chi-square analysis for trend). Reproduced with permission from Barbash, et al.[108]

patients assigned to each of the treatment strategies. However, at the time of hospital discharge patients in the invasive strategy had normal exercise responses more frequently (30 vs 26%), greater peak exercise LVEF (55 ± 14% vs 53 ± 14%), greater exercise—rest change in LVEF (3.7 ± 6.7% vs 2.7 ± 7.2%) and greater peak exercise infarct zone regional EF (53 ± 31% vs 50 ± 33%) than patients assigned to the conservative strategy. At 6-week follow-up these differences between treatment strategies were no longer evident. When data were restricted to those collected at comparable work loads, similar differences in hospital discharge exercise performance between invasive vs conservative strategy patients were observed. Thus, there is a small transient difference in exercise global and regional LV performance associated with an invasive as opposed to conservative strategy after thrombolytic therapy. These differences were noted at the time of hospital discharge but not at 6 weeks, and are unlikely to confer clinical benefit.

Intracranial hemorrhage

De Jaegere and associates[110] in Rotterdam, The Netherlands, evaluated 2,469 patients with AMI treated with a thrombolytic agent registered in 61 hospitals during a period of 18 months. Most patients (73%) were treated with streptokinase. Intracranial hemorrhage was observed in 24 patients corresponding to an incidence rate of 1%. The median time interval between the start of thrombolytic therapy and the first clinical signs of intracranial bleeding was 16 hours. In total, 16 (66%) of the 24 patients died as a result of cerebral hematoma. To determine clinical predictive factors, a case-control study was conducted. For every patient with intracranial hemorrhage, two control patients who received thrombolytic therapy because of AMI in the same hospital and in the same period were selected. Detailed clinical characteristics of 22 of the 24 patients as well as of 7 other patients with documented intracerebral bleeding from the European Cooperative Study Group and of 2 patients who sustained intracranial hemorrhage outside the registry were compared with 62 control patients. The results of multivariate logistic regression analysis indicate patients taking an oral anticoagulant before admission, patients with a total body weight <70 kg and those older than 65 years of age are at highest risk for intracranial hemorrhage during thrombolytic therapy.

PERCUTANEOUS TRANSLUMINAL CORONARY ANGIOPLASTY

Eckman and associates[111] from Boston, Massachusetts, reviewed the usefulness of angioplasty early in the course of AMI without preceding thrombolytic therapy. The English-language literature was searched from 1983 through October 1991. Twenty-three articles describing a total of 4,368 patients were found. After duplicate patient series were eliminated, weighted average short- and long-term mortality rates were calculated for the remaining 2,073 patients in 10 series and for selected clinical subsets. Average hospital mortality for patients with AMI having direct angioplasty was 8.3%. Patients in cardiogenic shock had the highest mortality; patients with 1-vessel CAD had the lowest. For patients in cardiogenic shock, data on direct angioplasty appeared superior to data for similar patients receiving thrombolytic therapy. Although few data exist, a survival advantage was also suggested for patients with a history of previous bypass surgery (hospital mortality, 11.1%). Direct angioplasty has an overall mortality similar to that of thrombolytic therapy. Patients who may benefit more from mechanical revascularization than from thrombolytic therapy include those at increased risk for thrombolytic therapy (uncontrolled hypertension, recent major surgery, cerebrovascular accident, prolonged cardiopulmonary resuscitation, or bleeding diathesis), and those with cardiogenic shock. The efficacy in several other patient subsets (age >65 years, previous CABG, prolonged delay before reperfusion) warrants further study.

To assess the changes in AMI following direct PTCA, O'Keefe and associates[112] from Kansas City, Missouri, evaluated 323 consecutive patients undergoing PTCA without antecedent thrombolytic therapy for AMI. LV function was evaluated using contrast ventriculography immediately pre-PTCA and at the time of predismissal follow-up PTCA (mean 7 days after AMI). The global EF increased from 53% to 59%. Multivariate correlates of improved global LV function included baseline EF ≤45%, and a patent infarct vessel at the time of predischarge follow-up PTCA. Systolic function in the infarct zone improved by a mean of 30%. Logistic regression analysis identified sustained infarct vessel patency and anterior AMI as multivariate correlates of improved regional function in the infarct zone. In patients presenting with baseline EF ≤40%, the mean EF increased from 28% to 42%. Long-term survival was compromised in patients with global EF fraction of ≤40% at the time of dismissal. Thus significant improvement in LV function can be expected in the majority of patients undergoing direct infarct PTCA. The myocardial salvage appears to be most significant in patients suffering large infarctions, and in those with sustained infarct vessel patency.

Recent evidence suggests that late reperfusion of an occluded infarct-related artery after AMI may convey a better prognosis than that produced by nonreperfusion. The clinical outcome of PTCA is a means of mechanical reperfusion in this particular setting has not been clearly delineated. Sabri and associates[113] from Richmond, Virginia, analyzed 97 patients with AMI undergoing PTCA of the occluded infarct-related artery 48 hours to 2 weeks (mean 8 ± 4 days) after onset of the AMI. The study consisted of 72 men (74%) (mean age 56.5 ± 12 years) and 25 women. Seventy-seven patients (79%) had a q-wave AMI and 20 patients (21%) a non-Q-wave AMI. Seventy-six patients (79%) had angina after AMI and 4 had previously undergone CABG. Clinical success was achieved in 85 patients (87%). Angiographic success was obtained in 90 of the 97 occluded arteries (93%) and was similar for all 3 major vessels: right coronary 97%, left anterior descending 93% and circumflex 85%. Major complications (AMI, emergency bypass and death) occurred in 3 patients (3.2%). Long-term follow-up (3.7 ± 0.8 years) revealed symptomatic recurrence in 20 (23%), whereas 51 (58%) remained asymptomatic. Most recurrences (16 of 20) were in the form of restenosis rather than reocclusion, with a high success rate for repeat dilatation (93%). These results indicate that mechanical reperfusion of an occluded infarct artery, performing PTCA 48 hours to 2 weeks after AMI, has a high success rate, a low complication rate and low symptomatic restenosis.

Eighty-one patients with cardiogenic shock complicating AMI were evaluated by Moosvi and associates[114] in Detroit, Michigan, to evaluate the effects of coronary revascularization either by PTCA or CABG or both on survival. Thirty-two patients had successful revascularization and 49 patients had unsuccessful or no revascularization. Revascularization was achieved by PTCA in 22 patients, CABG in 2 and PTCA followed by CABG in 8. No significant differences were noted between the two groups with regard to baseline clinical or hemodynamic variables. Intraaortic balloon counterpulsation was used in 27 (84%) of the 32 patients in the group with revascularization and in 19 (39%) of the 49 patients without revascularization. The in-hospital survival was better in the patients with (56%) than in patients without revascularization (8%). At a mean follow-up period of 21 ± 15 months, this survival difference persisted. The mean time from the onset of shock to revascularization differed significantly between survivors and nonsurvivors, being 12.4 ± 15 hours in survivors and 58.5 ± 93 hours in nonsurvivors, in the group with revascularization. In the revascularization group, the in-hospital survival rate was 77% when revascularization was performed within 24 hours but only 10% when it was performed after 24 hours. Thus, these data indicate that the combination of successful coronary revascularization and intraaortic balloon pumping is associated with improved survival in patients with cardiogenic shock complicating AMI. Improvements in survival is most evident if revascularization is performed early, especially within 24 hours of the onset of cardiogenic shock.

Brodie and associates[115] from Greensboro, North Carolina, examined the importance of a patent infarct-related artery (IRA) for hospital and late survival in 383 patients with AMI treated with direct coronary angioplasty. At hospital discharge, 317 of 348 patients (91%) had a patent IRA and mean follow-up LVEF was 58%. Cardiac survival after hospital discharge at 1, 3 and 6 years was 99, 95 and 90%. Patency of the IRA was the most important determinant of hospital mortality: patent versus occluded IRA, 5 vs 39% mortality. Follow-up LVEF was the most important determinant of late cardiac mortality: follow-up LVEF ≥45 versus <45%, 2 versus 24% mortality. Patency of the IRA was not a significant predictor of late cardiac mortality in the group as a whole: patent versus occluded IRA, 4.7 versus 6.5% mortality. In the subgroup of patients with depressed initial LVEF 45%, patency was a significant predictor of late cardiac mortality: patent versus occluded IRA, 9.2 versus 40% mortality. Patients with a patent IRA had better recovery of LV function than patients with an occluded IRA (follow-up LVEF 58.5 versus 47.6%). When late cardiac mortality was adjusted for differences in follow-up LVEF, patency was no longer a significant predictor of late mortality. The results indicate patency of the IRA is the most important determinant of hospital survival, and LV function (measured after recovery) is the most important determinant of late cardiac survival. Patency of the IRA is important for preservation of LV function, but is not an independent determinant of late cardiac survival.

Early restenosis after successful PTCA without antecedent thrombolytic therapy in patients with AMI was assessed by performing in-hospital cardiac catheterization in 62 (88%) of 70 consecutive patients in a study carried out by Morishita and colleagues[116] from Kyoto, Japan. Specific attention was focused on the effectiveness of the intracoronary administration of urokinase in cases with angiographic residual thrombus after successful direct PTCA. The following 2 treatment regimens were used: PTCA alone (43 patients) and PTCA followed by the intracoronary infusion of *urokinase* (27 patients). The rate of early restenosis (reobstruction < 30 days post-PTCA) was higher after successful direct PTCA alone (28%) than after direct PTCA followed by intracoronary urokinase (5%). Bleeding complications were no different between the 2 groups. These findings suggest that intracoronary urokinase can be effective in reducing early restenosis in patients with angiographic residual thrombus after successful direct PTCA. Therefore early restenosis may be related to residual intracoronary thrombus.

Experimental and observational clinical studies of acute coronary occlusion have suggested that late reperfusion prevents infarct expansion and facilitates myocardial healing. Topol and colleagues in the Thrombolysis and angioplasty myocardial infarction study group[117] in Cleveland, Ohio, assessed whether infarct vessel patency could be achieved in late-entry patients and what benefit, if any, can be demonstrated. In a double-blind fashion, 197 patients with 6 to 24 hours of symptoms and electrocardiographic ST elevation were randomly assigned to a tissue-type plasminogen activator (100 mg over 2 hours) or placebo. Coronary angiography within 24 hours was used to determine infarct vessel patency status. Patients with infarct-related occluded arteries were then eligible for a second randomization to either angioplasty (34 patients) or no angioplasty (37 patients). Ventricular function and cavity size were reassessed at 1 month by gated blood pool scintigraphy and at 6 months by repeat cardiac catheterization. The primary end point, infarct vessel patency, was 65% for plasminogen activator patients compared with 27% in the placebo group. There were no differences between these groups in EF or infarct zone regional wall motion at 1 or 6 months. At 6 months, infarct vessel patency was 59% in both groups. In the placebo group, there was a significant increase in end-diastolic volume from acute phase of 127 ml to 159 ml at 6-month follow-up, but no increase in cavity size for the plasminogen activator group patients. Coronary angioplasty was associated with an initial 81% recanalization success and improved ventricular function at 1 month, but by late follow-up no advantage could be demonstrated for this procedure, and there was a 38% spontaneous recanalization rate in the patients assigned to no angioplasty. The study demonstrates that it is possible to achieve infarct vessel recanalization in the majority of late-entry patients with either thrombolytic therapy or angioplasty. Thrombolytic intervention had a favorable effect on prevention of cavity dilatation and LV remodeling, but there are no late benefits on systolic function after thrombolysis or coronary angioplasty.

From June 1988 to March 1991, Juliard and associates[118] from Paris, France, managed an unselected cohort of 150 consecutive patients with AMI (<6 hours) according to a strategy designed to ensure early patency of the infarct-related artery in the maximum number of patients. The following procedures were used: (1) intravenous thrombolysis, which was the usual treatment (n = 103), followed in 98 cases by emergency coronary angiography 90 minutes after the beginning of thrombolysis. This identified 31 thrombolysis failures (32%) and led to 19 rescue angioplasties (18 successes). All patients were then scheduled for predischarge angiography. (2) Direct angioplasty, which was performed in 40 patients because of contraindications to thrombolysis (n = 23), cardiogenic shock (n = 3), diagnostic doubt (n = 7). Success (defined as Thrombolysis in Myocardial Infarction [TIMI] flow >1, with a residual stenosis 50% in the infarct-related artery) was achieved in 36 of 40 patients (90%). (3) The 7 remaining patients were given conventional medical treatment because of advanced age, contraindications to thrombolysis and angioplasty, or spontaneous reperfusion (confirmed by emergency angiography). In all, emergency angioplasty was performed in the acute phase in 39% of the 150 patients in this nonselected cohort. Despite the logistic burden involved, this strategy achieved a low in-hospital mortality rate (7 of 150 patients [4.7%]; 1.9% in those treated with thrombolysis) and a high infarct-related artery patency rate (both in the acute phase [88%] and at hospital discharge [93% of those with a predischarge angiogram]), whereas only a minimal number of patients (3.3%) had no benefit from early recanalization therapy. In conclusion, an aggressive revascularization strategy used during the acute phase in all patients with AMI (<6 hours) achieves high in-hospital patency and low in-hospital mortality.

The European Cooperative Study Group[119] in Rotterdam, the Netherlands, conducted 2 randomized trials in patients with suspected AMI to assess the effect of 100 mg single-chain recombinant tissue-type plasinogen activator (TPA, alteplase) on enzymatic infarct size, LV function, morbidity and mortality relative to placebo (alteplase/placebo trial) and to assess the effect of immediate (PTCA) in addition to alteplase (alteplase/PTCA trial). One-year follow-up results were reported. In the alteplase/placebo trial, 721 patients with chest pain of less than 5 hours and extensive ST-segment elevation were allocated at random to 100 mg alteplase or placebo over 3 hours. In the alteplase/PTCA trial, 367 similar patients received alteplase and subsequently were allocated at random to immediate coronary angiography and PTCA of the infarct-related vessel or control. All patients received aspirin and intravenous heparin. In the alteplase/placebo trial, mortality during the first year was reduced by 36% with alteplase. Revascularization was performed more frequently after alteplase, and more patients in the alteplase group were in New York Heart Association functional class I or II. Reinfarction tended to occur more frequently after alteplase than after placebo. In the alteplase/PTCA trial, reinfarction was less common after immediate PTCA, and revascularization procedures were less frequent. However, this benefit was offset by a high rate of immediate reocclusion and early recurrent ischemia and by higher mortality at 1 year (9 vs 5%) in the invasive group. In a multivariate analysis of 1,043 hospital survivors, mortality after discharge was related to coronary anatomy, LV function, age and previous infarction but not to initial treatment allocation. Reinfarction after hospital discharge tended to be more common after alteplase and related to coronary anatomy. Benefit from treatment with alteplase, heparin, and aspirin is not diminished at 1 year. Routine immediate PTCA does not confer additional benefit. Prognosis after hospital discharge mainly is determined by coronary anatomy and residual LV function and is unrelated to initial treatment assignment.

The value of routine administration of intravenous thrombolytic agents during PTCA therapy of AMI has not been determined. Therefore, O'Neill and colleagues[120] in Royal Oak, Michigan, prospectively randomized 122 patients with evolving AMI to PTCA therapy with or without adjunctive intravenous streptokinase therapy. Patients with electrocardiographic ST segment elevation who presented within 4 hours of symptom onset, had no contraindication to thrombolytic therapy, and were not in cardiogenic shock were enrolled. They were treated immediately with intravenous heparin (10,000 units) and oral aspirin (325 mg) and randomized to treatment with placebo or streptokinase (1.5 M units) administered intravenously over 30 minutes. Patients then were taken immediately to the catheterization laboratory, and those with suitable coronary anatomy underwent immediate PTCA. Subsequent clinical course, serial radionuclide ventriculography, and 6-month repeat angiography were analyzed. A total of 106 patients were treated with PTCA. Use of PTCA was similar for placebo (92%) and streptokinase (83%) groups. PTCA was successful in 95% of patients, with no difference in placebo (93%) and streptokinase (98%) groups. Serial radionuclide ventriculography demonstrated no difference in 24-hour or 6-week EF values for placebo and streptokinase groups, respectively. Contrast ventriculography demonstrated improvement in immediate versus 6-month values for the overall group. No differences in 6-month values were present for placebo and streptokinase groups, respectively. Coronary angiography was performed in 75% of the 90 patients eligible for restudy. Arterial patency was 87% at 6 months, and coronary restenosis was present in 38% of patients. No differences in chronic patency or restenosis were detected for the 2 treatment groups. Although adjunctive intravenous streptokinase therapy did not improve outcome, it did complicate the hospital course. Hospitalization was longer (9 vs 4 days) and more costly ($25,000 vs $20,000). Transfusion rate was higher (39% vs 8%) and need for emergency CABG was greater (10% vs 2%) for the streptokinase-treated patients. Adjunctive intravenous streptokinase therapy does not enhance early preservation of ventricular function, improve arterial patency rates, or lower restenosis rates after PTCA therapy of AMI. Hospital course is longer, more expensive, and more complicated. For these reasons, PTCA therapy of AMI should not be routinely performed with adjunctive intravenous streptokinase therapy.

Vacek and colleagues[121] from Kansas City, Missouri, studied the outcomes of patients with AMI who were treated either with direct PTCA or thrombolytics followed by PTCA. Two patient cohorts were analyzed: a previously reported (in regard to short-term follow-up) group of 371 patients who now have long-term follow-up (mean 3.4 years) of survival and event-free survival, and a second group of 202 patients who have been treated subsequently. Both 1-year and 2-year survival were significantly better in the group that was treated with thrombolytics first. Event-free survival (no AMI, CABG, repeat PTCA) was better overall for the group that was treated with thrombolytics first. The more recently treated group of patients also showed benefit in regard to both survival and event-free survival over a short-term follow-up period (mean 39 weeks) for patients who were treated initially with thrombolytics as compared with those who were treated with direct PTCA. Although the initial cohort was very similar to the treatment groups except for age (mean age for the direct PTCA group was 62 ± 12 years vs 57 ± 11 years for thrombolytics first group), several differences existed in the more recent treatment groups. The patients who were more recently treated with direct PTCA were older, had lower mean EF, had more extensive CAD, and were more likely to have had prior CABG. In the initial cohort of 371 patients 58% received direct PTCA, and 42% received initial treatment with thrombolytics. These percentages were 33 and 67, respectively, in the group of more recently treated patients. Thus, it was concluded that 1) the initial short-term benefit of initial thrombolytic therapy for AMI over direct PTCA is maintained over a long-term follow-up period, 2) short-term benefit is confirmed for a separate group of recently treated patients, 3) a change in treatment allocation has occurred in practice, and 4) a possible persistent bias toward treatment of patients who are sicker or who are at greater risk for AMI with direct PTCA may exist.

Despite recent clinical trials of PTCA in AMI, specific groups of patients that may benefit from adjunctive or alternative therapy have yet to be adequately characterized. In an investigation by Jaski and associates[122] from San Diego, California, the in-hospital outcome of 151 consecutive patients treated for AMI with urgent PTCA of the infarct-related artery was studied to identify a subgroup of patients at high risk. Patients were divided into 2 groups based on the angiographic presence of either single-vessel (n = 86) or multivessel (n = 65) CAD. Despite PTCA of only the infarct-related artery and similar baseline clinical characteristics such as age, peak serum creatine kinase concentration, LVEF, and time from the onset of chest pain to arrival at the hospital, the group with multivessel disease had a lower rate of successful PTCA (75% vs 92%), with higher incidences of persistent total occlusion of the infarct-related artery (14% vs 3%) and procedural complications during PTCA (28% vs 1%). In addition, the group with multivessel disease had a higher rate of urgent (≤ 24 hours) CABG (13% vs 2%) and a trend toward a higher in-hospital mortality rate (6% vs 1%). By stepwise logistic regression, only the presence of single-vessel versus multivessel disease was predictive of PTCA success. The location of the infarct-related artery was not associated with any differences in outcome. It was concluded from these data that urgent PTCA of the infarct-related artery only as treatment for AMI has a lower success rate and higher associated risk in patients with multivessel disease. This may be due to their greater ischemic burden and/or a fundamental biochemical or pathologic difference in the involved lesions. Thus in patients with multivessel CAD, alternative revascularization, improved mechanical hemodynamic support, or both may be warranted to achieve a better success rate and reduce complications and mortality.

In survivors of AMI, the restoration of anterograde flow in the infarct artery, even if accomplished beyond the time for myocardial salvage, may reduce the frequency of subsequent arrhythmic events and sudden death. Boehrer and associates[123] from Dallas, Texas, identified prospectively 12 subjects (8 men and 4 women, aged 39 to 69 years) with a first AMI, signal-averaged electrocardiographic late potentials, and an occluded infarct artery. Seven (group I) had successful coronary angioplasty 6 to 15 days after AMI, and 5 (group II) were managed conservatively. Follow-up signal-averaged electrocardiography was performed 3 to 7 months later. From baseline to follow-up, the 7 group I subjects had a significant change in QRS duration (117 ± 13 [mean + SD] to 102 ± 10 ms), root-mean-square voltage (10.4 ± 4.7 to 31.0 ± 7.6 uV), and low-amplitude signal duration (47.5 ± 8.5 to 32.4 ± 5.2 ms). No group I patient had a late potential at follow-up. In contrast, the 5 group II patients showed no change in QRS duration or low-amplitude signal duration from baseline to follow-up, and all 5 had a late potential at follow-up. At follow-up, the root-mean-square voltage was significantly greater and the low-amplitude signal and QRS durations significantly less in group I than in group II. Thus, in the patients, the mechanical restoration of anterograde perfusion in an occluded infarct artery 1 to 2 weeks after AMI caused the resolution of signal-averaged electrocardiographic late potentials.

References

1. Hansen O, Johansson BW, Gullberg B: Circadian distribution of onset of acute myocardial infarction in subgroups from analysis of 10,791 patients treated in a single center. Am J Cardiol 1992 (Apr 15); 69:1003–1008.
2. ISIS-2 (Second International Study of Infarct Survival) Collaborative Group: Morning peak in the incidence of myocardial infarction: experience in the ISIS-2 trial. Euro Heart J 1992 (May); 13:594–598.
3. Gillis AM, Peters RW, Mitchell B, Duff HJ, McDonald M, Wyse DG: Effects of left ventricular dysfunction on the circadian variation of ventricular premature complexes in healed myocardial infarction. Am J Cardiol 1992 (Apr 15); 69:1009–1014.
4. Bigger JT Jr, Fleiss JL, Rolnitzky LM, Steinman RG: Stability over time of heart period

variability in patients with previous myocardial infarction and ventricular arrhythmias. Am J Cardiol 1992 (Mar 15); 69:718–723.

5. Lombardi, F, Sandrone G, Mortara A, La Rovere MT, Colombo E, Guzzetti S, Malliani A. Circadian variation of spectral indices of heart rate variability after myocardial infarction. Am Heart J 1992 (June); 123:1521–1529.

6. Hirai T, Fujita M, Yamanishi K, Ohno A, Miwa K, Sasayama S: Significance of preinfarction angina for preservation of left ventricular function in acute myocardial infarction. Am Heart J 1992 (July); 124:19–24.

7. Huhtasaari F, Asplund K, Lundberg V, Stegmayr B, Wester PO: Tobacco and myocardial infarction: Is snuff less dangerous than cigarettes? Br Med J 1992 (Nov 21); 305:1252–1256.

8. Salonen J, Nyyssönen K, Korpela H, Tuomilehto J, Seppänen R, Salonen R: High Stored Iron Levels Are Associated With Excess Risk of Myocardial Infarction in Eastern Finnish Men. Circulation 1992 (September);86:803–811.

9. Hebert PR, Buring JE, O'Connor GT, Rosner B, Hennekens CH: Occupation and risk of nonfatal myocardial infarction. Arch Intern Med 1992 (Nov);152:2253–2257.

10. Buring JE, O'Connor GT, Goldhaber SZ, Rosner B, Herbert PN, Blum CB, Breslow JL, and Hennekens CH: Decreased HDL_2 and HDL_3 Cholesterol, Apo A-I and Apo A-II, and Increased Risk of Myocardial Infarction. Circulation 1992 (January);85:22–29.

11. Stampfer MJ, Malinow R, Willett WC, Newcomer LM, Upson B, Ullmann D, Tishler PV, Hennekens CH: A prospective study of plasma homocyst(e)ine and risk of myocardial infarction in US physicians. JAMA 1992 (Aug 19):268:877–881.

12. Kereiakes DJ, Gibler WB, Martin LH, Pieper KS, Anderson LC, and the Cincinnati Heart Project Study Group. Relative importance of emergency medical system transport and the prehospital electrocardiogram on reducing hospital time delay to therapy for acute myocardial infarction: A preliminary report from the Cincinnati Heart Project. Am Heart J 1992 (April);123:835–840.

13. Ridker PM, Manson JE, Goldhaber SZ, Hennekens CH, Buring JE: Comparison of delay times to hospital presentation for physicians and nonphysicians with acute myocardial infarction. Am J Cardiol 1992 (July 1);70:10–13.

14. Goldbert RJ, Gurwitz J, Yarzebski J, Landon J, Gore JM, Alpert JS, Dalen PM, Dalen JE: Patient delay and receipt of thrombolytic therapy among patients with acute myocardial infarction from a community-wide perspective. Am J Cardiol 1992 (Aug 15);70:421–425.

15. Birkhead JS: Time delays in provision of thrombolytic treatment in six district hospitals. Br Med J 1992 (Aug 22);305:445–448.

16. Towbin JA, Bricker T, Garson A Jr: Electrocardiographic criteria for diagnosis of acute myocardial infarction in childhood. Am J Cardiol 1992 (June 15):69:1545–1548.

17. Giroud D, Li JM, Urban P, Meier B, Rutishauser W: Relation of the site of acute myocardial infarction to the most severe coronary arterial stenosis at prior angiography. Am J Cardiol 1992 (Mar 15);69:729–732.

18. Van Rugge FP, Van Der Wall EE, Van Dijkman PRM, Louwerenburg HW, De Roos A, Bruschke AVG: Usefulness of ultrafast magnetic resonance imaging in healed myocardial infarction. Am J Cardiol 1992 (Nov 15);70:1233–1237.

19. Gurwitz JH, Col NF, Avorn J: The exclusion of the elderly and women from clinical trials in acute myocardial infarction. JAMA 1992 (Sept 16);168:1417–1422.

20. Wenger NK: Exclusion of the elderly and women from coronary trials: Is their quality of care compromised? JAMA 1991 (Sept 16);168:1460–1461.

21. Maynard C, Litwin PE, Martin JS, Weaver DW: Gender differences in the treatment and outcome of acute myocardial infarction. Arch Intern Med 1992 (May);152:972–976.

22. Krumholz HM, Douglas PS, Lauer MS, Pasternak RC: Selection of patients for coronary angiography and coronary revascularization early after myocardial infarction: Is there evidence for a gender bias? An Intern Med 1992 (May 15); 116:785–790.

23. Rost K, Smith GR: Return to work after an initial myocardial infarction and subsequent emotional distress. Arch Intern Med 1992 (Feb);152:381–385.

24. Petretta M, Bonaduce D, Bianchi V, Vitagliano G, Conforti G, Rotondi F, Themistoclakis S, Morgano G: Characterization and prognostic significance of silent myocardial ischemia on predischarge electrocardiographic monitoring in unselected patients with myocardial infarction. Am J Cardiol 1992 (Mar 1);69:579–583.

25. Rich MW, Bosner MS, Chung MK, Shen J, McKenzie JP: Is age an independent predictor of early and late mortality in patients with acute myocardial infarction? Am J Med 1992 (Jan);92:7–13.

26. Steinberg JS, Regan A, Sciacca RR, Bigger JT Jr, Fleiss JL, Salvatore DE, Fosina M, Rolnitzky LM: Predicting arrhythmic events after acute myocardial infarction using the signal-averaged electrocardiogram. Am J Cardiol 1992 (Jan 1);69:13–21.

27. Connolly SJ, Cairns JA: Comparison of one-, six- and 24-hour ambulatory electrocardiographic monitoring for ventricular arrhythmia as a predictor of mortality in survivors of acute myocardial infarction. Am J Cardiol 1992 (Feb 1);69:308–313.

28. Rodriguez LM, Oyarzun R, Smeets J, Brachmann J, Schmitt C, Brugada P, Geelen P, Lipcsei G, Albert A, Wellens HJJ: Identification of patients at high risk for recurrence of sustained ventricular tachycardia after healing of acute myocardial infarction. Am J Cardiol 1992 (Feb 15);69:462–464.

29. Bhandari AK, Widerhorn J, Sager PT, Leon C, Hong R, Kotlewski A, Hackett J, Rahimtoola SH: Prognostic significance of programmed ventricular stimulation in patients surviving complicated acute myocardial infarction: A prospective study. Am Heart J 1992 (July);124:87–96.

30. Wilson AC, Kostis JB: The prognostic significance of very low frequency ventricular ectopic activity in survivors of acute myocardial infarction. Chest 1992 (Sept);102:732–736.

31. Schechtman KB, Kleiger RE, Boden WE, Capone RJ, Schwartz DJ, Roberts R, Gibson RS. The relationship between 1-year mortality and infarct location in patients with non-Q wave myocardial infarction. Am Heart J 1992 (May);123:1175–1181.

32. Berger CJ, Murabito JM, Evans JC, Anderson KM, Levy D: Prognosis after first myocardial infarction: Comparison of Q-wave and non-Q-wave myocardial infarction in the Framingham heart study. JAMA 1992 (Sept 23/30)268:1545–1551.

33. Moss AJ: Q-wave vs non-Q-wave myocardial infarction: An oversimplified dichotomy. JAMA 1992 (Sept. 23/30)268:1595–1596.

34. Gottlieb S, Moss AJ, McDermott M, Eberly S: Interrelation of left ventricular ejection fraction, pulmonary congestion and outcome in acute myocardial infarction. Am J Cardiol 1992 (Apr 15):69:977–984.

35. Case RB, Moss AJ, Case N, McDermott M, Eberly S: Living alone after myocardial infarction: Impact on prognosis. JAMA 1992 (Jan 22/29);267:515–519.

36. Berkman LF, Leo-Summers L, Horwitz RI: Emotional support and survival after myocardial infarction: A prospective, population-based study of the elderly. An Intern Med 1992 (Dec 15);117:1003–1009.

37. Frasure-Smith N, Lesperance F, Juneau M: Differential long-term impact of in-hospital symptoms of psychological stress after non-Q-wave and Q-wave acute myocardial infarction. Am J Cardiol 1992 (May 1) 69:1128–1134.

38. Udvarhelyi IS, Gatsonis C, Epstein AM, Pashos CL, Newhouse JP, McNeil BJ: Acute myocardial infarction in the Medicare population: Process of care and clinical outcomes. JAMA 1992 (Nov 11);268:2530–2536.

39. Behar S, Reicher-Reiss H, Abinader E, Agmon J, Friedman Y, Barzilai J, Kaplinsky E, Kauli N, Kishon Y, Palant A, Peled B, Rabinovich B, Reisin L, Schlesinger Z, Zahavi I, Zion M, Goldbourt U. The prognostic significance of angina pectoris preceding the occurrence of a first acute myocardial infarction in 4166 consecutive hospitalized patients. Am Heart J 1992 (June);123:1481–1486.

40. Boehrer JD, Lange RA, Willard JE, Hillis LD: Influence of collateral filling of the occluded infarct-related coronary artery on prognosis after acute myocardial infarction. Am J Cardiol 1992 (Jan 1);69:10–12.

41. Behar S, Reicher-Reiss H, Abinader E, Agmon J, Barzilai J, Friedman Y, Kaplinsky E, Kauli N, Kishon Y, Palant A, Peled B, Reisin L, Schlesinger Z, Zahavi I, Zion M, Goldbourt U, Spring Study Group: Long-term prognosis after acute myocardial infarction in patients with left ventricular hypertrophy on the electrocardiogram. Am J Cardiol 1992 (Apr 15);69:985–990.

42. Ruberman W, Crow R, Rosenberg C, Rautaharju P, Shore R, Pasternack B: Intermittent ST Depression and Mortality After Myocardial Infarction. Circulation 1992 (April);85:1440–1446.

43. Berning J, Launbjerg J, Appleyard M: Echocardiographic algorithms for admission and

predischarge prediction of mortality in acute myocardial infarction. Am J Cardiol 1992 (June 15);69:1538–1544.

44. Launbjerg J, Berning J, Fruergaard P, Appleyard M: Sensitivity and specificity of echocardiographic identification of patients eligible for safe early discharge after acute myocardial infarction. Am Heart J 1992 (October);124:846–853.

45. Bolognese L, Rossi L, Sarasso G, Prando MD, Bongo AS, Dellavesa P, Rossi P. Silent versus symptomatic dipyridamole-induced ischemia after myocardial infarction: Clinical and prognostic significance. J Am Coll Cardiol 1992 (April);19:953–959.

46. Rodriguez LM, Smeets J, O'Hara GE, Geelen P, Brugada P, Wellens HJJ: Incidence and timing of recurrences of sudden death and ventricular tachycardia during antiarrhythmic drug treatment after myocardial infarction. Am J Cardiol 1992 (June 1);69:1403–1406.

47. Pfisterer M, Kiowski W, Burckhardt D, Follath F, Burkart F: Beneficial effect of amiodarone on cardiac mortality in patients with asymptomatic complex ventricular arrhythmias after acute myocardial infarction and preserved but not impaired left ventricular function. Am J Cardiol 1992 (June 1);69:1399–1402.

48. Eldar M, Sievner Z, Goldbourt U, Reicher-Reiss H, Kaplinsky E, Behar S, Spring Study Group: Primary ventricular tachycardia in acute myocardial infarction: Clinical characteristics and mortality. An Intern Med 1992 (July 1);117:31–36.

49. O'Hara GE, Brugada P, Rodriguez LM, Brito M, Mont L, Waleffe A, Kulbertus H, Wellens HJJ: Incidence, pathophysiology and prognosis of exercise-induced sustained ventricular tachycardia associated with healed myocardial infarction. Am J Cardiol 1992 (Oct 1);70:875–878.

50. Sweeney MO, Moss AJ, Eberly S: Instantaneous cardiac death in the posthospital period after acute myocardial infarction. Am J Cardiol 1992 (Dec 1);70:1375–1379.

51. Goldberg RJ, Zevallos JC, Yarzebski J, Alpert JS, Gore JM, Chen Z, Dalen JE: Prognosis of acute myocardial infarction complicated by complete heart block (the worcester heart attack study). Am J Cardiol 1992 (May 1);69:1135–1141.

52. Berger PB, Ruocco NA Jr, Ryan TJ, Frederick MM, Jacobs AK, Faxon DP, and the TIMI Investigators. Incidence and prognostic implications of heart block complicating inferior myocardial infarction treated with thrombolytic therapy: results from TIMI II. J Am Coll Cardiol 1992 (September);20:533–40.

53. Gacioch GM, Ellis SG, Lee L, Bates ER, Kirch M, Walton JA, Topol EJ. Cardiogenic shock complicating acute myocardial infarction: The use of coronary angioplasty and the integration of the new support devices into patient management. J Am Coll Cardiol 1992 (March);19:647–53.

54. Bengtson JR, Kaplan AJ, Pieper KS, Wildermann NM, Mark DB, Pryor DB, Phillips HR III, Califf RM. Prognosis in cardiogenic shock after acute myocardial infarction in the interventional era. J Am Coll Cardiol 1992 (December);20:1482–9.

55. Lehmann KG, Francis CK, Dodge HT, TIMI Study Group: Mitral regurgitation in early myocardial infarction: Incidence, clinical detection, and prognostic implications. An Intern Med 1992 (July 1);117:10–17.

56. Tcheng JE, Jackman JD, Nelson CL, Gardner LH, Smith LR, Rankin JS, Califf RM, Stack RS: Outcome of patients sustaining acute ischemic mitral regurgitation during myocardial infarction. An Intern Med 1992 (July 1);117:18–24.

57. Sharma SK, Seckler J, Israel DH, Borrico S, Ambrose JA: Clinical, angiographic and anatomic findings in acute severe ischemic mitral regurgitation. Am J Cardiol 1992 (Aug 1);70:277–280.

58. Parry G, Goudevenos J, Adams PC, Reid DS: Septal rupture after myocardial infarction: Is very early surgery really worthwhile. Eur Heart J (Mar);13:373–382.

59. Lemery R, Smith HC, Giuliani ER, Gersh BJ: Prognosis in rupture of the ventricular septum after acute myocardial infarction and role of early surgical intervention. Am J Cardiol 1992 (July 15);70:147–151.

60. Muehrcke DD, Daggett WM Jr, Buckley MJ, Akins CW, Hilgenberg AD, Austen WG: Post-infarct ventricular septal defect repair: Effect of coronary artery bypass grafting. An Thoracic Surgeons 1992 (Nov);54:876–883.

61. Westaby S, Parry A, Ormerod O, Gooneratne P, Pillai R: Thrombolysis and postinfarction ventricular septal rupture. J Thorac Cardiovasc Surg 1992 (Dec);104:1506–1509.

62. Muehrcke DD, Blank S, Daggett WM: Survival after repair of postinfarction ventricular

septal defects in patients over the age of 70. Journal of Cardiac Surgery 1992 (Dec);7:290–300.

63. López-Sendón J, González A, López de Sá E, Coma-Canella I, Roldán I, Dominiguez F, Maqueda I, Jadraque LM. Diagnosis of subacute ventricular wall rupture after acute myocardial infarction: sensitivity and specificity of clinical, hemodynamic and echo-cardiographic criteria. J Am Coll Cardiol 1992 (May);19:1145–53.

64. Komeda M, David TE, Malik A, Ivanov J, Sun Z: Operative risks and long-term results of operation for left ventricular aneurysm. Ann Thorac Surg (Jan);53:22–29.

65. Taylor GJ, Katholi RE, Womack K, Moses HW, Woods WT: Increased incidence of silent ischemia after acute myocardial infarction. JAMA 1992 (Sept 16);268:1448–1450.

66. Singh RB, Rastogi SS, Verma R, Laxmi B, Singh R, Ghosh S, Niaz MA: Randomized controlled trial of cardioprotective diet in patients with recent acute myocardial infarction: Results of one year follow up. Br Med J 1992 (Apr 18);304:1015–1019.

67. Lewin B, Robertson IH, Cay EL, Irving JB, Campbell M: Effects of self-help post-myocardial-infarction rehabilitation on psychological adjustment and use of health services. Lancet 1992 (Apr 15);339:1036–1040.

68. Antman EM, Lau J, Kupelnick B, Mosteller F, Chalmers TC: A comparison of results of meta-analyses of randomized control trials and recommendations of clinical experts: Treatments for myocardial infarction. JAMA 1992 (July 8);268:240–248.

69. Olsson G, Wikstrand J, Warnold I, Cats VM, McBoyle D, Herlitz J, Hjalmarson A, Sonnenblick EH: Metoprolol-induced reduction in postinfarction mortality: Pooled results from five double-blind randomized trials. Euro Heart J 1992 (Jan);13:28–32.

70. Wong S-C, Greenberg H, Hager WD, Dwyer EM Jr. Effects of diltiazem on recurrent myocardial infarction in patients with non-Q wave myocardial infarction. J Am Coll Cardiol 1992 (June);19:1421–5.

71. Lamas GA, Pfeffer MA, Hamm P, Wertheimer J, Rouleau JL, Braunwald E: Do the results of randomized clinical trials of cardiovascular drugs influence medical practice? N Engl J Med 1992 (July 23);327:241–247.

72. Gotzsche CO, Sogaard P, Ravkilde J, Thygesen K: Effects of captopril on left ventricular systolic and diastolic function after acute myocardial infarction. Am J Cardiol 1992 (July 15);70:156–160.

73. Pfeffer MA, Braunwald E, Moye LA, Basta L, Brown EJ Jr, Cuddy TE, Davis BR, Geltman EM, Goldman S, Flaker GC, Klein M, Lamas GA, Packer M, Rouleau J, Rouleau JL, Rutherford J, Wertheimer JH, Hawkins CM: Effect of captopril on mortality and morbidity in patients with left ventricular dysfunction after myocardial infarction: Results of the survival and ventricular enlargement trial. N Engl J Med 1992 (Sept 3);327:669–677.

74. Swedberg K, Held P, Kjekshus J, Rasmussen K, Ryden L, Wedel H: Effects of the early administration of enalapril on mortality in patients with acute myocardial infarction: Results of the Cooperative New Scandinavian Enalapril Survival Study II (CONSENSUS II). N Engl J Med 1992 (Sept 3);327:678–684.

75. Kroon C, ten Hove WR, de Boer A, Kroon JM, van der Pol JMJ, Harthoorn-Lasthuizen EJ, Shoemaker HC, van der Meer FJM, Cohen AF: Highly Variable Anticoagulant Response After Subcutaneous Administration of High-Dose (12,500 IU) Heparin in Patients With Myocardial Infarction and Healthy Volunteers. Circulation 1992 (November);86:1370–1375.

76. Antman E, Berlin J: Declining Incidence of Ventricular Fibrillation in Myocardial Infarction, Implications for the Prophylactic Use of Lidocaine. Circulation 1992 (September);86:764–773.

77. Cardiac Arrhythmia Suppression Trial II Investigators: Effect of the antiarrhythmic agent moricizine on survival after myocardial infarction. N Engl J Med 1992 (July 23);327:227–233.

78. Ceremuzynski L, Kleczar E, Krzeminska-Pakula M, Kuch J, Nartowicz E, Smielak-Korombel J, Dyduszynski A, Maciejewicz J, Zaleska T, Lazarczyk-Kedzia E, Motyka J, Paczkowska B, Sczaniecka O, Yusuf S. Effect of amiodarone on mortality after myocardial infarction: A double-blind, placebo-controlled, pilot study. J Am Coll Cardiol 1992 (November);20:1056–62.

79. Horner S: Efficacy of Intravenous Magnesium in Acute Myocardial Infarction in Reducing Arrhythmias and Mortality, Meta-Analysis of Magnesium in Acute Myocardial Infarction. Circulation 1992 (September);86:774–779.

80. Doorey AJ, Michelson EL, Topol EJ: Thrombolytic therapy of acute myocardial infarction: Keeping the unfulfilled promises. JAMA 1992 (Dec 2);268:3108–3114.

81. Lau J, Antman EM, Jimenez-Silva J, Kupelnick B, Mosteller F, Chalmers TC: Cumulative meta-analysis of therapeutic trials for myocardial infarction. N Engl J Med 1992 (July 23);327:248–257.

82. Cerqueira MD, Maynard C, Ritchie JL, Davis KB, Kennedy JW. Long-term survival in 618 patients from the Western Washington Streptokinase in Myocardial Infarction trials. J Am Coll Cardiol 1992 (December);20:1452–9.

83. Hildebrandt P, Torp-Pedersen C, Joen Tomas, Iversen E, Jensen G, Jeppesen D, Melchior T, Schytten H-J, Ringsdal V, Jensen J, Steensgaard-Hansen F, Granborg J, Hassager C, Weiss M, Ermer W: Reduced infarct size in nonreperfused myocardial infarction by combined infusion of isosorbide dinitrate and streptokinase. Am Heart J 1992 (November);124:1139–1144.

84. Great Group: Feasibility, safety, and efficacy of domiciliary thrombolysis by general practitioners: Grampian region early anistreplase trial. Br Med J 1992 (Sept 5);305:548–553.

85. Wall TC, Califf RM, George BS, Ellis SG, Samaha JK, Kereiakes DJ, Worley SJ, Sigmon K, Topol EJ, for the TAMI-7 Study Group. Accelerated plasminogen activator dose regimens for coronary thrombolysis. J Am Coll Cardiol 1992 (March);19:482–9.

86. Hackett D, Andreotti F, Haider AW, Brunelli C, Shahi M, Fussell A, Buller N, Foale R, Lipkin D, Caponnetto S, Davies G, Maseri A. Bolus Dose-Escalation Study of Tissue-Type Plasminogen Activator (Best) Investigators. Effectiveness and safety of a single intravenous bolus injection of tissue-type plasminogen activator in acute myocardial infarction. Am J Cardiol 1992 (June 1);69:1393–1398.

87. Hsia J, Kleiman N, Aguirre F, Chaitman BR, Roberts R, Ross AM, for the HART Investigators. Heparin-induced prolongation of partial thromboplastin time after thrombolysis: Relation to coronary artery patency. J Am Coll Cardiol 1992 (July);20:31–35.

88. De Bono DP, Simoons ML, Tijssen J, Arnold AER, Betriu A, Burgersdijk C, Bescos LL, Mueller E, Pfisterer M, Van de Werf F, Zijlstra F, Verstraete M: Effect of early intravenous heparin on coronary patency, infarct size, and bleeding complications after alteplase thrombolysis: Results of a randomized double blind European cooperative study group trial. Br Heart J 1992 (Feb);67:122–128.

89. Neuhaus K-L, Von Essen R, Tebbe U, Vogt A, Roth M, Riess M, Niederer W, Forycki F, Wirtzfeld A, Maeurer W, Limbourg P, Merx W, Haerten K. Improved thrombolysis in acute myocardial infarction with front-loaded administration of alteplase: Results of the rt-PA-APSAC Patency Study (TAPS). J Am Coll Cardiol 1992 (April);19:885–91.

90. Carney RJ, Murphy GA, Brandt TR, Daley PJ, Pickering E, White HJ, McDonough TJ, Vermilya SK, Teichman SL, for the RAAMI Study Investigators. Randomized angiographic trial of recombinant tissue-type plasminogen activator (alteplase) in myocardial infarction. J Am Coll Cardiol 1992 (July);20:17–23.

91. Arnout J, Simoons M, de Bono D, Rapold HJ, Collen D, Verstraete M. Correlation between level of heparinization and patency of the infarct-related coronary artery after treatment of acute myocardial infarction with alteplase (rt-PA). J Am Coll Cardiol 1992 (September);20:513–9.

92. Anderson JL, Becker LC, Sorensen SG, Karagounis LA, Browne KF, Shah PK, Morris DC, Fintel DJ, Mueller HS, Ross AM, Hall SM, Askins JC, Doorey AJ, Grines CL, Moreno FL, Marder VJ, for the TEAM-3 Investigators. Anistreplase versus alteplase in acute myocardial infarction: comparative effects on left ventricular function, morbidity and 1-day coronary artery patency. J Am Coll Cardiol 1992 (October);20:753–66.

93. Kalbfleisch J, Thadani U, Littlejohn JK, Brown G, Magorien R, Kutcher M, Taylor G, Maddox WT, Campbell WB, Perry J Jr, Spann JF, Vetrovec G, Kent R, Armstrong PW: Evaluation of a prolonged infusion of recombinant tissue-type plasminogen activator (Duteplase) in preventing reocclusion following successful thrombolysis in acute myocardial infarction. Am J Cardiol 1992 (May 1);69:1120–1127.

94. Sakamoto T, Yasue H, Ogawa H, Misumi I, Masuda T: Association of patency of the infarct-related coronary artery with plasma levels of plasminogen activator inhibitor activity in acute myocardial infarction. Am J Cardiol 1992 (Aug 1);70:271–276.

95. Gressin V, Louvard Y, Pezzano M, Lardoux H: Holter recording of ventricular arrhythmias during intravenous thrombolysis for acute myocardial infarction. Am J Cardiol 1992 (Jan 15);69:152–159.

96. Hohnloser H, Zabel M, Olschewski M, Kasper W, Just H. Arrhythmias during the acute phase of reperfusion therapy for acute myocardial infarction: Effects of B-adrenergic blockade. Am Heart J 1992 (June);123:1530–1535.

97. Schechter M, Rabinowitz B, Beker B, Motro M, Barbash G, Kaplinsky E, Hod H. Additional ST segment elevation during the first hour of thrombolytic therapy: An electrocardiographic sign predicting a favorable clinical outcome. J Am Coll Cardiol 1992 (December);20:1460–4.

98. Karagounis L, Sorensen SG, Menlove RL, Moreno F, Anderson JL, for the TEAM-2 Investigators. Does thrombolysis in myocardial infarction (TIMI) perfusion grade 2 represent a mostly patent artery or a mostly occluded artery? Enzymatic and electrocardiography evidence from the TEAM-2 study. J Am Coll Cardiol 1992 (January);19:1–10.

99. Mueller H, Cohen L, Braunwald E, Forman S, Feit F, Ross A, Schweiger M, Cabin H, Davison R, Miller D, Solomon R, Knatterud G, for the TIMI Investigators: Predictors of Early Morbidity and Mortality After Thrombolytic Therapy of Acute Myocardial Infarction, Analyses of Patient Subgroups in the Thrombolysis in Myocardial Infarction (TIMI) Trial, Phase II. Circulation 1992 (April);85:1254–1264.

100. Ranjadayalan K, Umachandran V, Timmis AD: Clinical impact of introducing thrombolytic and aspirin therapy into the management policy of a coronary care unit. Am J Med 1992 (Mar);92:233–238.

101. Kleiman NS, Terrin M, Mueller H, Chaitman B, Roberts R, Knatterud GL, Solomon R, McMahon RP, Braunwald E, and the TIMI Investigators. Mechanisms of early death despite thrombolytic therapy: Experience from the Thrombolysis in Myocardial Infarction Phase II (TIMI II) study. J Am Coll Cardiol 1992 (May);19:1129–35.

102. Williams DO, Braunwald E, Knatterub G, Babb J, Bresnahan J, Greenberg MA, Raizner A, Wasserman A, Robertson T, Ross R, and TIMI Investigators: One-Year Results of the Thrombolysis in Myocardial Infarction Investigation (TIMI) Phase II Trial. Circulation 1992 (February);85:533–542.

103. Ellis SG, Mooney MR, George BS, Ribeiro da Silva EE, Talley JD, Flanagan WH, Topol EJ, for the Treatment of Post-Thrombolytic Stenoses Study Group: Randomized Trial of Late Elective Angioplasty Versus Conservative Management for Patients With Residual Stenoses After Thrombolytic Treatment of Myocardial Infarction. Circulation 1992 (November);86:1400–1406.

104. Ruocco NA Jr., Bergelson BA, Jacobs AK, Frederick MM, Faxon DP, Ryan TJ, for the Thrombolysis in Myocardial Infarction Investigators. Invasive versus conservative strategy after thrombolytic therapy for acute myocardial infarction in patients with antecedent angina. A report from Thrombolysis in Myocardial Infarction Phase II (TIMI II). J Am Coll Cardiol 1992 (December);20:1445–51.

105. Pedretti R, Laporta A, Etro MD, Gementi A, Bonelli R, Anza C, Colombo E, Maslowsky F, Santoro F, Caru B: Influence of thrombolysis on signal-averaged electrocardiogram and late arrhythmic events after acute myocardial infarction. Am J Cardiol 1992 (Apr 1);69:866–872.

106. Malik M, Kulakowski P, Idemuyiwa O, Poloniecki J, Staunton A, Millane T, Farrell T, Camm AJ: Effect of thrombolytic therapy on the predictive value of signal-averaged electrocardiography after acute myocardial infarction. Am J Cardiol 1992 (July);70:21–25.

107. Moreno FLL, Karagounis L, Marshall H, Menlove RL, Ipsen S, Anderson JL: Thrombolysis-related early patency reduces ECG late potentials after acute myocardial infarction. Am Heart J 1992 (September);124:557–564.

108. Barbash GI, White HD, Modan M, Van de Werf F, for the Investigators of the International Tissue Plasminogen Activator/Streptokinase Trial. Antecedent angina pectoris predicts worse outcome after myocardial infarction in patients receiving thrombolytic therapy: Experience gleaned from the International Tissue Plasminogen Activator/Streptokinase Mortality Trial. J Am Coll Cardiol 1992 (July);20:36–41.

109. Zaret BL, Wackers FJT, Terrin ML, Ross R, Weiss M, Slater J, Morrison J, Bourge RC, Passamani E, Knatterud G, Braunwald E: Assessment of global and regional left ventricular performance at rest and during exercise after thrombolytic therapy for acute myocardial infarction: Results of the Thrombolysis in Myocardial Infarction (TIMI) II Study. Am J Cardiol 1992 (Jan 1);69:1–9.

110. de Jaegere PP, Arnold AA, Balk AH, Simoons ML. Intracranial hemorrhage in association

with thrombolytic therapy: Incidence and clinical predictive factors. J Am Coll Cardiol 1992 (February);19:289–94.

111. Eckman MH, Wong JB, Salem DN, Pauker SG: Direct angioplasty for acute myocardial infarction: A review of outcomes in clinical subsets. An Intern Med 1992 (Oct 15);117:667–676.

112. O'Keefe, JH Jr, Rutherford BD, McConahay DR, Johnson WL Jr, Giorgi LV, Shimshak TM, Ligon RW, McCallister BD, Hartzler GO: Myocardial salvage with direct coronary angioplasty for acute infarction. Am Heart J 1992 (January);123:1–6.

113. Sabri MN, Disciascio G, Cowley MJ, Goudreau E, Warner M, Kohli RS, Bajaj S, Kelly K, Vetrovec G. Immediate and long-term results of delayed recanalization of occluded acute myocardial infarction-related arteries using coronary angioplasty. Am J Cardiol 1992 (Mar 1);69:575–578.

114. Moosvi AR, Khaja F, Villaneuva L, Gheorghiade M, Douthat L, Goldstein S. Early revascularization improves survival in cardiogenic shock complicating acute myocardial infarction. J Am Coll Cardiol 1992 (April);19:907–14.

115. Brodie BR, Stuckey TD, Hansen CJ, Cooper TR, Weintraub RA, Lebauer EJ, Katz JD, Kelly TA: Importance of a patent infarct-related artery for hospital and late survival after direct coronary angioplasty for acute myocardial infarction. Am J Cardiol 1992 (May 1);69:1113–1119.

116. Morishita H, Hattori R, Aoyama T, Kawai C, Yui Y. The intracoronary administration of urokinase following direct PTCA for acute myocardial infarction reduces early restenosis. Am Heart J 1992 (May);123:1153–1156.

117. Topol E, Califf R, Vandormael M, Grines C, George B, Sanz M, Wall T, O'Brien M, Schwaiger M, Aguirre F, Young S, Popma J, Sigmon K, Lee K, Ellis S, and the Thrombolysis and Angioplasty in Myocardial Infarction-6 Study Group: A Randomized Trial of Late Reperfusion Therapy for Acute Myocardial Infarction. Circulation 1992 (June);85:2090–2099.

118. Juliard JM, Steg PG, Himbert D, Cohen-Solal A, Aumont MC, Gourgon R: A patency-oriented strategy for early management of acute myocardial infarction using emergency coronary angiography and selective coronary angioplasty. Am J Cardiol 1992 (June 1);69:1383–1388.

119. Arnold A, Simoons M, Van de Werf F, de Bono D, Lubsen J, Tijssen J, Serruys P, Verstraete M: Recombinant Tissue-Type Plasminogen Activator and Immediate Angioplasty in Acute Myocardial Infarction. Circulation 1992 (July);86:111–120.

120. O'Neill WW, Weintraub R, Grimes CL, Meany B, Brodie BR, Friedman HZ, Ramos RG, Gangadharan V, Levin RN, Choksi N, Westveer DC, Strzelecki M, Timmis GC: A Prospective, Placebo-Controlled, Randomized Trial of Intravenous Streptokinase and Angioplasty Versus Lone Angioplasty Therapy of Acute Myocardial Infarction. Circulation 1992 (December);86:1710–1717.

121. Vacek JL, Rosamond TL, Kramer PH, Crouse LJ, Robuck OW, White JL, Beauchamp GD: Direct angioplasty versus initial thrombolytic therapy for acute myocardial infarction: Long-term follow-up and changes in practice pattern. Am Heart J 1992 (December);124:1411–1418.

122. Jaski BE, Cohen JD, Trausch J, Marsh DG, Bail GR, Overlie PA, Skowronski EW, Smith SC Jr: Outcome of urgent percutaneous transluminal coronary angioplasty in acute myocardial infarction: Comparison of single-vessel versus multivessel coronary artery disease. Am Heart J 1992 (December);124:1427–1433.

123. Boehrer JD, Glamann B, Lange RA, Willard JE, Brogan WC III, Eichhorn EJ, Grayburn PA, Anwar A, Hillis LD: Effect of coronary angioplasty on late potentials one to two weeks after acute myocardial infarction. Am J Cardiol 1992 (Dec 15);70:1515–1519.

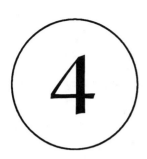

Arrhythmias, Conduction Disturbances, and Cardiac Arrest

As cause of left ventricular dysfunction

Grogan and associates[1] from Rochester, Minnesota, evaluated 10 patients aged 22 to 80 years (median 57) with severe LV dysfunction and AF with rapid ventricular response. Because most patients were unaware of their arrhythmia, duration was usually unknown. All patients had heart failure symptoms; 9 presented with New York Heart Association class III or IV disability, and 1 with class II disability. Initial LVEF ranged from 12 to 30% (median 25). No patient had symptomatic CAD (4 underwent angiography). Myocarditis and infiltrative processes were excluded by biopsy in 5 patients. All patients were considered initially to have idiopathic dilated cardiomyopathy with secondary AF. Ventricular rate was controlled in all patients, with sinus rhythm restored in 5. At follow-up (median 30 months, range 3 to 56), all patients were asymptomatic. LVEF after treatment ranged from 40 to 64% (median 52). It is concluded that in some patients initially considered to have idiopathic dilated cardiomyopathy, AF with rapid ventricular response may be the primary cause rather than the consequence of severe LV dysfunction. LV dysfunction may be completely reversible with ventricular rate control.

Left atrial echo contrast

The prevalence and clinical significance of LA spontaneous echo contrast were investigated by Liang-Miin Tsay and associates[2] from Taiwan, Republic of China, in 103 consecutive patients with chronic nonrheumatic AF using transesophageal echocardiography. LA spontaneous echo contrast was visualized in 25 of 103 patients (24.3%). Age, sex, LA diameter, LV diastolic and systolic dimensions, LV EF, and the percentage of lone AF were not significantly different between patients with and without LA spontaneous echo contrast; however, those with LA spontaneous echo contrast were less likely to have moderate or severe MR. LA thrombi were observed in 7 patients (6.8%), and all 7 thrombi were found in the atria with spontaneous echo contrast. History of cerebral ischemia or peripheral embolism, or both, was significantly more frequent in patients with than without LA spontaneous echo contrast (84 vs 18%). The presence of LA spontaneous echo contrast was highly specific (94%) and predictive for thromboembolic events (positive and negative predictive) values of 84 and 82%, respectively). Thus, transesophageal echo-detected LA spontaneous echo contrast is frequently found in patients with chronic nonrheumatic AF. This phenomenon may represent a precursor of thrombus formation, and its presence is associated with an increased thromboembolic risk.

Predictors of thromboembolism

To identify those patients with nonrheumatic AF who are at high risk and those at low risk for arterial embolism, the Stroke Prevention in Atrial Fibrillation Investigators[3] from multiple medical centers performed a cohort study of patients assigned to placebo in a randomized clinical trial. Five hundred and sixty-eight in-patients and out-patients with nonrheumatic AF were assigned to placebo therapy at 15 US medical centers from 1987 to 1989 in the Stroke Prevention in Atrial Fibrillation Study. The patients were followed for a mean of 1.3 years. Recent (within 3 months) CHF, a history of systemic hypertension, and previous arterial thromboembolism were each significantly and independently associated with a substantial risk for thromboembolism (> 7% per year). The presence of these 3 independent clinical variables (recent CHF, history of hypertension, previous thromboembolism) defined patients with rates of thromboembolism of 2.5% per year (no risk factors), 7.2% per year (1 risk factor), and 18% per year (2 or 3 risk factors). Nondiabetic patients without these risk factors, comprising 38% of the cohort, had a low risk for thromboembolism (1.4% per year). Patients without clinical risk factors who were under 60 years of age had no thromboembolic events. Patients with AF at high risk (7% per year) and low risk (> 7% per year) for thromboembolism can be identified by readily available clinical variables.

To identify echocardiographic features of arterial thromboembolism in patients with nonrheumatic AF and to determine whether these add to clinical variables for risk stratification, the Stroke Prevention in Atrial Fibrillation Investigators[4] assigned 568 in-patients and out-patients with nonrheumatic AF to placebo therapy at 15 US medical centers from 1987 to 1989 in the Stroke Prevention and Atrial Fibrillation Study. Patients were followed for a mean of 1.3 years. M-mode and 2-dimensional echocardiograms performed at study entry and interpreted by local cardiologists were the measurement mode. The predictive value of 14 echocardiographic variables for later ischemic stroke or systemic embolism was assessed by multivariate analysis. LV dysfunction from 2-D echocardiograms and the size of the left atrium from M-mode echocardiograms were the strongest independent predictors of later thromboembolism. Multivariate analysis of these 2 independent echocardiographic predictors with the 3 independent clinical predictors of thromboembolism (history of hypertension, recent CHF, previous thromboembolism) identified 26% of the cohort with a low risk for thromboembolism (1.0% per year). Compared with risk stratification using clinical variables alone, echocardiographic results altered thromboembolic risk stratification in 18% of the entire cohort and in 38% of those without clinical risk factors. Both LV and LA variables are significant predictors of thromboembolism in patients with nonvalvular AF. The results challenge traditional views of the pathogenesis of ischemic stroke in patients with AF and suggest that standard echocardiography contributes to risk stratification, differentiating the 1/3 of patients without clinical risk factors who are at increased risk for stroke from the remainder who may not need antithrombotic prophylaxis.

The purpose of this study by Corbalán and associates[5] from Santiago, Chile, was to define the risk factors for systemic embolism in patients with recently diagnosed paroxysmal AF. Studied were 63 consecutive patients with symptomatic nonvalvular paroxysmal AF who performed a clinical and noninvasive cardiac, peripheral vascular, and neurologic evaluation that included 2-dimensional echocardiography, 24-hour Holter monitoring, and computed tomographic brain scan. Patients with predisposing clinical conditions for systemic embolism (valvular heart disease or CAD) or paroxysmal AF (sick sinus disease, preexcitation, or thyroid dysfunction) were excluded. At entry 34 patients had idiopathic paroxysmal AF and 29 had hypertension. Fourteen patients had a recent systemic embolic complication: 9 had a recent occlusive nonlacunar cerebrovascular accident, 2 had transient ischemic attacks, and 3 had peripheral systemic emboli that required surgery. In addition, 5 patients had evidence of old cerebrovascular accident on the computed tomographic scan (group 1). Forty-four patients had no systemic embolism (group 2). Results of univariate analysis showed that patients in group 1 were older (72 ± 9 vs 63 ± 13 years), had a higher incidence of hypertension (70% vs 35%), and had an increased LA diameter (4.1 ± 0.7 vs 3.6 ± 0.5 cm). Multiple stepwise logistic regression analysis showed that a history of hypertension and LA enlargement on 2-dimensional echocardiography were significant independent risk factors for systemic embolism in patients with symptomatic nonvalvular paroxysmal AF.

Review of management

Pritchett[6] from Durham, North Carolina, provided a superb review of management of AF.

Quinidine

The findings in clinical trials of antiarrhythmic drug efficacy and safety are frequently difficult to compare, since study design often has an important effect on trial outcome. To explore this problem further, Reimold and associates[7] from Boston, Massachusetts, and Philadelphia, Pennsylvania, compared 3 designs—randomized control, nonrandomized control and uncontrolled—collectively enrolling 2415 patients in 21 trials reporting on the role of quinidine in the prevention of chronic AF. The proportion of patients remaining in sinus rhythm at 3, 6, and 12 months after cardioversion was calculated by means of Kaplan-Meier techniques, and the data were pooled for each trial design. For the randomized control trials the difference in the absolute percentage of patients remaining in sinus rhythm in the quinidine and control groups was 24% at each of the 3 follow-up intervals. Contrary to findings in the randomized control trials, the magnitude of the treatment benefit in nonrandomized trials was smaller and declined markedly over time. The percentage of patients remaining in sinus rhythm in the uncontrolled trials was intermediate to the percentages in the other 2 trial designs. When the data from all 3 trial designs were pooled, the crude mortality rate was 2.0% in quinidine-treated patients and 0.6% in control patients. Sudden cardiac death or VF was the cause of death in 13 of 19 patients for whom the cause of death was known, highlighting the potential risk of quinidine-induced proarrhythmia. Although quinidine is effective in maintaining sinus rhythm, estimates of the treatment effect vary among trial types. Because antiarrhythmic therapy with quinidine for suppression of AF has not been shown to reduce the risk of mortality, the decision to institute therapy should be guided strongly by patient symptoms.

Clonidine

To determine whether clonidine can slow ventricular rate in patients with rapid AF, Roth and associates[8] from Tel Aviv, Israel, performed a randomized, controlled trial with 4-hour follow-up period involving 18 hemodynamically stable patients with rapid AF. Exclusion criteria included acute or terminal illness, current use of antiarrhythmic agents, calcium-antagonists, or beta-blockers; excessive systemic hypertension, pulmonary valvular, or pericardial disease; and electrolyte imbalance. Patients were randomly assigned to receive either no treatment (control group) or clonidine, 0.075 mg orally, at baseline and after 2 hours if heart rate did not decrease by at least 20%. BP was measured in the same arm for 4 consecutive hours and a full 12-lead electrocardiogram was performed. Heart rate decreased to below 100 beats/min in 8 of 9 patients receiving clonidine compared with 2 of 9 patients in the control group. The difference in the mean decreases in heart rate was 38 beats/min. Six patients who were treated with clonidine and 1 patient in the control group reverted to normal sinus rhythm. Systolic BP decreased slightly in both groups, without significant differences. Clinical follow-up was uneventful. Low-dose clonidine was an easy, efficient, and effective treatment for patients with rapid AF who were hemodynamically stable.

Propafenone

Early postoperative AF is a frequent complication of major cardiovascular surgery. To assess the effectiveness of intravenous propafenone in this setting, Gentili and associates[9] from Rome, Italy, studied 50 patients who developed AF within 48 hours after open-heart surgery. Intravenous propafenone (2 mg/kg in 10 minutes) was administered 15 minutes after the onset of arrhythmia. Sinus rhythm was restored in 35 patients (70%) after a mean time of 22 ± 6 minutes after the beginning of the infusion. The conversion was obtained in 28 of 32 patients (88%) who had CABG and in 7 of 18 patients (39%) who had valvular or septal surgery. In those whose arrhythmia did not convert to sinus rhythm, the ventricular rate was reduced from 142 ± 14 beats/min to 108 ± 9 beats/min. In patients whose arrhythmia was converted to sinus rhythm, mean cardiac index increased from a mean baseline value of 2.7 ± 0.4 L/min/m² to 3.4 ± 0.1 L/min/m², while it remained virtually unchanged in those whose arrhythmia did not convert. No significant side effects were observed. It was concluded that intravenous propafenone is effective in converting to sinus rhythm the majority of patients with AF complicating open-heart surgery. Heart rate was reduced in those who did not convert to sinus rhythm and no side effects nor hemodynamic deterioration were observed in any case.

Theophylline

Dattilo and associates[10] from Boise, Idaho, and Seattle, Washington, investigated the effect of theophylline on AV conduction in AF by determining ventricular response rates at rest and during exercise treadmill tests in 8 patients aged 64 ± 2 years with chronic AF. Tests were performed before and after 7 days of oral theophylline treatment (plasma level, 87.7 ± 7.8 umol/L). There was no significant change in baseline ventricular rate or duration of exercise, but the maximum ventricular rate with theophylline treatment was 12% ± 2% higher than that with placebo (176 ± 7 vs 158 ± 9 beats per minute), and, during each stage of exercise, the ventricular rate with theophylline exceeded that with placebo. The increased heart rate during theophylline administration occurred without a significant difference in the exercise-induced increase in circulating plasma catecholamine levels. The authors concluded that treatment with theophylline may contribute to difficulties with rate control in acutely ill patients with coexisting AF.

Amiodarone

To study efficacy and safety of low-dose amiodarone for maintenance of sinus rhythm after electrical cardioversion of AF or flutter, Gosselink and associates[11] from Groningen, The Netherlands, studied 89 consecutive patients with chronic AF or atrial flutter and eligible for cardioversion in a non-randomized trial with mean duration of follow-up for 21 months. The patients had failed previous treatment aimed at maintaining sinus rhythm. During follow-up 1 patient was withdrawn because of side effects; all others were available for follow-up. Before cardioversion, patients received 600 mg of amiodarone daily during a 4-week loading period. After conversion, the daily maintenance dose was 204 ± 66 mg. The main outcome measures were arrhythmia recurrence and adverse effects causing drug discontinuation. During loading, 15 patients (16%) converted, and after electrical cardioconversion, 90% of all patients had sinus rhythm. Actuarially, 53% of these patients were still in sinus rhythm after 3 years. In patients with compromised LV function, 93% maintained sinus rhythm after 6 months. One patient died due to CHF. Intolerable side effects occurred in 1 patient. No proarrhythmia was observed. Logistic regression analysis revealed that amiodarone was ineffective in patients with MS or chronic arrhythmia. Low-dose amiodarone is effective for maintaining sinus rhythm in patients with difficult to treat chronic AF or flutter and is associated with a low incidence of serious side effects.

Proarrhythmia

To review data on the type, mechanism, and prevalence of the proarrhythmic effect of drugs used to treat AF or atrial flutter, Falk[12] from

Boston, Massachusetts, reviewed relevant articles from the early 1960s to the present. From this review, Falk concluded that antiarrhythmic therapy aimed at stabilizing the atrium may have adverse effects on the ventricle including torsade de pointes and, less commonly, sustained VT. Different antiarrhythmic agents appear to have differing potentials for this proarrhythmic response, which is most common with class 1A agents. Other proarrhythmic responses to atrial antiarrhythmic agents include the acceleration of the ventricular response either by enhancing atrioventricular nodal or bypass tract conduction or by converting AF to flutter with 1:1 conduction. Calcium-channel blocking agents and, less commonly, digoxin may perpetuate the duration of paroxysmal AF, and virtually all agents can cause sinus node dysfunction or atrioventricular block. Although drug therapy for AF or flutter is generally well tolerated, the potential exists for uncommon but serious proarrhythmic effects. Knowledge of the risk factors and symptoms of these adverse reactions will help to further reduce this risk.

His bundle ablation

Incessant supraventricular tachyarrhythmia may lead to a reversible impairment of LV function. Heinz and associates[13] from Vienna, Austria, investigated in 10 patients (aged 64 ± 13 years) who underwent radiofrequency His bundle ablation for control of drug refractory, chronic AF (n = 9) and recurrent AF (n = 1). LV function was assessed by 2-dimensional guided M-mode echocardiography within 24 hours (baseline) and 49 ± 18 days (follow-up) after successful ablation, both during VVI pacing at 70 beats/min. Fractional shortening increased from 28 ± 9% at baseline to 35 ± 8% at follow-up. This increase in fractional shortening was due to a significant reduction of end-systolic diameter from 41 ± 10 to 36 ± 10 mm, whereas there was no appreciable change in end-diastolic diameter (56 ± 7 to 55 ± 10 mm). These changes were substantially greater in patients with baseline impairment of LV function (fractional shortening < 27%). Fractional shortening increased by 12% in patients with normal LV function (n = 5) and by 44% in those with impaired LV function at baseline (n = 5). The greater increase in fractional shortening in patients with preexisting LV impairment was due to a more pronounced decline in end-systolic dimensions (−11.9%) compared with that of patients with normal LV function at baseline (−9.21%). End-diastolic diameter showed no significant change in either group (−3.53% and −0.58%). These data show that chronic, rapid AF and flutter may lead to impairment of LV systolic function, which is reversible on control of the tachycardia by radiofrequency His ablation. The recovery of LV mechanics is substantially greater in patients with the more profoundly depressed LV function at initial evaluation.

Aspirin

Recent randomized trials have consistently demonstrated the marked efficacy of warfarin in reducing the risk of stroke caused by nonrheumatic AF. These trials have provided conflicting evidence on the effect of aspirin. Singer and associates[14] from Boston, Massachusetts, reported the aspirin analysis from the Boston Area Anticoagulation Trial in Atrial Fibrillation study, a trial in which control patients could choose to take aspirin. There were 2 strokes in 446 person-years with warfarin (annual rate of 0.45%); 8 strokes in 206 person-years with aspirin, most at 325 mg per day (annual rate of 3.9%); and 6 strokes in 271 person-years among patients taking neither aspirin nor warfarin (annual rate of 2.8%). Simultaneously controlling for the other significant determinants of stroke in the Boston Area Anticoagulation Trial in Atrial Fibrillation study (age, mitral annular calcification, and clinical heart disease), the relative incidence rate ratio of stroke were: 1) warfarin versus aspirin = 0.135; 2) aspirin versus (no aspirin and no warfarin) = 1.95; and 3) warfarin versus (no aspirin and no warfarin) = 0.263. This treatment received analysis argues that warfarin is strikingly more effective than aspirin in preventing stroke in nonrheumatic AF.

Warfarin

Nonrheumatic AF is common among the elderly and is associated with an increased risk of stroke. Ezekowitz and associates[15] for the Veterans Affairs Stroke Prevention in Nonrheumatic Atrial Fibrillation Investigators investigated whether anticoagulation with Warfarin would reduce this risk. They conducted a randomized, double-blind, placebo-controlled study to evaluate low-intensity anticoagulation with warfarin (prothrombin-time ratio, 1.2 to 1.5) in 571 men with chronic nonrheumatic AF; 525 patients had not previously had a cerebral infarction, whereas 46 patients had previously had such an event. The primary end point was cerebral infarction; secondary end points were cerebral hemorrhage and death. Among the patients with no history of stroke, cerebral infarction occurred in 19 of the 265 patients in the placebo group during an average follow-up of 1.7 years (4.3% per year) and in 4 of the 260 patients in the warfarin group during an average follow-up of 1.8 years (0.9% per year) (Figure 4-1). The reduction in risk with warfarin therapy was 0.79. The annual event rate among the 228 patients over 70 years of age was 4.8% in the placebo group and 0.9% in the warfarin group (risk reduction, 0.79). The only cerebral hemorrhage occurred in a 73-year-old patient in the warfarin

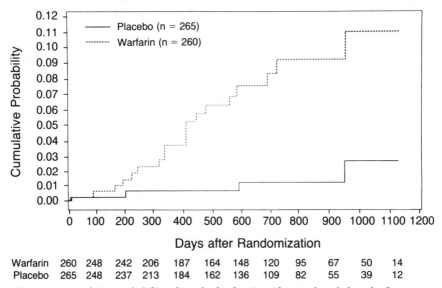

Fig. 4-1. Cumulative Probability of Cerebral Infarction. The numbers below the figure are the numbers of patients at risk for a cerebral infarction at each point. There was a significant reduction in risk in the warfain group as compared with the placebo group (risk reduction, 0.79; P = 0.001) Reproduced with permission from Ezekowitz, et al.[15]

group. Other major hemorrhages, all gastrointestinal, occurred in 10 patients; 4 in the placebo group, for a rate of 0.9% per year, and 6 in the warfarin group, for a rate of 1.3% per year. There were 37 deaths that were not preceded by a cerebral end point—22 in the placebo group and 15 in the warfarin group (risk reduction, 0.31). Cerebral infarction was more common among patients with a history of cerebral infarction (9.3% per year in the placebo group and 6.1% per year in the warfarin group) than among those without such a history. Low-intensity anticoagulation with warfarin prevented cerebral infarction in patients with nonrheumatic AF without producing an excess risk of major hemorrhage. This benefit extended to patients over 70 years of age.

Warfarin vs Aspirin

Flaker and colleagues[16] in Columbia, Missouri; Jacksonville, Florida; Seattle, Washington; New York, New York; San Antonio, Texas studied the relationship between cardiac mortality and antiarrhythmic drug administration from 1,330 patients enrolled in the Stroke Prevention in Atrial Fibrillation Study, a randomized clinical trial comparing warfarin, aspirin and placebo for the prevention of ischemic stroke or systemic embolism in patients with nonvalvular AF. Patients who received antiarrhythmic drug therapy for AF in this study were compared with patients not receiving antiarrhythmic agents. The relative risk of cardiac mortality, including arrhythmic death, in patients receiving antiarrhythmic drug therapy was determined and adjusted for other cardiac risk factors. In patients receiving antiarrhythmic drug therapy, cardiac mortality was increased 2.5-fold and arrhythmic deaths were increased 2.6-fold. Among patients with a history of CHF, those given antiarrhythmic medications had a relative cardiac risk of 4.7 compared with that of patients not so treated and the relative risk of arrhythmic death in the treated group was 3.7 (Figure 4-2). Patients without a history of CHF had no increased risk of cardiac mortality during antiarrhythmic drug therapy. After exclusion of 23 patients with documented ventricular arrhythmias and adjustment for other variables predictive of cardiac death, patients receiving antiarrhythmic drugs were not at increased risk of cardiac death or arrhythmic death. However, in patients with a history of CHF who received antiarrhythmic drug therapy, the relative risk of cardiac death was 3.3 and that of arrhythmic death was 5.8 compared with the risk in patients not taking antiarrhythmic medications. Therefore, although antiarrhythmic drug therapy was not randomly determined in this trial, the data suggest that in patients with AF and a history of CHF, the risk of such therapy may outweigh the potential benefit of maintaining sinus rhythm.

SUPRAVENTRICULAR TACHYCARDIA WITH AND WITHOUT SHORT P-R INTERVAL SYNDROME

Natural history of preexcitation

To examine the natural history of preexcitation occurring on the routine electrocardiogram, Krahn and associates[17] from Winnipeg, Canada, performed a longitudinal cohort study of 3,983 originally healthy

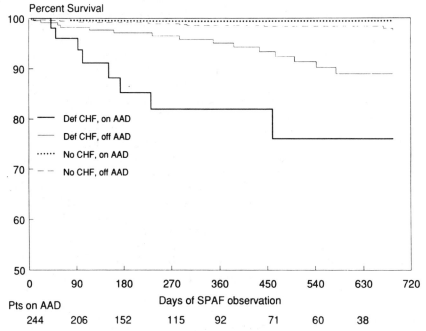

Fig. 4-2. Survival to cardiac-related death in patients with and without heart failure (CHF) at entry. AAD = antiarrhythmic drug therapy; Def = definite history of; Pts = patients; SPAF = Stroke Prevention in Atrial Fibrillation. Reproduced with permission from Flaker, et al.[16]

men followed prospectively for 40 years. Nineteen male study members with preexcitation occurring during routine examination in the 40-year follow-up of the Manitoba Follow-up Study were identified. Ten study members were found to have preexcitation at enrollment for a prevalence of 2.5/1,000. A delta wave was first detected during follow-up in an additional 9 study patients. Seventeen of 19 study members did not have the delta wave at some later time, and preexcitation was intermittently present in most of these members. Over time there was a loss of preexcitation, with 15 of 19 study members no longer exhibiting a delta wave by the end of follow-up. Five of 11 study members with symptoms had physician confirmation of an arrhythmia. Fourteen study members remain alive, and none of the 5 deaths was attributed to preexcitation. Preexcitation found on routine electrocardiogram in the originally healthy male study group did not confer excess morbidity or mortality, even in those study members who developed symptomatic arrhythmias. Most preexcitation was intermittent and disappeared over time.

Causing pounding in the neck

Gursoy and associates[18] from Aalst, Belgium, and Barcelona, Spain, studied 244 consecutive patients who were referred for electrophysiologic evaluation and who gave a history of palpitations, and they were asked if they felt any sort of rapid and regular pounding in the neck during the palpitations. The symptoms were correlated during the electrophysiologic study when an arrhythmia was observed or induced or when the patient felt palpitations. Of the 244 patients interviewed about their symptoms, rapid, regular pounding in the neck was felt by all but 4 of the 54 patients with AV nodal reentrant tachycardia but was not felt by any of the other 190 patients with other arrhythmias. In another phase of the study, hemodynamic measurements and right atrial angiograms were obtained during sinus rhythm and during tachycardias in 23 patients: 12 with AV nodal reentrant tachycardia, 8 with circus-movement tachycardia mediated by an AV accessory pathway, and 3 with both forms of tachycardia. The group with reentrant tachycardia had significantly higher mean and peak RA pressures during tachycardia than the group with circus-movement tachycardia. An analysis of the RA wave forms during tachycardia revealed distinct A and V waves during circus-movement tachycardia, whereas only a single wave (a-V fusion) was present during AV nodal reentrant tachycardia. Thus, rapid pounding in the neck is common during AV nodal reentrant tachycardia and seems to be a useful clinical marker in differential diagnosis of patients with palpitations. It can also be useful in patients with documented preexcitation on the surface electrocardiogram who describe neck pounding, since the presence of concomitant AV nodal reentrant tachycardia should be carefully sought in this group. Slow, irregular neck pounding can occur in patients with VT and AV dissociation.

Causing syncope

Syncope in patients with SVT has been suggested to be an ominous finding, predictive of rapid rates during SVT. Leitch and colleagues[19] in Ontario, Canada, induced SVT in the supine position and after passive head-up tilting to 60° in 13 patients with AV node reentry, 8 patients with AV reentry, and 1 patient with atrial tachycardia. Tilt testing was also performed in sinus rhythm for 30 minutes. Mean age was 38 years, and 11 patients had a history of syncope. The cycle length of tachycardia when upright was shorter than when supine (297 compared with 375 msec), and mean blood pressure fell to a greater extent after the onset of tachycardia (fall in mean BP, 53 compared with 24 mm Hg). Mean BP correlated significantly with tachycardia cycle length when supine but not when tilted upright. Syncope occurred in 7 patients during upright tachycardia. These 7 patients had a greater fall in mean BP with upright tachycardia then the 15 patients without syncope (fall in mean BP, 70 compared with 45 mm Hg), but there was no difference in the tachycardia cycle length. Six of the 7 patients with tachycardia-induced syncope also had syncope with tilt testing in sinus rhythm compared with 4 of the 15 patients without tachycardia-induced syncope. These data support the view that syncope during SVT is related to vasomotor factors and does not predict a more rapid tachycardia rate.

Sotalol

Huikuri and associates[20] from Oulu, Finland, studied the efficacy of intravenous sotalol (1 mg/kg) for suppressing inducibility of SVT with different electrophysiologic mechanisms in 30 consecutive patients referred for an electrophysiologic study because of paroxysmal SVT. Orthodromic SVT using accessory atrioventricular connection was inducible in 14 patients, atrioventricular nodal reentrant SVT in 8, and intraatrial SVT in 8 before administration of sotalol. Isometric handgrip exercise facilitated the inducibility of SVT in 8 patients who were noninducible at rest. After intravenous sotalol, 7 of 14 patients (50%) with orthodromic

SVT, 8 of 8 with atrioventricular nodal reentrant SVT, and 8 of 8 with intraatrial reentrant SVT became noninducible into sustained SVT. Isometric exercise facilitated the inducibility of only 3 nonsustained SVT runs after sotalol infusion, and exercise did not reverse the prolongation of refractory periods of the atrium, AV node, accessory pathway and ventricle caused by sotalol. During a mean follow-up period of 18 ± 7 months, none of the 14 patients who remained noninducible into sustained SVT during the stress test after intravenous sotalol and tolerated long-term oral sotalol therapy had recurrence of symptomatic SVT. Thus, sotalol is efficacious for suppressing SVT with AV nodal or intraatrial reentrant mechanism, but less efficacious in patients with accessory AV pathway. The B-blocking and cellular antiarrhythmic effects of sotalol are not significantly reversed by exercise.

Sotalol is a B blocker with class III activity. Few investigators have reported its use in pediatric patients. From August 1985 to May 1990, Maragnes and associates[21] from Vancouver, Canada, treated 66 patients (mean age 9 years; range 9 days to 24 years), including 14 infants aged < 3 months with oral sotalol alone (n = 46) or in association with digoxin (n = 20). SVT was present in 38 patients (20 with documented preexcitation), AF in 10 and atrial ectopic tachycardia in 7. Three patients had other types of SVT. Tachycardia was of ventricular origin in 6 patients and both of supraventricular and ventricular origin in the remaining 2. Mean dose of oral sotalol was 135 mg/m^2/day given in 2 doses. Congenital heart disease was present in 28 patients, 14 with previous cardiac surgery, mostly at the atrial level. Prior treatment with 1 or more antiarrhythmic agent had been unsuccessful in 83% of patients. Mean duration of treatment was 13.3 months (range 2 months to 5 years). Overall, treatment was successful in 79% of cases. Highest rate of success was observed in patients with supraventricular reentrant tachycardia with or without preexcitation (89%) and in those with atrial ectopic tachycardia (85.5%). Atrial flutter could be controlled in 60% of cases. Sotalol seemed less effective in VT with a complete control of the arrhythmia being achieved in only 17%; however, it decreased the number of runs of VT and the number of VPCs in 50% of patients. There were no adverse effects in 89% of patients. Two patients with previous sick sinus syndrome had worsening of their bradycardia necessitating implantation of a pacemaker in 1. Sotalol is a very effective drug for the treatment of the various pediatric arrhythmias, in particular supraventricular arrhythmias, without significant adverse effects.

Nadolol

Mehta and Chidambaram[22] from Johnson City, Tennessee, evaluated the efficacy and safety of oral nadolol for treatment of SVT in 27 children with a median age of 5.5 years. An unsuccessful trial of digoxin therapy occurred in 15 and intravenous nadolol was given to 7 patients during electrophysiologic study with 5 having an excellent response and 2 a partial response defined as a 25% decrease in tachycardia rate. Six of these patients had a similar response to oral nadolol. Twelve patients received both propranolol and nadolol. Among 6 patients, intravenous propranolol was successful in 4 and unsuccessful in 2; all 6 had a similar response to oral nadolol. With oral propranolol tachycardia was well controlled in 4 patients and persistent in 2; 5 of 5 patients had a similar response to oral nadolol. Oral nadolol was used to treat 26 patients; the arrhythmia was well controlled in 23, 2 had recurrent tachycardia and 1 had tachycardia at a 25% slower rate. The effective dose ranged from .25 to 2.5 mg/kg body weight given once daily with a median dose of 1 mg/kg/day. During follow-up of 3 to 36 months compliance and tolerance were excellent, excluding 2 patients with reactive airway disease who developed wheezing and 3 who had side effects necessitating a change in therapy. This drug appears safe and effective in a small group. Further studies are indicated to assess its place in pediatric antiarrhythmic therapy.

Flecainide

Concerns about the safety and efficacy of class IC antiarrhythmic agents have arisen as a result of the recent Cardiac Arrhythmia Suppression Trial. Hughes and associates[23] from Cleveland, Ohio, studied 110 consecutive patients treated with flecainide between July 1988 and July 1989 who had normal or mildly impaired LV function and symptomatic supraventricular arrhythmias. Follow-up data were obtained on 102 patients for a mean of 14 months. The average duration of flecainide therapy was 13 months. Tachyarrhythmias treated included AF/atrial flutter, AV reentry, and AV nodal reentry. Flecainide provided effective antiarrhythmic therapy in 62% of the patients and was discontinued in 38% of the patients. LA size did not predict treatment failure. Two patients developed proarrhythmic events (nonsustained VT). There were no deaths during the follow-up period. In conclusion, flecainide provides safe and effective therapy for supraventricular tachyarrhythmias in patients with normal or mildly impaired LV function.

Diltiazem

Diltiazem has electrophysiologic effects similar to those of verapamil. Dougherty and associates[24] for the IV Diltiazem Study Group examined its efficacy and safety in 4 doses for treatment of induced SVT and compared with those of placebo in 87 patients (25 with AV nodal reentry tachycardia, 60 with AV reentry associated with an accessory AV connection, and 2 with atrial tachycardia). Conversion to sinus rhythm occurred in 4 of 14 patients (29%) with 0.05 mg/kg of diltiazem, 16 of 19 (84%) with 0.15 mg/kg, 13 of 13 (100%) with 0.25 mg/kg, and 14 of 17 (82%) with 0.45 mg/kg compared with 6 of 24 (25%) treated with placebo. Conversion rates in groups receiving doses of 0.15 to 0.45 mg/kg of diltiazem were superior to that in the placebo group. Time to conversion was 3.0 ± 2.6 minutes in responding diltiazem patients compared with 5.9 ± 6.1 minutes in responding to control patients. Diltiazem administration resulted in significant lengthening of SVT cycle length, AH interval, and AV nodal effective refractory period and block cycle length. The most frequent adverse response to diltiazem was hypotension (7 of 63 patients); however, only 4 patients had symptoms related to hypotension. Thus, intravenous diltiazem in doses of 0.15, 0.25 and 0.45 mg/kg is an effective and safe treatment for the acute management of SVT.

Adenosine vs Verapamil

In a study carried out by Hood and Smith[25] from Auckland, New Zealand, the safety and efficacy of verapamil and adenosine in the acute termination of SVT were compared in a randomized double-crossover trial. Of 32 eligible patients with either spontaneous or induced narrow complex tachycardia, 7 (22%) patients experienced conversion to sinus rhythm with carotid sinus massage. The other 25 patients were randomly assigned to receive either adenosine (n = 14) or verapamil (n = 11). Relative drug efficacies were 100% for adenosine versus 73% for verapamil. Adenosine given at ≤ 120 μg/kg caused conversion in 12 (86%) of 14 patients. The other 2 patients required 20 mg adenosine for conversion. After conversion the systolic BP increased significantly in the adenosine group but not in the verapamil group. Reinitiation of tachycardia occurred in 2 (14%) of 14 patients randomized to the adenosine group. Serious adverse hemodynamic effects were observed in 1 (9%) of 11 patients randomized to verapamil. The incidence of conversion arrhythmias was similar in both treatment groups (adenosine 57% and verapamil 50%).

Radiofrequency catheter ablation

Keim and associates[26] in Gainesville, Florida, and New York, New York, utilized adenosine to assess completeness of accessory pathway ablation in 16 patients with an accessory pathway who had surgical ablations (n = 8), or catheter ablations with radiofrequency energy (n = 8). Before ablation, no accessory pathway was sensitive to adenosine. Twelve patients with pre-excitation showed high grade AV node block with maximal pre-excitation on the administration of adenosine during atrial pacing. Four patients with a concealed accessory pathway demonstrated high grade AV block without evidence of latent anterograde accessory pathway conduction. Preablation ventriculoatrial block was not observed in any of the 16 patients in response to adenosine during ventricular pacing. Immediately after accessory pathway ablation, all patients developed AV and ventriculoatrial block with the administration of adenosine during atrial and ventricular pacing, respectively. These findings were confirmed during follow-up study 1 week later. AV block during atrial and ventricular pacing with adenosine affords a reliable and immediate assessment of successful pathway ablation.

Lesh and associates[27] in San Francisco, California, have used percutaneous catheter ablation of 109 accessory pathways with use of radiofrequency energy attempted in 100 consecutive patients. Patient age ranged from 3 to 67 years. The patients had been treated for recurrent tachycardia with a mean of 3 ± 0.2 antiarrhythmic agents that proved ineffective or caused unacceptable side effects. In seven patients, previous attempts at accessory pathway ablation with use of direct current shock had been unsuccessful. Forty-five (41%) of the pathways were left free wall, 43 (40%) were septal and 21 (19%) were right free wall. Eighty-nine (89%) of 100 patients had successful radiofrequency ablation at the time of hospital discharge. In all but 12 patients, the ablation was accomplished during the first therapeutic effort. Complications resulting from the procedure occurred in 4 patients (4%). However, no patient developed AV block or had other cardiac arrhythmias. During a mean follow-up period of 10 months, nine patients had some return of accessory pathway conduction, and a repeat ablation procedure was successful in all five. Therefore, catheter ablation using radiofrequency energy may be performed on accessory pathways in all locations. The procedure is effective and safe, less costly and more convenient than cardiac surgery, and can be considered as an alternative to lifelong medical therapy in any patient with symptomatic accessory pathway-mediated tachycardia.

Kay and colleagues[28] in Birmingham, Alabama designed a study to evaluate the safety and efficacy of selective catheter ablation of the slow pathway using radiofrequency energy applied along the tricuspid annulus near the coronary sinus ostium as definitive therapy for A-V nodal reentrant tachycardia. Among 34 consecutive patients who were prospectively enrolled in the study, the slow pathway was selectively ablated in 30, and the fast pathway was ablated in 4. Antegrade conduction over the fast pathway remained intact in all 30 patients after successful selective slow pathway ablation. There was no statistically significant change in the atrio-His interval or A-V Wenckebach rate after selective ablation of the slow pathway. However, the antegrade effective refractory period of the fast pathway decreased from 348 msec before ablation to 309 msec after selective slow pathway ablation. Retrograde conduction remained intact in 26 of 30 patients after selective ablation of the slow pathway. The retrograde refractory period of the ventriculoatrial conduction system was 285 msec before and 280 msec after slow pathway ablation in patients with intact retrograde conduction. There were 3 complications in 2 patients, including an episode of pulmonary edema and the development of spontaneous A-V Wenckebach block during sleep in 1 patient after slow pathway ablation and the late development of complete A-V block in another patient after fast pathway ablation. Over a mean follow-up period of 322 days, A-V nodal reentrant tachycardia recurred in 3 patients, all of whom were successfully treated in a second ablation session. Radiofrequency ablation of the slow A-V pathway is highly effective and is associated with a low rate of complications.

AV nodal reentrant tachycardia, the most common form of SVT, results from conduction through a reentrant circuit comprising fast and slow AV nodal pathways. Antiarrhythmic-drug therapy is not consistently successful in slowing this rhythm disturbance. Catheter ablation of the fast pathway with radiofrequency current eliminates AV nodal reentrant tachycardia, but it can produce heart block. Jackman and associates[29] from Oklahoma City, Oklahoma, hypothesized that catheter ablation of the site of insertion of the slow pathway into the atrium would eliminate AV nodal reentrant tachycardia while leaving normal (fast pathway) AV nodal conduction intact (Figure 4-3). Eighty patients with symptomatic AV nodal reentrant tachycardia were studied. Retrograde slow-pathway conduction (in which the earliest retrograde atrial potential was recorded at the posterior septum, close to the coronary sinus) was present in 33 patients. The retrograde atrial potential was preceded by a potential consistent with activation of the atrial end of the slow pathway (A_{sp}). In 46 of the 47 patients without retrograde slow-pathway conduction, a potential with the same characteristics as the A_{sp} potential was recorded during sinus rhythm. Radiofrequency current delivered through a catheter to the A_{sp} site (in the posteroseptal right atrium or coronary sinus) abolished or modified slow-pathway conduction in 78 patients, eliminating AV nodal reentrant tachycardia without affecting normal AV nodal conduction. In the single patient without A_{sp}, the application of radiofrequency current to the proximal coronary sinus ablated the fast pathway and AV nodal reentrant tachycardia. AV block occurred in 1 patient (1.3%) with left BBB, after inadvertent ablation of the right BB. AV nodal reentrant tachycardia has not recurred in any patient during a mean ($\pm$ SD) follow-up of 15.5 $\pm$ 11.3 months. Electrophysiologic study 4.3 $\pm$ 3.3 months after ablation in 32 patients demonstrated normal atrioventricular nodal conduction without AV nodal reentrant tachycardia. Catheter ablation of the atrial end of the slow pathway using radiofrequency current, guided by A_{sp} potentials, can eliminate AV nodal reentrant tachycardia with very little risk of AV block.

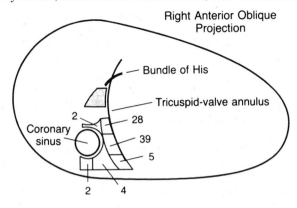

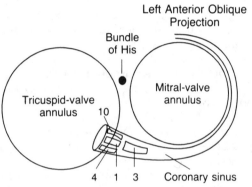

Fig. 4-3. Schematic Representation of the Septum as Viewed Fluoroscopically in the Right and Left Anterior Oblique Projections, Showing the 98 Sites of Successful Slow-Pathway Ablation in the 78 Patients. Numbers indicate the number of sites of successful ablation in each region. During selective retrograde fast-pathway conduction, the earliest atrial activation was recorded in the anterior septum, near the bundle of His (shaded region). During selective retrograde slow-pathway conduction, the earliest atrial potential was recorded in the posterior septum or proximal coronary sinus (unshaded regions). Reproduced with permission from Jackman, et al.[29]

In a study by Chen and associates[30] from Taipei, Taiwan, Republic of China, to evaluate and compare in patients with WPW syndrome, 114 patients with accessory pathway-mediated tachyarrhythmias underwent catheter ablation. Electrophysiologic parameters were similar in patients undergoing direct-current (group 1, 52 patients with 53 accessory pathways) and radiofrequency (group 2, 62 patients with 75 accessory pathways) ablation. Immediately after ablation, 50 of 53 accessory pathways (94%) were ablated successfully with direct current, but 2 of the 50 accessory pathways had early return of conduction and required a second ablation; 72 of 75 accessory pathways (96%) were ablated successfully with radiofrequency current. In the 3 accessory pathways in which radiofrequency ablation was unsuccessful, a later direct-current ablation was successful. During follow-up (group 1, 14 to 27 months; group 2, 8 to 13 months), none of the patients with successful ablation had a recurrence of tachycardia. Complications in direct-current ablation included transient hypotension (2 patients); accidental A-V block (1 patient), and pulmonary air trapping (2 patients); complications in radiofrequency ablation included cardiac tamponade (1 patient) and suspicious aortic dissection

(1 patient). Myocardial injury and proarrhythmic effects were more severe in direct-current ablation. The length of the procedure and the radiation exposure time were significantly shorter in direct-current (3.5 ± 0.2 hours, 30 ± 4 minutes) than in radiofrequency (4.1 ± 0.4 hours, 46 ± 9 minutes) ablation. Findings in this study confirm the impression that radiofrequency ablation is associated with fewer complications than direct-current ablation and radiofrequency ablation with a large-tipped electrode catheter is an effective and relatively safe nonsurgical method for treatment of WPW syndrome.

Walsh and associates[31] from Boston, Massachusetts, described 12 young pages, aged 10 months to 19 years, with drug-resistant ectopic atrial tachycardia treated with direct transcatheter ablation of the ectopic focus using radiofrequency energy. All had depressed LV contractility by echocardiographic criteria involving shortening fractions of 10–26%. The ectopic focus was mapped to the left atrium in 7 cases and to the right atrium in 5. Local activation at the ectopic site preceded the onset of the surface P wave by 20–60 msec. Tachycardia terminated .5–13 second into a successful RF application. The procedure eliminated tachycardia in 11 of 12 patients, all of whom were discharged in sinus rhythm without medication after a median hospital stay of 48 hours. Ablation was unsuccessful in 1 patient with diffuse dysplasia of the anterior right atrium who eventually did well after surgery for resection of abnormal atrial tissue. Transient depression of sinus node function was noted in 1 patient who had successful ablation of a focus in close proximity to the sinus node but normal sinus node function returned within 72 hours. No other complications were encountered. During follow-up of 3 to 21 months, 1 patient had recurrence of a slower and less-sustained atrial ectopic tachycardia that was successfully eliminated at a second ablation session. All others remained in sinus rhythm and all 12 subjects recovered normal ventricular function. These authors report outstanding results of radiofrequency ablation for ectopic tachycardia in young patients. These early results are extremely encouraging for this resistant type of arrhythmia.

Case and associates[32] from Charleston, South Carolina, attempted catheter ablation for incessant medically resistant SVT in 7 infants and children whose average age was 10 months (range 1 to 27 months). Diagnosis included reentrant SVT in 6 and atrial ectopic tachycardia in 1. A total of 9 catheter ablation procedures were performed in these 7 patients with the atrial approach employed in 8 of the 9 procedures. Catheter ablation was totally successful in 5 of the 7 patients, partially successful in 1 and unsuccessful in 1. The combination of catheter ablation and surgical ablation was successful in controlling tachycardia in all patients; with at least 5 months follow-up no patient has had a recurrence of SVT or reappearance of a delta wave. This initial experience with catheter ablation in infants and small children demonstrates that this procedure is a promising alternative to surgical ablation, even in young patients.

Haissaguerre and co-workers[33] in Bordeaux, France, described a new technique for catheter ablation of left lateral accessory pathways by radiofrequency energy applied at the epicardium through the coronary sinus wall using a unipolar configuration. In an overall group of 212 patients with left lateral accessory pathways, multiple endocardial ablation attempts of the accessory pathways were unsuccessful in 8 patients. The mean cumulative duration of previous attempts was 12 hours, using DC shocks and/or radiofrequency energy applied both at the atrial and/or ventricular accessory pathway insertions. Epicardial accessory pathway insertion was determined by bipolar and unipolar unfiltered distal electrograms by scanning the coronary sinus with a steerable 6F or 7F catheter with a 4-mm distal electrode. The local atrial to ventricular electrogram amplitude ratio was 0.3–1.6. At the ablation site, the catheter tip was slightly deflected toward the annulus to increase both the ventricular component of electrograms and contact with the epicardium. In 4 patients, epicardial electrogram timings were earlier than endocardial ones. The accessory pathway was ablated in 7 of the 8 patients with 20-30 W applied for 10-60 seconds. No complications occurred except a marked nonspecific pain during radiofrequency energy application; however, the catheter remained adherent to the coronary sinus wall, and its withdrawal was performed during a new radiofrequency application to decrease the risk of coronary sinus rupture. After ablation, echocardiograms, coronary artery angiograms, and levophase coronary sinus angiograms showed no abnormality in all patients except 2 who had a probable mural thrombus in the coronary sinus. Accessory pathway conduction remained abolished for 1–10 months of follow-up in 7 patients. Radiofrequency catheter ablation of left lateral accessory pathways can be achieved effectively and relatively safely via the mid or distal coronary sinus when endocardial approaches are unsuccessful.

Surgical ablation of accessory pathway

Yeh and associates[34] from Taipei, Taiwan, performed a predischarge electrophysiologic study in 113 patients with the WPW syndrome who had undergone surgical ablation of the accessory pathway. The study was performed 5 to 20 (mean 10 ± 3) days after surgery. There were 82 male and 31 female patients (aged 4 to 58 years, mean 36 ± 13). Sixty-one patients (54%) had manifest, 52 (46%) had concealed and 12 (11%) had multiple accessory pathways. All but 1 patient had AV reentrant tachycardia incorporating single or multiple accessory pathways during the control electrophysiologic study. The accessory pathways were located in the LV free wall in 60% of cases, RV free wall in 22%, posteroseptum in 13%, and anteroseptum in 5%. The predischarge electrophysiologic study showed that the accessory pathway was capable of anterograde and retrograde conductions in 4 patients (all with manifest WPW syndrome). Four patients showed induction of supraventricular tachycardia, including 2 with AV reentrant tachycardia, and 2 with AV nodal reentrant tachycardia. Recurrence of supraventricular tachycardia was noted in 5 patients during a follow-up of 28 ± 26 months. Of these 5 patients, 2 had inducible and 3 had no inducible SVT during the predischarge electrophysiologic study. Thus, the predischarge electrophysiologic study could predict late outcome with recurrence of preexcitation or SVT in patients who had undergone surgical ablation of the accessory pathway with an overall predictive accuracy of 95% (107 of 113 patients), negative predictive value of 96% (103 of 107), and positive predictive value of 67% (4 of 6).

Surgery for cardiac dysrhythmias is infrequently reported in infants and children as compared with the frequent reports in adults. Crawford and associates[35] from Charleston, South Carolina, reviewed 55 infants and small children ≤ 5 years of age operated on from July 1, 1984, to December 31, 1991, for WPW syndrome (41 patients), AV node reentry (2 patients), atrial automatic tachycardia (2 patients), and VT (9 patients). Ages ranged from 3 weeks to 71 (mean, 29) months. Associated congenital heart defects were present in 5 (10%). Indications for surgery included failure of medical therapy, life-threatening dysrhythmias, and more recently, failure of catheter ablation. There were no hospital or late deaths. One patient sustained perioperative central nervous system injury. Surgery was successful in 52 of 55 (94.5%) (WPW, 38/41 (93%); atrioventricular node reentry, 2/2; atrial automatic tachycardia, 3/3; VT, 9/9). Ventricular function returned to normal in all 12 patients in whom it was abnormal before operation. Thus, surgical ablation is highly successful in the management of various forms of refractory or life-threatening dysrhythmias in infants and small children. Catheter ablation techniques require significant fluoroscopic time, are more difficult in infants, and as yet do not have adequate long-term follow-up. Accordingly, surgery may continue to play a role in this particular group of patients.

VENTRICULAR ARRHYTHMIAS

Prognosis

Andresen and associates[36] from Berlin and Munchen, Germany, analyzed long-term clinical outcome of 60 prospectively studied patients with documented sustained ventricular tachyarrhythmias that were not inducible during baseline programmed ventricular stimulation: 39 had nonfatal cardiac arrest due to noninfarction VF and 21 had mild hemodynamically compromising sustained VT. LVEF was 55 ± 14% in the VF group and 50 ± 13% in the VT group. Patients were discharged without conventional antiarrhythmic drugs and received only empirical B-blocker therapy. During a mean follow-up period of 21 ± 16 months (mean ± SD), 10 of 60 patients (17%) died suddenly. The actuarial incidence of sudden death at 1 and 4 years was similar in both groups (VF group, 10 and 20%; VT group, 16 and 16%). The actuarial incidence of sudden cardiac death was significantly higher in patients with LVEF ≤ 40% than in those with > 40% (1-year incidence in VF group, 40 vs 9%; VT group, 50 vs 0%). Multivariate regression analysis identified LVEF ≤ 40% and previous myocardial infarction as the only independent predictor of sudden cardiac death. The occurrence of frequent ventricular pairs during Holter monitoring was the only independent predictor of sustained VT recurrences. It is concluded that patients with sustained ventricular tachyarrhythmia in whom arrhythmia was noninducible during baseline ventricular stimulation and not treated with antiarrhythmic therapy have a favorable outcome if LVEF is high. However, reduced LVEF identifies a subgroup at high risk of sudden cardiac death. Patients with mild hemodynamically compromising sustained VT have a similar risk of dying suddenly as those resuscitated earlier from cardiac arrest.

To evaluate the prevalence and prognostic significance of asymptomatic complex or frequent VPCs detected during ambulatory electrocardiographic monitoring, Bikkina and associates[37] from Framingham and Boston, Massachusetts, performed a cohort study with a follow-up period of 4 to 6 years. The participants were surviving patients of the original Framingham Heart Study cohort and offspring of original cohort members (2,727 men and 3,306 women). The measurement was a 1-hour ambulatory electrocardiogram. The age-adjusted prevalence of complex or frequent arrhythmia (more than 30VPCs per hour or multiform VPCs, ventricular couplets, VT, or R-on-T VPCs) was 12% in the 2,425 men without clinically evident CAD and 33% in the 302 men with CAD. The corresponding values in women (3,064 without CAD and 242 with CAD) were 12% and 26%. After adjusting for age and traditional risk factors for CAD in a Cox proportional hazards model, men without CAD who had complex or frequent ventricular arrhythmias were at increased risk for both all-cause mortality and the occurrence of AMI or death from CAD. In men with CAD and in women with and without CAD, complex or frequent arrhythmias were not associated with an increased risk for either outcome. Thus, in men who do not have clinically apparent CAD, the incidental detection of ventricular arrhythmias is associated with a 2-fold increase in the risk of all-cause mortality and AMI or death due to CAD.

Electrophysiologic reproducibility

Although electrophysiologic studies are often used to assess antiarrhythmic drug efficacy in patients with VT, the reproducibility of these studies during therapy has not been definitively established. Ferrick and associates[38] from Bronx, New York, performed confirmation studies during drug therapy in 64 patients (51 men, mean age 63 years) with sustained ventricular arrhythmias induced during initial study to assess the reproducibility of drug effect. All patients had CAD. The stimulation protocol used included the serial introduction of up to 3 premature ventricular stimuli during sinus rhythm and with ventricular pacing at 2 pacing rates. Rapid ventricular pacing techniques were also used. Antiarrhythmic drug efficacy was confirmed in 77% of patients. Sustained VT was induced at repeat electrophysiologic study in 19% of patients during antiarrhythmic therapy that was previously thought to be effective. In summary, electrophysiologic study results during antiarrhythmic therapy exhibit significant day-to-day variability. Sustained VT can be induced during antiarrhythmic therapy that was previously defined as effective by programmed stimulation in a substantial number of patients.

From unsuspected cardiomyopathy or myocarditis

Wiles and associates[39] from Charleston, South Carolina, performed endomyocardial biopsy in 33 patients ages 6 to 27 years with a median of 12.5 years presenting with ventricular ectopic rhythm but a structurally normal heart by exam and noninvasive studies. Normal myocardial histologic features were found in 16 (48%) whereas 14 (42%) had changes similar to those seen with dilated cardiomyopathy and 3 (9%) had lymphocytic myocarditis. Presenting clinical symptoms, electrocardiogram, exercise treadmill testing, and invasive electrophysiologic study failed to predict the biopsy results. There was no difference among groups in LV shortening fraction but patients with abnormal histology did show an increase in end-diastolic dimension by echocardiography. These data suggest that endomyocardial biopsy may be indicated to diagnose unsuspected myocarditis in young patients with unexplained abnormal ventricular ectopic rhythm and apparently normal hearts by exam and noninvasive testing. Some of these patients may benefit from steroid therapy.

In arrhythmogenic right ventricular dysplasia

Ventricular tachyarrhythmias are the major clinical manifestation of arrhythmogenic RV disease. Although antiarrhythmic therapy has been widely advocated, there is only limited information available on the efficacy of antiarrhythmic drugs in these patients. Wichter and co-workers[40] in Munster, Germany, retrospectively and prospectively analyzed the short- and long-term efficacies of various antiarrhythmic agents in 81 patients with arrhythmogenic RV disease. In 42 patients with inducible VT during programmed ventricular stimulation, the following efficacy rates were obtained: class Ia and Ib drugs 6%; class Ic drugs 12%; B-blockers 0%; sotalol 68%; amiodarone 15%, verapamil 0%; and drug combinations 15%. Only one of the 10 patients not responding to sotalol was treated effectively by amiodarone, whereas the remaining nine patients proved to be drug refractory toward all other drugs tested and underwent nonpharmacological therapy. During a follow-up of 34 months, three of the 31 patients discharged on pharmacological therapy had nonfatal recurrences of VT after 0.5, 51, and 63 months, respectively. In 39 patients with noninducible VT during programmed ventricular stimulation, the following efficacy rates were observed: class Ia and Ib drugs 0%; class Ic drugs 17%; B-blockers 29%; sotalol 83%; amiodarone 25%; verapamil 50%; and drug combinations 9%. During a follow-up of 14 months, four of 33 patients discharged on antiarrhythmic drugs had nonfatal relapses of their clinical ventricular arrhythmia. Thus, in arrhythmogenic RV disease, sotalol proved to be highly effective in patients with inducible as well as noninducible VT. Patients with inducible VT responding to sotalol are likely to not respond to other antiarrhythmic drugs and should be considered for nonpharmacological therapy without further drug testing. Amiodarone did not prove to be more effective than sotalol and may not be an alternative because of frequent side effects during long-term therapy, especially in young patients. Verapamil and B-blockers were effective in a considerable number of patients with noninducible VT and may be a therapeutic alternative in this subgroup. Class I agents appear to be rarely effective in the treatment of both inducible and noninducible VT in arrhythmogenic RV disease.

In hemodialysis patients

Sforzini and associates[41] from several medical centers found a high prevalence of ventricular arrhythmias, the frequency of which rose significantly during and after dialysis, among 127 randomly selected patients on hemodialysis. These patients have now been followed up for 4 years. Only age and CAD correlated independently with mortality. Although ventricular arrhythmias are often associated with cardiac disease in patients on chronic hemodialysis, they do not seem to predict overall mortality.

In patients having noncardiac surgery

To determine the incidence, clinical predictors and prognostic importance of perioperative ventricular arrhythmias, O'Kelly and associates[42] for the Study of Perioperative Ischemia Research Group studied a consecutive sample of 230 men with known CAD (46%) or at high risk of CAD (54%) undergoing major noncardiac surgical procedures. The authors recorded cardiac rhythm throughout the preoperative (mean = 21 hours), intraoperative (mean = 6 hours), and postoperative (mean = 38 hours) periods using continuous ambulatory electrocardiographic monitoring. Adverse cardiac outcomes were noted by physicians blinded to information about arrhythmias. Frequent or major ventricular arrhythmias (> 30 VPCs per hour, VT) occurred in 44% of the patients: 21% preoperatively, 16% intraoperatively, and 36% postoperatively (Figure 4-4). Compared with the preoperative baseline, the severity of arrhythmia increased in only 2% of patients intraoperatively but in 10% postoperatively. Preoperative ventricular arrhythmias were more common in smokers, those with a history of CHF, and those with electrocardiographic evidence of myocardial ischemia. Preoperative arrhythmias were associated with the occurrence of intraoperative and postoperative arrhythmias. Nonfatal AMI or cardiac death occurred in 9 men; these outcomes were not significantly more frequent in those with prior perioperative arrhythmias, albeit with wide CIs. Almost half of all high-risk patients undergoing noncardiac surgery have frequent ventricular ectopic beats or nonsustained VT. The results suggest that these arrhythmias, when they occur without other signs or symptoms of AMI, may not require aggressive monitoring or treatment during the perioperative period.

Moricizine

A fine review on moricizine was provided by Clyne and associates[43] from Boston, Massachusetts.

To assess the efficacy and toxicity of moricizine in treating patients with serious ventricular arrhythmias and inducible sustained VT, Damle and associates[44] from New York, New York, performed an uncontrolled

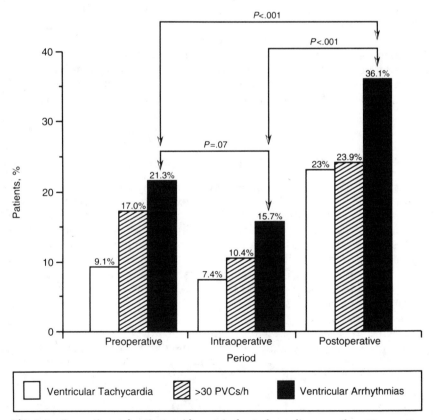

Fig. 4-4. Proportions of patients with ventricular tachycardia, more than 30 premature ventricular contractions (PVCs) per hour, or either, by time period. Reproduced with permission of Sforzini, et al.[42]

clinical trial involving 26 patients with sustained ventricular arrhythmias or hemodynamically significant nonsustained VT, most of whom failed therapy with at least one class I antiarrhythmic agent. The patients were treated with moricizine, 400 to 1000 mg/day. Efficacy was assessed by the results of programmed ventricular stimulation done during moricizine therapy. Seven of the 26 patients (27%) developed life-threatening ventricular proarrhythmia during moricizine loading. Three patients had incessant sustained VT, 2 had incessant nonsustained VT, 1 had new sustained VT, and 1 had new cardiac arrest. One of these patients died of intractable VF. No clinical or electrophysiologic variables clearly identified those at risk for proarrhythmia. Only 3 of 26 patients (12%) became noninducible on moricizine. Moricizine has a low rate of efficacy and carries a considerable risk for life-threatening proarrhythmia in patients with serious ventricular arrhythmias and inducible VT who have failed therapy with other class I antiarrhythmia agents.

To assess the short-term efficacy and safety of moricizine in patients receiving electrophysiologically guided therapy for sustained ventricular arrhythmias refractory to treatment with class 1A antiarrhythmic agents, Powell and associates[45] from Boston, Massachusetts, studied 21 patients (18 of whom had CAD) with a mean LVEF of 32% ± 11% who presented with sustained VT (13 patients), syncope (4 patients), or cardiac arrest. The patients were treated with moricizine 743 ± 85 mg/day. Electrophysiologic tests were performed in the drug-free state and after administration of moricizine unless sustained arrhythmias occurred. Sustained VT was inducible in the absence of antiarrhythmic drugs in 20 patients and was not suppressed by moricizine in any patient. Four patients had 6 episodes of spontaneous VT while receiving moricizine. A probable proarrhythmic response occurred in 4 patients. In patients with compromised LV function caused by CAD in whom class 1A antiarrhythmics were ineffective, moricizine was ineffective in suppressing sustained ventricular arrhythmias and resulted in proarrhythmic effects in some patients.

Propafenone and Mexiletine

Yeung-Lai-Wah and colleagues[46] in Vancouver, Canada, explored the potential efficacy of combined antiarrhythmic therapy with propafenone and mexiletine for control of sustained VT in 16 patients. Sixteen patients with sustained VT had their clinical arrhythmia induced by programmed stimulation. Procainamide and propafenone alone failed to prevent induction of VT in each patient. Mexiletine was subsequently added to propafenone and programmed stimulation was repeated. With combination therapy, VT was noninducible in three patients (19%). A fourth who had presented with polymorphic VT had slow bundle branch reentry. In the other 12 patients, tachycardia cycle length increased from 262 ± 60 ms at baseline to 350 ± 82 ms with propafenone and to 390 ± 80 ms with propafenone plus mexiletine. Hemodynamic deterioration requiring defibrillation occurred in 6 patients at baseline study, in 5 taking propafenone and in 2 taking both drugs. The combination of propafenone and mexiletine is effective in suppressing the induction of VT in some patients refractory to procainamide and propafenone alone, and in those in whom VT could still be induced, the heart rate was slower and hemodynamically better tolerated.

Metoprolol

Antiarrhythmic drug therapy guided by invasive electrophysiologic testing is now widely used in patients with symptomatic, sustained ventricular tachyarrhythmias. Steinbeck and associates[47] from Berlin, Germany, conducted a prospective, randomized trial in 170 patients to investigate whether this approach would improve long-term outcome. Patients whose arrhythmia was inducible by programmed electrical stimulation were assigned to treatment with electrophysiologically guided drug therapy based on serial testing (61 patients) or with metoprolol (54 patients). Electrophysiologically guided therapy consisted of serial testing of antiarrhythmic agents to identify the first one that rendered the arrhythmia noninducible. The 55 patients whose arrhythmia was noninducible during the initial electrophysiologic test were also treated with metoprolol. During a mean (± SD) follow-up period of 23 ± 17 months, recurrent, nonfatal arrhythmia occurred in 44 patients and sudden death due to cardiac factors in 27. The incidence of symptomatic arrhythmia and sudden death combined was virtually the same in the 2 groups with inducible arrhythmia after 2 years of observation (electrophysiologically guided therapy vs. metoprolol therapy, 46% vs 48%). The outcome was more favorable in the patients with noninducible arrhythmia at base line (75% had neither adverse event after 2 years) than in those with inducible arrhythmia who were assigned to metoprolol therapy. Only 6 of the 29 patients (21%) with inducible arrhythmia that became noninducible during drug therapy had recurrent arrhythmia or sudden death, as compared with 21 of the 32 patients (66%) with arrhythmia that continued to be inducible. A multivariate regression analysis identified continued inducibility of the arrhythmia as an independent predictor of recurrent arrhythmia or sudden death. As compared with metoprolol therapy, electrophysiologically guided antiarrhythmic drug therapy did not improve the overall outcome of patients with sustained VT. However, effective suppression of inducible arrhythmia by antiarrhythmic drugs was associated with a better outcome than was lack of suppression.

Sotalol

In an investigation by Kus and associates[48] from Montreal, Canada, the efficacy of oral sotalol in preventing sustained VT induction by invasive electrophysiological testing was assessed in 22 patients (60 ± 9 years) with prior myocardial infarction. Programmed stimulation consisted of 2 basic drives followed by up to 3 extrastimuli at 2 RV sites. At baseline, sustained monomorphic VT was inducible in all patients. With sotalol (360 ± 172 mg/day), it was no longer inducible in 10 patients; in 12 others, it remained inducible and its cycle length was minimally prolonged (322 ± 42 to 345 ± 44 msec). Sotalol markedly prolonged sinus cycle length, uncorrected QT interval, and RV effective and functional refractory periods, but had little effect on ventricular conduction time either in sinus rhythm or with RV pacing. There was no significant difference in drug dose or in electrophysiologic effect of drug that related to efficacy, nor was there any correlation between drug-induced prolongation of VT cycle length and its effects. Six patients received oral sotalol over the long-term without spontaneous recurrence of VT (follow-up 23 ± 18 months). These results demonstrate that sotalol is effective (45%) against sustained VT induction at moderate doses and is well tolerated over a long-term in the setting of remote myocardial infarction. However, its electrophysiologic effects as measured at invasive testing are not predictive of efficacy against VT induction.

In a study by Hohnloser and associates[49] from Freiburg, Germany, the antiarrhythmic and hemodynamic effects of sotalol (160 to 480 mg/day), a beta-blocking agent that prolongs ventricular repolarization, were examined in 38 patients with complex symptomatic ventricular ectopic activity. During ambulatory monitoring, 24 patients (63%) exhibited a reduction of > 75% in single VPCs and > 90% reduction in repetitive arrhythmia. In contrast to the effects of other agents, LVEF as determined by radionuclide angiography was not impaired, increasing slightly from 45 ± 14% to 47 ± 14% during therapy. Antiarrhythmic drug efficacy did not correlate with baseline EF or sotalol-induced changes in ventricular function. Late follow-up studies disclosed that antiarrhythmic efficacy and tolerance were maintained in the majority of patients. Repeat radionuclide angiography at 6 months revealed no late drug-induced depression of LV function. Sotalol appears to be an effective and well-tolerated agent for treatment of complex ventricular ectopic activity, even in the setting of compromised cardiac function.

Freedman and colleagues[50] in Salt Lake City, Utah, and New York, New York, examined the effect of sotalol on the signal-average ECG in patients with spontaneous and inducible sustained VT and correlated these findings with an effect of sotalol on tachycardia inducibility and tachycardia rate. Signal-averaged ECGs were obtained before therapy in 30 patients with spontaneous and inducible VT, and both electrophysiologic study and a signal-averaged ECG were repeated during therapy with d,l-sotalol. During sotalol therapy, the signal-averaged QRS duration decreased by 3 ± 7 ms in the 11 patients with no inducible tachycardia during therapy, whereas it increased by 4 ± 6 ms in the 19 patients with inducible tachycardia during therapy. In the latter group, there was a significant positive correlation between prolongation of tachycardia cycle length and prolongation of the late potential duration by sotalol. Sotalol can alter QRS and late potential durations as measured by the signal-averaged ECG. Prolongation of QRS duration or late potential duration may reflect a slowing of conduction caused by sotalol that interferes with this agent's antiarrhythmic efficacy and slow VT.

Amiodarone

In a study by Summitt and associates[51] from Ann Arbor, Michigan, the effects of 2 regimens for the initiation of amiodarone therapy were compared in 92 patients with inducible sustained VT at baseline electrophysiologic testing. Two groups of 46 patients each received a total of 17 gm of oral amiodarone before follow-up electrophysiologic testing. Group A (standard dose) received 1200 mg/day for 14 days, and group B (high dose) received 2400 mg/day for 7 days. Amiodarone suppressed the induction of sustained VT in 6 subjects (13%) in group A versus 10 (22%) in group B. In individuals who continued to have inducible VT after amiodarone loading, the mean increase in cycle length of induced VT was similar in group A and group B. The mean increase in sinus cycle length, AH and HV intervals, paced QRS duration, and ventricular refractory periods was also not significantly different between the 2 groups. Side effects developed in 10 (22%) patients in group B but were serious only in 1, and 1 patient required a reduction in dosage. Thus compared to the 14-day standard-dose regimen, the 7 day high-dose regimen was

well tolerated and had similar effects on VT inducibility and electrophysiologic variables. Its use may significantly shorten the duration of hospitalization in patients with life-threatening inducible VT who are undergoing
loading with amiodarone on an inpatient basis.

Magnesium

England and associates[52] from Boston, Massachusetts, and Baltimore,
Maryland, performed a study to determine whether magnesium administration is effective in reducing post-operative morbidity and mortality after
cardiac surgery. Over a 6-year period, 100 patients electively scheduled for
cardiac surgery involving cardiopulmonary bypass were studied. Fifty
patients were randomized to receive an intravenous infusion of magnesium chloride, 2 g, and 50 patients to receive placebo intraoperatively after
the termination of cardiopulmonary bypass. Magnesium-treated patients
had a significantly decreased frequency of postoperative ventricular dysrhythmias (8 [16%] of 50) compared with placebo-treated patients (17
[34%] of 50). Patients who were normomagnesemic postoperatively had
new supraventricular dysrhythmias less frequently than patients who
were hypomagnesemic postoperatively (8 [17%] of 48 vs 19 [37%] of 52).
Compared with placebo-treated patients, magnesium-treated patients
had significantly higher postoperative cardiac indices in the intensive
care unit (2.8 ± 0.1 vs 2.5 ± 0.1 L/min per m²). Patients with postoperative
total and ultrafilterable hypomagnesemia had postoperative ventricular
dysrhythmias and required prolonged mechanical ventilatory support
more frequently than patients without postoperative hypomagnesemia.
Total and ultrafilterable hypomagnesemia are prevalent findings in cardiac surgery patients, and postoperative hypomagnesemia is strongly
associated with clinically important morbidity. Magnesium administration decreased the frequency of postoperative ventricular dysrhythmias
and increased the stroke volume and thereby cardiac index in the early
postoperative period.

Effects of antiarrhythmic agents on blood lipids

Elevated levels of cholesterol and apoprotein B (apo B), the essential
carrier protein for LDL, are major lipid risk factors for premature CAD.
Antiarrhythmic agents are frequently prescribed to patients with CAD
and associated cardiac arrhythmias. As part of another study, Boden and
colleagues[53] in Rochester, New York, retrospectively investigated the effect
of antiarrhythmic agents on blood lipids. The study population consisted
of 1,567 postinfarction patients on whom the investigators prospectively
collected serial blood samples for lipid and apoprotein determinations
and recorded the concomitant medications the patients were receiving
at three follow-up time periods. The lipids, analyzed at a central core
laboratory, included total cholesterol, triglycerides, HDL, and apoproteins
A-I, A-II, and apo B. The difference in the group mean lipid values for
patients receiving and not receiving type Ia antiarrhythmic agents (quinidine, procainamide, and disopyramide) was elevated by the two-sample
t test, and multiple linear regression analyses were performed to adjust
for relevant covariates. Patients using type Ia antiarrhythmic agents at
the 30-month postinfarction contact had 9% lower cholesterol, 22% lower
triglycerides, 6% lower apo A-I, 10% lower apo A-II, and 13% lower apo
B levels than patients not on these medications. These lower lipid levels
were found after adjustment for age, sex, diabetes, smoking status, con-

comitant medications, and a variety of clinical factors relating to the severity of CAD. The HDL levels were similar in those receiving and not receiving type Ia agents. Patients on type Ia antiarrhythmic agents had significantly and meaningfully lower cholesterol, triglyceride, apo A-II, and apo B levels than patients not receiving these agents. The mechanism of this hypolipidemic effect is undefined, but the mechanism may be related to an alteration by these agents of ionic membrane currents at the hepatocyte level.

Radiofrequency catheter ablation

Radiofrequency energy has been used safely and successfully to eliminate accessory pathways in patients with the WPW syndrome and the substrate for AV nodal reentrant tachycardia. However, this form of ablation has had only limited success in eliminating VT in patients with structural heart disease. In contrast, direct-current catheter ablation has been used successfully to eliminate VT in patients with and without structural heart disease. The purpose of a study by Klein and co-workers[54] in Indianapolis, Indiana was to test whether radiofrequency energy can safely and effectively ablate VT in patients without structural heart disease. Sixteen patients (9 women and 7 men; mean age, 38 years) without structural heart disease who had VT underwent radiofrequency catheter ablation to eliminate the VT. Two patients presented with syncope, 9 with presyncope, and 5 with palpitations only. Mean duration of symptoms was 7 years. Radiofrequency catheter ablation successfully eliminated VT in 15 of 16 patients. Sites of VT origin included the high RV outflow tract (12 patients), the RV septum near the tricuspid valve (3 patients), and the LV septum (1 patient). The only ablation failure was in a patient whose VT arose from a region near the His bundle. An accurate pace map, early local endocardial activation, and firm catheter contact with endocardium were associated with successful ablation. Radiofrequency ablation did not cause arrhythmias, produced minimal cardiac enzyme rise, and resulted in no detectable change in cardiac function by Doppler echocardiography. Radiofrequency catheter ablation of VT in patients without structural heart disease is effective and safe and may be considered as early therapy in these patients.

Surgical subendocardial resection

Introduction of the automatic implantable cardioverter defibrillator (AICD) has dramatically affected the surgical treatment of malignant ventricular tachyarrhythmias. Geha and associates[55] from Cleveland, Ohio, and New Haven, Connecticut, reviewed their 8-year experience with electrophysiologically directed subendocardial resection of LV scars in selected patients with malignant ventricular tachyarrhythmias. During the period, 348 consecutive patients were treated surgically for these arrhythmias (electrophysiologically directed subendocardial resection since 1983 and AICD since 1986). All patients undergoing subendocardial resection had organized VT as a result of AMI and most had LV aneurysms; of those undergoing AICD or AICD/CABG, 60% had VT, 15% had VF, and 25% had both or were noninducible. The 30-day mortality rate was 2.5% (3/197) for AICD, 5.4% (5/93) for AICD/CABG, and 8.6% (5/58 for subendocardial resection; these mortality figures are not significantly different. Late deaths in all groups were predominantly due to CHF, and actuarial survival as well as freedom from sudden death was similar between the groups at 4 years. Recurrent VT occurred in 167 of 282 (59%) of long-term survivors of AICD or AICD/CABG during follow-up and in 9 of 53 (17%) of those with subendocardial resection. Forty-eight percent of survivors of AICD or AICD/CABG required antiarrhythmic medications, whereas only 11% of those with SEr required antiarrhythmics. Long-term survival in each group is much higher than that reported for comparable patients with severe LV dysfunction treated medically. In those patients with organized VT and LV aneurysm who are judged able to survive the procedure, subendocardial resection offers a high likelihood of cure rather than simple prevention of sudden death.

In an investigation by Mittleman and associates[56] from Worcester, Massachusetts, the results of surgical therapy performed in 51 consecutive patients with VT were reviewed to determine short- and long-term predictors of success of such therapy in preventing recurrences of life-threatening ventricular arrhythmias. Of 41 patients (80%) who survived surgery, 40 had postoperative programmed stimulation and, of these patients, 78% (n = 31) had no inducible VT on no antiarrhythmic therapy. This group had a very low incidence of arrhythmia recurrence, with only 1 nonfatal episode of VT after a mean follow-up of 41 ± 30 months. In contrast, 2 of the 9 patients (22%) who had inducible arrhythmias postoperatively had cardiac arrest. Multivariate analysis identified 2 significant predictors of perioperative mortality in these patients: increased duration of cardiopulmonary bypass time and increased baseline pulmonary capillary wedge pressure. It was concluded that 1) patients who do not have inducible VT after arrhythmia surgery have a very low incidence of recurrent arrhythmia and 2) prolonged time of cardiopulmonary bypass and increased pulmonary capillary wedge pressure are predictive of perioperative mortality.

In an investigation by Niebauer and associates[57] from Ann Arbor, Michigan, the results in 33 patients with VT treated by endocardial resection were evaluated, with special emphasis on the presence of single or multiple morphologies preoperatively and intraoperatively. Multiple VT morphologies were induced in 16 patients and a single VT morphology was induced in the remaining 17. Intraoperative programmed stimulation failed to induce VT in 8 patients and visually-directed endocardial resection was performed. The remaining patients underwent map-guided resection. The surgical success rate did not correlate with any morphologic characteristics of the VT, such as BBB pattern or axis. In addition, concordance of VT morphologies preoperatively and intraoperatively before resection did not correlate with the surgical success rate. However, patients in whom multiple morphologies of VT were induced intraoperatively had a significantly higher success rate (100%) compared with those patients in whom only a single morphology was induced intraoperatively (50%). Long-term follow-up was maintained in 26 patients. VT recurred in 2 patients and VF recurred in 2 others who did not have inducible VT 1 week after endocardial resection. It was concluded that neither the preoperative morphologic characteristics of VT nor discordance between the morphologies of VT induced preoperatively and in the operating room influenced the outcome of endocardial resection. However, the surgical success rate is higher when multiple morphologies of VT are inducible in the operating room than when only 1 VT morphology is inducible.

CARDIAC ARREST

Review

A fine review of sudden cardiac death was reported in *Current Problems in Cardiology*, November 1992, by Gilman and Naccarelli.[58]

Definitions

To determine the effect of different case and survival definitions of out-of-hospital cardiac arrest on survival rate calculations, Valenzuela and associates[59] from Tucson, Arizona, analyzed a 22-month case series of nontraumatic, out-of-hospital cardiac arrests which involved a consecutive sample of 372 patients found without palpable pulse or spontaneous respiration. The main outcome measures were survival rate after cardiac arrest, calculated using 3 case definitions of arrest and 2 definitions of survival. Twenty percent of all patients survived to hospital admission and 6% survived to hospital discharge (Table 4-1). Twenty-six percent of adults whose collapse was witnessed survived to hospital admission, and 10% survived to hospital discharge. Patients whose collapse was witnessed and who experienced initial VF survived to hospital admission in 38% and to hospital discharge in 15% of cases. The survival rate after out-of-hospital cardiac arrest varies widely depending on the case and survival definitions selected (Figure 4-5).

Successful resuscitation

To determine factors related to mortality within hospital after successful resuscitation from VF outside hospital by a mobile coronary care unit manned by a physician, Dickey and Adgey[60] from Belfast, Northern Ireland, performed a retrospective review of records of patients resuscitated and

TABLE 4-1. *Out-of-Hospital Cardiopulmonary Arrest.* Reproduced with permission from Valenzuela, et al.[59]

| | Patient Populations | | |
	All Arrests	Witnessed Arrests	Witnessed Ventricular Fibrillation
No. of cases	372	217	118
Age, y (± SD)	64.1 (± 19.4)	67.2 (± 15.0)	66.0 (± 13.1)
Sex, M/F	228/144	124/93	79/39
Witnessed, No. (%)	220 (59)	217 (100)	118 (100)
Bystander CPR, No. (%)	111 (30)	87 (40)	53 (45)
Previous MI, No. (%)	68 (18)	43 (20)	30 (25)
Cardiac history, No. (%)	160 (43)	103 (47)	65 (55)
First response, mean (± SD), min ≤4 min, %	4.1 (± 1.5) 65	4.1 (± 1.6) 65	4.1 (± 1.6) 70
Medic response, mean (± SD), min ≤8 min, %	5.1 (± 2.0) 95	5.1 (± 2.1) 95	5.1 (± 2.0) 97
Survival to admission, No. (%)	75 (20)	57 (26)	45 (38)
Survival to discharge, No. (%)	22 (6)	21 (10)	18 (15)

*CPR represents cardiopulmonary resuscitation; MI, myocardial infarction. Witnessed indicates collapse was observed by bystanders; bystander CPR, basic CPR initiated by lay bystanders; previous MI, history of previous MI; and cardiac history, history of cardiac disease other than MI.

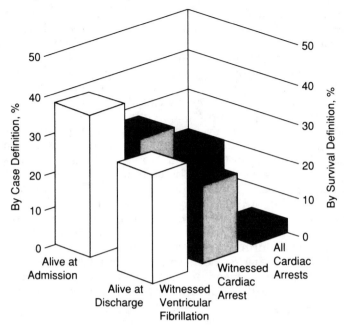

Fig. 4-5. Survival after out-of-hospital cardiac arrest as a function of case definition and survival definition. The case definitions are as follows: all arrests, all cases meeting study entry criteria; witnessed arrest, witnessed cardiac arrest in adults; and witnessed ventricular fibrillation, witnessed cardiac arrest in adults, with initial monitored cardiac rhythm of ventricular fibrillation. The survival definitions are as follows: alive at admission, vital signs present, patient admitted to cardiac care unit; and alive at discharge, patient discharged alive from initial hospitalization for cardiac arrest. Reproduced with permission from Valenzuela, et al.[59]

admitted to hospital between 1 January 1966 and 31 December 1987. A total of 281 patients (277 male), aged 14-82 years (mean 58) successfully resuscitated from VF outside hospital of whom 182 (65%) developed VF before the arrival of the mobile coronary care unit were studied. The aetiology of VF was AMI in 194 patients (69%), ischemic heart disease without infarction in 71 (25%), and other or unknown in 16 (6%). The main outcome measure was deaths occurring within the hospital. There were 91 deaths in the hospital (32%). Factors on univariate analysis significantly associated with increased mortality were patient age > 60 years, previous AMI or cerebrovascular disease, prior digoxin or diuretic treatment, collapse without prior chest pain or with pain lasting 30 minutes or less, defibrillation delayed by ≥ 5 min, ≥ 4 shocks required to correct FV, LV failure or pulmonary edema and cardiogenic shock after successful defibrillation, and coma on admission to hospital. On multivariate analysis the most important factors (in rank order) were cardiogenic shock after defibrillation, coma on admission to hospital, age ≥ 60 years, and the requirement for 4 or more shocks to correct VF.

Alcohol intake

To assess the relation between alcohol intake and sudden cardiac death (death within 1 hour of the onset of symptoms), Wannamethee and Shaper[61] performed a prospective study of a cohort of 7,735 men aged 40-59 years at screening and followed them up for 8 years. The main outcome measures were all deaths from CAD with particular reference to those that were sudden. During the follow-up period there were 217 deaths from CAD of which 117 (54%) were sudden. Although heavy drinkers (more than 6 drinks daily) did not show a high incidence rate of fatal heart attack, they showed the highest incidence rate of sudden cardiac death. This was seen in both manual and non-manual workers and was most clearly seen in older (50-59) men. Death from CAD was more likely to be sudden in heavy drinkers than in other drinking groups; this phenomenon was seen irrespective of the presence or degree of pre-existing CAD. The positive association between heavy drinking and the incidence of sudden death was most apparent in men without pre-existing CAD, with heavy drinkers showing an increase of 60% compared with occasional or light drinkers after adjustment for age, social class, and smoking, heavy drinkers free of pre-existing CAD had a marginally significantly higher incidence rate of sudden death than other drinkers combined. Additional adjustment for systolic BP reduced the risk to 1.7. This study suggests that heavy drinking is associated with an increased risk of sudden death. Studies that do not take pre-existing CAD into account are likely to underestimate the adverse effects of heavy drinking on the incidence of sudden death because the effects are not as evident in men with pre-existing CAD.

Heart rate variability in survivors

Reduced heart rate variability is associated with increased risk of cardiac arrest in patients with CAD. Huikuri and associates[62] from Oulu, Finland, and Miami, Florida, compared the power spectral components of HR variability and their circadian pattern in 22 survivors of out-of-hospital cardiac arrest not associated with AMI with those of 22 control patients matched with respect to age, sex, previous AMI, EF, and number of narrowed coronary arteries. Survivors of cardiac arrest had significantly lower 24-hour average standard deviation of RR intervals than control patients (29 ± 10 vs 51 ± 15 ms), and the 24-hour mean high frequency spectral area was also lower in survivors of cardiac arrest than in control patients (13 ± 7 ms^2 × 10 vs 28 ± 14 ms^2 × 10). In a single cosinor analysis, a significant circadian rhythm of heart rate variability was observed in both groups with the acrophase of standard deviation of RR intervals and high-frequency spectral area occurring between 3 and 6 a.m. which was followed by an abrupt decrease in heart rate variability after arousal. The amplitude of the circadian rhythm of heart rate variability is observed in the morning after awakening, corresponding to the time period at which the incidence of sudden cardiac death is highest.

In permanently paced patients

Permanent cardiac pacing is well established for the improvement of prognosis and quality of life in patients with severe bradycardia. However, sudden cardiac death still remains an unresolved problem, as it occurs in approximately 20–30% of paced patients. Zehender and colleagues[63] in Freiburg, Germany directed a 2-year follow-up study at prospectively assessing prevalence, circumstances, and mechanisms of sudden cardiac death in 2,021 permanently paced patients. During the observation period, 220 patients expired with a mean pacing interval of 51 months. Lethal cerebrovascular events occurred in 30% and sudden death in 22% which were the 2 most frequently reported modes of death. Nonsudden and sudden death mortality rate were highest during the first year. Mortality was unrelated to the patient's activity status at the time of death. Sudden cardiac death occurred more often in male patients and patients < 60 years of age. Patients with severe bradycardia, severe AV block, or AF with low ventricular rate before pacemaker implantation were more likely to suffer from sudden cardiac death than patients with previous syncopal attacks. The highest incidence of sudden death was observed in patients with bifascicular and trifascicular BBB. In this group, 35% of patients died suddenly during the follow-up period compared with 18% of patients without BBB. In a subsequent study in 90 consecutive patients with various types of BBB, undersensing of up to 13% of VPCs occurred in patients with bifascicular block. Pacing-induced tachyarrhythmias and VF were documented in 10% of undersensed VPCs as well as in the setting of AF associated with ventricular arrhythmias. Young age, male sex, and a severely diseased heart indicated by the presence of bifascicular and trifascicular BBB are the strongest predictive clinical parameters for sudden cardiac death, especially in the first year after the pacemaker implantation.

Cardiopulmonary resuscitation—review

A fine review of cardiopulmonary resuscitation appeared in the October 8, 1992, issue of the *New England Journal of Medicine.* The article was by James T. Niemann[64] of Los Angeles, California.

Epinephrine ± norepinephrine

Recent studies suggest that doses of epinephrine of 0.1 mg/kg of body weight or higher may improve myocardial and cerebral blood flow and also survival in patients having cardiac arrest. Such studies have called into question the traditional dose of epinephrine (0.007 to 0.014 mg per kg) recommended for advanced cardiac life support. Stiell and associates[65] from Ottawa, Canada, randomly assigned 650 patients who had had cardiac arrest either in or outside the hospital to receive up to 5 doses of high-dose (7 mg) or standard-dose (1 mg) epinephrine at 5-minute intervals according to standard protocols for advanced cardiac life support. Patients who collapsed outside the hospital received no advanced-life-support measures other than defibrillation before reaching the hospital. There was no significant difference between the high-dose group (n = 317) and the standard-dose group (n = 333) in the proportions of patients who survived for 1 hour (18% vs 23%, respectively) or who survived until hospital discharge (3% vs 5%). Among the survivors, there was no significant difference in the proportions who remained in the best category of cerebral performance (90% vs 94%) and no significant difference in the median Mini-Mental State score (36 vs 37). The exploration of clinically important subgroups, including those with out-of-hospital arrest (n = 335) and those with in-hospital arrest (n = 315), failed to identify any patients who appeared to benefit from high-dose epinephrine and suggested that some patients may have worse outcomes after high-dose epinephrine. High-dose epinephrine was not found to improve survival or neurologic outcomes in adult victims of cardiac arrest.

Experimental and uncontrolled clinical evidence suggests that intravenous epinephrine in doses higher than currently recommended may improve outcome after cardiac arrest. Brown and associates[66] for the Multicenter High-Dose Epinephrine Study Group from multiple US medical centers conducted a prospective multicenter study comparing standard-dose epinephrine with high-dose epinephrine in the management of cardiac arrest outside the hospital. Adult patients were enrolled in the study if they remained in VF, or if they had asystole or electromechanical dissociation, at the time the first drug was to be administered to treat the cardiac arrest. Patients were randomly assigned to receive either 0.02 mg of epinephrine per kilogram of body weight (standard-dose group, 632 patients) or 0.2 mg/kg (high-dose group, 648 patients), both given intravenously. In the standard-dose group 190 patients (30%) had a return of spontaneous circulation, as compared with 217 patients (33%) in the high-dose group; 136 patients (22%) in the standard-dose group and 145 patients (22%) in the high-dose group survived to be admitted to the hospital. Twenty-six patients (4%) in the standard-dose group and 31 (5%) in the high-dose group survived to discharge from the hospital. Ninety-two percent of the patients discharged in the standard-dose group and 94% in the high-dose group were conscious at the time of hospital discharge. None of the differences in outcome between the groups were statistically significant. In this study, the authors were unable to demonstrate any difference in the overall rate of return of spontaneous circulation, survival to hospital admission, survival to hospital discharge, or neurologic outcome between patients treated with a standard dose of epinephrine and those treated with a high dose.

To determine the relative efficacy of high- vs standard-dose catecholamines in initial treatment of prehospital cardiac arrest, Callaham and associates[67] from San Francisco, California, administered high-dose epinephrine (HDE, 15 mg), high-dose norepinephrine bitartrate (NE, 11 mg), or standard-dose epinephrine (SDE, 1 mg) for advanced cardiac life support doses of epinephrine. Of 2,694 patients with cardiac arrest during the study, resuscitation was attempted in 1,062 patients. Of this total, 816 patients met study criteria and were enrolled. In the entire cardiac arrest population, 63% of the survivors were among the 11% of patients who were defibrillated by first responders. The 3 drug treatment groups were similar for all independent variables. Thirteen percent of patients receiving HDE regained a pulse in the field vs 8% of those receiving SDE, and 18% of HDE patients were admitted to the hospital vs 10% of SDE patients who were admitted to the hospital. Similar trends for NE were not significant. There were 18 survivors; 1.7% of HDE patients and 2.6% of NE patients were discharged from the hospital compared with 1.2% of SDE patients, but this was not significant. There was a nonsignificant trend for Cerebral Performance Category scores to be worse for HDE (3.2) and NE patients (3.7) than for SDE patients (2.3). No significant complications were identified. High-dose epinephrine did not produce longer hospital or critical care unit stays. High-dose epinephrine significantly improves the rate of return of spontaneous circulation and hospital admission in patients who are in prehospital cardiac arrest without increasing complications. No benefit of NE compared with HDE was identified.

Sudden infant death syndrome

Sudden Infant Death Syndrome (SIDS) (the abrupt and unexplained death of an apparently healthy infant) is the second leading cause of infant mortality in the USA and the 8th leading cause of years of potential life lost. The *Morbidity and Mortality Weekly Report* of July 17, 1992, carried a piece which summarized race and regions specific data for SIDS during 1980–1988.[68] The analysis examined death certificate data from public-use mortality data tapes compiled by the Center for Disease Control's National Center for Health Statistics and included infants aged ≤ 364 days at the time of death from SIDS who were born to US residents. Neonatal deaths were defined as deaths among infants aged < 28 days; postneonatal deaths were those among infants aged 28–364 days. Rates of SIDS were calculated by dividing the number of SIDS cases in a year by the number of live-born infants in that calendar year. From 1980–1988, 47,932 infants born to US residents died from SIDS. During that time, overall SIDS rates declined 3.5% for white infants and 19.2% for black infants. In addition, throughout the 9-year period, SIDS rates were higher for black infants than for white infants. The black-to-white rate ratio declined from 2.2 in 1980 to 1.8 in 1988. Of all SIDS cases, 92.4% in 1980 and 93.2% in 1988 were postneonatal deaths. Autopsy rates for deaths diagnosed as resulting from SIDS increased from 82.3% in 1980 to 92.5% in 1988.

LONG Q-T INTERVAL SYNDROME

Genetics

Recombinant DNA technologies have facilitated the development of a set of polymorphic DNA markers covering the human genome. General linkage analysis in families predisposed to inherited disease is now feasible. Linkage analysis can help identify a disease gene even when relatively little is known about the disorder. Using this approach, Keating[69] in Salt Lake City, Utah, identified linkage between a gene that causes the long QT syndrome and DNA markers on chromosome 11. The identification of the chromosomal location of the long QT locus is the first step in defining the specific mutations that cause this disease.

Clinical features in carriers vs noncarriers

The familial long-QT syndrome is characterized by a prolonged QT interval on the electrocardiogram, ventricular arrhythmias, and sudden death. It is not certain, however, that the length of the QT interval is a sensitive or a specific diagnostic criterion. Recently, Vincent and associates[70] from Salt Lake City, Utah, identified genetic markers on chromosome 11 that distinguished between carriers and noncarriers of the gene for the long-QT syndrome in 3 families. They compared the clinical features of carriers and noncarriers and assessed the diagnostic accuracy of the QT interval. The authors obtained medical histories and electrocardiograms from 199 family members. QT intervals corrected for heart rate (QT_c) were determined independently by 2 blinded investigators. Carriers of the long-QT gene (83 subjects) and noncarriers (116 subjects) were distinguished by genetic-linkage analysis. Fifty-two carriers of the long-QT genes (63%) had a history of syncope, whereas 4 (5%) had a history of aborted sudden death. The QT_c intervals of the gene carriers ranged from 0.41 to 0.59 seconds (mean, 0.49). By contrast, the QT_c intervals of the noncarriers ranged from 0.38 to 0.47 second (mean, 0.42) (Figure 4-6). On average, carriers of the gene for the long-QT syndrome had longer QT_c intervals than noncarriers, but there was substantial overlap (in 126 of 199 subjects, or 63%). The use of a QT_c interval above 0.44 second as a diagnostic

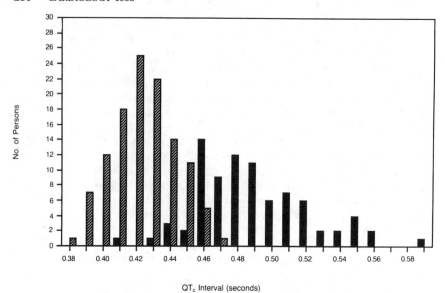

Fig. 4-6. Distribution of QT_c Intervals among Carriers (Solid Bars) and Noncarriers (Hatched Bars) of the Long-QT Gene in All Three Kindreds Studied. The number of persons of either sex who had a given QT_c interval is shown. Spouses are not included. Reproduced with permission from Vincent, et al.[70]

criterion resulted in 22 misclassifications among the 199 family members (11%). QT_c intervals of 0.47 second or longer in males and 0.48 second or longer in females were completely predictive but resulted in false negative diagnoses in 40% of the males and 20% of the females. In families affected by the long-QT syndrome, measurement of the QT_c interval may not permit an accurate diagnosis. DNA markers make it possible to make a genetic diagnosis in some families, but not all gene carriers have symptoms.

Late potentials

Tobé and associates[71] in Groningen, The Netherlands, determined the incidence of late potentials and their relation to QT prolongation in a family with a high incidence of sudden death during sleep at a young age and bradycardia-dependent QT prolongation and compared the findings with those in family members without QT prolongation. Six (67%) of the 9 family members with QT prolongation had late potentials on the signal-averaged electrocardiogram compared with 1 of 13 normal subjects. Positive predictive accuracy of the signal-averaged electrocardiogram for the detection of subjects with QT prolongation was 86% and the negative predictive accuracy was 80%. During exercise testing, the QT interval normalized, whereas late potentials did not change. Exercise testing did not reveal the presence of CAD as a possible cause of late potentials. Thus, compared with family members with a normal QT interval, patients with a long QT interval have a high incidence of late potentials; late potentials persist despite normalization of the QT interval and high heart rates and late potentials are not causes by CAD in these subjects. The detection of late potentials might be a new aid in the detection and risk stratification of patients with the long QT syndrome.

Beta-blocker and pacing

Eldar and associates[72] in San Francisco, California, reviewed current experience using a combination of beta-adrenergic blocking agents and long-term cardiac pacing to treat patients with the idiopathic long QT syndrome. Patients with the idiopathic long QT syndrome are at high risk for sudden cardiac death. Before combination therapy, 20 of the 21 study patients experienced cardiac arrest (n = 8) or syncope (n = 18) and 11 had documented polymorphous VT. Nine of these patients had not responded to isolated beta-blocker therapy and 5 had not responded to isolated left cervicothoracic sympathectomy. All patients were treated with combined beta-blocker therapy and long-term cardiac pacing at a rate designed to normalize the QT interval. Cardiac pacing at rates of 70 to 125 beats/min resulted in shortening the QT and corrected QT intervals from 517 ± 78 and 541 ± 62 ms to 404 ± 37 and 479 ± 41 ms, respectively. The mean follow-up interval after institution of pacing was 55 ± 45 months. The only sudden death occurred in a patient who had discontinued beta-blocker therapy. Syncope occurred in 4 patients, two of whom had interrupted pacemaker function due to lead fracture. Pacemaker problems, partly attributable to the specific rate required for QT interval shortening and to avoidance of T wave sensing were relatively common. No patient who continued the combination therapy died, but 10% of these patients had a recurrence of symptoms. Therefore, these data suggest that combination therapy with a beta-blocker and cardiac pacing appear to be a highly effective primary therapy for symptomatic patients with the long QT syndrome and in whom other therapies have been unsuccessful. This type of therapy might also provide excellent adjunctive therapy for patients who require insertion of an automatic internal defibrillator.

SYNCOPE

A good review of syncope was published by Kapoor[73] in the JAMA, November 11, 1992.

In an investigation by Brignole and associates[74] from Borzonasca, Italy, between 1982 and 1988, they observed 312 patients who were affected by syncope or presyncope and whose spontaneous symptoms could be reproduced by means of carotid sinus massage; no other definite cause of syncope could be identified. The clinical outcome during a 2 to 8 year follow-up period (mean 44 ± 24 months) was assessed in 262 of these patients (mean age 71 ± 11 years; 183 men) and compared with that of a group of 55 patients who were affected by unexplained syncope (control patients) who were matched 4:1 for age and sex with carotid sinus hypersensitivity patients. Carotid sinus hypersensitivity patients had an overall mortality rate of 7.3 per 100 person-years (cardiovascular 66%; sudden death 9%); overall predicted cumulative survival rates at 1, 3, 5, and 7 years were 92%, 80%, 66%, and 53%. Survival was similar in control patients: mortality rate was 5.8 per 100 person-years (cardiovascular 82%; sudden death 18%); cumulative survival rates at 1, 3, 5, and 7 years were 85%, 80%, 74%, and 69%. Standardized mortality rate of the general population with similar age and sex distribution, as calculated by means of Italian Istituto Centrale di Statistica death-rate data (1987 edition) was 8 per 100 person-years. Of 13 clinical variables, age, sex, abnormal electrocardiogram, and heart failure (but not carotid sinus hypersensitivity type or related arrhythmias) were independently linked to mortality in carotid sinus hypersensitivity patients. In the vasodepressor form of carotid sinus hypersensitivity, patients were younger than those with other forms of carotid sinus hypersensitivity and the percentage of women was higher. In conclusion, the long-term outcome for carotid sinus hypersensitivity patients is similar to that observed in patients with unexplained syncope and in the general population; outcome in independent of carotid sinus hypersensitivity type.

PACING AND PACEMAKERS

Bernstein and Parsonnet[75] from Newark, New Jersey, conducted a survey of physicians who implant permanent cardiac pacemakers to identify practice patterns related to pacemaker-implantation frequency, hospital and implantation-facility characteristics, indications for pacing and pulse-generator replacement, preferences regarding device types, pacing modes, follow-up methods and frequency, and type and frequency of pacing-related complications. Questionnaires were sent to 11,414 potential physician respondents and 6 pacemaker manufacturers. Implanters' opinions were solicited regarding such issues as the importance of various device features and capabilities, the appropriateness of practice guidelines, and the efficacy of quality-assurance measures. In 1989, 89,445 primary pacemaker implantations and 21,055 pulse-generator replacements were performed by approximately 7,919 physicians at about 3,400 U.S. centers. Typically, a pacemaker manufacturer's sales representative played an active role in 80% of cases. Since the last survey, which examined pacing practices in 1985, primary implantations of dual-chamber pacemakers increased from 22 to 32%, and the proportion of adaptive-rate pacemakers increased from 1 to 40% of primary implants. The "typical" implanter used bipolar electrode systems in 90% of cases, single-chamber pacemakers in 70%, and the introducer method in 95% of lead placements. Significant differences in practice patterns were found among subsets of the survey respondents. Surgeons tended to work alone, use simpler, single-chamber pacemakers, and leave follow-up to others. Electrode stability tended to be better among implanters in nonacademic environments. The quadrennial survey continues to provide useful information on an easily identifiable and traceable patient population, but the process would be greatly simplified by the adoption of a "universal" reporting system such as that used in Europe.

In a study by Gwinn and associates[76] from Charleston, South Carolina, 38 patients (ages 40 to 77 years, mean 63) followed in a pacemaker clinic underwent exercise treadmill tests to determine chronotropic incompetence. There were 28 men and 10 women. Twenty-seven patients had A-V block and 11 patients had sick sinus syndrome. All patients were exercised to fatigue. None of the patients were receiving beta-blockers or other drugs that could reduce heart rate. Maximum heart rate and percent predicted maximum heart rate were used as an index of chronotropic incompetence. Chronotropic incompetence was defined as inability to achieve a percent predicted maximum heart rate of $> 80\%$. The overall incidence of chronotropic incompetence was 58% (22 of 38 patients). The relationship between chronotropic incompetence and the time to pacemaker implantation was evaluated: in patients who had pacemakers for < 2 years, the mean maximum heart rate was 125 ± 22 beats/min compared with 112 ± 24 beats/min for patients who had pacemakers implanted for > 4 years. Similarly, the mean percent predicted maximum heart rate decreased from 77 ± 13% to 69 ± 15% in patients with pacemakers < 2 years versus those with pacemakers for > 4 years. Fifty-three percent of the patients with a pacemaker < 2 years old were chronotropic incompetent versus 70% of the patients with a pacemaker > 4 years old. These data suggest that chronotropic incompetence worsens with time after pacemaker input. To further support this, 8 patients with A-V block underwent a second stress test an average of 2 years following the first. In every case, both the maximum heart rate and percent predicted maximum heart rate decreased on the repeat stress test; mean maximum heart rate decreased from 133 ± 12 to 106 ± 26 beats/min and mean percent predicted maximum heart rate fell from 82 ± 7% to 66 ± 17%. This demonstrates a worsening of chronotropic incompetence over a relatively short period of time (approximately 2 years). Thus it was concluded that there is a marked incidence of chronotropic incompetence in this pacemaker population that includes a large percentage (71%) of patients with A-V block. Chronotropic incompetence is progressive and worsens over a short time after pacemaker implantation. Therefore chronotropic competent patients requiring pacemakers should be considered for a sensor-driven pacemaker at the initial implant because of the possibility of progressive chronotropic incompetence.

Johns and associates[77] from Nashville, Tennessee, reported on placement of 23 epicardial pacing leads in 12 patients age 3 weeks to 18 years with 8 atrial and 15 ventricular leads. Ventricular pulse width thresholds did not change over time whereas atrial pulse width thresholds improved significantly. At 6 months the mean pulse width threshold at 2.5 V for the atrial and ventricular leads was 0.1 ± .03 and 0.19 ± .09 ms respectively. The thresholds were slightly lower at 12 and 18 months. At most recent follow-up all atrial leads sensed appropriately at 2.5 mV and all ventricular leads at 5 mV. These encouraging results indicate the usefulness of epicardial leads in pediatric patients. These are an attractive option for infants and children who may require life-long pacing and in whom intravenous pacing may run a significant risk for thrombotic complications.

CARDIOVERTERS/DEFIBRILLATORS

Saksena and the Guardian Multicenter Investigators Group[78] evaluated a second-generation implantable pacemaker-cardioverter-defibrillator in 200 patients with sustained VT, VF or prior cardiac arrest. The device permits demand ventricular pacing for bradyarrhythmias and for long QT interval or tachycardia suppression, using programmable energy shocks for conversion of VT and VF, and is used with conventional pacing and defibrillation leads. VT/VF recognition is based on the ventricular electrogram rate and requires reconfirmation before shock delivery. Two hundred patients were enrolled and followed for 0 to 23 months. Epicardial lead system implantation was performed with the use of an anterolateral thoracotomy, median sternotomy, and subxiphoid or subcostal approach. Perioperative mortality was 5.5%. Implantation defibrillation threshold ranged from 3 to 30 joules. VT/VF sensing threshold ranged from 0.7 to 1.8 mV and the tachycardia detection interval from 288 to 416 ms. Reprogramming of implant variables was necessary for reliable electrocardiographic sensing, programmed shock therapy, and tachycardia detection rate. Device activation for potential shock delivery occurred in 111 patients with actual shock delivery after VT/VF reconfirmation in 66 patients. During follow-up, there was a 1% arrhythmia mortality rate, 6.5% cardiac mortality rate and 10.5% total mortality rate (Figure 4-7).

Newman and associates[79] from San Francisco, California, compared the actuarial survival of 60 consecutive recipients of the implanted cardioverter defibrillator (ICD) with 120 matched concurrent medically treated patients using a case-control design. All ICD patients and controls presented with either sustained VT or VF. Controls were matched in ICD recipients according to 5 variables: age, LVEF, arrhythmia at presentation, underlying heart disease and drug therapy status. Mean ages were 58 and 59 years with ICD patients and controls, and the average EFs were 36 and 35%. CAD was present in 75 and 79% of ICD patients and controls, respectively. During follow-up, sudden deaths were fewer in ICD recipients than in controls (5 vs 10%). At 1 and 3 years, actuarial survival was 0.89 versus 0.72 and 0.65 vs 0.49 for ICD recipients and controls. The 5-year actuarial survival curves were significantly different by the Cox proportional hazards model. It is concluded that in this retrospective case-control study, the use of the ICD in the management of patients at risk for sudden death results in improved probability of survival.

Kim and co-workers[80] in the Bronx, New York, compared the outcomes of patients treated with implantable defibrillators with LVEF ≥ 30% and < 30%. Of 68 consecutive patients treated with implantable defibrillators, 40 patients (group 1) had LVEF ≥ 30%, and 28 patients (group 2) had LVEF < 30%. Sudden death, surgical mortality, nonsudden arrhythmia-related death (death within 24 hours after an arrhythmic event despite initial termination of the arrhythmia by the implantable defibrillator), total arrhythmia-related death (including sudden death, surgical death, and nonsudden arrhythmia-related death), and total cardiac death were

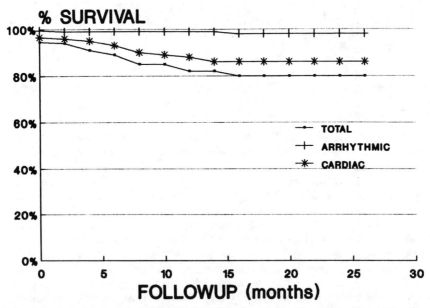

Fig. 4-7. Long-term survival of the study patients assessed with a Kaplan-Meier life table survival analysis. Arrhythmic, cardiac and total deaths are plotted over the follow-up period of 2 years. Reproduced with permission from Saksena, et al.[78]

compared between the 2 groups. Surgical mortality was 4% (0% in group 1, 11% in group 2). During the follow-up of 31 months, actuarial survival rates free of events were 97%, 97% and 97% in group 1 and 96%, 91% and 82% in group 2 at 12, 24, and 36 months, respectively, for sudden death; 97%, 97%, and 97% in group 1 and 85%, 81% and 72% in group 2 at 12, 24, and 36 months, respectively, for sudden death and surgical mortality; 97%, 97%, and 97% in group 1 and 82%, 78%, and 70% in group 2 at 12, 24, and 36 months, respectively, for total arrhythmia-related death; and 95%, 95%, and 95%, in group 1 and 82%, 69%, and 57% in group 2 at 12, 24, and 36 months, respectively, for total cardiac death. Four of 7 nonsudden cardiac death during the initial 36-month follow-up period were causally related to arrhythmia (three surgical deaths and one arrhythmia-related nonsudden death). The outcome of patients treated with implantable defibrillators is strongly influenced by the degree of LV dysfunction. In group 1 patients, surgical mortality, sudden death, and total cardiac death are rare. In group 2, sudden death rate may not be markedly different from that of group 1 patients. However, the risk of therapy is high. Many nonsudden cardiac deaths are causally related to arrhythmia. Therefore, the survival rate free of total arrhythmia-related death is significantly lower in group 2 (70% vs 97% in group 1 at 3 years). Further studies are needed to determine the roles of defibrillator therapy and therapies in various clinical setting.

Successful defibrillation by an implantable cardioverter-defibrillator depends on its ability to deliver shocks that exceed the defibrillation threshold. Epstein and co-investigators[81] in Birmingham, Alabama, designed a study to identify clinical characteristics that may predict the finding of an elevated defibrillation threshold and to describe the outcome of patients with high defibrillation thresholds. The records of 1,946 patients from 12 centers were screened to identify 90 patients with a defibrillation threshold ≥ 25 J. Excluding 3 patients who received defibrillators that delivered > 30 J, there were 81 men and 6 women with a mean age of 59 years, a mean LV EF of 0.32, and a 76% prevalence of CAD. Sixty-one patients were receiving antiarrhythmic drugs, and 45 were receiving amiodarone. Seventy-one patients received a cardioverter-defibrillator. Death occurred in 27 patients—19 of the 71 with a defibrillator, and 8 of the 16 without a defibrillator. Actuarial survival for all patients at 5 years was 67%. Actuarial survival rates at 2 years for patients with and without a defibrillator were 81% and 36%, respectively. Survival at 5 years for the defibrillator patients was 73%; no patient without a defibrillator has lived longer than 32 months. Actuarial survival free of arrhythmic death in the defibrillator patients at 5 years was 84%. Although the only variable to predict survival was defibrillator implantation, it is entirely possible that in this retrospective analysis, clinical selection decisions to implant or not to implant a defibrillator differentiated patients destined to have better or worse outcomes, respectively. Antiarrhythmic drug use may be causally related to the finding of an elevated defibrillation threshold. When patients with high defibrillation thresholds receive a defibrillator, arrhythmic death remains an important risk. Vigorous testing to optimize patch location can potentially benefit patients by enhancing the margin of safety for effective defibrillation.

Shock delivery of an implantable defibrillator may cause a change in the amplitude of endocardial electrograms and impair the detection of VF. Jung and colleagues[82] in Bonn, Germany, evaluated the effects of shock discharges on the amplitude of endocardial electrograms in 5 patients undergoing implantation of a cardioverter-defibrillator in combination with a new nonthoracotomy lead system. At implant, bipolar endocardial electrograms were recorded before each shock application, during VF, during redetection of VF in case the applied shock was ineffective, and at intervals of 5, 10, 20, 30, 60, and 120 seconds after each shock delivery. The amplitude of the endocardial electrograms decreased from 10 mV during sinus rhythm to 6 mV during initial VF and declined to 2 mV during redetection of VF. At predischarge testing, failure of redetection of VF could be documented in 2 patients, requiring rescue external defibrillation in both cases to restore sinus rhythm. These findings demonstrate that the implantable cardioverter-defibrillator did not ensure reliable redetection of VF in patients using the implanted nonthoracotomy lead system. Thus, the potential risk of sudden cardiac death may persist in these patients despite defibrillator therapy.

The quantitative benefit of implantable cardioverter-defibrillator therapy in patients with malignant ventricular tachyarrhythmia with different degrees of LV dysfunction is unclear. Thus, Mehta and associates[83] from Passaic and Newark, New Jersey, evaluated patterns of implantable cardioverter-defibrillator use and survival in 112 patients with moderate to severe LV dysfunction. Group 1 included 57 patients with moderate LV dysfunction (defined as LVEF > 30%) and group 2 comprised 55 patients with severe LV dysfunction (defined as EF ≤ 30%). The follow-up period ranged from 1 to 78 months. Age, incidence of CAD, and presenting arrhythmia in the 2 groups were similar. The mean LVEF in group 1 was 45 ± 8% and in group 2 was 22 ± 6%. At 3 years of follow-up 65% of the patients in group 1 and 71% in group 2 had similar implantable cardioverter-defibrillator activation for presumed VT. Survival was calculated by means of actuarial analysis. Arrhythmia or sudden death mortality at 4 years of follow-up was similar at 5% in group 1 and 9% in group 2. Cardiac mortality was higher in patients with severe LV dysfunction reaching levels of statistical significance at 2 years of follow-up. At 2 years of follow-up it was 12% in group 1 and 40% in group 2, and at 4 years of follow-up it was 15% in group 1 and 43% in group 2. In both groups there was no difference in cardiac mortality in patients who did and did not have appropriate implantable cardioverter-defibrillator shocks. It was concluded that the observed incidence of long-term implantable cardioverter-defibrillator use is comparable in patients with moderate and severe LV dysfunction. However, cardiac mortality is higher in patients with severe LV dysfunction regardless of device use. The long-term clinical outcome of implantable cardioverter-defibrillator device users and nonusers in these 2 subgroups with different degrees of LV dysfunction is comparable. This can be related to elimination of arrhythmic mortality by the implantable cardioverter-defibrillator in patients with LV dysfunction and recurrent ventricular tachyarrhythmias.

MISCELLANEOUS

Transient electrocardiographic changes and arrhythmias are known to be acute manifestations of cardiotoxicity secondary to cancer therapy with antiacyclines or cardiac irradiation. Despite the known risk of late cardiac dysfunction in survivors of childhood cancer therapy, the risk of clinically important electrocardiographic abnormalities and arrhythmias after treatment is unknown. Larsen and associates[84] from Philadelphia, Pennsylvania, recorded standard 12-lead and 24-hour ambulatory electro-

TABLE 4-2. *Arrhythmias Detected by 24-Hour Electrocardiography in Survivors of Childhood Cancer. Reproduced with permission from Larsen, et al.*[84]

	Supraventricular Premature Complexes	Supraventricular Tachycardia	Ventricular Premature Complexes	Ventricular Couplets	Ventricular Tachycardia
Anthracyclines (1–199 mg/m²)	8/14 (57%)*	0/14 (0%)	4/14 (29%)	0/14 (0%)	0/14 (0%)
Anthracyclines (200–299 mg/m²)	17/28 (61%)*	2/28 (7%)*	9/28 (36%)	1/28 (4%)†	0/28 (0%)
Anthracyclines (300–399 mg/m²)	16/21 (76%)*	0/21 (0%)	14/21 (67%)*	0/21 (0%)	0/21 (0%)
Anthracyclines (≥ 400 mg/m²)	5/10 (50%)*	0/10 (0%)	7/10 (70%)*	1/10 (10%)†	0/10 (0%)
Cardiac irradiation	15/24 (63%)*	1/24 (4%)*	12/24 (50%)*	0/24 (0%)	1/24 (4%)†
Both anthracyclines and irradiation	27/37 (73%)*	0/37 (0%)	23/37 (62%)*	3/37 (8%)*	3/37 (8%)*
All patients	(66%)*	(2%)*	(52%)*	(4%)*	(3%)*

*$p < 0.001$; †$p < 0.01$ (probabilities compared with that in normal subjects).

cardiograms in 73 patients who received anthracyclines alone, 24 who received cardiac irradiation alone, and 27 who received both anthracyclines and cardiac irradiation. The mean age of the patients was 15 years. Mean cumulative anthracycline dose was 282 mg/m² in patients who received anthracyclines alone and 244 mg/m² in patients who received both anthracyclines and cardiac irradiation. Analysis of the 12-lead and 24-hour electrocardiograms demonstrated increased frequency of QTc prolongation, supraventricular premature complexes, SVT, VPCs, couplets and VT when compared with an age-matched healthy population (Table 4-2). Most patients had abnormalities limited to single supraventricular or VPCs; however, potentially serious ventricular ectopic activation, including ventricular pairs and VT, were noted in patients with cumulative doses > 200 mg/m². Electrocardiographic abnormalities and arrhythmias are not limited to the acute phase of treatment with anthracyclines and cardiac irradiation. Survivors of childhood malignancy who received anthracyclines or cardiac irradiation, or both, probably should undergo ambulatory electrocardiographic monitoring as part of their follow-up to detect potentially life-threatening arrhythmias.

References

1. Grogan M, Smith HC, Gersh BJ, Wood DL: Left ventricular dysfunction due to atrial fibrillation in patients initially believed to have idiopathic dilated cardiomyopathy. Am J Cardiol 1992 (June 15); 69:1570–1573.

2. Liang-Miin Tsai, Jyh-Hong Chen, Ching Jing Fang, Li-Jen Lin, Chi-Ming Kwan: Clinical implications of left atrial spontaneous echo contrast in nonrheumatic atrial fibrillation. Am J Cardiol 1992 (Aug 1); 70:327–331.

3. Stroke Prevention in Atrial Fibrillation Investigators: Predictors of thromboembolism in atrial fibrillation: I. Clinical features of patients at risk. An Intern Med 1992 (Jan 1); 116:1–5.

4. Stroke Prevention in Atrial Fibrillation Investigators: Predictors of thromboembolism in atrial fibrillation: II. Echocardiographic features of patients at risk. An Intern Med 1992 (Jan 1); 116:6–12.

5. Pritchett ELC: Management of atrial fibrillation. N Engl J Med 1992 (May 7); 326:1264–1271.

6. Corbalan R, Arriagada D, Braun S, Tapia J, Huete I, Kramer A, Chavez A: Risk factors for systemic embolism in patients with paroxysmal atrial fibrillation. Am Heart J 1992 (July); 124:149–153.

7. Reimold SC, Chalmers TC, Berlin JA, Antman EM: Assessment of the efficacy and safety of antiarrhythmic therapy for chronic atrial fibrillation: Observations on the role of trial design and implications of drug-related mortality. Am Heart J 1992 (October); 124:24–932.

8. Roth A, Kaluski E, Felner S, Heller K, Laniado S: Clonidine for patients with rapid atrial fibrillation. An Intern Med 1992 (Mar 1); 116:388–390.

9. Gentili C, Giordano F, Alois A, Massa E, Bianconi L. Efficacy of intravenous propafenone in acute atrial fibrillation complicating open-heart surgery. Am Heart J 1992 (May); 123:1225–1228.

10. Dattilo GL, Eriksson CE Jr, Vestal RE: Increased ventricular response rate during exercise in patients with atrial fibrillation treated with theophylline. Arch Intern Med 1992 (Apr); 152:797–803.

11. Gosselink ATM, Crijns HJGM, Van Gelder IC, Hillige H, Wiesfeld ACP, Lie KI: Low-dose amiodarone for maintenance of sinus rhythm after cardioversion of atrial fibrillation or flutter. JAMA 1992 (June 24); 267:3289–3293.

12. Falk: Proarrhythmia in patients treated for atrial fibrillation or flutter. An Intern Med 1992 (July 15); 117:141–150.

13. Heinz G, Siostrzonek P, Kreiner G, Gossinger H: Improvement in left ventricular systolic function after successful radiofrequency His bundle ablation for drug refractory, chronic atrial fibrillation and recurrent atrial flutter. Am J Cardiol 1992 (Feb 15); 69:489–492.

14. Singer DE, Hughes RA, Gress DR, Sheehan MA, Oertel LB, Maraventano SW, Blewett DR, Rosner B, Kistler JP, for the BAATAF Investigators: The effect of aspirin on the risk of stroke in patients with nonrheumatic atrial fibrillation: The BAATAF study. Am Heart J 1992 (December); 124:1567–1573.

15. Ezekowitz MD, Bridgers SL, James KE, Carliner NH, Colling CL, Gornick CC, Krause-Steinrauf H, Kurtzke JF, Nazarian SM, Radford MJ, Rickles FR, Shabetai R, Deykin D: Warfarin in the prevention of stroke associated with nonrheumatic atrial fibrillation. N Engl J Med 1992 (Nov 12); 327:1406–1412.

16. Flaker GC, Blackshear JL, McBride R, Knonmal RA, Halperin JL, Hart RG, on behalf of the Stroke Prevention in Atrial Fibrillation Investigators. Antiarrhythmic drug therapy and cardiac mortality in atrial fibrillation. J Am Coll Cardiol 1992 (September); 20:527–32.

17. Krahn AD, Manfreda J, Tate RB, Mathewson FAL, Cuddy TE: The natural history of electrocardiographic preexcitation in men: The Manitoba follow-up study. An Intern Med 1992 (Mar 15); 116:456–460.

18. Gursoy S, Steurer G, Brugada J, Andries E, Brugada P: Brief report: The hemodynamic mechanism of pounding in the neck in atrioventricular nodal reentrant tachycardia. N Engl J Med 1992 (Sept 10); 327:772–774.

19. Leitch JW, Klein GJ, Yee R, Leather RA, Kim YO: Syncope Associated with Supraventricular Tachycardia An Expression of Tachycardia Rate or Vasomotor Response? Circulation 1992 (March); 85:1064–1071.

20. Huikuri HV, Koistinen J, Takkunen JT: Efficacy of intravenous sotalol for suppressing inducibility of supraventricular tachycardias at rest and during isometric exercise. Am J Cardiol 1992 (Feb 15); 69:498–502.

21. Maragnes P, Tipple M, Fournier A: Effectiveness of oral sotalol for treatment of pediatric arrhythmias. Am J Cardiol 1992 (Mar 15); 69:751–754.

22. Mehta AV and Chidambaram B: Efficacy and Safety of Intravenous and Oral Nadolol for Supraventricular Tachycardia in Children. J Am Coll Cardiol (March 1) 1992; 19:630–635.

23. Hughes MM, Trohman RG, Simmons TW, Castle LW, Wilkoff BL, Morant VA, Maloney JD: Flecainide therapy in patients treated for supraventricular tachycardia with near normal left ventricular function. Am Heart J 1992 (February); 123:408–412.

24. Dougherty AH, Jackman WM, Naccarelli GV, Friday KJ, Dias VC: Acute conversion of paroxysmal supraventricular tachycardia with intravenous diltiazem. Am J Cardiol 1992 (Sept 1); 70:587–592.

25. Hood MA and Smith WM. Adenosine versus verapamil in the treatment of supraventricular tachycardia: A randomized double-crossover trial. Am Heart J 1992 (June); 123:1543–1549.

26. Keim S, Curtis AB, Belardinelli L, Epstein ML, Staples ED, Lerman BB. Adenosine-induced atrioventricular block: A rapid and reliable method to assess surgical and radiofrequency catheter ablation of accessory atrioventricular pathways. J Am Coll Cardiol 1992 (April); 19:1005–12.

27. Lesh MD, Van Hare GF, Schamp DJ, Chien W, Lee MA, Griffin JC, Langberg JJ, Cohen TJ, Lurie KG, Scheinman MM. Curative percutaneous catheter ablation using radiofrequency energy for accessory pathways in all locations: Results in 100 consecutive patients. J Am Coll Cardiol 1992 (May); 19:1303–9.

28. Kay G, Epstein A, Dailey S, Plumb V: Selective Radiofrequency Ablation of the Slow Pathway for the Treatment of Atrioventricular Nodal Reentrant Tachycardia, Evidence for Involvement of Perinodal Myocardium Within the Reentrant Circuit. Circulation 1992 (May); 85:1675–1688.

29. Jackman WM, Beckman KJ, McClelland JH, Wang X, Friday KJ, Roman CA, Moulton KP, Twidale N, Hazlitt HA, Prior MI, Overholt ED, Lazzara R: Treatment of supraventricular tachycardia due to atrioventricular nodal reentry by radiofrequency catheter ablation of slow-pathway conduction. N Engl J Med 1992 (July 30); 327:313–318.

30. Chen S-A, Tsang W-P, Hsia C-P, Wang D-C, Chiang C-E, Yeh H-I, Chen J-W, Ting C-T, Kong C-W, Wang S-P, Chiang BN, Chang M-S: Catheter ablation of accessory atrioventricular pathways in 114 symptomatic patients with Wolff-Parkinson-White syndrome—A comparative study of direct-current and radiofrequency ablation. Am Heart J 1992 (August); 124:356–365.

31. Walsh EP, Saul P, Hulse JE, Rhodes LA, Hordof AJ, Mayer JE, Lock JE: Transcatheter ablation of ectopic atrial tachycardia in young patients using radiofrequency current. Circulation (October) 1992; 86:1138–1146.

32. Case CL, Gillette PC, Oslizlok PC, Knick BJ, Blair HL: Radiofrequency catheter ablation of incessant, medically resistant supraventricular tachycardia in infants and small children. J Am Coll Cardiol (November 15) 1992; 20:1405–1410.

33. Haissaguerre M, Gaita F, Fischer B, Egloff P, Lemetayer P, Warin JF: Radiofrequency Catheter Ablation of Left Lateral Accessory Pathways Via the Coronary Sinus. Circulation 1992 (November); 86:1464–1468.

34. Yeh SJ, Wang CC, Lin FC, Chang JP, Chang CH, Wu D: Usefulness of predischarge electrophysiologic study in predicting late outcome after surgical ablation of the accessory pathway in the Wolff-Parkinson-White syndrome. Am J Cardiol 1992 (Apr 1) 69:909–912.

35. Crawford FA Jr, Gillette PC, Case CL, Zeigler V: Surgical management of dysrhythmias in infants and small children. An Surg 1992 (Sept) 318–326.

36. Andresen D, Steinbeck G, Broggemann T, Haberl R, Fink L, Schroder R: Prognosis of patients with sustained ventricular tachycardia and of survivors of cardiac arrest not inducible by programmed stimulation. Am J Cardiol 1992 (Nov 15); 70:1250–1254.

37. Bikkina M, Larson MG, Levy D: Prognostic implications of asymptomatic ventricular arrhythmias: The Framingham Heart Study. An Intern Med 1992 (Dec 15); 117:990–996.

38. Ferrick KJ, Luce J, Miller S, Mercando AD, Kim SG, Roth JA, Fisher JD: Reproducibility of electrophysiologic testing during antiarrhythmic therapy for ventricular arrhythmias secondary to coronary artery disease. Am J Cardiol 1992 (May 15); 69:1296–1299.

39. Wiles HB, Gillette PC, Harley RA, Upshur JK: Cardiomyopathy and myocarditis in children with ventricular ectopic rhythm. J Am Coll Cardiol (August) 1992; 20:359–362.

40. Wichter T, Borggrefe M, Haverkamp W, Chen X, Breithardt G: Efficacy of Antiarrhythmic Drugs in Patients with Arrhythmogenic Right Ventricular Disease, Results in Patients with Inducible and Noninducible Ventricular Tachycardia. Circulation 1992 (July); 86:29–37.

41. O'Kelly B, Browner WS, Massie B, Tubau J, Ngo L, Mangano DT: Ventricular arrhythmias in patients undergoing noncardiac surgery. JAMA 1992 (July 8); 268:217–221.

42. Sforzini, Latini R, Mingardi G, Vincenti A, Redaelli B: Ventricular arrhythmias and four-year mortality in hemodialysis patients. Lancet 1992 (Jan 25); 339:212–213.

43. Clyne CA, Estes NAM III, Wang PJ: Moricizine. N Engl J Med 1992 (July 23); 327:255–260.

44. Damle R, Levine J, Matos J, Greenberg S, Brooks R, Frumkin W, Goldberger J, Kadish

AH: Efficacy and risks of moricizine in inducible sustained ventricular tachycardia. An Intern Med 1992 (Mar 1); 116:375–381.

45. Powell AC, Gold MR, Brooks R, Garan H, Ruskin JN, McGovern BA: Electrophysiologic response to moricizine in patients with sustained ventricular arrhythmias. An Intern Med 1992 (Mar 1); 116:382–387.

46. Yeung-Lai-Wah JA, Murdock CJ, Boone J, Kerr CR. Propafenone-mexiletine combination for the treatment of sustained ventricular tachycardia. J Am Coll Cardiol 1992 (September); 20:547–51.

47. Steinbeck G, Andresen D, Bach P, Haberl R, Oeff M, Hoffmann E, Von Leitner ER: A comparison of electrophysiologically guided antiarrhythmic drug therapy with beta-blocker therapy in patients with symptomatic, sustained ventricular tachyarrhythmias. N Engl J Med 1992 (Oct 1); 327:987–992.

48. Kus T, Campa MA, Nadeau R, Dubuc M, Kaltenbrunner W, Shenasa M: Efficacy and electrophysiologic effects of oral sotalol in patients with sustained ventricular tachycardia caused by coronary artery disease. Am Heart J 1992 (January); 123:82–89.

49. Hohnloser SH, Zabel M, Krause T, Just H. Short- and long-term antiarrhythmic and hemodynamic effects of d, l-sotalol in patients with symptomatic ventricular arrhythmias. Am Heart J 1992 (May); 123:1220–1224.

50. Freedman RA, Karagounis LA, Steinberg JS. Effects of sotalol on the signal-averaged electrocardiogram in patients with sustained ventricular tachycardia: Relation to suppression of inducibility and changes in tachycardia cycle length. J Am Coll Cardiol 1992 (November); 20:1213–9.

51. Summitt J, Morady F, Kadish A: A comparison of standard and high-dose regimens for the initiation of amiodarone therapy. Am Heart J 1992 (August); 124:366–373.

52. England MR, Gordon G, Salem M, Chernow B: Magnesium administration and dysrhythmias after cardiac surgery: A placebo-controlled, double-blind, randomized trial. JAMA 1992 (Nov 4); 268:2395–2402.

53. Boden W, Moss A, Oakes D: Hypolipidemic Effect of Type Ia Antiarrhythmic Agents in Postinfarction Patients. Circulation 1992 (June); 85:2039–2044.

54. Klein L, Shih H, Hackett K, Zipes D, Miles W: Radiofrequency Catheter Ablation of Ventricular Tachycardia in Patients Without Structural Heart Disease. Circulation 1992 (May); 85:1666–1674.

55. Geha AS, Elefteriades JA, Hsu J, Biblo LA, Hoch DH, Batsford WP, Rosenfeld LE, Carlson MD, Johnson NJ, Waldo AL: Strategies in the surgical treatment of malignant ventricular arrhythmias: An 8-year experience. An Surg 1992 (Oct 1); 309–317.

56. Mittleman RS, Candinas R, Dahlberg S, Vander Salm T, Moran JM, Huang SKS: Predictors of surgical mortality and long-term results of endocardial resection for drug-refractory ventricular tachycardia. Am Heart J 1992 (November); 124:1226–1232.

57. Niebauer MJ, Kirsh M, Kadish A, Calkinsa H, Morady F: Outcome of endocardial resection in 33 patients with coronary artery disease: Correlation with ventricular tachycardia morphology. Am Heart J 1992 (December); 124:1500–1506.

58. Gilman JK, Naccarelli GV: Sudden cardiac death. Current Problems in Cardiology 1992 (Nov); 11.

59. Valenzuela TD, Spaite DW, Meislin HW, Clark LL, Wright AL, Ewy GA: Case and survival definitions in out-of-hospital cardiac arrest: Effect on survival rate calculation. JAMA 1992 (Jan 8); 267:272–274.

60. Dickey W, Adgey AAJ: Mortality within hospital after resuscitation from ventricular fibrillation outside hospital. Br Heart J 1992 (Apr); 67:334–338.

61. Wannamethee G, Shaper AG: Alcohol and sudden cardiac death. Br Heart J 1992 (Nov); 68:443–448.

62. Huikuri HV, Linnaluoto MK, Seppanen T, Airaksinen KEJ, Kessler KM, Takkunen JT, Myerburg RJ: Circadian rhythm of heart rate variability in survivors of cardiac arrest. Am J Cardiol 1992 (Sept 1); 70:610–615.

63. Zehender M, Buchner C, Meinertz T, and Just H: Prevalence, Circumstances, Mechanisms, and Risk Stratification of Sudden Cardiac Death in Unipolar Single-Chamber Ventricular Pacing. Circulation 1992 (February); 85:596–605.

64. Niemann JT: Cardiopulmonary resuscitation. N Engl J Med 1992 (Oct 8); 327:1075–1080.

65. Stiell IG, Hebert PC, Weitzman BN, Wells GA, Raman S, Stark RM, Higginson AJ, Ahuja J, Dickinson GE: High-dose epinephrine in adult cardiac arrest. N Engl J Med 1992 (Oct 8); 327:1045–1050.

66. Brown CG, Martin DR, Pepe PE, Stueven H, Cummins RO, Gonzalez E, Jastremski M, Multicenter High-Dose Epinephrine Study Group: A comparison of standard-dose and high-dose epinephrine in cardiac arrest outside the hospital. N Engl J Med 1992 (Oct 8); 327:1051–1055.

67. Callaham M, Madsen D, Barton CW, Saunders CE, Pointer J: A randomized clinical trial of high-dose epinephrine and norepinephrine vs standard-dose epinephrine in prehospital cardiac arrest. JAMA 1991 (Nov 18); 268:2667–2672.

68. Sudden infant death syndrome—United States, 1980–1988. MMWR 1992 (July 17); 41:515–517.

69. Keating M: Linkage Analysis and Long QT Syndrome, Using Genetics to Study Cardiovascular Disease. Circulation 1992 (June); 85:1973–1986.

70. Vincent GM, Timothy KW, Leppert M, Keating M: The spectrum of symptoms and QT intervals in carriers of the gene for the long-QT syndrome. N Engl J Med 1992 (Sept 17); 327:846–852.

71. Tobé TJM, DeLangen CDJ, Bink-Boelkens MTE, Mook PH, Viersma J-W, Lie KI, Wesseling H. Late potentials in a bradycardia-dependent long QT syndrome associated with sudden death during sleep. J Am Coll Cardiol 1992 (March); 19:541–9.

72. Eldar M, Griffin JC, Van Hare GF, Witherell C, Bhandari A, Benditt D, Scheinman MM. Combined use of beta-adrenergic blocking agents and long-term cardiac pacing for patients with the long QT syndrome. J Am Coll Cardiol 1992 (October); 20:830–7.

73. Kapoor WN: Evaluation and management of the patient with syncope. JAMA 1992 (Nov 11); 268:2553–2560.

74. Brignole M, Oddone D, Cogorno S, Menozzi C, Gianfranchi L, Bertulla A: Long-term outcome in symptomatic carotid sinus hypersensitivity. Am Heart J 1992 (March); 123:687–692.

75. Bernstein AD and Parsonnet V: Survey of cardiac pacing in the United States in 1989. Am J Cardiol 1992 (Feb 1); 69:331–338.

76. Gwinn N, Leman R, Kratz J, White JK, Zile MR, Gillette P. Chronotropic incompetence: A common and progressive finding in pacemaker patients. Am Heart J 1992 (May); 123:1216–1219.

77. Johns JA, Fish FA, Burger JD, Hammon JW: Steroid-eluting epicardial packing leads in pediatric patients: encouraging early results. J Am Coll Cardiol (August) 1992; 20:395–401.

78. Saksena S, Poczobutt-Johanos M, Castle LW, Fogoros RN, Alpert BL, Kron J, Pacifico A, Griffin J, Ruskin JN, Kehoe RF, Yee R, Dorian P, Kerr CR, Luceri RM, Poliseno M, for the Guardian Multicenter Investigators Group. Long-term multicenter experience with a second-generation implantable pacemaker-defibrillator in patients with malignant ventricular tachyarrhythmias. J Am Coll Cardiol 1992 (March); 19:490–9.

79. Newman D, Sauve MJ, Herre J, Langberg JJ, Lee MA, Titus C, Franklin J, Scheinman MM, Griffin JC: Survival after implantation of the cardioverter defibrillator. Am J Cardiol 1992 (Apr 1); 69:899–903.

80. Kim S, Fisher J, Choue C, Gross J, Roth J, Ferrick K, Brodman R, Furman S: Influence of Left Ventricular Function on Outcome of Patients Treated With Implantable Defibrillators. Circulation 1992 (April); 85:1304–1310.

81. Epstein AE, Ellenbogen KA, Kirk KA, Kay GN, Dailey SM, Plumb VJ, and the High Defibrillation Threshold Investigators: Clinical Characteristics and Outcome of Patients With High Defibrillation Thresholds, A Multicenter Study. Circulation 1992 (October); 86:1206–1216.

82. Jung W, Manz M, Moosdorf R, Luderitz B: Failure of an Implantable Cardioverter-Defibrillator to Redetect Ventricular Fibrillation in Patients With a Nonthoracotomy Lead System. Circulation 1992 (October); 86:1217–1222.

83. Mehta D, Saksena S, Krol RB: Survival of implantable cardioverter-defibrillator recipients: Role of left ventricular function and its relationship to device use. Am Heart J 1992 (December); 124:1608–1614.

84. Larsen RL, Jakacki RI, Vetter VL, Meadoes AT, Silber JH, Barber G: Electrocardiographic changes and arrhythmias after cancer therapy in children and young adults. Am J Cardiol 1992 (Jul 1); 70:73–77.

Systemic Hypertension

GENERAL TOPICS

Ambulatory vs office blood pressure

Bottini and associates[1] from Augusta, Georgia, compared blood pressures collected by 2 indirect methods on the same patients during a hypertensive research project. Data obtained on patients in a typical clinical setting were provided and 24-hour diastolic pressures obtained by the automated method demonstrated no regression to a lower mean, while BP obtained casually in the office exhibited such regression. The 95% confidence interval of repeated measures for casual office BP on a patient in a research setting (35/17 mm Hg) or in typical clinic practice (26/19 mm Hg) were similar, while the range of the mean 24-hour automated BP monitoring, (21/11 mm Hg) was smaller and demonstrated less variability. The magnitudes of the differences in BP obtained on separate occasions in the same subjects were significantly lower with automated vs casual BP determination methods (7.9/4.6 vs 13.7/7.4 mm Hg for both systolic and diastolic pressures). The agreement between BP obtained by the 2 methods (19/12 mm Hg) was found to be similar to the repeatability of automated BP monitoring alone, and superior to that for data recorded casually in the office (35/17 mm Hg). Thus the variability in the mean 24-hour automated BP is less than that for casual office BP. The variability of BP measured on an individual may be much greater than that reported for populations of hypertensive patients, and must be considered when applying epidemiologic group data to a specific patient.

Ambulatory BP has generally been reported to be lower than office BP, but population-based data are lacking. To better characterize ambulatory and office BP relations, Pearce and associates[2] from Minneapolis, Minnesota, and Chicago, Illinois, explored the interrelations of BPs measured in the office by mercury sphygmomanometry, 24-hour ambulatory

BP measured with a portable device, and echocardiographic LV mass in a random sample of 50 men aged 51 to 72 years drawn from a much larger pool. Office BP was based on the mean of 10 measurements performed over 5 visits. Among all participants, mean 24-hour ambulatory and mean office BPs were highly correlated: r (systolic/diastolic) = .90/.79; and both mean 24-hour and mean awake ambulatory BPs were significantly higher than mean office BPs (Figures 5-1 and 5-2). For the subsample not receiving antihypertensive therapy, mean ambulatory and office

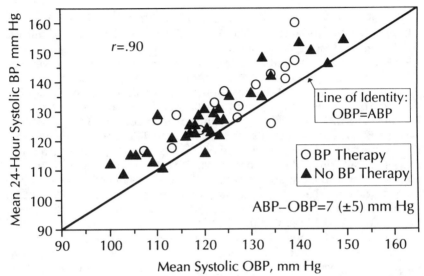

Fig. 5-1. The relationship between systolic office blood pressure (OBP) and 24-hour systolic ambulatory blood pressure (ABP). BP indicates blood pressure. Reproduced with permission from Pearce, et al.[2]

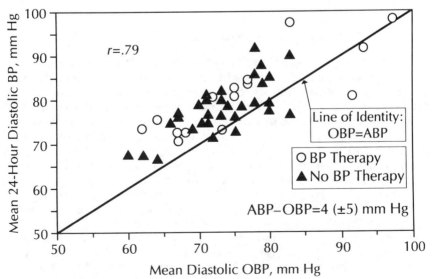

Fig. 5-2. The relationship between diastolic office blood pressure (OBP) and 24-hour diastolic ambulatory blood pressure (ABP). BP indicates blood pressure. Reproduced with permission from Pearce, et al.[2]

BPs were similar in terms of their associations with Penn LV mass index. No association between BP and LV mass observed among the subjects receiving antihypertensive medication. The authors concluded that a single session of 24-hour ambulatory BP monitoring is unlikely to improves the determination of usual BP in older white men beyond that achievable with BP carefully measured over 5 separate office visits; and that white coat hypertension is rare in this population.

Diurnal blood pressure profile

Staessen and associates[3] from Leuven and Hasselt, Belgium, London, UK, and Dublin, Ireland, studied 399 subjects to determine the diurnal BP rhythm and found that 370 (93%) did indeed have a significant diurnal BP rhythm. The nocturnal BP fall was normally distributed and averaged 16 ± 9 mm Hg systolic and 14 ± 7 mm Hg diastolic (mean ± SD). The amplitude of the diurnal BP curve followed a positively skewed distribution, with a mean of 16 ± 5 mm Hg for systolic BP and 14 ± 4 mm Hg for diastolic BP. The daily BP maximum occurred at 15:54 ± 4:47 for systolic BP and at 15:11 ± 4:20 for diastolic BP. Thirty-four subjects were reexamined after a median interval of 350 days. The test for the presence of a significant diurnal rhythm was discordant in only 2 subjects. Repeatability (twice the standard deviation of the differences between paired recordings expressed as a percentage of the mean) varied from 11 to 25% for the 24 hours, daytime, and overnight BP, and from 76 to 138% for the parameters describing the diurnal BP rhythm. In 9 subjects with an initial night/day ratio of mean BP <0.78, the nighttime BP was significantly increased at the repeat examination, whereas the opposite tendency was observed in 9 subjects with an initial ratio >0.87. In conclusion, the distribution of nocturnal BP fall is unimodal. The reproducibility of the ambulatory BP is satisfactory for the level of BP and for the presence of a diurnal BP rhythm, but not for the parameters of the diurnal BP curve. Thus, one 24-hour recording is insufficient to fully characterize an individual's diurnal BP profile.

Early morning pressure rise

The marked increase in cardiovascular events that occur in the early morning hours could be related to a significant rise in BP at this time but there is uncertainty as to whether this rise in BP occurs before, at, or after awakening. Khoury and associates[4] from Dallas, Texas, took automatic BP and pulse measurements on 15 normotensive subjects and 3 times on 11 untreated hypertensive subjects starting before the onset of sleep and at 10 minute intervals for 1 hour before and 60 to 90 minutes after awakening (Figures 5-3 and 5-4). In random order, all subjects either remained supine or immediately arose and ambulated on the first 2 occasions. The hypertensives had a third study involving ingestion of 10 mg nifedipine after awakening and remaining supine for the next 60 minutes. The BP and pulse changed little before and after awakening if the subjects remained supine. They rose rapidly and significantly immediately upon arising. The rise in pressure upon arising was blunted by the prior ingestion of nifedipine. The early morning rise in BP and pulse is mainly related to arising from bed. Possible ways to reduce the abrupt rise in BP and the increase in cardiovascular events that occur after arising are suggested.

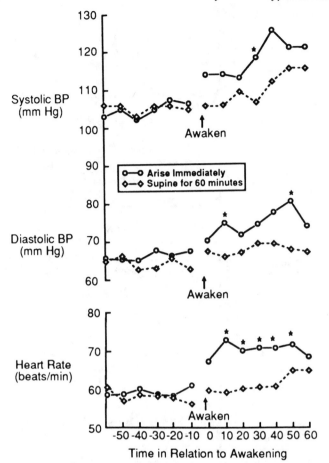

Fig. 5-3. Mean levels of systolic and diastolic blood pressure and heart rate in 15 normotensive subjects measured every 10 min for 1 h prior to awakening and for 1 h after awakening while either supine or ambulatory. *P<.05 from supine levels. Reproduced with permission from Khoury, et al.[4]

Isolated systolic elevation

To assess the association between isolated systolic hypertension (ISH) and subclinical disease in adults aged 65 years and above, Psaty and associates[5] from multiple USA medical centers used Medicare eligibility lists to obtain a representative sample of 5,201 community-dwelling elderly persons for the Cardiovascular Health Study, a National Heart, Lung, and Blood Institute—sponsored cohort study of risk factors for CAD and stroke. In a cross-sectional analysis of baseline data, the authors excluded 3,012 participants who were receiving anti-hypertensive medications, had clinical cardiovascular disease, or had a diastolic BP of at least 90 mm Hg. Among the 2,189 men and women in the analysis, 195 (9%) had ISH (systolic BP 160 mm Hg) and 596 (23%) had borderline ISH (systolic BP 140-159 mm Hg). Systolic BP was associated with myocardial infarction by electrocardiogram. Borderline and definite ISH were strongly associated with LV mass. While there was little association with cardiac systolic

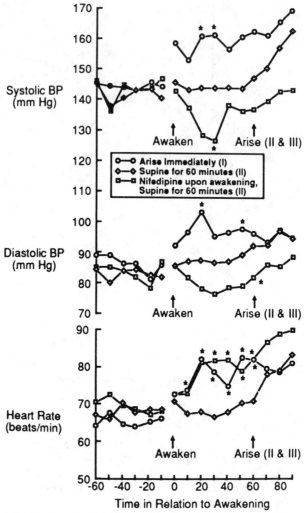

Fig. 5-4. Mean levels of systolic and diastolic blood pressure and heart rate in 11 hypertensive subjects measured every 10 min during the hour prior to awakening and for 90 min after awakening while either remaining supine for 60 min (◇) arising immediately (O), or remaining supine for 60 min after ingestion of nifedipine and then arising (□). *P<.05 from supine levels. Reproduced with permission from Khoury, et al.[4]

function, borderline and definite ISH were associated with cardiac diastolic function. Isolated systolic hypertension was also strongly associated with cardiac diastolic function. Isolated systolic hypertension was also strongly associated with increased intima-media thickness of the carotid artery. While cohort analyses of future repeated measures will provide a better assessment of risk, both borderline and definite ISH were strongly related to a variety of measures of subclinical disease in elderly men and women.

Isolated systolic hypertension occurs with increased prevalence in the elderly population. It is characterized by reduced vascular compliance, often combined with increased peripheral resistance. These changes are not specific to patients with systolic hypertension, occurring, perhaps to a lesser extent, in the normotensive aging population also. Systolic hypertension is associated with a risk of cardiovascular mortality and morbidity that possibly exceeds that associated with systolic-diastolic hypertension. Until the recent report of the Systolic Hypertension in the Elderly Program, however, the benefit of treatment of this population was undocumented. Mann[6] from New York, New York, reviewed the findings of the Systolic Hypertension in the Elderly Program, which demonstrated that lowering of BP with a diuretic, combined, when necessary, with a beta blocker, reduced the rate of AMI and stroke. Other agents may also be effective in lowering BP, although their ability to reduce cardiovascular morbidity and mortality in the population remains undocumented. The results suggest that pharmacologic treatment be considered for patients >60 years whose systolic BP remains 160 mm Hg (with a diastolic BP <90 mm Hg). Whether treatment should be recommended for all patients with systolic hypertension, or, alternatively, for only those at higher risk for cardiovascular events, remains controversial.

Predisposing factor

Shea and associates[7] from New York, New York, studied the characteristics of the medical care received by patients with hypertensive emergency and urgent hypertension, the most severe forms of uncontrolled hypertension to identify risk factors for severe, uncontrolled hypertension. Using a case-controlled study design, the authors interviewed 93 patients with severe, uncontrolled hypertension who presented in the hospital emergency room and 114 control patients with hypertension. Both groups were seen at 2 New York City hospitals from 1989–1991. All the patients were black or Hispanic. Multiple logistic-regression models were used to adjust for age, sex, race or ethnic background, education, smoking status, alcohol-related problems, and use of illicit drugs during the previous year. After additional adjustment for lack of health insurance, severe, uncontrolled hypertension was found to be more common among patients who had no primary care physician and among those who did not comply with treatment for their hypertension. Lack of health insurance was marginally associated with severe, uncontrolled hypertension after adjustment for lack of a primary care physician and noncompliance with antihypertensive treatment.

Ventricular arrhythmias

Circadian patterns have been observed for various cardiovascular functions and events including sudden cardiac death. Siegel and associates[8] from San Francisco, California, examined whether ventricular arrhythmias could be a pathophysiologic explanation for the increase in prevalence of sudden cardiac death observed between 6 A.M. and noon. Hypertensive men 35 to 70 years of age and without a history of symptomatic cardiac disease were withdrawn from diuretic treatment and received 1 month of oral electrolyte repletion with both 40 mmol of potassium chloride and 400 mg of magnesium oxide daily. Then continuous 24-hour Holter monitoring was performed and ventricular arrhythmias were classified by 6-hour time intervals. The interval from 6 A.M. to noon revealed a higher prevalence of complex or frequent ventricular arrhythmias than the interval from midnight to 6 A.M., as well as a higher mean number of VPCs per hour. The differences were statistically significant and amounted to increases of about one third. Ventricular arrhythmias during the other two 6-hour periods were intermediary in frequency. It is concluded that the increase in sudden cardiac death noted in the morning might be related, at least in part, to an increase in frequency of ventricular arrhythmias.

Most studies on the relation between ventricular ectopic activity and systemic hypertension have been performed in patients with elevation of diastolic BP. There are no data on the prevalence of characteristics of ventricular ectopic activity in patients with isolated systolic hypertension. Accordingly, Kostis and associates[9] from New Brunswick, New Jersey, performed 24-hour ambulatory electrocardiograms in 238 patients with isolated systolic hypertension who participated in the Systolic Hypertension in the Elderly Program (SHEP) and in a group of 100 age- and sex-matched normotensive control subjects. All subjects were ≥60 years of age. Their systolic BP varied from 160 to 219 mm Hg and their diastolic BP was <90 mm Hg. Two readings at 2 baseline visits were averaged (4 readings) to obtain baseline BP. Electrocardiographic exclusion criteria were AF or atrial flutter, AV block, multifocal VPCs or bradycardial <50 beats per minute on the 12-lead electrocardiogram. Twenty-four hour ambulatory electrocardiograms were obtained at baseline before medication was begun. The findings are summarized in Table 5-1 and in Figures 5-5 and 5-6. Compared with normotensive control subjects, patients with isolated systolic hypertension had greater weight, body-mass index, systolic and diastolic BP, and were older by 2 years. Patients with isolated systolic hypertension had greater weight, body-mass index, systolic and diastolic BP and were older by 2 years. Patients with isolated systolic hypertension had more VPCs (412 ± 1612/24 hours) than normotensive

TABLE 5-1. *Ventricular Ectopic Activity and Left Ventricular Mass in Patients with Isolated Systolic Hypertension and in Normotensive Control Subjects. Reproduced with permission from Kostis, et al.[9]*

	SHEP (n = 226)	Control (n = 98)	p Value
Ventricular Ectopic Activity			
VPCs/24 hours	412 ± 1,612	179 ± 479	0.048
VPC pairs/24 hours	2.6 ± 14.8	1.8 ± 9.7	NS
No. (%) with VPCs	190 (84%)	76 (78%)	NS
No. (%) with > 10 VPCs	151 (67%)	51 (52%)	0.009
No. (%) of repetitive forms	52 (23%)	15 (15%)	NS
Left Ventricular Mass			
	(n = 95)	(n = 38)	
Left ventricular mass	262 ± 90	234 ± 81	0.104
Left ventricular mass index (g/m)	162 ± 51	144 ± 47	0.064
No. (%) with left ventricular hypertrophy	(76%)	(45%)	0.001

NS = not significant; SHEP = Systolic Hypertension in the Elderly Program; VPC = ventricular premature contractions.

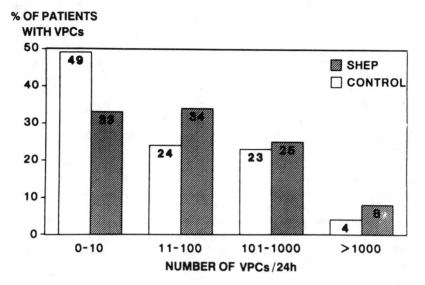

Fig. 5-5. Frequency distribution of ventricular premature contractions (VPCs) per 24 hours in patients with isolated systolic hypertension and normotensive control subjects. SHEP = Systolic Hypertension in the Elderly Program. Reproduced with permission from Kostis, et al.[9]

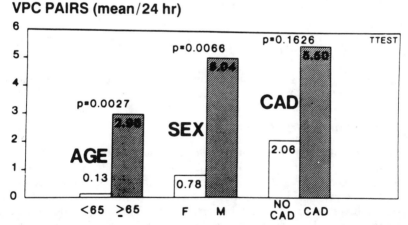

Fig. 5-6. Frequency of ventricular premature contraction pairs on 24-hour ambulatory electrocardiography in patients with isolated systolic hypertension by age, sex and history of coronary artery disease (CAD). Reproduced with permission from Kostis, et al.[9]

controls (179 ± 479/24 hours). Sixty-seven percent of the patients with isolated systolic hypertension and 52% of normal controls had greater than 10 VPCs per 24 hours. In isolated systolic hypertension, the number of VPCs correlated with age, male gender, and CAD. The number of VPC pairs was also related to age and male gender. Body weight was positively related to both LV mass and LV mass correlated for height but not with ventricular ectopic activity. A relation between LV mass and ventricular ectopic activity was seen for pairs and VPCs in the SHEP group and for pairs and for VPCs in the total cohort. A relation between baseline serum potassium and cardiac arrhythmias was not observed. There were no significant differences between ventricular ectopic activity and patients who had been taking antiarrhythmic medications before randomization and those who had not. By multivariate analysis considering age and male gender were significant determinants of the number of VPCs in the SHEP cohort. Repetitive forms (VPC pairs and nonsustained VT) were independently related to age, male gender and baseline systolic BP. When gender was removed from the model, age and CAD were related to total VPCs, and age, CAD and baseline systolic BP were related to the presence of repetitive forms.

Hypertensive patients with the electrocardiographic pattern of LV hypertrophy and strain are at increased risk of sudden death. It has been suggested that ventricular arrhythmias may be responsible. Pringle and associates[10] from Glasgow, Scotland, studied the prevalence and significance of ventricular arrhythmias in 90 hypertensive patients with LV hypertrophy and strain by taking 48-hour ambulatory electrocardiographic monitoring, electrocardiographic signal-averaging and programmed ventricular stimulation. Complex ventricular ectopic activity (Lown grade ≥3) was detected in 59 patients (66%). Eleven patients (12%) had episodes of nonsustained VT. There were no sustained arrhythmias either on ambulatory electrocardiographic monitoring or induced by programmed ventricular stimulation. Only 1 patient had ventricular late potentials recorded by the signal-averaged electrocardiogram. Therefore, there was little to suggest an underlying arrhythmogenic substrate in these patients. In conclusion, whereas ventricular arrhythmias occur often in patients with LV hypertrophy associated with systemic hypertension, their significance, if any, remains to be established.

Effect on heart—review

A fine review article[11] on the heart in systemic hypertension appeared in the October 1, 1992, issue of *The New England Journal of Medicine*.

Left ventricular hypertrophy

To assess the prevalence of symptomatic and silent myocardial ischemia in patients with hypertensive LV hypertrophy, Pringle and associates[12] from Glasgow, Scotland, performed a cross-sectional study of 90 patients (68 men and 22 women; mean age 57 [range 25-79]) with LV hypertrophy due to essential hypertension. A 48-hour ambulatory ST segment monitoring was performed in all patients, exercise electrocardiography (n = 79), stress thallium scintigraphy (n = 80) and coronary arteriography (n = 35). Forty-three patients had at least 1 episode of ST segment depression on ambulatory electrocardiographic monitoring. The median number of episodes was 16 (range 1 to 84) with a median duration of 8.6 (range 2 to 17) min. Over 90% of these episodes were clinically silent. Twenty-six patients had positive exercise electrocardiography and 48 patients had reversible thallium perfusion defects despite chest pain during exercise in only 5 patients. Eighteen of the thirty-five patients who had coronary arteriography had important CAD. Seven of these patients gave no history of chest pain. Symptomatic and silent AMI are common in hypertensive patients with LV hypertrophy, even in the absence of epicardial CAD.

Ghali and associates[13] from Chicago, Illinois, measured all-cause and cardiac mortality in a cohort of 785 patients, most of whom were black and had systemic hypertension, to determine the association between echocardiographically determined LV hypertrophy and mortality in patients with and without CAD. LV hypertrophy, based on LV mass corrected for body surface area was present in 194 of 381 patients (51%) with CAD and in 162 of 404 patients (40%) without CAD. Patients with LV hypertrophy had worse survival than those without hypertrophy in both the group with CAD and the group without CAD. After adjustment was made for age at baseline, sex, and hypertension, the relative risk for death from any cause in patients with hypertrophy compared with patients without hypertrophy was 2.14 among those with CAD and 4.14 among those without CAD. Echocardiographically determined LV hypertrophy is an important prognostic marker in patients with or without CAD.

Silent myocardial ischemia

Siegel and associates[14] from San Francisco, California, studied the prevalence, characteristics and circadian pattern of silent myocardial ischemia, and its association with ventricular arrhythmias in hypertensive men aged 35 to 70 years (mean 61) without clinical cardiac disease. Participants were withdrawn from diuretic treatment and received 1 month of oral electrolyte repletion with 40 mmol of potassium chloride, and 400 mg of magnesium oxide daily. Twenty-four-hour Holter monitoring was then performed. Episodes of silent myocardial ischemia occurred in 50 of 186 men (27%) and lasted from 2 to 289 minutes (mean 30 and median 18). Statistical analysis comparing the interval from midnight to 6 a.m. with each of the other three 6-hour time intervals revealed that participants were less likely to have silent myocardial ischemia in this period than at other times of the day. There was little difference in the proportion of men with a frequent or complex ventricular arrhythmia during the entire day or within 1 hour of the silent myocardial ischemic episode (or during a comparable time period) comparing those with to those without silent myocardial ischemia. These findings indicate that silent myocardial ischemia occurs in approximately 25% of an older population of hypertensive men without history of symptomatic cardiac disease. The circadian pattern of frequency of silent ischemic events in men free of clinical cardiac disease is similar to that reported for patients with cardiac disease and coincides with that reported for sudden death. There was no significant association between silent myocardial ischemia and ventricular arrhythmias.

TREATMENT

Blood pressure lowering—how much?

Fletcher and Bulpitt[15] from London, United Kingdom, asked the question "How far should blood pressure be lowered?" How far should the diastolic BP be lowered below 85 mm Hg is unclear. In most studies the intended diastolic BP has been 90 mm Hg, and little is known about outcome with treated pressures below 80 mm Hg. The Systolic Hypertension in the Elderly Program trial provides evidence that even in elderly patients, many of whom had CAD, diastolic pressures could safely be lowered to below 70 mm Hg, although such low levels of diastolic BP could safely be lowered to <70 mm Hg, although such low levels of diastolic BP were in the presence of raised systolic BP. When systolic BP is not high, we do not know the optimal levels to which we can reduce BP. The ongoing prospective trial has randomly assigned patients whose initial diastolic pressure is in the range of 90 to 100 mm Hg and whose average systolic pressure is 155 mm Hg to intensive or nonintensive lowering of BP. The trial will provide important evidence on the benefits or adverse effects of reducing BP <80 mm Hg. Rapid reductions in BP should probably be avoided. In particular, a large and sudden decrease in pressure that is unrelated to treatment may be predictive of a poor prognosis.

To examine the association between the level of treated BP and the incidence of AMI, McCloskey and associates[16] from Seattle, Washington, conducted a population-based case-control study of 912 members of a health maintenance organization who were receiving standard clinical treatment for systemic hypertension. The authors found a J-shaped relation between the most recently measured diastolic BP and the risk of AMI, the lowest risk occurring at 84 mm Hg. The relative risk of AMI at 60 mm Hg was 2.07 and at 100 mm Hg, 1.45. Treated systolic pressure bore a linear relation to the risk of infarction. The authors concluded that the optimum target range for diastolic BP in hypertensive patients may be 84 to 90 mm Hg. Levels outside this range may be associated with increased risk of AMI.

Non-pharmacologic interventions

Kostis and associates[17] from New Brunswick, New Jersey, compared the effects of nonpharmacologic therapy, propranolol monotherapy, and placebo on BP, metabolic, exercise, and quality of life variables in a 12-week, randomized, placebo-controlled trial of 79 male patients with hypertension. A significant reduction in diastolic BP was observed with both nondrug therapy (-8.0 ± 1.08 mm Hg) and propranolol (-9.5 ± 1.46 mm Hg) compared to placebo (-0.1 ± 2.01 mm Hg). However, only patients receiving nonpharmacologic therapy showed a reduced body mass index, lower total and LDL serum cholesterol levels, and increased exercise tolerance compared to both propranolol and placebo. Patients receiving nondrug therapy felt more energetic and reported improved sexual satisfaction after treatment. Reductions in BP in the nondrug treatment group were related to both weight reduction and improved fitness. It was concluded that nondrug therapy is effective in controlling BP in men with mild hypertension and is associated with improvements in weight, lipoprotein levels, and exercise tolerance compared to both propranolol and placebo. Quality of life assessments further support the use of nondrug therapy in this context.

To test the short-term feasibility and efficacy of 7 nonpharmacologic interventions in persons with high normal diastolic BP, the Trials of Hypertension Prevention Collaborative Research Group[18] performed a randomized, controlled, multi-center trial involving 16,821 screenees, 2,182 men and women, aged 30 to 54 years, with diastolic BP from 80 through 89 mm Hg. Of these, 50 did not return for follow-up BP measurements. Three lifestyle change groups (weight reduction, sodium reduction, and stress management) were each compared with unmasked, nonintervention controls over 18 months. Four nutritional supplement groups (calcium, magnesium, potassium, and fish oil) were each compared singly, in double-blind fashion, with placebo controls over 6 months. The main outcome measures were change in diastolic BP from baseline to final follow-up and also changes in systolic BP and intervention compliance measures. Weight reduction intervention produced weight loss of 3.9 kg, diastolic BP change of −2.3 mm Hg, and systolic BP change of −2.9 mm Hg. Sodium reduction interventions lowered urinary sodium excretion by 44 mmol/24 h, diastolic BP by 0.9 mm Hg, and systolic BP by 1.7 mm Hg. Despite good compliance, neither stress management nor nutritional supplements reduced diastolic BP or systolic BP significantly. Weight reduction is the most effective of the strategies tested for reducing BP in normotensive persons. Sodium reduction is also effective. The long-term effects of weight reduction and sodium reduction, alone and in combination, require further evaluation.

Blaufox and associates[19] from 4 USA medical centers measured plasma renin activity at baseline and 6 months in a trial of nonpharmacologic therapy of mild systemic hypertension to determine whether plasma renin activity predicts the diastolic BP response to nonpharmacologic therapy. The study was a randomized controlled trial of volunteers from the general community with diastolic BP between 90 and 100 mm Hg of all antihypertensive therapy at baseline, treated in special research clinics (n = 593). The subjects were randomly assigned to usual, weight loss, or low sodium/high potassium diet and then randomly assigned to receive placebo, chlorthalidone, or atenolol. Renin was analyzed as plasma renin activity and as a renin index (logarithm of 24-hour urinary sodium excretion times logarithm of plasma renin activity) (593 patients at baseline and 6 months) to correct for varied sodium intakes. The diastolic BP was measured using the random zero device. Change in diastolic BP at 6 months could be predicted from baseline plasma renin activity or renin index. The diastolic BP was decreased after 6 months of therapy by 2 mm Hg for each unit increase in baseline plasma renin activity and by 0.16 mm Hg for each unit increase in baseline renin index. Patients in the highest renin index quartile had a greater diastolic BP response to atenolol therapy, and patients in the lowest renin index quartile had a greater diastolic BP response to chlorthalidone therapy. Weight loss diet achieved a greater reduction in diastolic BP in patients with higher baseline renin index and had an additive effect on diastolic BP response in both of the drug groups. Patients on a weight loss diet receiving placebo in the highest baseline renin index quartile had a reduction in diastolic BP of 12.4 mm Hg, compared with 4.4 mm Hg in the lowest baseline renin index quartile. A low sodium/high potassium diet had a lesser effect than a weight loss diet on pharmacologic therapy. As with the weight loss diet, patients on a low sodium/high potassium diet in the highest baseline renin index quartile had a greater reduction in diastolic BP than patients in the lowest baseline renin index quartile. These data suggest a significant relation between baseline levels of plasma renin index and the likelihood of success of nonpharmacologic treatment of hypertension.

An effect of diet in determining BP is suggested by epidemiological studies, but the role of specific nutrients is still unsettled. Ascherio and co-workers[20] in Boston, Massachusetts, examined the relation of various nutritional factors with hypertension prospectively among 30,681 predominantly white US male health professionals, 40–75 years old, without diagnosed hypertension. During 4 years of follow-up, 1,248 men reported a diagnosis of hypertension. Age, relative weight, and alcohol consumption were the strongest predictors for the development of hypertension. Dietary fiber, potassium, and magnesium were each significantly associated with lower risk of hypertension when considered individually and after adjustment for age, relative weight, alcohol consumption, and energy intake. When these nutrients were considered simultaneously, only dietary fiber had an independent inverse association with hypertension. For men with a fiber intake of <12 g/day, the relative risk of hypertension was 1.57 compared with an intake of >24 g/day. Calcium was significantly associated with lower risk of hypertension only in lean men. Dietary fiber, potassium, and magnesium were also inversely related to baseline systolic and diastolic BP and to change in BP during the follow-up among men who did not develop hypertension. Calcium was inversely associated with baseline BP but not with change in BP. No significant associations with hypertension were observed for sodium, total fat, or saturated, transunsaturated, and polyunsaturated fatty acids. Fruit fiber but not vegetable or cereal fiber was inversely associated with incidence of hypertension. These results support hypotheses that an increased intake of fiber and magnesium may contribute to the prevention of hypertension.

Hydrochlorothiazide ± potassium ± magnesium vs hydrochlorothiazide + triamterene vs chlorthalidone

To investigate the patterns of electrolyte abnormalities resulting from thiazide administration and whether they cause ventricular arrhythmias, and to help resolve the controversy over whether clinicians should routinely prescribe potassium-conserving therapy to all patients treated with thiazides, Siegel and associates[21] from San Francisco, California, performed a double-blind, randomized controlled trial involving 233 hypertensive men aged 35 to 70 years. Participants were withdrawn from prior diuretic therapy and were replenished with oral potassium chloride and magnesium oxide. They were then randomized to 2 months of treatment with (1) hydrochlorothiazide; (2) hydrochlorothiazide with oral potassium; (3) hydrochlorothiazide with oral potassium and magnesium; (4) hydrochlorothiazide and triamterene; (5) chlorthalidone; or (6) placebo. The main outcome measures were ventricular arrhythmias on 24-hour Holter monitoring and serum and intracellular potassium and magnesium levels. Of the 233 participants, 212 (91%) completed the study. Serum potassium levels were 0.4 mmol/L lower in the hydrochlorothiazide group than in the placebo group, and this mean difference was not affected by supplementation with potassium, with potassium and magnesium, or with triamterene. However, the supplements did prevent the occasional occurrence of marked hypokalemia; all 12 of the men who developed serum postassium levels of 3.0 mmol/L or less were among the 90 who received diuretics without supplementation. Similarly, the overall proportion of men with ventricular arrhythmias was not affected by randomized treatment, but there was a twofold increase in the proportion with arrhythmias among the 12 men with serum potassium levels of 3.0 mmol/L or less. Serum magnesium and intracellular potassium and magnesium levels were not reduced by hydrochlorothiazide, nor were they related to ventricular arrhythmias. Most hypertensive patients, treatment with 50 mg/d of hydrochlorothiazide does not cause marked hypokalemia or ventricular arrhythmias. However, because some individuals will develop hypokalemia after starting diuretic therapy, serum potassium levels should be monitored and potassium-sparing strategies should be used when indicated.

Chlorthalidone or atenolol

The Trial of Antihypertensives Interventions and Management (TAIM) was a multicenter double-blind placebo-controlled clinical trial of drug and diet combinations for the treatment of mild systemic hypertension among 878 participants, aged 21 to 65 years, 110% to 160% ideal weight, and baseline diastolic BP 90 to 100 mm Hg. The drugs used were placebo, chlorthalidone (25 mg/daily) or atenolol (50 mg/daily). The diets studied were usual, weight loss, sodium reduction/potassium increase. Trial end points were 6-month diastolic BP change, cardiovascular risk change, and quality of life change. Wassertheil-Smoller and associates[22] from multiple medical centers summarized the final results of the trial. Either drug combined with weight loss produced the greatest BP reduction of 15 mm Hg, compared to 8 mm Hg on placebo/usual diet. Adding sodium restriction to either drug did not enhance BP lowering effect. Drugs out-performed diet in terms of antihypertensive effect. However, those on placebo and assigned to weight reduction who lost more than 4.5 kg and those on sodium restriction who reduced sodium to less than 70 mEq daily lowered BP to a similar extent as those on either of the 2 drugs alone. Cardiovascular risk at 6 months relative to baseline ranged from 0.85 in weight loss/atenolol subgroup to 1.04 in the usual diet/chlorthalidone subgroup. Blacks were more responsive to chlorthalidone plus weight loss and whites to atenolol plus weight loss. Quality of life, as measured by scales of distress and well-being, was favorably affected by weight reduction. Although there were few side effects of the drugs and most patients improved on most parameters, sexual complaints were worsened among those on chlorthalidone and usual diet compared to placebo. This was ameliorated by adding weight reduction to chlorthalidone. The authors concluded that from the perspective of all 3 endpoints, BP, cardio-vascular risk, and quality of life, weight loss added to either drug provides the most beneficial regimen.

Wassertheil-Smoller and associates[23] from several USA medical centers examined the effect of weight loss, alone and in combination with drugs, on diastolic BP change in the Trial of Antihypertensive Interventions and Management (TAIM), a randomized, multicenter, placebo-controlled clinical trial of drug and diet combinations in the treatment of mild hypertension among 787 patients. Diastolic BP drop (11.6 mm Hg) at 6 months among those patients who were randomized to weight reduction and placebo drug treatment was greater among those who lost 4.5 kg or more, than the 7-mm Hg drop for those who lost less than 2.25 kg or for the placebo-treated control group, and it was statistically equivalent to the reduction achieved by 25 mg of chlorthalidone or 50 mg of atenolol (11.1- and 12.4-mm Hg drop, respectively). Weight loss potentiated effects of drugs, with reductions of 18.4 mm Hg, for those patients who were taking atenolol and had a 4.5-kg or more weight loss, and of 15.4 mm Hg, for those patients who were taking chlorthalidone and had at least a 2.25-kg weight loss. The authors concluded that effective weight loss (≥4.5 kg) lowers BP similarly to low-dose drug therapy and potentiates drug effects, with the apparent 4.5-kg threshold being lowered to 2.25 kg for those patients who receive chlorthalidone.

Doxazosin

Shieh and associates[24] from Palo Alto, California, and Taipei, Republic of China, Taiwan, evaluated metabolic changes associated with doxazosin treatment of systemic hypertension in 10 patients with mild hypertension (mean BP 150 ± 3/100 ± 1 mm Hg) and a plasma triglyceride concentration >1.50 mmol/L. The BP was lower after 4 to 6 months of doxazosin which was also associated with a significantly lower plasma insulin response to a 75 g oral glucose load, and lower plasma TG and cholesterol concentrations. In addition, insulin-mediated glucose uptake was significantly greater after doxazosin treatment. These data suggest that doxazosin treatment of patients with mild hypertension is associated with changes in insulin and lipid metabolism that should decrease the risk of CAD.

Atenolol + enalapril

Ketelhut and colleagues[25] in Todtmoos, Germany, and New Orleans, Louisiana, designed a study to evaluate the long-term effects of combination therapy with an angiotensin-converting enzyme inhibitor and a beta-adrenergic blocking agent on the relation between the decrease in arterial pressure at rest and during exercise and decrease in LV mass. Several antihypertensive drugs, including angiotensin-converting enzyme inhibitors and beta-blockers have been shown to reduce LV hypertrophy, but little is known about combination therapy and the time course of their influence on LV mass. Twenty-one patients with previously untreated essential hypertension were treated with a low dose combination of 50 mg of atenolol and 10 mg of enalapril once daily for 39 months. Cardiovascular findings were assessed by 2-dimensionally guided M-mode echocardiography in the pretreatment phase and after 6 and 39 months of combination therapy. Combination therapy reduced arterial pressure at rest from 161/108 to 130/86 mm Hg and exercise arterial pressure at 100 Watts from 192/112 to 167/95 mm Hg. After 6 months of treatment, significant decreases in interventricular septal thickness, posterior wall thickness and LV mass index were demonstrated on the echocardiogram (Figure 5-7). Following 39 months of therapy, reductions in these values were 28%, 29% and 40%, respectively. Long-term treatment with combination therapy of atenolol and enalapril produced significant reductions in arterial pressure at rest and during exercise associated with reductions in LV mass. The changes in LV mass occurred gradually and continued throughout the treatment period of >3 years. Despite the marked reduction in LV mass, LV pump function was well preserved during rest and exercise.

Atenolol vs enalapril vs hydrochlorothiazide vs isradipine

There is little information about the relative effectiveness of different drug regimens in systemic hypertension. Silagy and associates[26] from Prahran Vic, Australia, compared the efficacy and tolerability of 50 mg of atenolol, 10 mg of enalapril, 25 mg of hydrochlorothiazide, and 2.5 mg of isradipine in the treatment of isolated systolic hypertension. After a 3-week placebo run-in phase, 24 subjects were randomized into a 4-period double-blind crossover study by use of an orthogonal latin square design. Treatment periods were of 6 weeks' duration with titration to a higher dose after 4 weeks in those not reaching goal BP. Each active treatment was followed by a 3-week placebo washout. Casual clinic and 24-hour ambulatory BP (Accutracker II) were measured at the end of each treatment phase. Routine biochemistry was also performed after the placebo run-in, at the end of each active treatment phase, and after the placebo

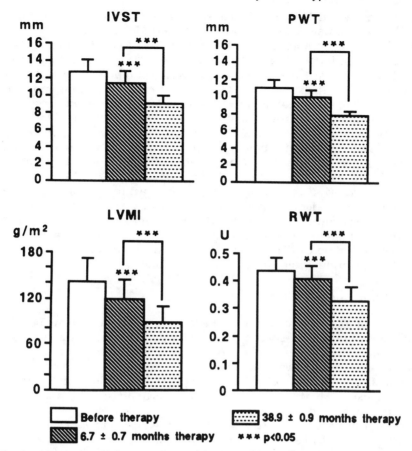

Fig. 5-7. Regression of left ventricular mass during long-term treatment with a combination of atenolol and enalapril. IVST = interventricular septal thickness; LVMI = left ventricular mass index; PWT = posterior wall thickness; RWT = relative wall thickness. Reproduced with permission from Ketelhut, et al.[25]

run-out. Of the 24 subjects entered (mean age 72.3 years, 38% men) 20 completed the whole study. Mean ± standard deviation of supine clinic and daytime ambulatory BP on entry were 181/79 ± 21/9 mm Hg and 165/82 ± 23/15 mm Hg, respectively. All drugs reduced mean casual and ambulatory BP significantly relative to placebo but only hydrochlorothiazide and enalapril produced a consistent hypotensive effect throughout the entire 24-hour period. Isradipine and enalapril exhibited a relatively greater effect on reducing systolic BP than either hydrochlorothiazide or atenolol. The frequency of adverse effects was similar except ankle edema was more frequent with isradipine, cough with enalapril, and breathlessness with atenolol. It is concluded that in the dosages used, both hydrochlorothiazide and enalapril provide suitable treatment for isolated systolic hypertension.

Nifedipine

Middlemost and associates[27] from Johannesburg, South Africa, treated 39 black patients with mild to moderate systemic hypertension for 1 year with various long-acting preparations of nifedipine, during which time serial changes in 24-hour ambulatory BP, exercise performance, LV mass index, and LV systolic function were evaluated. Mean 24-hour ambulatory BP decreased from $156 \pm 15/99 \pm 8$ to $125 \pm 10/79 \pm 6$ mm Hg at 1 year. LV mass index decreased from 130 ± 40 to 114 ± 39 g/m^2 at 6 weeks and to 95 ± 32 at 1 year. There was a significant reduction in septal and posterior wall thickness from 11.0 ± 2.0 to 9.3 ± 2.0 mm and from 10.9 ± 2.0 to 9.3 ± 2.0 mm, respectively. Cardiac index and fractional shortening changed insignificantly from 2.9 ± 0.7 to 2.9 ± 0.6 liters/min/m^2, and from 35 ± 5 to $36 \pm 6\%$ respectively. At 1 year, using a modified Bruce protocol, exercise time increased from 691 ± 138 to 845 ± 183 seconds; peak exercise and 1 minute post-effort systolic BP decreased from 240 ± 26 to 200 ± 21 mm Hg and from 221 ± 27 to 169 ± 32 mm Hg, respectively. It is concluded that in the treatment of black patients with mild to moderate hypertension, the marked and sustained antihypertensive action of long-acting nifedipine documented by 24-hour ambulatory BP monitoring is associated with LV mass regression with no adverse effect on cardiac function together with a reduction in exercise systolic BP and a prolongation of exercise time.

Atenolol vs nifedipine

To compare the effects of atenolol and nifedipine on mood and cognitive function in elderly hypertensive patients, Skinner and associates[28] from Stanford and Palo Alto, California, performed a randomized, double-blind, cross-over trial involving 31 volunteers (7 women and 24 men) aged 60 to 81 years of age with mild to moderate systemic hypertension. Six volunteers withdrew at early phases of the study for reasons unrelated to adverse drug reactions. The participants had 2 weeks of placebo, 2 to 6 weeks of titration with atenolol or nifedipine, and 4 weeks of treatment followed by similar periods with the other drug. Psychometric tests designed to assess mood and cognitive function were performed. In the group first treated with nifedipine, the summed recall score on the Buschke selective reminding test (a test of verbal learning and memory) decreased by 9.3 words, or 9%, during nifedipine treatment compared with placebo. The group first treated with atenolol showed no improvement in summed recall scores when results seen during atenolol therapy and placebo administration were compared; however, this group had an improvement of 16.1 words, or of 16%, when the atenolol score was compared with the nifedipine score. In the group first treated with nifedipine, 6 of 11 patients (55%) showed a decrease of 5 words or more during nifedipine therapy compared with placebo, whereas only 1 of the 14 patients (7%) in the group first treated with atenolol showed a similar decrease. On the digit symbol test (a psychomotor test), patients treated first with atenolol tended to improve, whereas patients treated first with nifedipine tended to decline. The difference between nifedipine and atenolol, in terms of the change from the score seen during placebo, was 4.3 codings. No statistically significant differences were seen between nifedipine and atenolol therapy regarding the other measures of psychomotor ability, sustained attention, motor performance, verbal fluency, or abstract reasoning, and no effects of either drug on mood or psychopathologic symptoms were noted. Although atenolol and nifedipine are generally free of gross effects on cognition or mood, nifedipine may subtly impair learning and memory in some elderly hypertensive patients.

Nicardipine

Dittrich and associates[29] from San Diego, California, analyzed in patients with mild to moderate systemic hypertension the effects of a sustained-release formulation of the calcium antagonist nicardipine on LV mass, Doppler transmitral velocity profiles, and plasma neurohumoral studies. A double-blind, placebo control phase in 28 patients was carried out for 6 weeks with a subgroup of 13 subsequently entering an open-label long-term phase for 1 year. Nicardipine produced a significant decrease in systolic and diastolic pressure over the 6-week phase (158 ± 15 to 142 ± 9 mm Hg, and 100 ± 5 to 89 ± 9 mm Hg, respectively). No significant differences in Doppler measures of mitral inflow or echocardiographic measures of LV function, wall thickness or mass were noted in the 6-week phase of the study. Although nicardipine increased both norepinephrine and renin values after the first dose, these levels had returned to baseline in most patients after 6 weeks. In addition, there was no evidence for stimulation of adrenomedullary activity because nicardipine had no effect on epinephrine or dopamine-B-hydroxylase levels at first dose or after 6 weeks. In the 13 patients treated for 1 year, systolic and diastolic pressure remained significantly decreased compared with pressure before therapy (135 ± 9 vs 147 ± 15 mm Hg, and 85 ± 6 vs 97 ± 9 mm Hg). Concomitantly, both septal and posterior wall thickness decreased significantly (12.4 ± 1.5 to 10.7 ± 1.7 mm, and 11.0 ± 1.4 to 9.9 ± 1.7 mm) over 1 year as did LV mass index (150 ± 28 to 127 ± 31 g/m²). Importantly, no change was noted in LV cavity size, demonstrating that LV mass reduction was due solely to regression of hypertrophy. Doppler mitral inflow patterns were minimally affected with an increase in atrial velocity time integral. These results demonstrate that regression of LV hypertrophy takes place with long-term antihypertensive therapy with nicardipine, and this may be possible, in part, because of the lack of sustained neurohumoral stimulation by this agent.

Nicardipine vs verapamil

In a double-blind, parallel, multicenter study reported by Gradman and associates[30], sustained release (SR) preparations of 2 calcium antagonists, nicardipine and verapamil, were compared for treatment of mild to moderate systemic hypertension. Two hundred eighteen patients with supine diastolic BP 95 to 114 mm Hg were randomly assigned to receive nicardipine-SR 45 mg twice daily (n = 73), nicardipine-SR 60 mg twice daily (n = 73) or verapamil-SR 240 mg once daily in the morning (n = 72). All 3 regimens significantly reduced supine and sitting systolic and diastolic BPs compared with baseline values. The efficacy of drugs became apparent after 2 weeks of therapy, and was sustained throughout the 12-week study. Reductions in sitting diastolic BP and supine and sitting systolic BPs were statistically greater with nicardipine-SR 60 mg twice daily compared with verapamil, and nicardipine-SR 45 mg twice daily was equivalent to verapamil. Asthenia and constipation occurred more frequently in patients treated with verapamil (9.7 and 11.1%, respectively, compared with 6.8 and 4.1% in either nicardipine group). Adverse events reported more frequently with nicardipine were headache (17.8% with nicardipine-SR 60 mg and 15.1% with nicardipine-SR 45 mg vs 13.9% with verapamil) and edema (15.1% in the nicardipine-SR 60 mg group, 8.2% with nicardipine-SR 45 mg vs 4.2% with verapamil). Verapamil, but not nicardipine, produced significant reductions in heart rate. SR preparations of calcium antagonists offer options for effective monotherapy of systemic hypertension. Side-effect profiles differ and may affect choice of therapy.

Isradipine vs diltiazem

Black and associates[31] from multiple USA medical centers compared the safety of isradipine, a new dihydropyridine calcium entry blocker, with an equal potent dose of diltiazem in 174 mild hypertensive patients (diastolic BP 95–105 mm Hg). After appropriate washout and placebo periods, patients were randomly assigned to receive either 1.25 mg isradipine twice daily (Group I) or 40 mg diltiazem thrice daily (Group D). If diastolic BP remained above 90 mm Hg, doses were increased to a maximum of 5 mg isradipine twice daily or 120 mg diltiazem thrice daily. Active therapy was given for a total of 12 weeks. Only 18 patients (9 from each group) did not complete the protocol. The patients were well-matched at baseline with a mean BP of 149/100 mm Hg for those who were randomized to isradipine and completed the protocol and 153/99 mm Hg for the diltiazem group. The responses to each drug were excellent with 72% of the isradipine patients and 73% of the diltiazem group having diastolic BP <90 mm Hg at the completion of the study. Of the 156 patients who completed the protocol, only 18 patients (10 in Group I and 8 in Group D) failed to respond. Both drugs were well-tolerated. No adverse reactions were reported by 68% of the patients in Group I and 65% of those in Group D. The most common side effect was headache (9.0% in Group I and 7.8% in Group D) followed by fatigue (5.2% in Group I and 3.9% in Group D). Age and race did not predict response to either agent but men responded slightly better to diltiazem than women. The authors concluded that isradipine and diltiazem are equally well tolerated and can be used successfully as a monotherapy to treat hypertension in a wide variety of patients.

Isradipine vs lisinopril

Bielen and associates[32] from Leuven, Belgium, compared the effects on cardiac structure and function of antihypertensive regimens with different effects on the renin-angiotensin system. In a 1-year study, 32 patients with essential hypertension were randomized to treatment with either the converting enzyme inhibitor lisinopril or the calcium antagonist isradipine; hydrochlorothiazide could be added. BP decreased significantly and similarly in the 2 treatment groups. LV mass was already significantly reduced after 16 weeks of treatment and remained decreased thereafter, with no difference in the response to the 2 treatment regimens. The change in LV mass was related to the decrease in systolic BP for the total study group and for each treatment group separately. During the 3 week run-out period on placebo, BP and LV mass increased again. Afterload decreased during active treatment, and fractional shortening of the LV internal diameter was significantly increased to a similar extent in both groups. The ratio of peak mitral flow velocities during atrial contraction and early filling was reduced after 1 year of active treatment in the total study group; this change was similar in both groups. The data suggest that the regression of LV mass during antihypertensive therapy is mainly related to the decrease in systolic BP.

Felodipine

Leenen and Holliwell[33] from Ottawa, Canada, studied 20 patients whose systemic hypertension was not controlled with chronic B-blocker therapy to evaluate the acute (first dose), short-term (4 weeks) and chronic (6 to 12 months) effects of the calcium antagonist felodipine on BP, LV anatomy and function and on plasma norepinephrine. The first dose of felodipine rapidly reduced total peripheral resistance and BP, associated with significant increases in heart rate, cardiac output and plasma norepinephrine. During chronic therapy, at the end of the dosing interval (12 hours), significant decreases in BP persisted with minimal changes in the other variables. However, even after 1 year of therapy BP after dosing again rapidly decreased associated with 50 to 100% increases in plasma norepinephrine and small increases in heart rate and cardiac output. Despite the marked decreases in systolic BP, LV wall thickness and mass showed only small decreases (LV mass - 17 ± 7 g/m² after 1 year) and significant LV hypertrophy persisted after 1 year. Both average systolic BP and plasma norepinephrine were significant determinants of LV mass over the duration of the study. It is concluded that during chronic treatment with the twice-daily tablet formulation of felodipine, major daily fluctuations in BP persist associated with persisting sympathetic hyperactivity. The latter may play a role in the modest regression of LV hypertrophy despite 30 to 40 mm Hg decreases in systolic BP for 1 year.

Clentiazem

To determine the hemodynamic and certain metabolic effects of clentiazem, a diltiazem congener, Frohlich and associates[34] from New Orleans, Louisiana, gave 10 untreated patients with essential hypertension the calcium antagonist in 3 successive doses totaling 1.0 mg/kg intravenously. Mean arterial pressure and total peripheral resistance progressively declined from 121 ± 3 mm Hg and 47 ± 2 U (mean) to 110 ± 3 mm Hg and 33 ± 1 U, respectively; heart rate remained unchanged. Cardiac output increased as a result of augmented cardiopulmonary volume produced by peripheral venoconstriction and norepinephrine release (from 258 ± 41 to 319 ± 42 pg/ml). Surprisingly, there was an immediate reduction in plasma aldosterone (10.4 ± 1.2 to 6.5 ± 1.0 ng/dl), serum potassium (4.3 ± 0.1 to 3.6 ± 0.1 mEq/dl) and calcium (9.5 ± 0.1 to 8.8 ± 0.1 mg/dl) concentrations, whereas epinephrine increased (21.2 ± 3.3 to 45.8 ± 5.9 pg/ml). Previous studies with diltiazem, conducted similarly, did not show these changes. Therefore, clentiazem reduced mean arterial pressure through a decrease in total peripheral resistance, and released epinephrine was associated with intracellular potassium influx (urinary potassium did not change). The inhibited aldosterone release was not compensated by altered renal blood flow, glomerular filtration or increased plasma renin activity. These findings underscore the concept that calcium antagonists are a remarkably heterogeneous antihypertensive group.

Nitroprusside or fenoldopam

Electrocardiograms are routinely obtained before and during the acute treatment of hypertensive emergencies. Little is known, however, about the frequency and significance of such changes or their relation to the treatment used. Gretler and associates[35] from Chicago, Illinois, analyzed

12-lead electrocardiograms from 21 patients admitted for hypertensive emergencies (average BP, 222 ± 4/140 ± 3 mm Hg). Patients were randomly assigned to treatment with sodium nitroprusside (n = 11) or the dopamine receptor agonist fenoldopam mesylate (n = 10). Electrocardiograms were obtained at baseline and within 30 minutes of reaching goal BP (diastolic BP, 100 to 110 mm Hg). There was no significant effect of either drug treatment on PR interval, QRS duration, QT interval, or R-wave amplitude, and no major ST-segment changes were noted. During treatment with either drug, the average T-wave amplitude decreased in all leads except aVR. New T-wave inversions in lead V_4 occurred in 2 and 4 patients after fenoldopam and nitroprusside treatment, respectively. There were no clinically apparent episodes of AMI in any patient. Even in the absence of obvious AMI, a decrease in T-wave amplitude, including T-wave inversion, occurs commonly during acute BP reduction in hypertensive emergencies, an observation that may be explained by the accompanying acute changes in cardiac chamber volumes.

Metaanalysis of effects on left ventricular mass

Dahlof and associates[36] from Goteborg, Sweden, evaluated via a meta-analysis all available studies as of December 1990 on the effect of antihypertensive pharmacologic therapy on LV structure examined by echocardiography. The authors applied preset inclusion criteria to the analysis. A total of 109 studies comprising 2,357 patients (28% previously untreated) with an average age of 49 years (range 30 to 71) were included. Overall LV mass was reduced by 11.9% in parallel with a reduction of mean arterial pressure of 14.9%. To differentiate between first-line therapies and to adjust for differences between studies, the authors performed ANCOVA. Angiotensin converting enzyme inhibitors reduced LV mass by 15%, B-blockers by 8%, calcium antagonists by 8.5%, and diuretics by 11.3%. When the authors calculated LV mass using the same formula for all studies the absolute reductions in grams were 44.7 g with angiotensin converting enzyme inhibitors, 22.8 g with B-blockers, 26.9 g with calcium antagonists, and 21.4 g with diuretics. Except for diuretics, predominately reduced ventricular diameter. In conclusion, this metaanalysis shows that angiotensin converting enzyme inhibitors, B-blockers, and calcium antagonists all reduce LV mass by reversing wall hypertrophy, and that the effect is most pronounced with angiotensin converting enzyme inhibitors. Conversely, diuretics reduce LV mass mainly through a reduction of LV volume. Based on these data, the authors hypothesize that angiotensin converting enzyme inhibitors are more effective than other first-line therapies in reducing LV mass.

References

1. Bottini PB, Carr AA, Rhoades RB, Prisant M: Variability of indirect methods used to determine blood pressure: Office vs mean 24-hour automated blood pressures. Arch Intern Med 1992 (Jan);152:139–144.
2. Pearce KA, Grimm RH JR, Rao S, Svendsen K, Liebson PR, Neaton JD, Ensrud K: Population derived comparisons of ambulatory and office blood pressures: Implications for the determination of usual blood pressure and the concept of white coat hypertension. Arch Intern Med 1992 (Apr);152:750–756.

3. Staessen J, Bulpitt CJ, O'Brien E, Cox J, Fagard R, Stanton A, Thijs L, Van Hulle S, Vyncke G, Amery A: The diurnal blood pressure profile: A population study. Am J Hypertens 1992 (June);5:386–392.

4. Khoury AF, Sunderajan P, Kaplan NM: The early morning rise in blood pressure is related mainly to ambulation. Am J Hypertens 1992 (June);5:339–344.

5. Psaty BM, Furberg CD, Kuller LH, Borhani NO, Rautaharju PM, O'Leary DH, Bild DE, Robbins J, Fried LP, Reid C: Isolated systolic hypertension and subclinical cardiovascular disease in the elderly: Initial findings from the cardiovascular health study. JAMA 1992 (Sept 9) 268:1287–1291.

6. Mann SJ: Systolic hypertension in the elderly: Pathophysiology and management. Arch Intern Med 1992 (Oct);152:1977–1984.

7. Shea S, Misra D, Ehrlich MH, Field L, Francis CK: Predisposing factors for severe, uncontrolled hypertension in an inner-city minority population. N Engl J Med 1992 (Sept 10);327:776–781.

8. Siegel D, Black DM, Seeley DG, Hulley SB: Circadian variation in ventricular arrhythmias in hypertensive men. Am J Cardiol 1992 (Feb 1);69:334–347.

9. Kostis JB, Lacy CR, Shindler DM, Borhani NO, Hall WD, Wilson AC, Krieger S, Chelton S: Frequency of ventricular ectopic activity in isolated systolic systemic hypertension. Am J Cardiol 1992 (Feb 15);69:557–559.

10. Pringle SD, Dunn FG, MacFarlane PW, McKillop JH, Lorimer AR, Cobbe SM: Significance of ventricular arrhythmias in systemic hypertension with left ventricular hypertrophy. Am J Cardiol 1992 (Apr 1);69:913–917.

11. Frohlich ED, Apstein C, Chobanian AV, Devereux RB, Dustan HP, Dzau V, Fauad-Tarazi F, Horan MJ, Marcus M, Massie B, Pfeffer MA, Re RN, Rocella EJ, Savage D, Shub C: The heart in hypertension. N Engl J Med 1992 (Oct 1);327:998–1008.

12. Pringle SD, Dunn FG, Tweddel AC, Martin W, MacFarlane PW, McKillop JH, Lorimer AR, Cobbe SM: Symptomatic and silent myocardial ischemia in hypertensive patients with left ventricular hypertrophy. Br Heart J 1992 (May);67:377–382.

13. Ghali JK, Liao Y, Simmons B, Castaner A, Cao G, Cooper RS: The prognostic role of left ventricular hypertrophy in patients with or without coronary artery disease. An Intern Med 1992 (Nov 15);117:831–836.

14. Siegel D, Cheitlin MD, Seeley DG, Black DM, Hulley SB: Silent myocardial ischemia in men with systemic hypertension and without clinical evidence of coronary artery disease. Am J Cardiol 1992 (Jul 1);70:86–90.

15. Fletcher AE and Bulpitt CJ: How far should blood pressure be lowered? N Engl J Med 1992 (Jan 23);326:251–254.

16. McCloskey LW, Psaty BM, Koepsell TD, Aagaard GN: Level of blood pressure and risk of myocardial infarction among treated hypertensive patients. Arch Intern Med 1992 (Mar);152:513–520.

17. Kostis JB, Rosen RC, Brondolo E, Taska L, Smith DE, Wilson AC: Superiority of nonpharmacologic therapy compared to propranolol and placebo in men with mild hypertension: A randomized, prospective trial. Am Heart J 1992 (February);123:466–474.

18. Trials of Hypertension Prevention Collaborative Research Group: The effects of nonpharmacologic interventions on blood pressure of persons with high normal levels: Results of the trials of hypertension prevention, Phase I. JAMA 1992 (Mar 4);267:1213–1220.

19. Blaufox MD, Lee HB, Davis B, Oberman A, Wassertheil-Smoller S, Hangford H: Renin predicts diastolic blood pressure response to nonpharmacologic and pharmacologic therapy. JAMA 1992 (Mar 4);267;1221–1225.

20. Ascherio A, Rimm EB, Giovannucci EL, Colditz GA, Rosner B, Willett WC, Sacks F, Stampfer MJ: A Prospective Study of Nutritional Factors and Hypertension Among US Men. Circulation 1992 (November);86:1475–1484.

21. Siegel D, Hulley SB, Black DM, Cheitlin MD, Sebastian A, Seeley DG, Hearst N, Fine R: Diuretics, serum and intracellular electrolyte levels, and ventricular arrhythmias in hypertensive men. JAMA 1992 (Feb 26);267:1083–1089.

22. Wassertheil-Smoller S, Oberman A, Blaufox MD, Davis B; Langford H: The trial of antihypertensive interventions and management (TAIM) study: Final results with regard to blood pressure, cardiovascular risk, and quality of life. Am J Hypertension 1992 (Jan);5:37–44.

23. Wassertheil-Smoller S, Blaufox MD, Oberman AS, Langford HG, Davis BR, Wylie-Rosett

J: The trial of antihypertensive interventions and management (TAIM) study: Adequate weight loss, alone and combined with drug therapy in the treatment of mild hypertension. Arch Intern Med 1992 (Jan);152:131–136.

24. Shieh SM, Sheu WHH, Shen DC, Fuh MMT, Chen YDI, Reaven GM: Glucose, insulin, and lipid metabolism in doxazosin-treated patients with hypertension. Am J of Hypertension 1992 (Nov);5:827–831.

25. Ketelhut R, Franz IW, Behr U, Toennesmann U, Messerli FH. Preserved ventricular pump function after a marked reduction of left ventricular mass. J Am Coll Cardiol 1992 (October);20:864–8.

26. Silagy CA, McNeil JJ, McGrath BP: Crossover comparison of atenolol, enalapril, hydrochlorothiazide and isradipine for isolated systolic systemic hypertension. Am J Cardiol 1992 (Nov 15);70:1299–1305.

27. Middlemost SJ, Sack M, Davis J, Skoularigis J, Wisenbaugh T, Essop MR, Sareli P: Effects of long-acting nifedipine on casual office blood pressure measurements, 24-hour ambulatory blood pressure profiles, exercise paramemters and left ventricular mass and function in black patients with mild to moderate systemic hypertension. Am J Cardiol 1992 (Aug 15);70:474–478.

28. Skinner MH, Futterman A, Morrisette D, Thompson LW, Hoffman BB, Blaschke TF: Atenolol compared with nifedipine: Effect on cognitive function and mood in elderly hypertensive patients. An Intern Med 1992 (Apr 15);116:615–623.

29. Dittrich HC, Adler J, Ong J, Reitman M, Weber M, Ziegler M: Effects of sustained-release nicardipine on regression of left ventricular hypertrophy in systemic hypertension. Am J Cardiol 1992 (June 15);69:1559–1564.

30. Gradman AH, Frishman WH, Kaihlanen PM, Wong SC, Friday KJ, Comparison of sustained-release formulations of nicardipine and verapamil for mild to moderate systemic hypertension. Am J Cardiol 1992 (Dec 15);70:1571–1575.

31. Black HR, Lewin AJ, Stein GH, MacCarthy EP, Hamilton JH, Hamilton BP, Madias NE, Kochar MS, Abrams AP, Isaacsohn JL, Gibbons ME, Matthews KP: A comparison of the safety of therapeutically equivalent doses of isradipine and diltiazem for treatment of essential hypertension. Am J Hypertens 1992 (Mar);5:141–146.

32. Bielen EC, Fagard RH, Lijnen PJ, Tjandra-Maga TB, Verbesselt R, Amery AK: Comparison of the effects of isradipine and lisinopril on left ventricular structure and function in essential hypertension. Am J Cardiol 1992 (May 1);69:1200–1206.

33. Leenen FHH, Holliwell DL: Antihypertensive effect of felodipine associated with persistent sympathetic activation and minimal regression of left ventricular hypertrophy. Am J Cardiol 1992 (Mar 1);69:639–645.

34. Frohlich ED, McLoughlin M, Ketelhut R: Hemodynamic and metabolic effects of intravenous clentiazem in hypertensive patients. Am J Cardiol 1992 (Jan 15);69:229–232.

35. Gretler DD, Elliott WJ, Moscucci M, Childers RW, Murphy MB: Electrocardiographic changes during acute treatment of hypertensive emergencies with sodium nitroprusside or fenoldopam. Arch Intern Med 1992 (Dec);152:2445–2448.

36. Dahlof B, Pennert K, Hansson L: Reversal of left ventricular hypertrophy in hypertensive patients: A metaanalysis of 109 treatment studies. Am J Hypertens 1992 (Feb);5:95–110.

6

Valvular Heart Disease

Third heart sound

The presence of third heart sounds in patients with valvular heart disease is often regarded as a sign of CHF, but it may also depend on the type of valvular disease. Folland and participants in the Veterans Affairs Cooperative Study on Valvular Heart Disease[1] assessed the prevalence of third heart sounds and the relation between third heart sounds and cardiac function in 1,288 patients with 6 types of valvular heart disease (Figures 6-1 and 6-2). The prevalence of third heart sounds was higher in patients with MR (46%) or AR (28%) than in those with AS (11%)

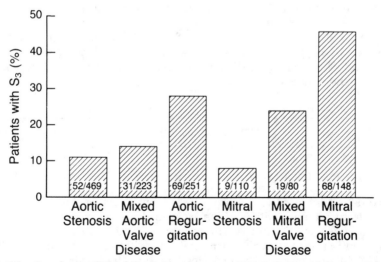

Fig. 6-1. Prevalence of Third Heart Sounds among 1281 Patients with Various Valvular Diagnoses. The numbers inside the bars are numbers of patients, S_3 was also present in 56 of 183 patients (31 percent) with multivalvular disease. Reproduced with permission from Folland, et al.[1]

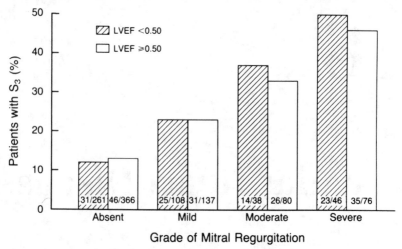

Fig. 6-2. Prevalence of Third Heart Sounds among 1112 Patients with Complete Data on Both the Degree of Visually Graded Mitral Regurgitation and the Left Ventricular Ejection Fraction (LVEF). The prevalence of S_3 varied directly and significantly (P<0.0001) with the severity of mitral regurgitation regardless of the LVEF. Within each grade the percentage of patients with S_3 was not statistically different whether the LVEF was ≥0.50 or <0.50 (P = 0.64 to 0.92). The relation was the same in 196 patients with visually graded mitral regurgitation for whom LVEF data were not available. This stepwise relation was not demonstrated for aortic regurgitation. Reproduced with permission from Folland, et al.[1]

or MS (8%). The LVEF was significantly lower when a third heart sound was detected in patients with AS (0.38 vs 0.56 in those without third heart sounds) or mixed aortic valve disease (0.40 vs 0.55). However, the EF was only slightly lower in patients with MR and third heart sounds (0.51 vs 0.57). The PA wedge pressure was higher when a third heart sound was detected in patients with aortic stenosis (18.6 mm Hg, vs. 12.1 mm Hg in those without third heart sounds). There was no association between the PA wedge pressure and third heart sounds in patients with MR. The prevalence of third heart sounds increased with the severity of MR. In patients with MR, third heart sounds are common but do not necessarily reflect LV systolic dysfunction or increased filling pressure. In patients with AS, third heart sounds are uncommon but usually indicate the presence of systolic dysfunction and elevated filling pressure.

MITRAL VALVE PROLAPSE

Morphologic observations

To determine if certain morphologic characteristics were present in hearts from patients with sudden cardiac death associated with MVP, Farb and associates[2] from Washington, D.C., and Nashville, Tennessee, compared hearts at necropsy from patients with sudden death and isolated MVP who were previously asymptomatic or had a history of cardiac arrhythmias (n = 27) with (1) hearts from patients with CHf and MR secondary to MVP (n = 14), and (2) hearts from persons dying from noncardiac causes in which MVP was an incidental finding (n = 19).

Patients who died suddenly were younger than both patients with MR/ CHF and incidental cases (37 ± 10 vs 65 ± 16 and 58 ± 21 years, respectively). Mitral valve annular circumference, anterior and posterior mitral valve leaflet lengths, posterior mitral valve thickness, and presence and extent of endocardial plaque were greater in hearts from patients with sudden death than hearts from those with incidental MVP. Hearts from patients with MR/CHF weighed significantly more, had greater left and right atrial cavity sizes and LV cavity diameter than hearts from both sudden death and incidental cases.

Electrocardiographic observations

A number of electrocardiographic findings associated with MVP have been reported. Bhutto and associates[3] from Chicago, Illinois, obtained electrocardiograms from 148 consecutive patients (32% men and 68% women, mean age 45 ± 18 years) referred for suspected MVP and with MVP documented by echocardiogram. The electrocardiograms were analyzed with respect to interventricular conduction disturbances, PR, QRS and QTc intervals, and T-wave abnormalities. The results were compared with electrocardiographic data from 116 patients matched for age and sex. The findings are summarized in Tables 6-1 and 6-2. In all other previous investigations examining electrocardiographic abnormalities in association with MVP, a comparison was not performed with results obtained from patients matched for age and sex who had no evidence of MVP on echocardiogram. In the present study, there was no significant difference in the frequency of a prolonged QTc interval between patients with and without MVP. Furthermore, the mean QTc interval of the 2 groups did not differ significantly. Similarly, there was no significant difference in the incidence of conduction disturbances of the bundle

TABLE 6-1. *Frequency of Electrocardiographic Abnormalities in Mitral Valve Prolapse. Reproduced with permission from Bhutto, et al.*[3]

| | No. of Pts. | Left BBB | Right BBB | | QTc Prolongation | T-Wave Inversion |
			Complete	Incomplete		
Controls	116	1 (0.8%)	2 (2%)	10 (9%)	23 (20%)	20 (17%)
MVP	148	0 (0%)	4 (3%)	9 (6%)	33 (22%)	57 (39%)*

*p <0.001, chi-square.
BBB = bundle branch block; MVP = mitral valve prolapse.

TABLE 6-2. *Electrocardiographic Intervals in Normal Patients and in Those with Mitral Valve Prolapse. Reproduced with permission from Bhutto, et al.*[3]

	No. of Pts.	PR (ms)	QRS (ms)	QT (ms)	QTc (ms)
Controls	116	157 ± 25	86 ± 11	360 ± 42	415 ± 28
MVP	148	160 ± 29	88 ± 13	369 ± 42	418 ± 35

Values represent mean ± SD.
MVP = mitral valve prolapse.

branches. Thus, these results indicate that MVP is not associated with electrocardiographic abnormalities other than inferior T-wave inversion.

Induction by dehydration

This study by Lax and associates[4] from Tucson, Arizona, was designed to investigate the hypothesis that MVP can be induced after diuresis in women without the abnormality who have characteristic body habitus. Fifteen tall, slim, healthy female volunteers with normal cardiac findings, echocardiogram, and history were investigated after mild diuresis with furosemide and after placebo. All subjects lost weight after furosemide and placebo administration; but mean weight loss was significantly greater after furosemide administration than after placebo administration. Echocardiography showed MVP in none of the 15 patients before treatment, in 7 after administration of placebo, and in 7 after administration of furosemide. Coaptation point prolapsed superior to the anulus in 7 subjects with echocardiographically determined MVP. LV end-diastolic dimensions decreased significantly after placebo or furosemide administration in individuals in whom MVP developed compared with the measurement in those in whom MVP did not develop. Murmurs characteristics of MVP disappeared in the rehydrated subjects and echocardiographic changes resolved in 2 of the 5 rehydrated individuals. Thus echocardiographically determined MVP can be induced by mild dehydration in women with phenotypic body habitus of MVP; changes may resolve with rehydration. Results suggest an explanation for variable physical examination findings in persons with MVP.

MITRAL REGURGITATION

Total 12-lead QRS voltage

Electrocardiographic criteria for diagnosing LV hypertrophy are known to be relatively nonspecific and insensitive. Several studies have described total 12-lead QRS voltage in various cardiac diseases, and most have found this criterion to be more sensitive than previously described criteria. Glick and Roberts[5] from Bethesda, Maryland, examined total 12-lead QRS voltage in 24 necropsy patients with chronic, pure, isolated MR, and compared its sensitivity to the Sokolow-Lyon and Romhilt-estes criteria for diagnosis of LV hypertrophy. The 24 patients ranged in age from 21 to 84 years (mean 42). Thirteen (54%) were women. All 24 patients had clinical evidence of MR for >5 months and none had clinical or hemodynamic evidence of associated MS, and none had evidence of aortic valve dysfunction. All 24 patients had been in New York Heart Association functional class III or IV CHF. The amplitude of the QRS was measured from the peak of the R wave to the nadir of either the Q wave or the S wave, whichever was deeper. The total 12-lead QRS amplitude in the 24 patients ranged from 111 to 364 mm (mean 220). The upper limit of normal for total QRS amplitude is probably 175 mm. Although the 12-lead QRS amplitude was more sensitive than the other 2 criteria examined, heart weight did not correlate with the total 12-lead QRS amplitude. Table

6-3 shows comparison of the total 12-lead QRS voltage and the patients with MR in the present study to those previously studied in the same laboratory.

Relation of chamber size to severity

LV and LA chamber sizes are frequently used to assist in assessing the severity of MR. To study the reliability of these measurements Burwash and associates[6] from Halifax, Canada, obtained 2-dimensional echocardiographic measurements of LV and LA size in 92 consecutive patients with MR present on both angiography and Doppler echocardiographic examinations performed within 2.8 ± 2.5 days of each other. The accuracy of chamber dimensions in identifying severe MR (angiographic grade 3 to 4+) was determined in the total population and the following patient subgroups: (1) isolated chronic MR with preserved LV function inclusive of all rhythms; (2) isolated chronic MR, preserved LV function and sinus rhythm; (3) isolated chronic MR with LV dysfunction; (4) chronic MR associated with other valvular disease; and (5) acute MR. Only in subgroup 2 were chamber sizes reliable in identifying severe MR (Table 6-4). Atrial dimensions provided the most accurate assessment with an LA volume >58 ml, anteroposterior dimension >45 mm and superoinferior dimension >55 mm, with sensitivities of 75, 75 and 88%, specificities of 83, 100

TABLE 6-3. *Comparison of the Sensitivity of Total QRS Voltage in Identifying Left Ventricular Hypertrophy of Various Etiologies. Reproduced with permission from Glick, et al.[5]*

	Normal (n = 17)*	Aortic Stenosis (n = 50)	Aortic Regurgitation (n = 30)	Hypertrophic Cardiomyopathy (n = 57)	Idiopathic Dilated Cardiomyopathy (n = 49)	Amyloid (n = 30)	Mitral Regurgitation (n = 24)
Age (years) (mean)	41–74 (54)	16–65 (48)	19–65 (45)	14–87 (49)	19–75 (48)	21–93 (58)	21–84 (42)
Heart weight (g) (range)	288–392	380–880	375–1110	290–1230	400–940	370–900	350–900
Mean	351	606	696	593	614	532	550
Total QRS voltage (mm) (range)	84–159	144–417	109–428	66–339	74–281	58–199	111–364
Mean	124	257	270	197	153	104	220
Patients with 12-lead QRS voltage > 175 mm	0 (0%)	47 (94%)	27 (90%)	30 (53%)	20 (41%)	2 (7%)	17 (71%)

*Patients with heart weights < 400 g.

TABLE 6-4. *Cardiac Dimensions in the Total Population (n = 92) with Mitral Regurgitation. Reproduced with permission from Burwash, et al.[6]*

Dimensions	Mild-Moderate MR (n = 47)	Severe MR (n = 45)	p Value
LA volume (ml)	69 ± 48	104 ± 61	0.004
LA anteroposterior (mm)	46 ± 9	51 ± 9	0.01
LA superoinferior (mm)	57 ± 10	65 ± 12	0.001
LA mediolateral (mm)	47 ± 9	55 ± 13	<0.001
LV anteroposterior (mm)	53 ± 9	55 ± 8	NS
LV mediolateral (mm)	47 ± 7	50 ± 7	NS
Fractional shortening (%)	23 ± 10	30 ± 11	0.002
Ejection fraction (%)	45 ± 18	56 ± 17	0.002

LA = left atrial; LV = left ventricular; MR = mitral regurgitation; NS = not significant.

and 83%, positive predictive values of 92, 100, and 93% and negative predictive values of 56, 60, and 71%, respectively. LV dimensions had excellent positive predictive values but lower sensitivities. Normalizing for body surface area did not improve the accuracy of uncorrected dimensions. Although increased LA and LV dimensions can identify severe MR, smaller dimensions do not exclude this diagnosis. With acute MR, atrial fibrillation, LV dysfunction or associated valvular disease, these dimensions are not reliable.

Quantification by echocardiography

Castello and associates[7] in St. Louis, Missouri, studied 80 consecutive patients undergoing both left ventriculography and single-plane transesophageal echocardiography with Doppler color flow mapping to compare the two techniques and their ability to detect and assess severity of MR. Only the mosaic aspect of the regurgitant jet was included in the measurements. Values for inter- and intraobserver variability for the maximum regurgitant area measurements were $10 \pm 9\%$ and $9 \pm 8\%$, respectively. The best correlation between angiography and Doppler color flow imaging was obtained with a maximal regurgitant area. A maximal regurgitant area <3 cm^2 predicted mild MR with a sensitivity of 96%, specificity of 100% and a predictive accuracy of 98%, whereas a maximal regurgitant area >6 cm^2 predicted severe MR with a sensitivity of 91%, specificity of 100% and a predictive accuracy of 98%. A strong, although inferior, correlation was found for the maximal regurgitant area/left atrial area ratio. A ratio $<20\%$ predicted mild MR with 94% accuracy, and a ratio $>35\%$ predicted severe MR with 85% accuracy. Thus, single-plane transesophageal echocardiography with Doppler color flow mapping is a useful technique for the diagnosis of MR. Minimal degrees of MR may be detected in approximately 62% of patients in whom no MR is detected by angiography.

Mitral valve repair

Freeman and colleagues[8] in Rochester, Minnesota, designed a study to delineate the utility and results of intraoperative transesophageal echocardiography in the evaluation of patients undergoing mitral valve repair for MR. Mitral valve reconstruction surgery offers advantages over prosthetic valve replacement and intraoperative assessment of valve competence after repair is important in evaluating the effectiveness of this procedure. Intraoperative transesophageal echocardiography was performed in 143 patients undergoing MV repair during a 23 month period. Before and after repair, the functional morphology of the mitral apparatus was defined by two-dimensional echocardiography. Doppler color flow imaging was used to clarify the mechanism of MR and to semiquantitate its severity. There was significant improvement in the mean MR grade by composite intraoperative transesophageal echocardiography after valve repair. Excellent results from initial repair were observed in 88% of patients. Significant residual MR was identified in 11 patients and 5 underwent prosthetic MVR, 5 had revision of the initial repair, and 1 patient had observation only. Among 100 patient with myxomatous mitral valves, the risk of grade ≥ 3 MR after initial repair was 2% in patients with isolated posterior leaflet disease compared with 23% in patients with anterior or bileaflet disease. Severe systolic anterior motion of the mitral apparatus causing grade 2 to 4 MR was present in 13 patients after cardiopulmonary bypass. In 8 patients, systolic anterior motion resolved immediately with correction of hyperdynamic hemodynamic status, resulting in grade ≤1 residual MR without further intervention. Transthoracic echocardiography before hospital discharge demonstrated grade ≤1 residual MR in 86% in 132 patients. A significant discrepancy in residual MR by predischarge transthoracic versus intraoperative transesophageal echocardiography was noted in 17 patients (13%). These data indicate that transesophageal echocardiography is useful in the intraoperative assessment of MV repair.

Effect of mitral ring on motion of anterior leaflet

Cohen and associates[9] from San Antonio, Texas, described the Doppler and 2-dimensional echocardiographic characteristics of systolic anterior motion of the chordal apparatus after mitral annuloplasty, 24 consecutive patients (19 men and 5 women; mean age, 55 years) with the use of serial Doppler and 2-dimensional echocardiography, which included preoperative transthoracic, intraoperative epicardial, and postoperative transthoracic examinations at 1 week after annuloplasty and every 3 months thereafter for up to 12 months. Systolic anterior leaflet motion of the mitral valve was not seen in this series; however, chordal systolic anterior motion was seen in 3 patients during surgery and in 1 additional patient at the time of the 1-week transthoracic examination. During subsequent studies at 3-month intervals, chordal systolic anterior motion was not present. The LV outflow tract velocities were normal in all patients with and without chordal systolic anterior motion. In conclusion, chordal systolic anterior motion should be differentiated from leaflet systolic anterior motion after mitral annuloplasty because the former is a transient, benign and relatively common finding.

Valve replacement

Standard mitral valve replacement in patients with chronic MR consistently results in a decrease in postoperative LV EF. This fall in EF performance has been attributed, at least in part, to unfavorable loading conditions imposed by the elimination of the low-impedance pathway for LV emptying into the LA. In contrast to standard mitral valve replacement in which the chordae tendineae are severed, however, mitral valve replacement with chordal preservation does not usually decrease LV EF performance despite similar removal of the low-impedance pathway. Rozich and co-investigators[10] in Charleston, South Carolina, studied the mechanisms responsible for this discordance in postoperative EF performance between mitral valve replacement with and without chordal preservation. Echocardiography and sphygmomanometer blood pressures were obtained in 15 patients with pure chronic MR before and 7–10 days after mitral valve surgery. These measurements were used to calculate LV volume, wall stress, and EF. Seven patients underwent mitral valve replacement with chordal transection, and 8 patients underwent mitral valve replacement with chordal preservation. Chordal transection resulted in no postoperative change in LV end-diastolic volume, a significant increase in LV end-systolic volume, a significant increase in end-systolic stress, and a significant decrease in EF, from 0.60 to 0.36. In contrast, patients who underwent mitral valve replacement with chordal preservation had a significant decrease in LV end-diastolic and end-systolic volumes. End-systolic wall stress actually fell and EF was unchanged instead of reduced (Figure 6-3). Mitral valve replacement with chordal transection resulted in a decrease in LV EF performance caused in part by an increase in end-systolic stress, which in turn increased end-systolic volume. Conversely, mitral valve replacement with chordal preservation resulted in a smaller LV size, allowing a reduced end-systolic stress and preservation of LV EF performance despite closure of the low-impedance LA ejection pathway.

MITRAL VALVE STENOSIS

Natural history

Gordon and associates[11] in Boston, Massachusetts, studied 52 patients with rheumatic MS with serial two-dimensional and Doppler echocardiography to determine the natural history of changes in mitral valve area and its relation to transmitral gradient and mitral valve morphology. During a 39 month observation period, the decline in valve area was 0.09 ±0.21 cm²/year. There were significant increases in total echocardiographic score, severity of mitral anulus calcification, and severity of MR. Patients with an echocardiographic score ≥8 had a more progressive course. Patients with a more progressive course also had a significantly greater initial mean gradient, peak gradient, and total echocardiographic score. Initial valve area did not correlate with the rate of stenosis progression. Among 22 patients with a net echocardiographic score <8 and a

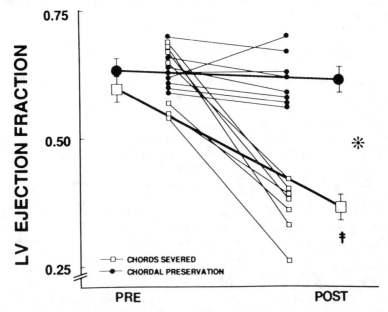

Fig. 6-3. Graph showing preoperative (pre) and postoperative (post) left ventricular (LV) ejection fraction for patients undergoing mitral valve replacement (MVR) with chordae tendineae severed (open squares) and MVR with chordae tendineae preserved (closed circles). Data for individual patients are represented by smaller symbols; mean ± SEM is represented by larger symbols. *p<0.05 vs. between two patient groups; ‡p<0.05 pre vs. post. MVR with chords severed resulted in a decrease in fraction ejection, but MVR with chords preserved did not. Reproduced with permission from Rozich, et al.[10]

peak mitral valve gradient <10 mm Hg, only 1 patient (5%) had a progressive course compared with 80% of those with a total echocardiographic score ≥8 and a gradient ≥10 mm Hg. Therefore, the rate of mitral valve narrowing in individual patients with rheumatic MS is variable. Patients whose valve disease progresses more rapidly are those with a greater mitral valve echocardiographic score and higher peak and mean transmitral gradients.

Closed transventricular mitral commissurotomy

Rihal and colleagues[12] in Rochester, Minnesota, determined the long-term outcome and multivariate predictors of late events in patients who underwent transventricular mitral commissurotomy at the Mayo Clinic in the early 1960s. Percutaneous balloon mitral valvuloplasty is an important new procedure for which long-term follow-up data are not available. Such data do exist for patients who have undergone transventricular mitral commissurotomy, a similar but older and more invasive procedure. Follow-up data with a mean duration of 14 years for 207 women and 60 men undergoing transventricular mitral commissurotomy were obtained from medical records, referring physicians, questionnaires and telephone interviews. Survival and survival free of repeat commissurotomy or mitral valve surgery were estimated with the Kaplan-Meier method. Cox proportional hazard method was used to determine predictors of survival and repeat mitral valve surgery. Postoperatively, 92% of patients had symptomatic improvement which was sustained for at least 3 to 4 years in 78%. At 10, 15 and 20 years postoperatively, 79%, 67%, and 55%, respectively, of patients were alive and 57%, 36% and 24%, respectively, were alive and free of a need for repeat mitral valve surgery. At 10 years, 90% of all patients were free of transient or fixed cerebrovascular events. In multivariate analyses, atrial fibrillation, age and male gender were independently associated with death, whereas mitral valve calcium, cardiomegaly and MR independently predicted the need for repeat mitral valve surgery. Thus, long-term results after transventricular mitral commissurotomy are excellent in selected patients with symptomatic MS. Because of similarities in patient selection and mechanisms of mitral valve dilation, similar favorable long-term outcomes may be expected after percutaneous balloon mitral valvuloplasty.

Percutaneous balloon valvuloplasty

In an investigation carried out by Fawzy and associates[13] from Riyadh, Saudi Arabia, percutaneous mitral balloon valvotomy using the Inoue balloon catheter was attempted in 60 consecutive patients with severe symptomatic MS. There were 10 children (mean age 13 years) and 50 adults (mean age 31 years). Forty patients were females and 20 were males; 53 were in sinus rhythm. The procedure was technically successfully performed in 57 (95%) patients. There were no deaths or thromboembolic complications. Balloon valvotomy was done using a 22 to 30 mm diameter catheter with the echocardiographic Doppler-guided stepwise mitral dilatation technique. After percutaneous mitral balloon valvotomy the mean LA pressure decreased from 23 ± 5.0 to 14 ± 4.0 mm Hg; the mean mitral valve gradient decreased from 15 ± 4.0 to 6.0 ± 2.0 mm Hg; the mitral valve area (Gorlin formula) increased from 0.7 ± 0.2 to 1.6 ± 0.4 cm². Mild MR developed in 6 patients (11%) and increased by 1 grade in another 5 patients (9%). No patient developed severe MR. Mitral valve area at mean follow-up of 4.8 months remained unchanged at 1.9 ± 0.3 cm². It was concluded that percutaneous mitral balloon valvotomy, using the Inoue balloon catheter, is safe and effective in the treatment of severe MS in children and adults without inducing significant MR.

Percutaneous balloon mitral valvotomy (PBMV) compares well with surgical commissurotomy, showing comparable improvement in symptoms and catheterization-proven valve area early after the procedure. Block and associates[14] from Boston, Massachusetts, reported the New York Heart Association class, mitral valve area calculated by echocardiography, and the results of transseptal cardiac catheterization 2 years after PBMV. The data are compared with the status immediately before and after PBMV. Forty-one patients returned to enter the study (mean follow-up time 24 ± 3 months). All patients were evaluated clinically by the same investigator who had seen them at the time of PBMV. Transseptal cardiac catheterization and echocardiographic analysis (2-dimensional and Doppler echocardiography) were performed on the same day. At follow-up, 17 patients were class I, 20 were class II, and 4 were class III. Although the mitral valve area calculated by cardiac catheterization increased significantly from immediately before to immediately after PBMV there was a decrease in the calculated mitral valve area at 2-year follow-up. Echocardiographic analysis did not show as large an increase in mitral area, immediately after PBMV, and no significant decrease in mitral valve area at 2 years (before PBMV planimetry 1.1 ± 0.1 cm^2; immediately after 1.8 ± 0.1; follow-up 1.6 ± 0.1. Doppler halftime measurements were similar. PBMV is effective therapy with good midterm results for selected patients with mitral stenosis.

Tuzcu and co-investigators[15] in Boston, Massachusetts, analyzed the immediate and long-term outcome of percutaneous balloon mitral valvotomy in 99 patients who were ≥65 years of age (81 women and 18 men). There were 84 patients in New York Heart Association class III or IV; 26 patients had previous surgical commissurotomy; 64 had one or more comorbidities; 73 had fluoroscopically visible mitral valve calcification; and 63 had echocardiographic score greater than 8. There were 3 procedural deaths, all occurring in the early experience. Pericardial tamponade occurred in 5 patients, thromboembolism in 3, and transient AV block in 1. After mitral valve valvotomy, mitral valve area was ≥1 cm^2 in 86 patients and ≥1.5 cm^2 in 56. A successful outcome (defined as mitral valve area ≥1.5 cm^2 without a >grade 2 increase in mitral regurgitation and without left-to-right shunt with a pulmonary-to-systemic flow ratio of ≥1.5) was achieved in 46 patients. The best multivariate predictor of success was the combination of echocardiographic score, Heart Association functional class, and inverse of mitral valve area. Mean follow-up was 16 months. Actuarial survival (79% vs 62%), survival without MVR (71% vs 41%) and survival without MVR and Heart Association class III or IV (54% vs. 38%) at 3 years were significantly better in the successful group of 46 patients than in the unsuccessful group of 53 patients. Low echocardiographic score was the only independent predictor of survival. Lack of mitral valve calcification and low Heart Association class, low mean LA pressure, and low PA pressure were the independent predictors of event-free survival. Percutaneous mitral valvotomy can be performed safely in selected patient greater than 65 years old with good immediate and long-term results. In addition to clinical examination, echocardiographic evaluation of the mitral valve and fluoroscopic screening for valvular calcium are the most important steps in patient selection for successful outcome.

Percutaneous retrograde nontransseptal balloon mitral valvuloplasty is a new technique developed by Stefanadis and co-workers[16] in Athens,

Greece, for opening a stenotic mitral valve. This technique is based on a new, externally steerable cardiac catheter that enters the LA retrogradely via the LV. The technique was used in 86 consecutive patients (18 men and 68 women; mean age, 51 years). Dilatation of the stenotic mitral valve was achieved in 85 of 86 patients. After the procedure, mitral valve area increased from 0.9 to 2.1 cm² and transmitral gradient decreased from 16 to 5 mm Hg. Major complications, such as cardiac perforation, embolic events, or death, were not encountered. Severe MR developed in 3 patients. In 2 patients, there was major injury of the femoral artery. The maintenance of the initial improvement was similar to that found in studies that used transseptal techniques. The restenosis rate during the 2-year follow-up was 15%. The immediate and long-term findings of this study indicate that retrograde percutaneous nontransseptal balloon mitral valvuloplasty is an effective and safe procedure with an acceptable major complication rate. Moreover, this new technique has the advantage that it does not involve puncture and dilatation of the atrial septum, although it may occasionally lead to arterial damage. Further studies will show whether it may really be considered as an alternative method or method of choice for percutaneous balloon mitral valvuloplasty.

In response to the increasing use of percutaneous balloon mitral commissurotomy, the National Heart, Lung, and Blood Institute established the Balloon Valvuloplasty Registry in November 1987. Between November 1, 1987, and October 31, 1989, 738 patients aged 18 or older underwent percutaneous balloon mitral commissurotomy at the clinical sites. Data were prospectively entered into the registry at the time consent was obtained, and the experience was reviewed by Dean and co-investigators[17] from Birmingham, Alabama. Serious complications occurred in 87 procedures, or 12%. Death in the laboratory occurred in 8 patients, or 1%. Within 30 days there were 24 cumulative deaths, 18 cardiac and six noncardiac. Univariate analysis revealed that older age, a history of cardiac arrest, cerebrovascular disease, dementia, renal insufficiency, cachexia, class IV congestive heart failure, use of an intra-aortic balloon pump, use of sympathomimetic amines, and a high echo score were associated with early death. Additional univariate predictors included a precommissurotomy mitral valve area of <0.7 cm². Left atrial pressure of >12mm Hg and a mitral valve area of <1.5 cm² after the procedure were also associated with higher 30-day mortality. Multivariate analysis identified higher echo score and smaller valve area before the procedure as the strongest predictors of early death. Centers that performed more than 25 procedures also had lower complication rates. Although percutaneous balloon mitral commissurotomy appears to be effective at relieving the hemodynamic effects of rheumatic MS, it does have risks. In properly selected patients, however, it appears to have low morbidity and a 30-day mortality. Individual center experience with the procedure also appears to have great impact on complications.

Desideri and associates[18] from Montreal, Canada, assessed late results after successful percutaneous mitral commissurotomy by prospective clinical and echocardiographic follow-up. Fifty-seven patients were followed for a mean of 19 ± 6 months (range 9 to 33) after the procedure. Mitral valve area (measured by Doppler half-time method) increased from 1.0 ± 0.2 to 2.2 ± 0.5 cm² immediately after commissurotomy, and then decreased to 1.9 ± 0.5 cm² at follow-up, whereas gradient did not change after its immediate postcommissurotomy reduction. Echocardiographic restenosis (mitral valve area ≤1.5 cm² with >50% reduction of initial gain) was seen in 12 of 57 patients (21%). Atrial shunting, detected by transthoracic color Doppler in 61% of patients immediately after the procedure (color flow jet through atrial septum), persisted in 30% at follow-up. Restenosis by univariate analysis correlated with age, smaller valve area after the procedure, and higher echocardiographic score. Multivariate analysis identified leaflet mobility and calcifications as the components of a score that was predictive for restenosis. Magnitude of shunt (pulmonary-to-systemic flow ratio >1.5), use of a Bifoil balloon (2 balloons on 1 shaft), and smaller valve area after the procedure were predictors by multivariate analysis of the persistence of atrial shunting. Clinical improvement persisted at long-term follow-up (mean New York Heart Association class 1.6 ± 0.6 vs 2.6 ± 0.6 before commissurotomy). Improvement of ≥1 functional class was seen in 75% of patients (80% of those without and 58% of those with restenosis); patients with a shunt did not differ from the entire group. Thus, percutaneous mitral commissurotomy provides excellent late (9 to 33 months) clinical results. Echocardiographic restenosis was identified in 20% of patients, and was related to age, valve morphology and a suboptimal result. Atrial shunting (small and clinically well-tolerated) was absent after long-term follow-up in 50% of patients; its persistence was related to the magnitude of the shunt, the size of the deflated balloon, and a suboptimal result.

In an investigation reported by Reid and associates[19] from Orange, California, echocardiographic data were analyzed in 555 patients undergoing mitral balloon commissurotomy. Patients were enrolled in the National Heart, Lung and Blood Institute Balloon Valvuloplasty Registry from 24 centers. There were 456 women and 99 men with a mean age of 54 years. Before mitral balloon commissurotomy the 2-dimensional echocardiographic variables of mitral valve thickness, mobility, calcification, and subvalvular disease were evaluated and assigned scores of 1 to 4. The mitral valve morphology score was related to mitral valve area measured after mitral balloon commissurotomy by cardiac catheterization. The leaflet mobility score was related to the immediate post-mitral balloon commissurotomy mitral valve area: 2.2 ± 0.8 cm^2 for grade 1, 1.9 ± 0.7 cm^2 for grade 2, 1.7 ± 0.7 cm^2 for grade 3 and 1.9 ± 0.9 cm^2 for grade 4. Results of the mitral valve area after mitral balloon commissurotomy showed a similar relationship for each echocardiographic variable. The total morphology score (sum of the 4 variables) showed a relationship to mitral valve area immediately after mitral balloon commissurotomy, which was persistent at 6 months after mitral balloon commissurotomy. Multiple regression analysis showed that mitral valve area after mitral balloon commissurotomy is predicted by pre-mitral balloon commissurotomy valve area, LA size, balloon diameter, cardiac output, and leaflet mobility. Total morphology score, leaflet thickness, calcium, and subvalvular disease were not important univariate or multivariate predictors of the results of mitral balloon commissurotomy. These data suggest that although mitral valve morphology, particularly leaflet mobility, relates to mitral valve area after mitral balloon commissurotomy, other variables such as the severity and duration of disease are also important and are influenced by the larger balloon sizes used in the procedure. Mitral valve morphology should not be used alone in the selection of patients for mitral balloon commissurotomy.

Percutaneous balloon mitral valvuloplasty is known to produce short-term hemodynamic and symptomatic improvement in many patients with MS. Comprehensive assessment of the clinical usefulness of balloon valvuloplasty requires evaluation of patients' long-term outcomes. Cohen and associates[20] from Boston, Massachusetts, performed balloon mitral valvuloplasty in 146 patients between October 1, 1985, and October 1, 1991. Base-line demographic, clinical, echocardiographic, and hemodynamic variables were evaluated in order to identify predictors of long-term event-free survival. Balloon mitral valvuloplasty was completed successfully in 136 (93%) of the patients in whom the procedure was attempted; it resulted in an increase in the mean (± SD) mitral-valve area from 1.0 ± 0.4 to 2.1 ± 0.9 cm² and a decrease in the mean transmitral pressure gradient from 14 ± 5 to 6 ± 3 mm Hg. The estimated overall 5-year survival rate was 76 ± 5%, and the estimated 5-year event-free survival rate (the percentage of patients without mitral-valve replacement, repeat valvuloplasty, or death from cardiac causes) was 51 ± 6%. According to multivariate Cox proportional-hazards analysis, the independent predictors of longer event-free survival were a lower mitral-valve deformity; range, 0 for a normal valve to 16 for a seriously deformed valve, lower LV end-diastolic pressure, and a lower New York Heart Association functional class. Patients with no risk factors for early restenosis or only 1 risk factor (echocardiographic score >8, LV end-diastolic pressure >10 mm Hg, or New York Heart Association functional class IV) had a predicted 5-year event-free survival rate of 60 to 84%, whereas patients with 2 or 3 risk factors had a predicted 5-year event-free survival rate of only 13 to 41%. Balloon mitral valvuloplasty as a treatment for selected patients with MS has good long-term results. The long-term outcome after this procedure can be predicted on the basis of patients' base-line characteristics.

Chen and associates[21] from Guangzhou, China, and Washington, D.C., reported results of the initial 85 patients who successfully underwent percutaneous mitral valvuloplasty (PMV) with the Inoue balloon catheter at their hospital between November, 1985, and November, 1988. The mean follow-up was 5 ± 1 year (range 43–79 months). Before and after PMV and at follow-up, mean diastolic mitral gradients by the catheter method were 17.5 ± 6.2, 3.1 ± 3.3 and 3.3 ± 3.4 mm Hg, respectively. Mean diastolic mitral gradients by the Doppler method were 18 ± 6, 8 ± 5 and 9 ± 5 mm Hg, respectively. Mitral valve areas by the echo-Doppler method were 1.1 ± 0.3, 2.0 ± 0.4 and 1.8 ± 0.5 cm², respectively. Phonocardiographic and vectorcardiographic studies, and cardiopulmonary exercise testing showed significant improvement after PMV and at follow-up. Functional status before PMV was New York Heart Association class IV in 2 patients, class III in 52, and class II in 31; at follow-up, the status was class I in 74, class II in 6, and class III in 5. All 5 patients (6.8%) in class III developed mitral restenosis; in all 5, severe mitral calcification and subvalvular fusion were found by 2-dimensional echocardiography. It is concluded that PMV with the Inoue balloon catheter can achieve excellent and sustained long-term results in relieving symptomatic, rheumatic MS in patients without severe mitral calcium and subvalvular fusion.

AORTIC VALVE STENOSIS

Rate of progression

Until recently the hemodynamic severity of valvular AS was evaluated only at cardiac catheterization. Now Doppler echocardiography allows a non-invasive and accurate assessment of AS severity and can be used to study its progression with time. Faggiano and associates[22] from Brescia,

Italy, assessed the progression of AS during a follow-up period of 6 to 45 months (mean 18) by serial Doppler examinations in 45 adult patients (21 men and 24 women, mean age 72 ± 10 years) with isolated AS. The following parameters were serially measured: LV outflow tract diameter and velocity by pulsed Doppler, peak velocity of aortic flow by continuous-wave Doppler, to calculate peak gradient by the modified Bernoulli equation, and aortic valvular area by the continuity equation. At the initial observation, 13 of 45 patients (29%) were symptomatic (1 angina, 1 syncope and 11 dyspnea); during follow-up, 25 (55%) developed new symptoms or worsening of the previous ones (5 angina, 3 syncope and 17 dyspnea); 11 underwent aortic valve replacement and 3 died from cardiac events. Baseline peak velocity and gradient ranged between 2.5 and 6.6 m/s, and 25 and 174 mm Hg, respectively; aortic area ranged between 0.35 and 1.6 cm². With time, mean peak velocity and gradient increased significantly from 4 ± 0.7 to 4.7 ± 0.8 m/s, and 64 ± 30 to 88 ± 30 mm Hg, respectively. A concomitant reduction in mean aortic area occurred (0.75 ± 0.3 to 0.6 ± 0.15 cm². The rate of progression of AS (− 0.72 to + 0.14 cm²/year, mean − 0.1 ± 0.13) was variable among patients and did not relate to age, sex, follow-up duration or symptoms. Patients with a reduction in LV systolic function had a faster progression than did those with normal systolic function. In conclusion, a significant progression of AS may occur and a mild or moderate stenosis can become critical after a few years. Doppler echocardiography appears to be the ideal method for follow-up and can add new insights to the natural history of the disease.

Coronary artery dimensions

Villari and co-workers[23] in Zurich, Switzerland, evaluated the effect of regression of myocardial hypertrophy on coronary artery dimensions in patients with aortic valve disease who underwent valve replacement. Cross-sectional area of the 3 major coronary arteries (LAD, LC and right) was determined by quantitative coronary arteriography in 15 patients with aortic valve disease before and 38 months after successful AVR. Twelve normal subjects served as controls. LV angiographic mass was calculated according to the method of Rackley. Cross section of the area of the LAD was larger in aortic valve disease than in controls. After valve replacement, cross sectional area of the LAD decreased but remained significantly larger than in controls. Cross section area of the right coronary artery in patients with aortic valve disease was not different from controls. LV muscle mass was significantly increased in aortic valve disease patients before and after valve replacement compared with controls. The appropriateness of coronary artery size with respect to muscle mass was evaluated by normalizing cross sectional area of the LAD coronary per 100 g of LV muscle mass. This index amounted to 11 mm²/100 g in controls, to 8 mm²/100 g in preoperative patients and 10 mm²/100 g in postoperative patients with aortic valve disease. In patients with aortic valve disease, cross sectional area of the proximal LAD and LC is increased, but this increase is not sufficient to keep cross sectional area per 100 g of LV mass within normal limits. The postoperative decrease muscle mass is associated with a decrease in the size of LAD and LC, whereas the size of the right coronary artery remains unchanged. In contrast to the preoperative state, the residually hypertrophied LV myocardium after aortic valve replacement is supplied by an enlarged but adequately sized LAD and LC.

Villari and associates[24] in Zurich, Switzerland, evaluated the effect of progression of LV hypertrophy on coronary artery dimensions in patients with AV disease. Cross-sectional area of the left coronary artery was larger in patients with AV disease than in control subjects, 13 vs. 8 mm², left circumflex artery 13 vs 6 mm², respectively. At the follow-up examination, cross-sectional area of the left coronary artery increased, LAD 17 mm² and left circumflex artery 15 mm². The cross-sectional area of the right coronary artery was not different in patients with AV disease from that in controls. LV muscle mass was larger in patients with AV disease both at baseline and after follow-up examination (269 g and 339 g, respectively) than in control subjects (136 g). The appropriateness of coronary artery size with respect to muscle mass was evaluated by normalizing cross-sectional area of the left coronary artery per 100 g of LV muscle mass. This index was 11 mm²/100 g in control subjects and decreased in subjects with AV disease from 10 mm²/100 at baseline to 9 mm²/100 g at the follow-up measurement. Therefore, in patients with AV disease, the progression of LV hypertrophy is associated with an increase in LAD and LC coronary artery dimensions, whereas the size of the right coronary artery remained unchanged. Despite the enlargement of the left coronary artery, the cross-sectional area of the left coronary artery per 100 g of LV muscle mass decreased. Thus, the increase in coronary artery size appears inadequate when the severity of LV hypertrophy increases in these patients.

Left ventricular function

In AS, the response of the LV to pressure overload varies from compensated hypertrophy to overt CHF. The determinants of LV adaptation are poorly understood. Carroll and co-workers[25] in Chicago, Illinois, compared LV function to assess the role of sex in 34 women and 29 men 60 years or older with both hemodynamic and echocardiographic data characteristic of severe AS and no important CAD. Despite a similar degree of LV outflow obstruction in women versus men (aortic valve area 0.54 vs 0.59 cm²), the LV of women had a greater fractional shortening, achieved a smaller end-systolic chamber size, and generated more pressure with a greater maximum positive dP/dt. The men had a lower cardiac index, higher mean PA pressure, and shorter ejection period. Women and men were equally symptomatic. Supernormal LV ejection performance was present in 41% of the women and only 14% of the men. This subgroup of women had a small, thick-walled chamber with low end-systolic wall stress. Subnormal ejection performance was present in 64% of the men and only 18% of the women. This subgroup of men had an increased chamber size and high end-systolic wall stress compared with control men. Greater LV mass was present in men compared with women. The investigators concluded that sex is a factor in LV adaptation to valvular AS in adults 60 years or older.

Percutaneous balloon valvuloplasty

Bernard and colleagues[26] in Besançon, France, assessed the long-term results of percutaneous aortic valvuloplasty and AVR in elderly patients in two similar nonrandomized series of patients ≥75 years of age treated by one or the other methods between January, 1986 and March, 1989. Forty-six patients, 23 men and 23 women, with a mean age of 80 years underwent percutaneous aortic valvuloplasty (group 1) and 23 additional patients, mean age of 78 years, underwent AVR with a bioprosthesis (group 2). All of these patients suffered from severe calcified AS. Clinical and hemodynamic status were similar in both groups. The mean follow-up period was 22 months in group 1 and 28 months in group 2. Three patients (7%) in group 1 died within 5 days after percutaneous aortic valvuloplasty and 24 patients (52%) died during the follow-up period. Sixteen of these patients died of recurrent CHF. Of 16 patients (35%) subsequently operated on at an average of 16 months after percutaneous aortic valvuloplasty, 2 died at operation. Only three group 1 patients (7%) were still alive at follow-up without subsequent AVR. In group 2, two patients (9%) died postoperatively and three patients (13%) died the follow-up period. All other patients (78%) were still alive and in New York Heart Association functional class I or II. The overall survival rate in group 1 was 75% at 1 year, 47% at 2 years, and 33% at 5 years. In group 2, survival rate was 83% at 1 and 2 years and 75% at 3 and 4 years. Thus, the results of percutaneous aortic valvuloplasty do not compare favorably with those of surgery in elderly patients (Figure 6-4).

AORTIC REGURGITATION

Congenitally bicuspid aortic valve

To investigate the morphology of congenitally bicuspid aortic valves causing pure aortic regurgitation, Sadee and associates[27] from Amsterdam, The Netherlands, studied 148 excised congenitally bicuspid aortic valves. Pure valve regurgitation was defined as grade 3–4/4 with a peak systolic pressure gradient <30 mm Hg. Three types were recognized: valves that were purely bicuspid (23%), bicuspid valves with a raphe (34%), and valves with an additional indentation of the free edge of the conjoined cusp (43%). In 14 cases pure valve regurgitation was present. Dilatation of the aortic root was present in 47 cases. The relative risk for AR when the aortic root was dilated (compared with no dilatation) was 3.99. The relative

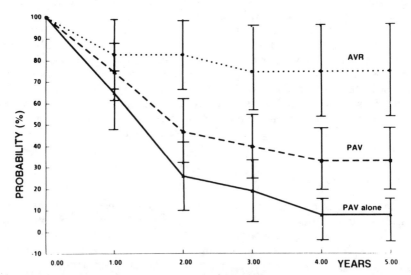

Fig. 6-4. Long-term survival rate. AVR = aortic valve replacement (group 2); PAV = percutaneous aortic valvuloplasty (group 1); PAV alone = patients who underwent percutaneous aortic valvuloplasty without subsequent operation (part of group 1). Reproduced with permission from Bernard, et al.[26]

risk for valve regurgitation when there was indentation of the conjoined cusp (comparex with no indentation) was 4.95. The mean age at operation in patients with pure AR was 56 years, which is significantly younger than that of patients with a congenitally bicuspid valve with combined valve stenosis and regurgitation (65 years). Congenitally bicuspid aortic valves with a central indentation of the free edge of the conjoined cusp seem particularly likely to develop pure aortic valve regurgitation. Patients with infective endocarditis were excluded from this study. The 148 patients included 99 men, mean age 64 (range 31–86) 49 women, mean age 65 (range 35–81). Of the 148 valves, 143 had some degree of calcium within the cusp. The 5 valves without calcium all belonged to the group of 14 valves with pure AR. Thus, only 14 of the 148 patients included in this study had pure AR. The remaining 134 appeared to have some degree of AS.

INFECTIVE ENDOCARDITIS

In the Netherlands

van der Meer and associates[28] from Rotterdam and Leiden, the Netherlands, conducted a nationwide prospective epidemiologic study of active bacterial endocarditis in the Netherlands during a 2-year period. All cases of hospitalized patients with suspected endocarditis in the Netherlands during that 2-year period were reported to the authors. While hospitalized, the patients were visited for an in-person interview and a review of the medical record. Of the 559 episodes, 438 met the criteria for endocarditis; these included 89 episodes of prosthetic valve endocarditis and 349 episodes of native valve endocarditis. Adjusted for age- and sex-specific population figures, the incidence was 19 per million person-years. The incidence increased significantly with age, and men were more often affected than women (266 and 172 cases, respectively). Rheumatic and congenital cardiac lesions formed most of the underlying heart diseases (Table 6-5). Mitral valve prolapse was present in only 29 patients with native valve endocarditis (8.3%). A history of intravenous drug abuse was present in 32 patients (7.3%). Viridans streptococci, staphylococci, and enterococci together constituted 86% of the isolated bacterial strains. Only 1.1% of the patients had culture-negative endocarditis. Overall case fatality was 19.7% and varied widely according to causative microorganism. The distribution of causal microorganisms, the case fatality rate, and the incidence rate of endocarditis are age related. Therefore, a meaningful comparison of data is only possible between population-based cohorts of patients with endocarditis.

In a hospital in India

Choudhury and associates[29] from Chandigarh, India, studied clinical data from 186 patients (133 males and 53 females) with 190 episodes of infective endocarditis occurring between January 1981, and July 1991. The patients were studied retrospectively at a large referral hospital in Northern India with the intention of highlighting certain essential differences from those reported in the West. The mean age was much lower (25 ± SD 12 years, range 2 to 75 years). Rheumatic heart disease was the

TABLE 6-5.   *Underlying Heart Disease in 349 Episodes of Native Valve Endocarditis.* Reproduced with permission from van der Meer, et al.*[28]

Valve	Heart Disease Previously Known, No.	
	Yes	No
Aorta (n=110 [31.5%])		
Bicuspid valve	0	2
Bicuspid valve+AOI/AOS	3	0
Sclerotic valve	3	4
Regurgitation	16	48
Regurgitation+stenosis	12	5
Stenosis	8	1
HOCM	7	1
Total	**49**	**61**
Mitral and aortic (n=36 [10.3%])		
Regurgitation and/or stenosis	23	13
Total	**23**	**13**
Congenital heart disease (n=38 [10.9%])		
Atrial septal defect	1	0
VSD	13	0
VSD+right-sided valvular disease	6	0
Patent arterial duct	4	1
Fallot's tetralogy	5	0
Other	8	0
Total	**37**	**1**
Mitral (n=125 [35.8%])		
Prolapse	1	0
Prolapse+regurgitation	23	4
Prolapse+stenosis	1	0
Regurgitation	46	43
Regurgitation+stenosis	3	1
Stenosis	2	1
Total	**76**	**49**
Right-sided (n=21 [6.0%])		
Tricuspid regurgitation	3	16
Pulmonary regurgitation	1	0
Pulmonary+tricuspid regurgitation	1	0
Total	**5**	**16**
Other (n=19 [5.4%])		
Right+left-sided valvular disease	7	5
Systolic murmur only	0	3
No murmur	0	2
BE accidental finding, previous heart disease unknown	0	2
Total	**7**	**12**

*AOI indicates aortic insufficiency (aortic regurgitation); AOS, aortic stenosis; HOCM, hypertrophic obstructive cardiomyopathy; VSD, ventricular septal defect; and BE, bacterial endocarditis.

most frequent underlying heart lesion accounting for 79 patients (42%). This was followed by congenital heart disease in 62 (33%) and normal valve endocarditis in 17 (9%). Twenty-four patients had either aortic regurgitation (n = 15) or mitral regurgitation (n = 9) of uncertain etiology. Prosthetic valve infection and mitral valve prolapse were present in only 2 patients each. A definite predisposing factor could be identified in only 28 patients (15%). Postabortal sepsis and sepsis related to childbirth accounted for 6 and 5 cases, respectively. Only 1 patient had history of intravenous drug abuse. Two-dimensional echocardiography showed vegetations in 121 patients (64%). Blood cultures were positive in only 87 (47%), with a total of 90 microbial isolates. Commonest infecting organisms were staphylococci (37 cases) and streptococci (34 cases). Except for a significantly higher number of patients with neurologic complications in the culture-negative group, there were no differences between patients with culture-positive and culture-negative ineffective endocarditis. Of the 190 episodes of IE, the patients had received antibiotics before admission in 110 (58%) instances. A significantly greater number of culture-negative patients had received antibiotics than did culture-positive patients (87 vs 23). Overall in-hospital mortality was 25%. There was a significantly higher number of neurologic complications in patients who died than in those who recovered (38 vs 14%). It is concluded that the spectrum of patients with IE that is seen is quite different from that seen in the West. Control of rheumatic fever on a national level, maintaining aseptic techniques during procedures related to childbirth including prophylactic antibiotics, and wider availability of sophisticated surgical techniques would go a long way in improving the outlook in these patients.

Transesophageal echocardiography

In this investigation by Birmingham and colleagues[30] from Madison, Wisconsin, the increment advantage of transesophageal echocardiography was determined by comparing results of paired transthoracic and transesophageal echocardiographic examinations performed in 61 patients for evaluation of suspected infective endocarditis. According to clinical and pathologic data, 31 of 61 (51%) patients had findings that were positive for infective endocarditis. Studies were graded as positive or negative for vegetations and were also graded for image quality. The sensitivity of transesophageal echocardiography in detecting vegetations was 88% versus 30% for transthoracic studies. For patients with aortic valve infective endocarditis, transesophageal sensitivity was 88% versus 25% for transthoracic sensitivity, because transesophageal echocardiography successfully separated vegetations from chronic valve disease caused by sclerosis or calcification. For patients with mitral valve infective endocarditis, transesophageal sensitivity was 100% versus 50% for transthoracic sensitivity, because transesophageal echocardiography distinguished vegetations from myxomatous changes or detected vegetations on prosthetic valves. Thus transesophageal echocardiography improves recognition of infective endocarditis, particularly in the presence of underlying valvular disease.

Duration of fever

Lederman and associates[31] from Cleveland, Ohio, reviewed the duration of fever among 123 patients treated for active infective endocarditis at their hospital between 1972 and 1984. One-half of the patients became afebrile within 3 days after initiation of antibiotic therapy and nearly three quarters were afebrile after 1 week of therapy. After 2 weeks of therapy, nearly 90% had defervesced. Endocarditis due to *Staphylococcus aureus* or gram-negative bacilli, and culture-negative endocarditis, were associated with prolonged fever. Microvascular phenomena, major vessel embolization, or vegetations seen on 2-D echocardiogram also were associated with prolonged fever. Multivariate analysis revealed that only microvascular phenomena or major vessel embolization were independently associated with longer duration of fever. Endocarditis-associated mortality among patients who remained febrile after 1 week of therapy was 18%, and this was greater than the 2% mortality among patients who defervesced. These data suggest that prolonged fever during treatment of infective endocarditis is often due to tissue infarction or vascular injury. Prolonged fever also identifies patients at higher risk of a fatal outcome.

Right-sided endocarditis in addicts

Hecht and Berger[32] from New York, New York, reported clinical, laboratory, and echocardiographic findings in 121 intravenous drug users with clinical and bacteriologic evidence of 132 episodes of active infective endocarditis. The presence of a right-sided valvular vegetation detected by 2-dimensional echocardiography was required for entry into the study. Staphylococcus aureus was the most common infecting organism (*82%, 108 of 132). Vegetations involved the tricuspid valve in 127 episodes, the pulmonic in 4, and both in 1; they ranged in size from 0.4 to 4.3 cm (mean, 1.5 ± 0.7 cm). Vegetations >1.0 cm were present in 106 cases (80%). Among patients with isolated native right-sided endocarditis who reached a definite end point in treatment, mortality was 7% (7 of 98). Vegetations >2.0 cm were associated with a significantly higher mortality compared with vegetations of 2.0 cm or less (33% compared with 1.3%). Overall, right-sided endocarditis has a favorable prognosis. Although complications and prolonged fever are common, most cases respond to medical therapy. The findings suggest that vegetation size may be an important predictor of outcome and that vegetations greater than 2.0 cm are associated with increased mortality.

Complications in non-opiate addicts

Tornos and associates[33] from Barcelona, Spain, described the incidence and clinical manifestations of long-term cardiac complications of active infective endocarditis involving native cardiac valves in non-opiate addicts. One hundred and twelve consecutive patients, survivors from a series of 140 non-addicted patients with a first episode of active, infective endocarditis on normal valves hospitalized from 1975–1990 were studied. Thirty-two patients had had valve replacement during the active phase of the infection and the remaining 80 patients received medical treatment alone. Relapse, recurrence, need for late cardiac surgery, and cardiac mortality were measured. Relapses occurred in 3 patients (2.7%) and recurrences in 5 patients (4.5%, incidence density at 15 years, 0.0030 per patient-year). Late cardiac surgery was needed by 47% of the patients treated medically during the active phase, and most had surgery in the first 2 years of follow-up (incidence density, 0.25 per patient-year at 2 years). Aortic valve involvement were associated with the need for late surgery in univariate analysis. Multiple logistic regression analysis showed aortic valve involvement to be an independent predictor of the need for late surgery. Only 2 of the 32 patients who had surgery during the active infection needed a second operation during follow-up. At the end of follow-up, the number of patients who had surgery after the onset of the infection was 86 (60% of the whole series). Cardiac death occurred in 16 patients; most deaths were sudden or postoperative and occurred in the first 2 years of follow-up (incidence density, 0.047 per patient-year at 2 years). Independent predictors of death were not found. Survival was 90% at 2 years, 88% at 5 years, 81% at 10 years, and 61% at 15 years (Figure

6-5). Survival after infective endocarditis is fair (81% probability of survival at 10 years), and the most common types of cardiac death are sudden and postoperative. Aortic valve involvement is an independent predictor of the need for late cardiac surgery (Figure 6-6). The rate of recurrences is not negligible (incidence density at 15 years, 0.0030 per patient-year).

Treatment with ceftriaxone

To evaluate the efficacy and safety of ceftriaxone sodium in the treatment of streptococcal endocarditis, Francioli and associates[34] from Lausanne, Switzerland, Lyons, France, Brussels, Belgium, and Bergdorf, Switzerland, performed an open, multi-center, noncomparative study with a follow-up of patients for 4 months to 5 years by treating 59 patients with defined criteria for streptococcal endocarditis. Cefriaxone sodium was administered at a once-daily dose of 2 g for 4 weeks. The main outcome measures were clinical outcome and microbiological cure rate. Among the 59 patients, 55 completed the treatment and were followed up for 4 months to 5 years. No patients showed evidence of relapse. Treatment was completely uneventful in 42 patients (71%). A cardiac valve was replaced in 4 patients (7%) receiving anti-microbial therapy and in 6 patients (10%) who had completed antimicrobial therapy. One of the 10 valves taken for culture at surgery was positive, but only for microorganisms that were different from the microorganism isolated before the treatment. The treatment had to be interrupted in 4 patients because of drug allergy. Other side effects were mild except for 2 cases of reversible neutropenia. The treatment was easy to administer: 27 patients (46%) had no permanent intravenous catheter at any time, 7 patients (12%) had such a catheter for less than 4 days. Twenty-three patients (39%) were

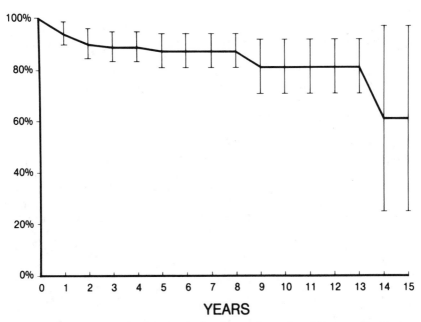

Fig. 6-5. Survival (Cardiac Mortality). Calculated survival rates for cardiac mortality (Kaplan-Meier) for 112 patients cured of endocarditis. 95% confidence intervals are indicated by bars. Number of patients alive at 0 years, 112; at 5 years, 53; at 10 years, 18; and at 15 years, 4. Reproduced with permission from Tornos, et al.[33]

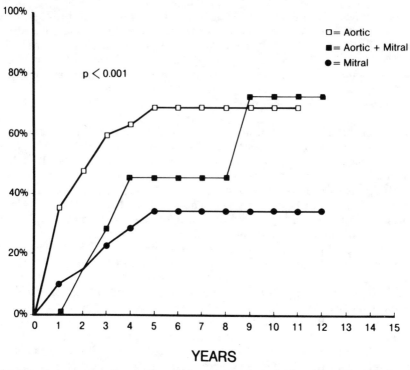

Fig. 6-6. Late surgery after aortic, mitral, or aortic plus mitral endocarditis. Calculated need of cardiac surgery (Kaplan-Meier) during follow-up for 80 patients cured of aortic, mitral, or combined endocarditis with medical treatment alone. Aortic valve involvement was significantly correlated with the need for late surgery. Reproduced with permission from Tornos, et al.[33]

discharged from the hospital less than 2 weeks after admission. Cefriaxone sodium administered at a once-daily dose of 2 g appears to be an effective and safe treatment of streptococcal endocarditis. In hospitals, this agent may be more convenient to administer than penicillin G with or without aminoglycosides. Some patients may even be treated as outpatients.

Aortic valve replacement

Haydock and associates[35] from Auckland, New Zealand, and Birmingham, Alabama, described a total of 108 patients hospitalized with active infective endocarditis on either a native aortic valve (n = 66) or a previously inserted replacement device (n = 42) who underwent AVR because they were too ill for hospital discharge. A nonstented aortic allograft valve was used in 78 patients and prosthetic (mechanical or bioprosthetic) valves in 30 patients. The survival rate was 82% at 1 month, 73% at 1 year, 64% at 5 years, and 36% at 15 years (Figure 6-7). It was better in patients with native valve endocarditis than prosthetic valve endocarditis. The incremental risk factors for death in the early phase postoperatively were older age at operation, higher New York Heart Association functional class, and a larger number of previous aortic valve procedures. There were 13 episodes of recurrent endocarditis, giving an actuarial freedom of 80% at 10 years. The hazard function for recurrent endocarditis had only a low constant phase when allograft valves were used, which contrasted with the existence of a high peaking early phase

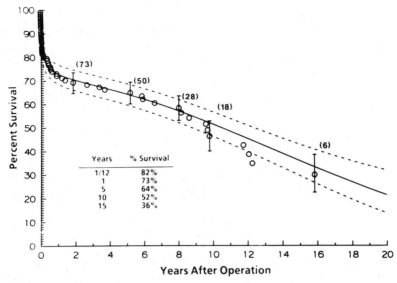

Fig. 6-7. Survival after aortic valve replacement for acute infectious endocarditis. The circles, representing deaths, are positioned at the time of death along the horizontal axis. The vertical bars represent 70% confidence limits (approximately 1 standard deviation) of the estimates. The numbers in parentheses are the number of patients at risk at that time after operation. The solid line is the parametric estimate of survival and is enclosed within its 70% confidence limits (dashed line). (See Appendix B for details.) Reproduced with permission from Haydock, et al.[35]

(in addition to the constant phase) when prosthetic devices were used. No risk factors for recurrent endocarditis were found in patients receiving a prosthesis, and "localized" versus "extensive" endocarditis was the only risk factor when an allograft was used. Reoperation was performed in 24 patients for a variety of reasons, and freedom from reoperation was 61% at 10 years. It is concluded that the allograft valve is the valve of choice when AVR is required for active endocarditis.

VALVE REPLACEMENT

St. Jude Medical vs Medtronic–Hall

To better define the merits of the fileaflet and tilting-disc valves, Fiore and associates[36] from St. Louis, Missouri, prospectively randomized 102 patients (mean age 57 years; range 11 to 85 years) to receive either the St. Jude (n = 55) or the Medtronic–Hall (n = 47) prostheses for mitral valve replacement between September, 1986 and May, 1991. The 2 groups were not different with respect to preoperative New York Heart Association class, incidence of mitral stenosis and insufficiency, angina score, extent of CAD, ventricular function, completeness of revascularization, or cross-clamp or bypass time. The hospital mortality (14.5% vs 10.6%, St. Jude vs Medtronic-Hall) and late mortality (7.3% vs 2.1%) were not significantly different. Follow-up was complete in 84 of 89 hospital survivors (94%) with a mean of 26 months (range, 1 to 60 months). The linearized rates of valve-related events and the 3-year actuarial survival demonstrated no significant differences between both cohorts. Comparison of the clinical outcome and echocardiographic parameters obtained at the time of follow-up demonstrated no significant differences between the 2 prostheses. These data indicate that the Medtronic–Hall and St. Jude mitral prostheses are similar with respect to their rates of valve-related complications and hemodynamic profiles. This study suggests that there is no difference between the St. Jude and Medtronic–Hall prostheses with regard to early clinical performance or hemodynamic results and therefore does not support the preferential selection of either prosthesis.

Bjork-Shiley strut fracture

The incidence of and factors that predispose to outlet strut fracture of Bjork–Shiley heart valves are still not known. To obtain such information van der Graaf and associates[37] from Rotterdam, the Netherlands, conducted a retrospective cohort study on all 2,303 patients in the Netherlands with a 60° convexo-concave (60° CC) or a 70° convexo-concave (70° CC) Bjork-Shiley heart valve. Patients were followed-up for a mean of 6.6 years (range 1–4271 days) (Figure 6-8). Forty-two cases of mechanical failure due to outlet strut fracture have been recorded—6 of the 7 patients with fracture of the aortic valve died, as did 18 of the 35 patients with fracture of the mitral valve. Multivariate analysis identified wide opening angle (70°), large valve size (≥29 mm diameter), and young age (<50 years) as risk factors for outlet strut fracture. For large 70° CC mitral valves the cumulative risk of outlet strut fracture after 8 years was 17.4%. Unlike previous findings, this excessive risk applied to late as well as to early batches of valves. In patients with a large 60° CC mitral valve the cumulative risk after 8 years was 4.2%. The incidence rate of outlet strut fracture in 60° CC and 70° CC valves (aortic and mitral) was constant over time. Overall survival since implantation was better for patients with 60° CC prostheses than for those with 70° CC prostheses; the adjusted hazard ratio for mortality for patients receiving a 70° CC prosthesis was 1.5. Together with the low (24%) necropsy rate, this ratio suggests that the reported incidence of strut fracture for the 70° CC valves is an underestimate. The data indicate that prophylactic replacement of 60° CC and 70° CC valves is advisable for selected groups of patients. Since the case-

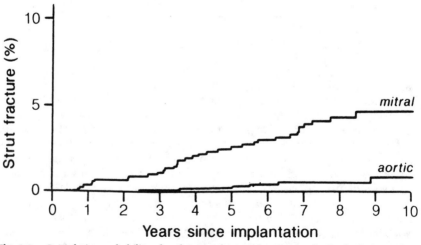

Fig. 6-8. Cumulative probability of outlet strut fracture in aortic and mitral valves. Reproduced with permission from Van der Graaf, et al.[37]

fatality rate is 50% for emergency replacement of faulty valves, patients suspected of Bjork–Shiley heart-valve failure should be referred without delay to a cardiothoracic center.

About 85,000 patients have undergone replacement of diseased heart valves with Bjork-Shiley convexo-concave valves. These prostheses are prone to fracture of the outlet strut, which leads to acute valve failure that is usually lethal. Should patients with these valves undergo prophylactic replacement to avoid fracture? The incidence of strut fracture varies between 0% and 1.5% per year, depending on valve opening angle (60° or 70°), diameter (<29 mm or ≥29 mm), and location (aortic or mitral). Other factors include the patient's life expectancy and the expected morbidity and mortality associated with reoperation. Birkmeyer and associates[38] from Hanover and Lebanon, New Hampshire, used decision analysis to identify the patients most likely to benefit from prophylactic reoperation. The incidence of outlet strut fracture was estimated from the data of 3 large studies on convexo-concave valves, and stratified by opening angle, diameter, and location (Table 6-6). A Markov decision analysis model was used to estimate life expectancy for patients undergoing prophylactic valve replacement and for those not undergoing reoperation. Prophylactic valve replacement does not benefit patients with convexo-concave valves that have low strut fracture risks (60° aortic valves and <29 mm, 60° mitral valves). For most patients with convexo-concave valves that have high strut fracture risks (≥29 mm, 70° convexo-concave), prophylactic valve replacement increases life expectancy. However, elderly patients with such valves benefit from prophylactic reoperation only if the risk of operative mortality is low. Patient age and operative risk are most important in recommendations for patients with convexo-concave valves that have intermediate strut fracture risks (<29 mm, 70° valves and ≥29 mm, 60° mitral valves). For all patients and their doctors facing the difficult decision on whether to replace convexo-concave valves, individual estimates of operative mortality risk that take account of both patient-specific and institution-specific factors are essential.

Thrombolysis for prosthetic thrombus

In a study carried out by Vasan and associates[39] from New Delhi, India, 16 patients with echocardiographic and cinefluoroscopic evidence of Björk-Shiley prosthetic valve obstruction (13 mitral valves and 3 aortic valves) were treated with intravenous streptokinase. Streptokinase was administered as an initial bolus of 250,000 units for 30 minutes, followed by an infusion of 100,000 units/hr. Serial cinefluoroscopy and echocardiography (M-mode, 2-dimensional and Doppler) were performed at 0, 24, 48,

TABLE 6-6. *Estimates of Annual Strut Fracture Incidence. Reproduced with permission from Birkmeyer, et al.*[38]

	Van der Graaf[1]			Lindblom/Ericsson[2,3*]			Combined fracture rate (95% CI) (% per year)
	Strut fractures	Follow-up (patient-years)	Fracture rate (% per yr)	Strut fractures	Follow-up (patient-years)	Fracture rate (% per year)	
Aortic valves							
70°, ≥29 mm	1	92	1·10	5	364	1·40	1·32 (0·48–2·86)
70°, <29 mm	3	651	0·46	9	3200	0·28	0·31 (0·16–0·54)
60°†	3	9230	0·03	6	4000	0·15	0·07 (0·03–0·13)
Mitral valves							
70°, ≥29 mm	10	454	2·20	13	1158	1·10	1·43 (0·90–2·14)
70°,•<29 mm	3	268	1·10	3	649	0·46	0·65 (0·24–1·42)
60°, ≥29 mm	22	4270	0·52	..	..	..	0·52 (0·32–0·78)
60°, <29 mm	0	2010	0	..†	..	..	0 (0–0·18)

*Modified to exclude Dutch centre at Leiden.
†Not stratified by size.

and 72 hours of treatment. The end-point of treatment was defined as near normalization of clinical, echocardiographic, and fluoroscopic parameters. Successful thrombolysis was achieved in all patients. The average duration of streptokinase therapy was 43 hours (range 2 to 72 hours). Two of 16 patients had minor systemic embolism during therapy. Short-term follow-up showed sustained benefit in 14 of 16 patients. Two patients have had rethrombosis of the mitral prosthetic valves and have undergone thrombectomy. This study demonstrates the feasibility, safety, and efficacy of thrombolytic therapy in the treatment of prosthetic valve thrombosis. It also emphasizes the role of serial Doppler echocardiography in guiding the duration of therapy and assessing its efficacy.

Durability of porcine bioprostheses

Burdon and associates[40] from Stanford, California, performed isolated AVR (n = 857) or MVR (n = 793) with a porcine valve prosthesis in 1,650 patients between 1971 and 1980. Follow-up (total = 12,012 patient years) extended to more than 15 years and was 96% complete. Patient age ranged from 16 to 87 years; mean age was 59 ± 11 years for the AVR cohort and 56 ± 12 years for the MVR cohort. The operative mortality rates were 5% ± 1% (± 70% confidence limits) and 8% ± 1%, respectively, for the aortic and mitral subgroups. Estimated freedom from structural valve deterioration after 10 and 15 years was significantly higher for the AVR than for the MVR subgroup (85% ± 0.4% and 63% ± 3% vs 78% ± 2% and 45% ± 3%, respectively). Reoperation-free actuarial estimates were also significantly greater for the AVR cohort: 83% ± 2% and 57% ± 3% vs 78% ± 2% and 43% ± 3% for MVR at 10 and 15 years, respectively. The mortality rate for reoperative AVR was 11% ± 1%; it was 8% ± 1% for reoperative MVR. Importantly, the estimates of freedom from valve-related death (including sudden, unexplained deaths) were relatively high at 10 and 15 years: 78% ± 2% and 69% ± 3% in the aortic cohort and 74% ± 2% and 63% ± 3% in the mitral cohort. Excluding sudden, unexplained deaths, these estimates were 81% ± 3% (aortic) and 73% ± 4% (mitral at 15 years. Thromboembolism-free rates were 84% ± 3% (aortic) and 78% ± 6% (mitral) at 15 years, and freedom from anticoagulant related hemorrhage was 96% ± 1% and 89% ± 2%, respectively. At the time of current follow-up, 13% of patients having AVR and 50% of patients having MVR were receiving warfarin sodium. The hazard functions for thromboembolism and prosthetic valve endocarditis were constant and remained <1%/per year over the entire follow-up period. Considering all 1,650 patients, multivariate (Cox model) regression analysis revealed that MVR (vs aortic) and younger operative age were the only significant, independent predictors of structural valve deterioration or reoperation. In the AVR subset, the only significant, independent predictor of reoperation was younger age; for the patients having MVR, younger age, female gender, and presence of angina were linked to a higher likelihood of reoperation. Valve-related mortality (including sudden, unexpected deaths) was associated with older age, advanced New York Heart Association class, and hepatic dysfunction for the patients having AVR; in the MVR cohort, the only significant independent determinants of valve-related mortality were older age and advanced New York Heart Association class. Despite the known finite durability of porcine bioprostheses, the long-term results reported herein with this first-generation porcine xenograft valve were generally satisfactory, particularly in patients >50 to 60 years of age.

Carpentier–Edwards parietal pericardial aortic valve

The Edwards Parietal pericardial aortic valve has unique design features that minimize cuspal stress and reduce abrasion wear. Wear tests and in vivo fluid dynamic tests have shown superior performance compared with other bioprostheses. Between August 1981 and July 1985, 719 Carpentier–Edwards pericardial aortic valves were used to replace native aortas in 10 U.S. medical centers without replacement of other cardiac valves, and these results were summarized by Frater and associates[41] from 5 U.S. medical centers. Patients were aged 18 to 90 years (mean 64). Men were 63% of the patients. Aortic stenosis was present preoperatively in 63.4% of patients. New York Heart Association functional classes III and IV were assigned to 62% of the patients. Valve sizes were 21 mm or less in 49% of patients. Concomitant procedures (most often CABG) were performed in 48% of patients. Hospital mortality was 5%. There was 1 valve-related death due to anticoagulant hemorrhage. Late mortality yielded 23 valve related deaths: endocarditis (13), anticoagulant hemorrhage (4), thromboembolism (3), structural (2), and pannus overgrowth (1). Freedom from valve-related death at 7 years was 95%. Regarding valve survival, cusp tears were not seen. There were 11 calcified valves and 8 explants (57 to 107 months). Seven-year freedom from all valve reoperation was 95%, with 11% of the patients receiving warfarin sodium, freedom of the total series from hemorrhage at 7 years was 93%, and from major thromboembolism, 96%. Echocardiographic follow-up of hemodynamics at 7 years yielded the following calculated effective orifice areas: 19 mm, 1 cm²; 21 mm, 1.3 cm²; and 23 mm, 1.4 cm². Average mean gradient for 19-mm valves was 15 mm Hg. New York Heart Association class improved in 78% of the patients. The Carpentier-Edwards pericardial valve, carefully studied by the Food and Drug Administration guidelines, is easy to use and has excellent hemodynamics. At 7-year follow-up there were no cusp tears and very little calcification. Intermediate-term performance is as good as or better than that of currently available devices, thus making this valve an outstanding bioprosthesis for the small aortic root.

Pregnancy afterwards

Maternal and fetal complications in a consecutive series of 60 pregnancies in 49 patients with prosthetic heart valves were prospectively evaluated by Born and colleagues[42] from São Paulo, Brazil, and New York, New York. Group 1 consisted of 40 pregnancies in 31 patients who were taking oral anticoagulants. No oral anticoagulation was used in 20 pregnancies in 19 patients (group 2). In group 1 there were 3 instances of acute valvular thrombosis during the 35 pregnancies in patients with mechanical prostheses, with 2 maternal deaths. There were 2 episodes of cerebral embolism, 1 in group 1 and 1 in group 2. Patients with isolated AVR had fewer maternal complications (2 of 13) than patients with isolated MVR (15 of 42). Severe bioprosthesis dysfunction occurred in 4 of 25 pregnancies (1 rupture and 3 stenosis) with 2 maternal deaths, 1 in the puerperium and the other in the postoperative period of cardiac surgery during pregnancy. When analyzing obstetric events, it was observed that 7 spontaneous abortions and 1 hydatidiform mole occurred. All spontaneous abortions occurred in group 1. The incidences of prematurity and low birth weight were significantly higher in group 1 than in group 2 (47% vs 11%, and 50% vs 11%, respectively). Moreover, there was a significant association between prematurity and the mother's New York Heart Association functional class (62% in classes III and IV vs 22% in classes I and II). There were 5 neonatal deaths, all in group 1. Three infants had warfarin-related congenital defects. It was concluded that pregnancy in patients with artificial valves is a high-risk situation for both the fetus and the mother.

Echocardiography

To assess the value and limitations of single-plane transesophageal echocardiography in the evaluation of prosthetic aortic valve function, Karalis and associates[43] from Philadelphia, Pennsylvania, studied 89 patients (69 mechanical and 20 bioprosthetic aortic valves) by combined transthoracic and transesophageal 2-dimensional and color flow Doppler echocardiography. In the assessment of AR, the transthoracic and transesophageal echocardiographic findings were concordant in 71 of 89 patients (80%). In 8 patients, the degree of AR was underestimated by the transthoracic approach; in each case the quality of the transthoracic echocardiogram was poor. In 10 patients, transesophageal echocardiography failed to detect trivial AR due to acoustic shadowing of the LV outflow tract from a mechanical valve in the mitral valve position. Transesophageal echocardiography was superior to transthoracic echocardiography in diagnosing perivalvular abscess, subaortic perforation, valvular dehiscence, torn or thickened bioprosthetic aortic valve cusps, and in clearly distinguishing perivalvular from AR. Transesophageal echocardiography correctly diagnosed bioprosthetic valve obstruction in 1 patient, but failed to diagnose mechanical valve obstruction in another. In conclusion, transesophageal echocardiography offers no advantage over the transthoracic approach in the detection and quantification of prosthetic AR unless the transthoracic image quality is poor. Transesophageal echocardiography is limited in detecting mechanical valve obstruction and in detecting AR in the presence of a mechanical prosthesis in the mitral valve position. However, it is superior to transthoracic echocardiography in identifying perivalvular pathology, differentiating perivalvular from valvular regurgitation and in defining the anatomic abnormality responsible for the prosthetic valve dysfunction. Combined transthoracic and transesophageal examination provides complete anatomic and hemodynamic assessment of prosthetic aortic valve function.

In this investigation by Stoddard and colleagues[44] from Louisville, Kentucky, 2-dimensional transesophageal echocardiographic findings are reported in 13 patients with structurally and functionally normal St. Jude Medical bileaflet mitral valve prostheses. Multiple mobile linear echogenic densities attached to the pivot of the prosthesis were present in 9 of 13 patients. These densities may represent fibrin strands. These mobile strands alternatively resolve and reform over a period of 5 to 14 months after MVR. No adverse clinical events were attributable to these prosthetic mitral valve strands. It was concluded that mobile strands are frequently attached to the structurally and functionally normal St. Jude Medical mitral valve prosthesis.

Melacini and associates[45] from Padova, Italy, performed echocardiographic and Doppler studies of 134 patients with a Hancock bioprosthesis in the mitral valve position during a follow-up period of 1–216 months. Among the xenografts, 57% were clinically normal and 43% had severe dysfunction. Among the normal bioprostheses, 35% had echocardiographically thickened mitral cusps (3 mm) with normal hemodynamic function; by setting the lower 95% confidence limit of valve area at 1.7 cm^2 these patients had a significantly smaller valve area than that of normal control subjects. Evaluation of all thickened normal mitral valves showed the highest incidence of thickening at 9 years after implantation. Valve replacement surgery was subsequently performed in 33 patients with dysfunctioning bioprostheses, and echocardiographic diagnosis was confirmed in 91% of explanted valves (bioprosthetic stenosis 21%, incompetence 46%, and combined stenosis and regurgitation 33%). In 2 valves that were found to be stenotic on echocardiographic examination, a calcium-related commissural tear was also observed at reoperation, and in another, a paravalvular leak was found. Dystrophic calcium, isolated (64%) or occasionally associated with fibrous tissue overgrowth (21%), was the main cause of failure. Pannus was present in prostheses with longer satisfactory function (168 ± 31 vs 124 ± 21 months). Long-term performance was evaluated by the Kaplan-Meier method for up to 18 years of follow-up. Freedom from structural valvular disfunction after MVR was 89% at 6 years, 77% at 8 years, 56% at 10 years, 31% at 12 years, 16% at 15 years, and 15% at 18 years.

Alton and associates[46] in Columbus, Ohio, studied 50 transthoracic and transesophageal echocardiographic studies in 37 patients with 47 Starr-Edwards prosthetic valves retrospectively. Six cases of surgically confirmed infective endocarditis were also studied. Vegetation or abscess formation, or both, was identified by transesophageal echocardiography in all six cases of infective endocarditis, but was found in only one of these cases by transthoracic echocardiography. Thrombus was detected by transesophageal echocardiography in 9 of 11 patients with transient ischemic attacks or stroke and in only 2 patients by transthoracic echocardiography with 3 confirmed at surgery. In 26 of the 30 patients with a mitral Starr-Edwards valve, the valve demonstrated trivial or mild "closing volume" early systolic or holosystolic leak on transesophageal echocardiography alone. Transthoracic evaluation identified significant MR in 6 of the 8 patients who had this finding on transesophageal echocardiography. These observations demonstrate the unique utility of transesophageal echocardiography in patients with Starr-Edwards prosthetic valve dysfunction, endocarditis, or thrombus formation and of its clear superiority over transthoracic echocardiography in these same patients.

RHEUMATIC FEVER DIAGNOSTIC GUIDELINES

The special Wriging Group of the Committee on Rheumatic Fever, Endocarditis, and Kawasaki Disease of the Council on Cardiovascular Disease in the Young of the American Heart Association reported in the October 21, 1992, JAMA a 1992 revision of the Jones Criteria for guidance in the diagnosis of acute rheumatic fever which were first published by T. Duckett Jones in 1944 and have been revised periodically since then by the American Heart Association[47]. The current guidelines are an update of these criteria. For the first time, the guidelines are designed to establish the initial attach of acute rheumatic fever. Major manifestations, minor manifestations, and supporting evidence of antecedent group A streptococcal infection are discussed. These updated guidelines expand on the available tools to diagnose streptococcal pharyngitis and clarify the available antibody tests for detecting antecedent group A streptococcal infection. At the present time echocardiography without accompanying auscultatory findings is insufficient to be the sole criterion for valvulitis in acute rheumatic fever. Finally, this article addresses overdiagnosis of rheumatic fever and lists exceptions to the Jones Criteria, including recurrent attacks in individuals with a history of rheumatic fever.

References

1. Folland ED, Kriegle BJ, Henderson WG, Hammermeister KE, Sethi GK, Participants in the Veterans Affairs Cooperative Study on Valvular Heart Disease. N Engl J Med 1992 (Aug 13); 327:458–462.
2. Farb A, Tang AL, Atkinson JB, McCarthy WF, Virmani R: Comparison of cardiac findings in patients with mitral valve prolapse who die suddenly to those who have congestive heart failure from mitral regurgitation and to those with fatal noncardiac conditions. Am J Cardiol 1992 (July 15); 70:234–239.
3. Bhutto ZR, Barron JT, Liebson PR, Uretz EF, Parrillo JE: Electrocardiographic abnormalities in mitral valve prolapse. Am J Cardiol 1992 (July 15); 70:265–266.
4. Lax D, Eicher M, Goldberg SJ: Mild dehydration induces echocardiographic signs of mitral valve prolapse in healthy females with prior normal cardiac findings. Am Heart J 1992 (December); 124:1533–1540.
5. Glick BN, Roberts WC: Usefulness of total 12-lead QRS voltage in diagnosing left ventricular hypertrophy in clinically isolated, pure, chronic, severe mitral regurgitation. Am J Cardiol 1992 (Oct 22); 70:1088–1092.
6. Burwash IG, Blackmore GL, Koilpillai CJ: Usefulness of left atrial and left ventricular chamber sizes as predictors of the severity mitral regurgitation. Am J Cardiol 1992 (Sept 15); 70:774–779.
7. Castello R, Lenzen P, Aguirre F, Labovitz AJ. Quantitation of mitral regurgitation by transesophageal echocardiography with Doppler color flow mapping: Correlation with cardiac catheterization. J Am Coll Cardiol 1992 (June); 19:1516–21.
8. Freeman WK, Schaff HV, Khandheria BK, Oh JK, Orszulak TA, Abel MD, Seward JB, Tajik AJ. Intraoperative evaluation of mitral valve regurgitation and repair by transesophageal echocardiography: incidence and significance of systolic anterior motion. J Am Coll Cardiol 1992 (September); 20:599–609.
9. Cohen DJ, Norris LP, Montemayor IE, O'Rourke RA, Zabalgoitia M: Systolic anterior motion of the chordal apparatus after mitral ring insertion. Am Heart J 1992 (September) 124:666–670.
10. Rozich JD, Carabello BA, Usher BW, Kratz JM, Bell AE, Zile MR: Mitral Valve Replacement With and Without Chordal Preservation in Patients With Chronic Mitral Regurgitation, Mechanisms for Differences in Postoperative Ejection Performance. Circulation 1992 (December); 86:1718–1726.
11. Gordon SPF, Douglas PS, Come PC, Manning WJ. Two-dimensional and Doppler echocardiographic determinants of the natural history of mitral valve narrowing in patients with rheumatic mitral stenosis: Implications for follow-up. J Am Coll Cardiol 1992 (April); 19:968–73.
12. Rihal CS, Schaff HV, Frye RL, Bailey KR, Hammes LN, Holmes DR Jr. Long-term follow-up of patients undergoing closed transventricular mitral commissurotomy: a useful surrogate for percutaneous balloon mitral valvuloplasty? J Am Coll Cardiol 1992 (October);20:781–6.
13. Fawzy ME, Ribeiro PA, Dunn B, Galal O, Muthusamy R, Shaikh A, Mercer E, Duran CMG: Percutaneous mitral valvotomy with the Inoue balloon catheter in children and adults: Immediate results and early follow-up. Am Heart J 1992 (February); 123:462–465.
14. Block PC, Palacios IF, Block EH, Tuzcu EM, Griffin B: Late (two-year) follow-up after percutaneous balloon mitral valvotomy. Am J Cardiol 1992 (Feb 15); 69:537–541.
15. Tuzcu EM, Block PC, Griffin BP, Newell JB, and Palacios IFL. Immediate and Long-term Outcome of Percutaneious Mitral Valvotomy in Patients 65 Years and Older. Circulation 1992 (March); 85:963–971.
16. Stefanadis C, Stratos C, Pitsavos C, Kallikazaros I, Triposkiadis F, Trikas A, Vlachopoulos C, Gavaliatsis I, Toutouzas P: Retrograde Nontransseptal Balloon Mitral Valvuloplasty, Immediate Results and Long-Term Follow-up. Circulation 1992 (May);85:1760–1767.

17. National Heart, Lung, and Blood Institute Balloon Valvuloplasty Registry: Complications and Mortality of Percutaneous Balloon Mitral Commissurotomy, A Report From the National Heart, Lung, and Blood Institute Balloon Valvuloplasty Registry. Circulation 1992 (June);85:2014–2024.

18. Desideri A, Vanderperren O, Serra A, Barraud P, Petitclerc R, Lesperance J, Dyrda I, Crepeau J: Long-term (9 to 33 months) echocardiographic follow-up after successful percutaneous mitral commissurotomy. Am J Cardiol 1992 (June 15); 69:1602–1606.

19. Reid CL, Otto CM, Davis KB, Labovitz A, Kisslo KB, McKay CR: Influence of mitral valve morphology on mitral balloon commissurotomy: Immediate and six-month results from the NHLBI Balloon Valvuloplasty Registry. Am Heart J 1992 (September); 124:657–665.

20. Cohen DJ, Kuntz RE, Gordon SPF, Piana RN, Safian RD, McKay RG, Baim DS, Grossman W, Diver DJ: Predictors of long-term outcome after percutaneous balloon mitral valvuloplasty. N Engl J Med 1992 (Nov 5); 327:1329–1335.

21. Chen CR, Cheng TO, Chen JY, Zhou YL, Mei J, Ma TZ: Long-term results of percutaneous mitral valvuloplasty with the Inoue balloon catheter. Am J Cardiol 1992 (Dec 1); 70:1445–1448.

22. Faggiano P, Ghizzoni G, Sorgato A, Sabatini T, Simoncelli U, Gardini A, Rusconi C: Rate of progression of valvular aortic stenosis in adults. Am J Cardiol 1992 (July 15); 70:229–233.

23. Villari B, Hess OM, Meier C, Pucillo A, Gaglione A, Turina M, and Krayenbuehl HP: Regression of Coronary Artery Dimensions after Successful Aortic Valve Replacement. Circulation 1992 (March); 85:972–978.

24. Villari B, Hess OM, Moccetti D, Vassalli G, Krayenbuehl HP. Effect of progression of left ventricular hypertrophy on coronary artery dimensions in aortic valve disease. J Am Coll Cardiol 1992 (November); 20:1073–9.

25. Carroll JD, Carroll EP, Feldman T, Ward DM, Lang RM, McGaughey D, Karp RB: Sex-Associated Differences in Left Ventricular Function in Aortic Stenosis of the Elderly. Circulation 1992 (October);86:1099–1107.

26. Bernard Y, Etievent J, Mourand J-L, Anguenot T, Schiele F, Guseibat M, Bassand J-P. Long-term results of percutaneous aortic valvuloplasty compared with aortic valve replacement in patients more than 75 years old. J Am Coll Cardiol 1992 (October);20:796–801.

27. Sadee AS, Becker AE, Verheul HA, Bouma B, Hoedemaker G: Aortic valve regurgitation and the congenitally bicuspid aortic valve: A clinico-pathological correlation. Br Heart J 1992 (June); 67:439–441.

28. van der Meer JTM, Thompson J, Valkenburg HA, Michel MF: Epidemiology of bacterial endocarditis in the Netherlands: I. Patient characteristics. Arch Intern Med 1992 (Sept); 152:1863–1868.

29. Choudhury R, Grover A, Varma J, Khattri HN, Anand IS, Bidwai PS, Wahi PL, Sapru RP: Active infective endocarditis observed in an Indian hospital 1981–1991. Am J Cardiol 1992 (Dec 1); 70:1453–1458.

30. Birmingham GD, Rahko PS, Ballantyne F III: Improved detection of infective endocarditis with transesophageal echocardiography. Am Heart J 1992 (March); 123:774–781.

31. Lederman MM, Sprague L, Wallis RS, Ellner JJ: Duration of fever during treatment of infective endocarditis. Medicine 1992; 71:52–57.

32. Hecht SR, Berger M: Right-sided endocarditis in intravenous drug users: Prognostic features in 102 episodes. An Intern Med 1992 (Oct 1); 117:560–566.

33. Tornos MP, Permanyer-Miralda G, Olona M, Gil M, Galve E, Almirante B, Soler-Soler J: Long-term complications of native valve infective endocarditis in non-addicts: A 15-year follow-up study. An Intern Med 1992 (Oct 1) 117:567–572.

34. Francioli P, Etienne J, Hoigne R, Thys JP, Gerber A: Treatment of streptococcal endocarditis with a single daily dose of ceftriaxone sodium for 4 weeks: Efficacy and outpatient treatment feasibility. JAMA 1992 (Jan 8); 267:264–267.

35. Haydock D, Barratt-Boyes B, Macedo T, Kirklin JW, Blackstone E: Aortic valve replacement for active infectious endocarditis in 108 patients: A comparison of freehand allograft valves with mechanical prostheses and bioprostheses. J Thorac Cardiovasc Surg 1992 (Jan); 103:130–139.

36. Fiore AC, Naunheim KS, D'Orazio S, Kaiser GC, McBride LR, Pennington G, Peigh PS,

Willman VL, Labovitz AJ, Barner HB: Mitral valve replacement: Randomized trial of St. Jude and Medtronic-Hall prostheses. Ann Thorac Surg 1992 (July); 54:68–73.

37. van der Graaf Y, de Waard F, van Herwerden LA, deFauw J: Risk of strut fracture of Bjork-Shiley valves. Lancet 1992 (Feb 1); 339:257–261.

38. Birkmeyer JD, Marrin CAS, O'Connor GT: Should patients with Bjork-Shiley valves undergo prophylactic replacement? Lancet 1992 (Aug 29); 340:520–523.

39. Vasan RS, Kaul U, Sanghvi S, Kamlakar T, Negi PC, Shivastava S, Rajani M, Venugopal P, Wasir HS. Thrombolytic therapy for prosthetic valve thrombosis: A study based on serial Doppler echocardiographic evaluation. Am Heart J 1992 (June); 123:1575–1580.

40. Burdon TA, Miller DC, Oyer PE, Mitchell RS, Stinson EB, Starnes VA, Shumway NE: Durability of porcine valves at fifteen years in a representative North American patient population. J Thorac Cardiovasc Surg 1992 (Feb); 103:238–252.

41. Frater RWM, Salomon NW, Rainer WG, Cosgrove DM III, Wickham E: The Carpentier-Edwards pericardial aortic valve: Intermediate results. Ann Thorac Surg 1992 (May); 53:764–771.

42. Born D, Martinez EE, Almeida PAM, Santos DV, Carvalho ACC, Moron AF, Miyasaki CH, Moraes SD, Ambrose JA: Pregnancy in patients with prosthetic heart valves: The effects of anticoagulation on mother, fetus and neonate. Am Heart J 1992 (August); 124:413–417.

43. Karalis DG, Chandrasekaran K, Ross JJ JR, Micklin A, Brown BM, Ren JF, Mintz GS: Single-plane transesophageal echocardiography for assessing function of mechanical or bioprosthetic valves in the aortic valve position. Am J Cardiol 1992 (May 15); 69:1310–1315.

44. Stoddard MF, Dawkins PR, Longaker RA: Mobile strands are frequently attached to the St. Jude Medical mitral valve prosthesis as assessed by two-dimensional transesophageal echocardiography. Am Heart J 1992 (September); 124:671–674.

45. Melacini P, Villanova C, Thiene G, Minarini M, Fasoli G, Bortolotti U, Ramuscello G, Scognamiglio R, Ponchia A, Volta SD: Long-term echocardiographic Doppler monitoring of Hancock bioprostheses in the mitral valve position. Am J Cardiol 1992 (Nov 1); 70:1157–1163.

46. Alton ME, Pasierski TJ, Orsinelli DA, Eaton GM, Pearson AC. Comparison of transthoracic and transesophageal echocardiography in evaluation of 47 Starr-Edwards prosthetic valves. J Am Coll Cardiol 1992 (December); 20:1503–11.

47. Special Writing Group of the Committee on Rheumatic Fever, Endocarditis, and Kawasaki Disease of the Council on Cardiovascular Disease in the Young of the American Heart Association: Guidelines for the diagnosis of rheumatic fever: Jones criteria, 1992 update. JAMA 1992 (Oct 21); 268:2069–2073.

Myocardial
Heart Disease

IDIOPATHIC DILATED CARDIOMYOPATHY

NHLBI workshop

Idiopathic dilated cardiomyopathy (IDC) is the primary indication for cardiac transplantation, with associated costs of approximately $177 million per year. Recognizing the economic implications of IDC, the increasing incidence, and the limited information on pathogenesis and prognosis, Manolio and associates[1] reported results of a workshop sponsored by the National Heart, Lung, and Blood Institute on the prevalence and etiology of IDC held on June 13 to 14, 1991. The difficulties of studying the disease were reviewed, including its relatively low prevalence, its potentially pluricausal nature, and the fact that it is often a diagnosis of exclusion. Still, it presents significant challenges to the cardiovascular scientific community, since the mechanism of myocardial damage and related etiologic and prognostic factors are virtually unknown. The development of more reliable measures of immune-mediated damage and noninvasive measures of impaired cardiac function present new research opportunities in this disorder. Standardized diagnostic criteria for use in observational and interventional trials were developed, and priorities for future research were proposed. Population-based registries and nested case-control studies, where feasible, are appropriate study designs for tracking incidence and prevalence, and for identifying risk factors, respectively. Interventional studies should focus on secondary prevention, through modifying immune-mediated damage in clinically evident IDC and through prevention of sudden death in patients with the disorder. Primary prevention trials must await the identification of modifiable risk factors and of appropriate and effective interventions.

Clinical course

To describe the prognosis of individuals with IDC in a population-based sample and to compare this with the prognosis of patients in a previous referral center case series with IDC, Sugrue and associates[2] from Rochester, Minnesota, followed 40 residents of Olmsted County, Minnesota, with IDC initially diagnosed between 1975 and 1984 and followed them through 1 July 1989 and 104 patients from a Mayo Clinic referral case series from 1960 to 1973. The authors measured survival of the population-based cohort at 1 year and 5 years. Survival at 1 year differed dramatically between the population-based cohort and the referral case series at 1 year (95% compared with 69%, respectively) and at 5 years (80% compared with 36%, respectively). Long-term survival for the population-based cohort was nonetheless impaired when compared with an age- and sex-matched cohort, that is, the 1980 Minnesota white population (8-year survival: observed, 58% compared with expected, 83%). Among community patients, older age and lower LVEF were independently associated with impaired survival (Figure 7-1). These population-based data challenge the clinical perception of the clinical course of IDC based on referral practice prognostic studies and suggest that the clinical course of this condition may be more favorable than previously recognized.

Familial variety

Dilated cardiomyopathy is characterized by an increase in cardiac ventricular size and impairment of cardiac ventricular function. Most cases are believed to be sporadic, and familial dilated cardiomyopathy is usually considered to be rare. Michels and associates[3] from Rochester, Minnesota, and Ann Arbor, Michigan, studied the proportion of cases of IDC that were familial in a large sequential series of patients whose first-degree relatives were investigated regardless of whether these relatives had cardiac symptoms. The authors studied the relatives of 59 index patients with IDC by obtaining a family history and performing a physical examination, electrocardiography, and 2-dimensional, M-mode, and Doppler echocardiography. A total of 315 relatives were examined. Eighteen relatives from 12 families were shown to have dilated cardiomyopathy. Thus, 12 of the 59 index patients (20.3%) had familial disease. There was no difference in age, sex, severity of disease, exposure to selected environmental factors, or electrocardiographic or echocardiographic features between the index patients with familial disease and those with nonfamilial disease. A noteworthy finding was that 22 of 240 healthy relatives (9.2%) with normal EFs had increased LV diameters during sys-

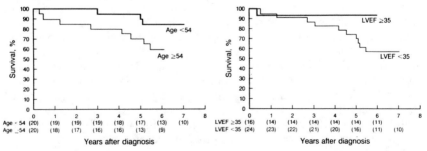

Fig. 7-1. The effect of age and ejection fraction on survival in the population-based cohort. Survival after initial diagnosis of idiopathic dilated cardiomyopathy among residents of Olmsted County, Minnesota, 1975 to 1984, stratified by age in years (left panel) and by ejection fraction (right panel). LVEF = left ventricular fraction. Reproduced with permission from Sugrue, et al.[2]

tole or diastole (or both), as compared with 2 of 112 healthy control subjects (1.8%) who were studied separately. Dilated cardiomyopathy was found to be familial in at least 1 in 5 of the patients in this study, a considerably higher percentage than in previous reports.

Ventricular thrombi

To determine the prevalence and natural history of LV thrombus in IDC, Falk and colleagues[4] from Boston, Massachusetts, prospectively performed 2-dimensional echocardiograms in 25 patients with IDC who were not receiving anticoagulation. Eighty-five echocardiograms were performed serially over a 9- to 30-month period (mean follow-up 21.5 months). An LV thrombus was present on initial echocardiogram in 11 (44%) patients, became present during follow-up in an additional 4, and disappeared in 2. Thrombus was significantly more common in patients with fractional shortening of ≤10% (12 of 15) than in those with a fractional shortening 11% to 25% (3 of 10). Five embolic events (4 cerebral) occurred over the follow-up period, 4 of which were associated with a previously visualized LV thrombus. Three of 15 thrombi that protruded into the LV cavity subsequently embolized. It was concluded that in nonanticoagulated patients with IDC, LV thrombus and thromboembolism are common. Echocardiography may be helpful in predicting which patients are at risk of thromboembolism.

Brain abnormalities

Dusleag and associates[5] from Graz, Austria, studied 20 patients with IDC aged <50 years (mean 41) and an age-matched group of 20 healthy volunteers. All subjects were free of cerebrovascular symptoms and risk factors for stroke. Magnetic resonance imaging of the brain, extracranial Doppler ultrasonography, heart catheterization and echocardiography were performed. In patients with IDC, a higher frequency of ventricular enlargement, cortical atrophy and white matter lesions was observed. Cerebral infarcts were found in 4 patients who showed clinically severe limitation of functional capacity (New York Heart Association class III or IV). The extent of cortical atrophy, and the duration of clinical evidence of IDC showed a significant correlation. The data indicate a high incidence of parenchymal abnormalities of the brain in young, neurologically asymptomatic patients with IDC.

Late potentials

To assess the incidence and clinical significance of ventricular late potentials in IDC, Denereaz and associates[6] from Geneva, Switzerland, studied 51 consecutive patients (44 men and 7 women, mean age 53 ± 11 years). Twenty-eight patients (55%) were in New York Heart Association functional class III or IV, 34 out of 51 (76%) had an LVEF of less than 40%, 10 out of 51 (20%) had a history of sustained VT, 24 out of 37 (65%) had runs of non-sustained VT during Holter monitoring and 15 out of 51 (29%) had a left BBB. A signal-averaged electrocardiogram (gain $10^6 \times$, bipolar chest leads, filters 100–300 Hz) was performed in all the patients; late potentials were considered present if the total filtered QRS duration was longer than 118 ms and the interval between the end of QRS and the voltage 40 μ V was more than 40 ms in the absence of left BBB (total filtered QRS duration >140 ms and interval between the end of QRS and the voltage 40 μ V >50 ms in the presence of left BBB). Ventricular late potentials were detected in 22 out of 51 patients (43%). Late potentials were present in 80% (8 out of 10) of patients with sustained VT but in only 34% (14 of 41) without sustained VT. This difference remained statistically significant even when patients with a left BBB were excluded from the analysis (4 out of 6 vs 4 out of 30). To identify patients with IDC and sustained VT, signal-averaging had a sensitivity of 80%, a specificity of 66%, a positive predictive value of 36% and a negative predictive value of 93%. It is concluded that, in IDC, the signal-averaged electrocardiogram allows the identification of patients with sustained VT, even in the presence of a left BBB.

With pulmonary hypertension

To ascertain whether pulmonary hypertension, as assessed noninvasively by continuous-wave Doppler or TR, can be an important independent factor in the prognosis of patients with ischemic or IDC, Abramson and associates[7] from Philadelphia, Pennsylvania, performed M-mode, 2-dimensional, and Doppler echocardiographic examinations on 108 patients with dilated cardiomyopathy and follow-up was obtained on all survivors for 28 years. The echocardiograms were obtained at entry and on survivors 1 year later. The main outcome measures were overall mortality, mortality due to myocardial failure, and hospitalization for CHF. Twenty-eight patients had a high velocity of TR (>2.5 m/s), and 80 patients had a low velocity (≤2.5 m/s). After 28 months of follow-up, the mortality rate was 57% in patients with a high velocity compared with 17% in patients with a low velocity (difference of 40%). Hospitalization for CHF occurred in 75% and 26% of patients, respectively (difference of 49%). Eighty-nine percent of patients with a high velocity either died or were hospitalized compared with only 32% of patients with a low velocity (difference of 57%). The peak velocity of TR was the only prognostic variable selected using stepwise logistic regression models for the 3 outcome events. Noninvasive assessment of pulmonary hypertension using continuous-wave Doppler of TR can predict morbidity and mortality in patients with ischemic or IDC.

Ventricular arrhythmias

Prevalence and characteristics of ventricular arrhythmias on Holter monitoring were evaluated by DeMaria and associates[8] on behalf of the Italian Multicenter Cardiomyopathy Study (SPIC) Group in 218 patients with invasively documented IDC to clarify their relation to pump dysfunction, and their prognostic role. Ventricular arrhythmias were observed in 205 patients (94%) and were high grade (ventricular pairs or VT) in 130 (60%). No simple or multiform VPCs were present in 88 patients (group 1; 41%), ventricular pairs in 63 (group 2; 32%), and VT in 67 (group 3; 27%). Only echocardiographic RV dimensions and prevalence of ventricular arrhythmias during effort (8% in group 1, 15% in group 2, and 14% in group 3) differed significantly between groups. Ventricular arrhythmias severity, and number of VPCs and VT episodes were not correlated to RV or LV dimensions and pump function indexes. During a mean follow-up of 29 ± 16 months, 27 patients died from cardiac events, and 16 received transplants. Three-year survival probability was lower in groups 2 (0.82) and 3 (0.81) than in group 1 (0.94). By Cox multivariate analysis, ventricular arrhythmia severity was a major independent predictor of prognosis after markers of ventricular dysfunction such as LVEF and stroke work index.

Dual-chamber pacing

Hochleitner and associates[9] from Vienna and Innsbruck, Austria, evaluated the long-term efficacy of physiologic dual-chamber (DDD) pacing in the treatment of end-stage IDC in a longitudinal study of up to 5 years in 17 patients. The considerable clinical improvement achieved after implantation of a pacemaker programmed for DDD pacing at an AV delay of 100 ms was maintained throughout the follow-up period or until death and was associated with a consistent decrease in New York Heart Association class and an increase in LVEF. Cardiothoracic ratio, heart rate and echocardiographic dimensions progressively decreased, and systolic and diastolic BP increased. Median survival time was 22 months. During follow-up, 4 patients received donor hearts, 9 had a sudden death at home without defined cause or after a thromboembolic event and 1 died from adenocarcinoma. Three patients survived the follow-up. No patient needed rehospitalization owing to a worsening of CHF after pacemaker implantation. An interruption of pacing in DDD mode for 2 to 4 hours was followed within the first months by a marked decrease in LVEF and an increase in cardiothoracic ratio and echocardiographic dimensions, but this response consistently decreased during follow-up. The data indicate that DDD pacing can be recommended as a useful tool in the long-term treatment of end-stage IDC, with progressive improvement in cardiac function and a reduction of LV dilatation.

MR or TR of long duration may so shorten the ventricular filling time in IDC that stroke volume is limited. Brecker and associates[10] from London, UK, assessed the effects of changing the AV interval during temporary or permanent dual-chamber DDD pacing in 12 IDC patients with short ventricular filling times due to TR or MR or both. The authors measured ventricular filling time and cardiac output with Doppler echocardiography and exercise capacity on a treadmill, at baseline and with the best AV delay during pacing. The durations of both MR and TR were significantly shorter at the shorter AV interval (mean reductions 85 ms and 110 ms, respectively). There were consequent increases in LV and RV filling times (65 ms and 90 ms). For each 50 ms reduction in AV delay, LV filling time increased by 35 ms in 6 subjects with presystolic MR and RV filling time by 30 ms in 9 subjects with presystolic TR. At the short AV interval, cardiac output was greater than baseline (by 1.1 1/min) and there were rises in exercise duration (104 s) and maximum oxygen consumption (2.1 ml kg^{-1} min^{-1}). There was a decrease in the Likert visual analogue score of breathlessness at peak exercise (8.6 vs 4.9). Although from a small sample, these findings suggest that DDD pacing with a short AV delay may have therapeutic potential in patients with IDC even in the absence of conventional indications for pacemaker implantation.

HYPERTROPHIC CARDIOMYOPATHY

Myosin mutations

Recently, 2 families with HC have been shown to have mutations in the cardiac B-myosin heavy chain gene located on the long arm of chromosome 14. Epstein and colleagues[11] in Bethesda, Maryland, performed linkage analysis of 5 newly ascertained pedigrees with more than 50 chromosomal markers detecting polymorphisms. Their findings confirmed the linkage to B-myosin heavy chain gene locus on chromosome 14 in one family and suggested linkage to the same gene in another kindred. Chromosome 14 markers were not linked to the disease gene in the other three kindreds, however, and a test for genetic heterogeneity was statistically significant. Moreover, markers for the B-myosin heavy chain gene identified affected individuals who were recombinants with respect to this gene and the disease phenotype in these three kindreds. These results provided conclusive evidence that HC in separate families is caused by mutations in disease genes at 2 or more locations in the genome.

Familial HC is characterized by a variable degree of myocardial hypertrophy and a wide range of symptoms. Different mutations in the B cardiac myosin heavy-chain gene have been identified in 3 affected families. Neither the proportion of cases attributable to myosin mutations nor the effect of different mutations on clinical outcome, however, are known. Using a ribonuclease protection assay, Watkins and associates[12] from Boston, Massachusetts, London, UK, and Taichung, Taiwan, screened the B cardiac myosin heavy-chain genes of probands from 25 unrelated families with familial HC. This assay is a sensitive method for detecting the presence and location of mutations. The authors further defined the mutations by analyzing their nucleotide sequences. The clinical features of HC were compared in families with various myosin mutations. Seven mutations in the B cardiac myosin heavy-chain gene were identified in 12 of the 25 families (Figure 7-2). All were missense mutations (i.e., causing the substitution of a single amino acid) clustered in the head and head-rod junction regions of the molecule. Six mutations resulted in a change in the charge of the amino acid. Patients with mutations that changed

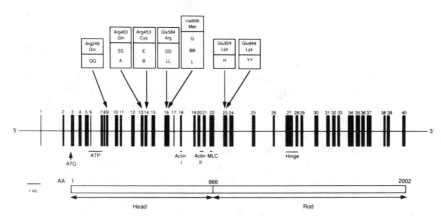

Fig. 7-2. Location and Identity of Missense Mutations in Families with Familial Hypertrophic Cardiomyopathy. A schematic diagram of the normal β cardiac myosin heavy-chain gene is shown in the center (5′ to 3′), and the location of the missense mutations is shown according to exon. The amino acid substitutions predicted by each mutation are shown in the top of each box, and the families with these mutations are designated by letters. Sequences that encode the initiation of transcription (ATG), ATPase activity (ATP), actin binding (Actin I and Actin II), myosin light-chain binding (MLC), and hinge function (Hinge) are indicated. The head and rod regions of the encoded polypeptide are shown at the bottom of the figure. Reproduced with permission from Watkins, et al.[12]

the charge of the altered amino acid (such as that from arginine to gluta-mine at nucleotide 403 or from arginine to cysteine at nucleotide 453) had a significantly shorter life expectancy (mean age at death, 33 years), whereas patients with the 1 mutation that did not produce a change in charge (VAl606Met) had nearly normal survival. However, patients with different mutations did not differ appreciably in their clinical manifesta-tions of familial HC. Different missense mutations in the B cardiac myosin heavy-chain gene can be identified in approximately 50% of families with HC. In those families, a definite genetic diagnosis can be made in all members. Since the location of a mutation or its DNA-sequence alteration (or both) appears to influence survival, the authors suggest that the precise definition of the disease-causing mutation can provide important prog-nostic information about affected members.

Clinical course

Patients with HC may present a wide spectrum of clinical and morphologic manifestations. Although many aspects of the natural history of HC are understood, the initial presentation and subsequent clinical course of certain subgroups are not yet well defined. To further our understanding in this regard, Hecht and associates[13] from Bethesda, Maryland, analyzed 241 middle-aged patients with HC (aged 35 to 55 years). Most patients (n = 210) had already had symptoms whereas the remaining 31 initially presented with no or minimal symptoms and were the focus of this investigation; 29 of these were followed for ≥2 years (range to 11.5 years, mean 8). A separate group of 30 moderately symptomatic age- and gender-matched patients with HC were selected as control subjects for morphologic comparisons. Of the 29 study patients with follow-up, 22 (76%) are presently free of important cardiac symptoms, but 3 showed progression of symptoms, and 4 have died suddenly. Annual mortality rate was 1.7%. Eighteen of the middle-aged asymptomatic patients with HC (58%) had localized LV hypertrophy, usually involving only the anterior ventricular septum; in contrast, only 9 of the 30 symptomatic control subjects (30%) had such localized hypertrophy. In conclusion, of those patients with HC who achieved middle-age without developing important cardiac symptoms, approxi-mately 75% remained asymptomatic during the ensuing average 8-year follow-up. However, such patients are not protected in absolute terms from unfavorable clinical events (despite relatively mild LV hypertrophy and in most cases absence of outflow obstruction). This is evidenced by the fact that approximately 25% eventually experienced symptomatic deterioration or sudden cardiac death.

Exercise limitation

Chikamori and associates[14] in London, UK, evaluated the relationship between exercise and systolic and diastolic function in patients with HC. Eighty one patients underwent two-dimensional echocardiography, technetium-99m equilibrium radionuclide angiography and maximal, symptom-limited, treadmill exercise testing with measurements of maxi-mal oxygen consumption. Thirty-six patients achieved ≤70% of age-pre-dicted maximal oxygen consumption. Patients with exercise limitation were more likely to be in New York Heart Association functional class II or III; there was no such relation between maximal oxygen consumption and the incidence and magnitude of rest LV outflow tract pressure gradient. In the 22 patients with LV outflow tract gradients, the ratios of peak ejection to peak filling rate and of atrial contribution to left atrial dimension were related to percent of the age-predicted maximal oxygen consumption. These ratios reflect impaired LV systolic performance and atrial systolic failure, respectively. Stepwise discriminant analysis revealed these two ratios to be the strongest predictors of patients with an LV outflow gradient whose maximal oxygen consumption was ≤70% of the age-predicted value. In 59 patients without a rest LV outflow tract gradient, peak filling rate and time to end-systole were related to the age-predicted maximal oxygen consumption. Stepwise discriminant analysis revealed that in those patients without an LV outflow tract gradient, reduced peak filling rate and prolonged time to end-systole best identified patients whose maximal oxygen consumption was ≤70% of the age-predicted value. These data indicate different mechanisms of exercise limitation in HC. In patients with an LV outflow tract gradient at rest, the main determinants of exercise limitation are impaired LV and LA systolic performance. In those without a gradient, diastolic function is a more important factor in limiting exercise ability.

Prognostic determinants

Patients with HC frequently have arrhythmias and hemodynamic abnormalities and are prone to sudden death and syncope. An important need exists for improved risk stratification and definition of appropriate investigation and therapy. Fananazapir and colleagues[15] in Bethesda, Maryland, examined the relation of 31 clinical, Holter, cardiac catheterization, and electrophysiological variables to subsequent cardiac events in 230 HC patients by multivariate analysis. Studies were for cardiac arrest, syncope, presyncope, VT on Holter, a strong family history of sudden death, and palpitations. Nonsustained VT on Holter was present in 115 patients. Sustained ventricular arrhythmia was induced in 82 patients. Seventeen cardiac events (8 sudden deaths, 1 cardiac arrest, and 8 syncope with defibrillator discharges) occurred during a follow-up of 28 months. The 1-year and 5-year event-free rates were 99% and 79%, respectively. Two variables were significant independent predictors of subsequent events: sustained ventricular arrhythmia induced at electrophysiologic study and a history of cardiac arrest or syncope. Only 2 of 66 patients without symptoms of impaired consciousness had a cardiac event. In contrast, nonsustained VT on Holter was associated with a worse prognosis only in patients with symptoms of impaired consciousness: 11 of 79 symptomatic patients with VT on Holter had events versus only 4 of 85 symptomatic patients without VT on Holter. Notably, none of 51 patients without symptoms of impaired consciousness in whom VT was not induced at electrophysiologic study had a cardiac event. In HC, VT on Holter is of benign prognostic significance in the absence of symptoms of impaired consciousness and inducible VT, and sustained VT induced at electrophysiologic study, especially when associated with cardiac arrest or syncope, identifies a subgroup at high risk for subsequent cardiac events.

Atrial fibrillation

It has been generally assumed that most patients with HC who develop AF have marked LV hypertrophy and subaortic obstruction. The morpho-

logic and functional features of this subset of patients with HC have not
been systematically investigated. Spirito and associates[16] from Bethesda,
Maryland, compared the LV morphology and functional profile of 46
patients with HC and chronic AF with those of 81 control patients with
HC and normal sinus rhythm. Contrary to expectations, LV hypertrophy
(assessed with 2-dimensional echocardiography) was substantially less
marked in the patients with AF than in the control patients, and prevalence of subaortic obstruction was similar in the 2 groups. Maximal LV
wall thickness and wall thickness index were lower in patients with AF
(18 ± 2 and 56 ± 7 mm, respectively) than in control patients (22 ± 6
and 67 ± 16 mm, respectively). Furthermore, mild LV hypertrophy (maximal LV wall thickness ≤17 mm confined to 1 ventricular segment) was
almost twice as frequent in patients with AF (63%) than in control patients
(36%). Subaortic obstruction was present in 9 patients with AF (20%) and
in 28 control patients (35%). In a subgroup of 22 patients with AF who
were followed for 4 to 10 years, 5 patients had marked LV wall thinning
(≥5 mm, range 5 to 14). In conclusion, these results demonstrate that
most patients with HC and chronic AF have the nonobstructive form
of HC, and relatively mild LV hypertrophy. In many of these patients,
progressive LV wall thinning is probably responsible for the mild LV
hypertrophy.

Ventricular tachycardia

Dritsas and associates[17] from London, UK, studied 69 patients with
HC by 2-dimensional and Doppler echocardiography and 72-hour Holter
monitoring to examine the relation between the degree of LV hypertrophy
and dysfunction and the occurrence of VT. Episodes of nonsustained VT
were detected in 20 patients (29%). Maximal wall thickness was not different between patients with (22 ± 5 mm) and without (21 ± 5 mm) VT.
Total hypertrophy score, calculated as the sum of 10 segmental wall
thicknesses, was also similar in both groups (157 ± 22 and 153 ± 32
mm, respectively). Furthermore, no significant differences were found
between the 2 groups in LV end-diastolic dimension (41 ± 7 vs 40 ± 6
mm), fractional shortening (33 ± 7 vs 34 ± 10%) and left atrial size (40
± 10 vs 41 ± 11 mm). An LV outflow tract gradient was detected in 25%
of patients with and 35% without VT. One or more Doppler indexes of
diastolic function were abnormal in 70% of patients, but no difference in
any of these indexes was found between those with and without VT. In
summary, the occurrence of VT in hypertrophic cardiomyopathy is not
related to the degree of LV hypertrophy, outflow tract gradient or dysfunction. This finding suggests a dissociation between the arrhythmogenic
substrate and echocardiographic features of the disease.

Developing outflow obstruction

Panza and associates[18] from Bethesda, Maryland, studied the development of subaortic obstruction in young patients with HC using serial
echocardiograms. Studies were carried out in 26 consecutive children
who showed no evidence of obstruction at their initial evaluation at a
mean age of 11 ± 3 years. After follow-up of 3–12 years, 7 of the 26 (27%)
developed evidence of obstruction with systolic anterior motion of the
mitral valve and increased LV outflow tract Doppler velocities averaging
3.8 ± .3 m/sec. Patients who developed obstruction had smaller transverse
dimensions of the LV outflow tract and more anteriorly displaced mitral

valve when initially evaluated than did patients without development of obstruction. In addition, the already reduced outflow tract dimension decreased further during follow-up and the mitral valve became even more anteriorly displaced within the LV cavity. These developmental changes were associated with increases in LV wall thickness, particularly of the basal anterior septum compared with control patients with HC who did not develop obstruction. This study demonstrates that subaortic obstruction can develop *de novo* in patients with HC during the adolescent years. The finding of marked thickening of basal anterior septum and reduction in LV outflow tract dimension highlights children who are at higher risk for development of obstruction and are useful markers in terms of follow-up and prognosis.

Dipyridamole effects

Recent studies have indicated that myocardial ischemia can occur and thus may play an important role in the pathophysiology of patients with HC. Therefore, Koga and associates[19] from Kurume, Japan, investigated whether or not dipyridamole—a selective coronary vasodilating agent—could favorably modify myocardial perfusion and the clinical manifestations in 20 patients with HC (19 nonobstructive and 1 mildly obstructive) with an average age of 50 years. Oral dipyridamole, 150 mg/day for 2 weeks, prevented reversible perfusion defects initially observed in 6 patients on baseline exercise thallium-201 scintigraphy and significantly increased the radiothallium clearance, while 1 patient developed new reversible perfusion defects. There were significant increases in echocardiographic fractional shortening and treadmill exercise time and reductions in cardiac size and supraventricular arrhythmias with dipyridamole therapy. These observations suggest that coronary vasodilation with dipyridamole may improve myocardial perfusion and cardiac function in HC patients.

Mitral valve prolapse

Petrone and associates[20] in Bethesda, Maryland, studied patients with HC to determine the frequency of MVP. It was possible to make assessments of the frequency and severity of MVP in 528 consecutive patients with HC studied by echocardiography. Patients ranged in age from 1 to 86 years; 335 of them were males. Unequivocal echocardiographic evidence of systolic MVP into the left atrium was identified in only 16 (3%) of the 528 patients. The MV excised at operation from three of the patients had morphologic characteristics of a floppy MV. The occurrence of clinically evident AF was common in patients with HC and MVP (56%). Therefore, in a large group of patients with HC, the association of echocardiographically documented MVP was uncommon. The presence of MVP in patients with HC appeared to predispose to AF.

Infective endocarditis

Roberts and associates[21] in Bethesda, Maryland, used clinical and morphologic findings in 11 patients with HC complicated by infective endocarditis to study severe MR or AR or both that necessitated valve replacement. In each of the 11 patients, there were changes in the operatively excised valve or valves characteristic of healed infective endocarditis.

The infection involved only the mitral valve in 7 patients, only the aortic valve in 3, and both valves in one patient. The evaluation of the operatively excised mitral valves indicated that the healed vegetations were located most commonly on the LV aspects of the anterior mitral leaflet, indicating that vegetation had formed at contact points of this leaflet with mural endocardium of the LV outflow tract (Figure 7-3). The infective endocarditis either worsened preexisting valve regurgitation or caused valve regurgitation and led to the development of cardiac dysfunction requiring valve replacement. Functional class improved in the nine patients surviving valve replacement. Thus, HC appears to predispose to infective endocarditis. Patients with HC should receive prophylactic antibiotic therapy during procedures that predispose to infective endocarditis.

Associated atherosclerotic coronary artery disease

The role of CAD in HC has not been thoroughly clarified. To assess the clinical and prognostic significance of these 2 coexistent diseases, Lazzeroni and associates[22] from Parma, Italy, studied 96 patients with HC (62 men, mean age 45 years) who underwent coronary arteriography and 2-dimensional echocardiography. Significant stenosis (>70%) of 1 or more coronary arteries was detected in 11 patients, all aged >45 years. This group, compared with the other group without significant CAD (n = 85), was characterized by an older age (59 ± 7 vs 42 ± 15 years), a greater prevalence of previous AMI (24 vs 9%), complex ventricular arrhythmias (100 vs 50%), non-obstructive forms (82 vs 46%), dilated (45 vs 7%) and hypocontractile LV (36 vs 6%) and higher mortality (36 vs 8%) during a mean follow-up of 3.6 years. It is concluded that CAD associated with HC is a complex clinical syndrome, difficult to diagnose clinically, that can reliably be recognized by coronary angiography. CAD seems to play an important role in modifying the pathophysiology, the natural history and the prognosis of HC.

Mitral valve abnormalities

To assess the possibility that the mitral valve itself may be involved in the disease process, Klues and co-workers[23] in Bethesda, Maryland,

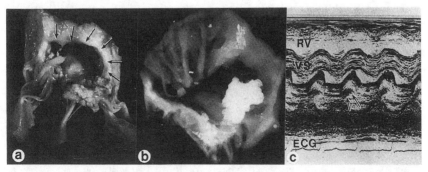

Fig. 7-3. (above). Patient 1. Operatively excised mitral valve. a, Leaflets, chordae tendineae and attached papillary muscles showing loss of tissue in the posterior leaflet and absence of chordae tendineae (arrows). A large deposit of calcium is present and is better seen in b, a radiograph of the excised valve. c, M-mode echocardiogram taken shortly before mitral valve replacement, showing thickening and impaired mobility of the anterior mitral leaflet and fluttering (arrows) of the posterior leaflet. ECG = electrocardiogram; RV = right ventricular cavity; VS = ventricular septum. Reproduced with permission from Roberts, et al.[21]

studied mitral valves from 94 patients with HC and 45 normal control subjects. The area of the mitral leaflets was increased in patients with HC compared with control subjects (13 versus 8 cm²). For the overall group of patients, this increase was largely caused by an increase in anterior leaflet length (2.2 for HC versus 1.8 cm for control subjects), because circumference did not differ between the 2 groups. Mitral leaflet area was increased in 55 of the 94 valves. In 12 of these 55 valves, both the anterior and posterior leaflets were enlarged; the other 45 valves had asymmetrical or segmental enlargement of either the anterior leaflet or a portion of posterior leaflet. In addition, 9 patients had a congenital malformation of the mitral apparatus in which one or both papillary muscles inserted directly into anterior mitral leaflet. Sixty-two (66%) of 94 mitral valves had a constellation of structural malformations, including increased leaflet area and elongation of the leaflets or anomalous papillary muscle insertion directly into anterior mitral leaflet. These findings expand the morphological definition of HC by demonstrating that the disease process is not confined to cardiac muscle but rather many patients also have structural abnormalities of the mitral valve that are unlikely to be acquired or secondary to mechanical factors.

Myofiber disorganization

The presence of numerous, abnormally arranged, cardiac muscle cells distributed widely throughout the hypertrophied LV wall has been considered a characteristic, morphologic feature of patients dying with HC and also probably a determinant of impaired LV compliance. The relation between such regions of myocardial cell disarray and the magnitude of wall thickness in the same areas of the LV wall has not been defined. Maron and associates[24] from Bethesda, Maryland, therefore, systematically compared LV wall thickness and the percent area of myocardium disorganized in the same tissue sections. No correlation was identified between wall thickness and the amount of myocardium disorganized in the same tissue sections, either when calculated separately for the ventricular septum, and anterolateral and posterior free walls, or when expressed for all 3 regions combined. Therefore, in patients with HC: (1) disorganized myocardial architecture is not confined to greatly thickened portions of the LV wall, but regions of the LV with normal or only mildly increased thickness may also be disordered; and (2) whereas both LV wall thickening and cellular disorganization are manifestations of the primary cardiomyopathic process, these 2 morphologic features do not appear to be directly related with regard to their extent and distribution within the LV wall. These observations will potentially enhance understanding of the relation between LV structure and compliance in HC.

Dual-chamber pacing

Although attempts have been made to treat patients with obstructive HC with RV pacing, the usual treatment for those refractory to medical therapy is cardiac surgery. To assess in detail the value of non-surgical therapy the effects of acute and long-term dual-chamber pacing were investigated by Jeanrenaud and associates[25] from Lausanne, Switzerland, in 13 patients with obstructive HC refractory to medical therapy. In the first part of the study, AV sequential pacing was found to reduce peak LV outflow pressure gradient in 12 of the 13 patients, from 82 to 47 mm Hg, without concomitantly reducing aortic BP or cardiac output (Figure

7-4). This effect was related to AV interval. In the second part of the study, a dual-chamber pacemaker was implanted in 8 patients and programmed to the optimum AV interval for the individual (50–90 ms). Patients were followed up for up to 62 months. Pacing resulted in a significant and long-lasting reduction in severity of angina pectoris (from New York Heart Association class 3 to 1) and dyspnea (from New York Heart Association class 3 to 2). Echocardiography showed no significant change in septal thickness or LV contractility but there was a trend to a spontaneous decrease in obstruction. In patients with obstructive HC, synchronized and ventricular pacing at optimum AV interval for the individual reduces the intraventricular pressure gradient and improves functional tolerance. Since the effect is longlasting, such pacing should be deemed an alternative therapy to surgery in selected cases.

Patients with obstructive HC with symptoms refractory to drugs (β-blockers or verapamil) are candidates for cardiac surgery (LV myectomy or MVR). Fananapazir and co-investigators[26] in Bethesda, Maryland, examined prospectively the ability of dual-chamber pacing to improve symptoms and relieve LV outflow obstruction in such patients. Forty-four consecutive patients with obstructive HC who had failed to benefit from pharmacotherapy underwent treadmill exercise tests, echocardiography, and cardiac catheterization before and 1.5–3 months after implantation of a dual-chamber pacemaker. Symptoms of angina, dyspnea, palpitations, presyncope, and syncope, New York Heart Association functional class status, and exercise durations were improved at follow-up evaluation. This was associated with significant reduction in LV outflow tract gradient and significant increases in cardiac output and systemic arterial pressure. Notably, when pacing was discontinued and comparisons were made in sinus rhythm, treadmill exercise durations were greater and LV outflow

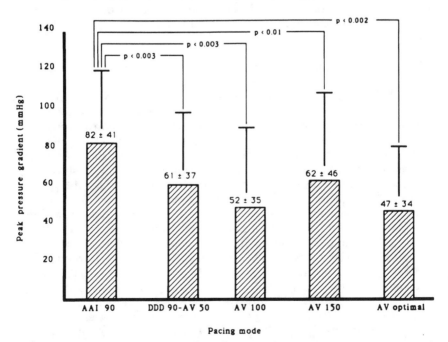

Fig. 7-4. Subaortic peak pressure gradient during atrial pacing at rate 90/min (AAI 90) and during dual-chamber pacing at the same rate (DDD 90) at AV intervals of 50, 100, or 150 ms, respectively, or at the optimum AV interval (AV optimum) for the individual. Values given as mean (SD). Reproduced with permission from Jeanrenaud, et al.[25]

tract gradients were less at the follow-up evaluation compared with the baseline study. Dual-chamber pacing is an effective alternative to surgery in most patients with obstructive HC with drug-refractory symptoms. The beneficial effects of pacing continue to be evident when pacing is acutely discontinued.

Dual-chamber DDD pacing relieves LV outflow obstruction in patients with HC. The reduction in LV outflow gradient persists in some patients after cessation of pacing. Twelve-lead and signal-averaged electrocardiograms were obtained before and after 12 weeks of DDD pacing in 18 patients with obstructive HC by McAreavey and Fananapazir[27] from Bethesda, Maryland, to determine whether the altered hemodynamic state after chronic pacing was accompanied by electrical changes. Hemodynamic studies were performed at baseline and at follow-up. Signal-averaged electrocardiograms were obtained using a Corazonix Predictor and bidirectional filters at 25 Hz to a noise level of 0.5 μV. At follow-up, LV outflow tract gradients were reduced significantly during DDD pacing and with cessation of pacing in sinus rhythm by 56 $\pm$ 10 and 47 $\pm$ 10 mm Hg, respectively. There was no simple relation between changes in LV outflow tract gradient and in the electrocardiogram. For example, amplitude of the R wave in $V_{5,6}$ was reduced by $\geq$0.5 mv in 4 patients, unchanged in 12 and increased in 2. Similarly, the S wave in leads $V_{1,2}$ was reduced in 7 patients, unchanged in 7 and increased in 4. The T wave became more negative ($\geq$0.1 mv) in leads II, III, aVF and $V_{5,6}$ in 13 patients and more positive in leads I and aVL in 12. The QRS was also altered by signal-averaged electrocardiographic criteria; duration of the total QRS and root-mean-square voltage of the QRS of the filtered Y axis increased (106 $\pm$ 12 to 112 $\pm$ 13 ms and 170 $\pm$ 82 to 195 $\pm$ 102 μV, respectively). In conclusion, chronic DDD pacing significantly reduces obstruction to LV outflow, and after discontinuation of chronic DDD pacing, there is evidence of altered mechanical as well as electrical myocardial state.

Myotomy–myectomy

To determine predictors of exercise benefit in patients with HC after operative relief of LV outflow tract obstruction, Diodati and associates[28] from Bethesda, Maryland, performed cardiac catheterization and exercise testing before and 6 months after operation in 30 patients. The increase in maximal oxygen consumption (VO_2max) during exercise testing was chosen as an index of exercise benefit. Univariate analysis showed a significant positive correlation of operative change in VO_2max with preoperative LV end-diastolic and pulmonary arterial wedge pressures, operative change in exercise duration, and operative reductions in LV end-diastolic and pulmonary arterial wedge pressures and resting LV outflow tract gradient, and a significant negative correlation with preoperative VO_2max and percent predicted VO_2max. Multivariate analysis by stepwise linear regression of only significant univariate variables selected only preoperative percent predicted VO_2max, and operative reduction in LV end-diastolic pressure and resting LV outflow tract gradient as significant predictors of postoperative change in VO_2max. Stepwise regression analysis, applied only to preoperative exercise and catheterization hemodynamic variables, selected only preoperative percent predicted VO_2max and preoperative LV end-diastolic pressure as predictors of improvement in exercise capacity. Thus, patients with obstructive hypertrophic cardiomyopathy, after failing medical therapy, are most likely to demonstrate improvement in exercise capacity if preoperative exercise testing demonstrates limited exercise capacity and if surgery achieves reduction in elevated resting LV outflow tract gradients and LV filling pressures.

Cohn and associates[29] from Boston, Massachusetts, reviewed long-term results of patients undergoing myotomy/myectomy of the ventricular septum for obstructive HC in 31 patients (15 women, 16 men, age 21–80 years [mean 55]) with mean New York Heart Association functional class III–IV CHF, who underwent radical myotomy/myectomy at their hospital from 1972–1991. Preoperative gradients by catheterization or echocardiography ranged from 26 to 240 mm Hg (average 96). There were no operative deaths. Two patients developed early postoperative complete heart block requiring a transvenous pacemaker. Clinical follow-up was 1 to 14 years (mean 6.5). All surviving patients were restudied by echocardiography and clinical examination. The mean post-operative functional class was II. Postoperative gradients ranged from 0 to 30 mm Hg (mean 4.5). There were 5 late deaths (low cardiac output in 2, stroke in 2, and acute respiratory failure in 1); 4 of 5 deaths occurred in patients with concomitant CAD. Survival at 10 years was 86 ± 9%. There were no reoperations for subaortic obstruction.

Grigg and associates[30] in Toronto, Ontario, Canada, have used intraoperative transesophageal Doppler echocardiography in decision making in 32 consecutive patients undergoing ventriculomyectomy with HC. The mean preoperative LV outflow gradient was 83 ± 39 mm Hg and the mean basal septal width was 24 ± 6 mm. Compared with transesophageal findings in 10 normal control subjects, the mitral leaflets were longer and the coaptation point was abnormal in the patients with HC. The coaptation point in the patient group was in the body of the leaflets at a mean of 9 ± 2 mm from the anterior leaflet tip, where it was at or within 3 mm of the leaflet tip pin the normal group. During early systole, the distal third to half of the anterior mitral leaflet angled sharply anteriorly and superiorly resulting in leaflet-septal contact and incomplete mitral leaflet coaptation in mid-systole. This led to the formation of a funnel composed of the distal parts of both leaflets allowing a jet of posteriorly directed MR to occur in mid- and late systole. The sequence of events in systole was eject/obstruct/leak. Transesophageal echocardiography was helpful in planning the extent of the resection, including the immediate result and excluding important complications. In successful surgical outcomes, the post-myectomy study showed (1) thinning of the septum with widening of the LV outflow tract to a width similar to that found in normal subjects; (2) disappearance of systolic anterior motion in the LV outflow tract color mosaic; and (3) marked reduction or abolition of MR. Thus, transesophageal echocardiography may be useful in patients with HC undergoing surgical myectomy.

Marwick and associates[31] in Cleveland, Ohio, determined the role of intraoperative echocardiography in planning the site and extent of myectomy and in ensuring adequate control of the LV outflow tract gradient. In 50 patients undergoing septal myectomy over a 5-year period, epicardial echocardiography was performed before cardiopulmonary bypass to help establish the extent of outflow tract obstruction, locate its site, and help plan the myectomy. In 30 patients, transesophageal echocardiography was used to corroborate data on outflow tract anatomy and examine the mitral valve. In 40 patients (80%), the initial myectomy resulted in a reduction of the maximal outflow tract gradient from 88 ± 45 to 24 ± 11 mm Hg, measured by epicardial continuous wave Doppler echocardiography. Ten patients (20%) were shown by postbypass intraoperative echocardiography to have an unsatisfactory result based on a persistent gradient >50 mm Hg (n = 7) or persistent MR of greater than moderate severity (n = 3). The postbypass two-dimensional echocardiogram was used to direct the surgeon toward the most likely site of continued obstruction, and the cardiopulmonary bypass was reinstituted to permit further myectomy (n = 9) or mitral valve repair (n = 1). After the second or subsequent period of cardiopulmonary bypass, the outflow tract gradient (26 ± 14 mm Hg) was substantially reduced and was not significantly different from the postbypass gradient in the group with initial surgical success. At postoperative follow-up 20 ± 37 weeks, the maximum measured outflow tract gradient (22 ± 21 mm Hg) showed no difference between patients with immediate surgical success and those requiring a second period of cardiopulmonary bypass for further resection. Intraoperative echocardiography proved useful in guiding the site and extent of septal myectomy, leading to more adequate surgical resection and persistence of satisfactory control of the outflow tract gradient into the early follow-up period of this study.

MYOCARDITIS

Mimicking acute myocardial infarction

Dec and associates[32] in Boston, Massachusetts, evaluated 34 patients with clinical signs and symptoms consistent with AMI who underwent RV endomyocardial biopsy during a 6.5 year period after angiographic identification of normal coronary arteries. Myocarditis was found on histologic study in 11 of these 34 patients. Cardiogenic shock requiring intraaortic balloon support developed within 6 hours of admission in 3 (27%) of the patients with myocarditis. The mean age of the group with myocarditis was 42 ± 5 years. A preceding viral illness had been present in 6 patients (54%). The electrocardiographic abnormalities were varied and included ST segment elevation (n = 6), T wave inversions (n = 3), ST segment depression (n = 2), and Q wave development (n = 2). The electrocardiographic abnormalities were seen in the anterior precordial leads most commonly, but were diffusely evident in three patients. LV function was normal in 6 patients and globally decreased in the remaining 5 patients whose ejection fractions ranged from 14% to 45%. Lymphocytic myocarditis was recognized in 10 patients and giant cell myocarditis in the remaining patient. All 6 patients whose LV function was normal on admission are alive and in functional class I presently. Among the 5 patients with impaired systolic function, ejection fraction normalized in 3 of the 4 patients who received immunosuppressive therapy within 3 months of treatment and in the one patient who received only supportive therapy. All patients who required intraaortic balloon pump support survived to discharge. One death, due to progressive CHF occurred at 18 months in the patient with giant cell myocarditis. Thus, myocarditis should be suspected in patients with an ischemic chest pain syndrome, especially when electrocardiographic abnormalities are present and are more extensive than can be explained with a single vascular distribution, segmental wall motion abnormalities are lacking or global LV dysfunction is present. The subsequent demonstration of normal coronary arteries should prompt consideration of RV endomyocardial biopsy.

ASSOCIATION WITH A CONDITION AFFECTING PRIMARILY
A NON-CARDIAC STRUCTURE(S)

HIV and/or AIDS

Abnormalities of cardiac structure and function are common in children infected with the human immunodeficiency virus (HIV). It is unclear, however, whether these abnormalities are attributable to the disease itself, associated infections, or possible cardiotoxic effects of the most commonly used treatment, zidovudine. Lipshultz and associates[33] from Boston, Massachusetts, performed echocardiography in 24 children with symptomatic HIV infection immediately before they started zidovudine therapy and a mean of 1.32 years after therapy began. Sixteen of these children were also studied a mean of 1.26 years before starting zidovudine treatment. Comparison groups included 27 age-matched children with symptomatic HIV infection who had not received zidovudine and 191 normal children. As compared with the normal children, the children treated with zidovudine had progressive LV dilatation and an increase in ventricular-wall stress at end-systole (a measure of ventricular afterload); dilatation and stress were significantly elevated both before and during zidovudine treatment. The ratio of ventricular thickness to internal dimension was below normal before zidovudine treatment began. After treatment with zidovudine, however, overall LV mass was increased, as was peak wall stress (a stimulus to ventricular hypertrophy). Ventricular contractility remained normal, but fractional shortening of the LV was decreased. No statistically significant differences were detected at follow-up in any of these measurements between HIV-infected children treated with zidovudine and those not so treated. Progressive LV dilatation occurred in children with symptomatic HIV infection. Compensatory hypertrophy also occurred but was inadequate to maintain peak systolic wall stress within the normal range. The progressive elevation of ventricular afterload due to dilatation resulted in depressed ventricular performance, but intrinsic ventricular contractility remained normal. Zidovudine did not appear to worsen or ameliorate these cardiac changes.

Castro and associates[34] from Rome, Italy, evaluated the frequency of heart involvement in AIDS patients during various stages of the disease. Between January 1988, to September 1991, they conducted a prospective study in 114 anti-HIV positive patients. The patients, whose mean age ($\pm$ SD) was 35 $\pm$ 5 years (range 20 to 54), were divided into 3 groups: anti-HIV positive asymptomatic (n = 31; 27%), AIDS related complex (ARC) group IV-A (n = 11; 10%), and AIDS subgroups IV-C1 (n = 62; 54%) and IV-D (n = 10.9%). Overall, 84 patients (74%) were i.v. drug abusers, 24 (21%) were homosexuals, and 6 (5%) were partners at risk. Zidovudine was administered to 94 patients (82%). Opportunistic infections and/or secondary malignancies were detected in 72 patients (63%). Electrocardiographic changes were of little clinical relevance (Table 7-1). Of 72 AIDS patients 47 (65.2%) presented a cardiac involvement: 12 subjects (16.6%) were affected by a dilated cardiomyopathy, 13 (18%) by pericardial effusion, 3 (4.1%) by MVP, 4 (5.5%) by myocarditis, 5 (6.9%) by bacterial endocarditis, and 10 (13.8%) by alterations of LV regional contractility. During a mean follow-up period of 44 months, 29 AIDS patients (40.2%) died. Death was attributed to a cardiac event in 4 patients; autopsy could be performed in 24 of the 29 patients who died. The results demonstrate that heart

TABLE 7-1. *Electrocardiographic alterations during HIV infection (n = 114). Reproduced with permission from De Castro, et al.*[34]

	No.	%
Ventricular repolarization abnormalities	20	17·5
LBBB/RBBB	5	4·3
AVB I	2	1·7
VEB/SVEB	27	23·6

LBBB = left bundle branch block; RBBB = right bundle branch block; AVB I = first grade atrioventricular block; VEB = ventricular ectopic beats; SVEB = supraventricular ectopic beats.

involvement is present in 45.6% of HIV-infected patients, but only in the end-stage of the disease (AIDS) and it is presumably due to opportunistic infections and/or secondary malignancies. The direct role of HIV in the genesis of cardiomyopathy remains uncertain and will be evaluated by further studies.

Jacob and associates[35] from Edinburgh, UK, performed echocardiography in 173 patients infected with human immunodeficiency virus (HIV): 119 were current or previous injection drug users, 38 were homosexuals, 10 were hemophiliac patients, and 6 were heterosexual. Of the 173 patients, 26 had abnormalities of ventricular size or function or both. The abnormality was (a) dilated cardiomyopathy in 13 patients; (b) LV dilatation without loss of function in a further 6 patients; and (c) isolated RV dilation in 7 patients. Follow-up echocardiograms were obtained in 71 patients, 18 of whom had myocardial dysfunction (103 echocardiograms, mean (SD) 2.5 (0.6) scans per patient, mean interval 200 (116) days, range 14–538 days). These showed that in 4 cases of isolated RV dilatation, 1 of isolated LV dilatation, and 2 with borderline LV dysfunction myocardial function subsequently reverted to normal. There was no excess of exposure to zidovudine in the patients with myocardial dysfunction. Similarly, patients with myocardial dysfunction had no serological evidence of excess secondary infection with Toxoplasma gondii and cytomegalovirus. There was a high prevalence and wide range of myocardial dysfunction in HIV positive patients. Dilated cardiomyopathy was a feature of advanced HIV disease and affected all major risk groups for HIV infection. In contrast, isolated dilatation of either ventricle occurred at an earlier stage of HIV infection and, particularly in the case of the RV, often was transient. Neither treatment with zidovudine nor infection with Toxoplasma gondii or cytomegalovirus seemed to be responsible for these findings.

Systemic lupus erythematosus

Sasson and associates[36] from Toronto, Canada, evaluated LV diastolic performance with pulsed-wave Doppler echocardiography in a cross-sectional population of 35 patients with systemic lupus erythematosus (SLE) in search of subclinical myocardial involvement. Such involvement is reported to occur infrequently, despite pathohistologic evidence of myocarditis in up to 70% of patients with SLE. Thirty-five consecutive patients with SLE were evaluated, 14 with active and 21 with inactive disease, and were compared with 30 age-matched healthy control subjects. Twenty-six patients were restudied at 7 months. All had normal LV systolic function, normal pericardial and valvular structures, and no significant valvular regurgitation on Doppler echocardiography. In SLE patients with active disease, indexes of LV diastolic function differed significantly from the inactive group and from control subjects, with marked prolongation of isovolumic relaxation time (104 ± 18 vs 74 ± 13 ms), as well as reduced peak early diastolic filling velocity (E) (0.69 ± 0.19 vs 0.83 ± 0.17 ms), reduced ratio of early to late diastolic flow velocity (E/A) (1.15 ± 0.53 vs 1.47 ± 0.35), and prolonged mitral pressure halftime (74 ± 14 vs 65 ± 8 ms). Similar significant differences were found between the active and inactive SLE patient groups. SLE patients with inactive disease differed from control subjects in only mild prolongation of mitral pressure halftime. Abnormal prolongation of isovolumic relaxation (>100 ms) was found to be the most useful marker of diastolic impairment, being present in 64% of SLE patients with active disease and in 14% of patients with inactive disease. LV diastolic function did not change appreciably in the 26 patients restudied at 7 months, although there was a trend for improvement in the 5 active patients who became inactive at follow-up. It is concluded that impaired LV diastolic function is common and persistent in patients with SLE, especially in those with active disease. This most likely represents myocardial involvement in the lupus process.

Cardiovascular manifestations occur in most patients with SLE and recent reports indicate an increasing frequency of cardiovascular morbidity and mortality. Sturfelt and associates[37] from Lund, Sweden, formed a prospective epidemiologically based study within a defined area in southern Sweden of 101 patients, 75 of whom were investigated according to a fixed protocol by echocardiography, Doppler echocardiography, electrocardiography at rest and at exercise, and myocardial scintigraphy. IgG anticardiolipin antibodies (IgG aCL) were determined by ELISA. Twenty of the 75 patients (27%) had valvular disease and 12 of these (60%) had increased concentrations of IgG aCL, compared with 12 of 55 (22%) without valvular disease. Pericardial effusion was detected in 14 patients (19%) during the study period. Mild pulmonary hypertension was found in 11 patients (16%), who also had increased frequency of IgG aCL. Myocardial infarction had occurred in 7 patients, 3 of whom were women <40 years of age. Echocardiography revealed regional hypokinesis or akinesis in 5 of the patients with AMI. Exercise testing revealed low work capacity in 13 of 54 patients (24%), the limiting symptoms being mainly exhaustion or musculoskeletal pain. An abnormal resting ECG was found in 9 of the patients participating in the exercise test. During exercise, abnormal ST-depression was observed in 8 patients, 2 of whom developed angina. Myocardial scintigraphy was performed in 6 of these patients, revealing reversible uptake defects in all. Prolonged glucocorticoid treatment was associated with valvular abnormalities as well as AMI. Valvular abnormalities and IgG aCL appeared to be risk factors for cerebral infarction.

Roldan and associates[38] in Albuquerque, New Mexico, attempted to better characterize valve disease SLE and to determine its association with antiphospholipid antibodies. Transesophageal echocardiography was performed on 54 patients with lupus, 22 of them with (group I) and 32 without (group II) antiphospholipid antibody. Transesophageal echocardiograms were also obtained in 10 patients with antiphospholipid syndrome (group III) and on 35 normal subjects (group IV). Patients in groups I and III had similar types and concentrations of antibodies.

Leaflet thickening was found in 50% of patients in group I, 47% of group II, 10% of group III and 9% of group IV. Leaflet thickening in patients with lupus was diffuse and usually involved the mitral and aortic valves and was associated with valvular regurgitation (73%) or valve masses (50%). Masses were observed in 41% of patients in group I, 25% in group II, 10% in group III, and in none of group IV patients. Most valve masses in patients with lupus were located near the base on the atrial side of the mitral valve or on the vessel side of the aortic valve and they had variable sizes or 0.2 to 0.85 cm², shapes, and echodensity. Valve regurgitation was found in 64% of patients in group I, 59% of group II, 10% of group III, and 20% of group IV patients. Moderate or severe regurgitation was noted in 27% of group I and 25% of group II patients. Thus, lupus valve disease is frequent (74%) regardless of the presence or absence or antiphospholipid antibodies. Therefore, antiphospholipid antibodies may not be a primary pathogenetic factor. The characteristic appearance of leaflet thickening and masses in patients with lupus may help in the recognition of this problem.

Acromegaly

Myocardial hypertrophy and interstitial fibrosis are common in acromegalic hearts and these findings may lead to LV dysfunction. Rossi and associates[39] from Rome, Italy, examined the transmitral flow pattern by pulsed-wave Doppler in 20 patients with active acromegaly and 9 with acromegaly cured by pituitary microsurgery. Control groups consisted of 25 normal subjects and 13 with systemic hypertension. The authors related Doppler indices of LV filling (E and A peak velocities and E/A ratio) to the duration of acromegalic disease, the growth hormone plasma levels and LV mass. The LV mass/body surface area was significantly greater in active acromegaly (187 ± 53 g/m²) and systemic hypertension groups (161 ± 48 g/m²) than in cured acromegaly (125 ± 35 g/m²) and the normal control group (109 ± 36 g/m²). No differences were found in the E peak velocity, A peak velocity, and E/A ratio in the groups with active acromegaly (E/A: 0.9 ± 0.2), cured acromegaly (E/A: 0.9 ± 0.3), and systemic hypertension (E/A: 0.8 ± 0.5). In the active acromegaly group, the E/A ratio was related to either LV mass or the duration of disease. In the cured acromegaly group, the E/A ratio was related to the duration of disease before surgery and not to LV mass. In conclusion, an impairment in LV filling may be present not only in the patients with active acromegaly but also in those successfully treated by surgery after a long duration of the disease, despite normal LV mass.

To examine the possible role of growth hormone as a pathogenetic factor in the development of myocardial hypertrophy in acromegaly, Lim and associates[40] from Ann Arbor, Michigan, and New Orleans, Louisiana, divided 16 patients with acromegaly into 2 groups: Group I (10 patients) had LV hypertrophy and Group II (6 patients) did not have LV hypertrophy. Therapy with octreotide acetate (SMS 201-995), a long-acting somatostatin analog (mean dose, 538 μg/d), was administered for 2 months. Plasma growth hormone and insulin-like growth factor I concentrations, hand volume, and echocardiographic LV dimensions and mass were measured at baseline and at 1 and 8 weeks after the start of therapy. Before octreotide therapy, both groups had similar hand volumes and similar growth hormone and insulin-like growth factor I hypersecretion. Both groups showed a reduction in growth hormone at 2 months (mean reduction, 13.7 μg/L in patients with LV hypertrophy and 14.1 μg/L in patients without LV hypertrophy. Plasma insulin-like growth factor I was also decreased (mean reduction, 305 μg/L in patients with LV hypertrophy and 304 μg/L in patients without LV hypertrophy. Reduction of growth hormone and insulin-like growth factor I hypersecretion in patients with LV hypertrophy was associated with a rapid decrease in LV mass (339 g to 299 g) within 1 week, which was sustained at 2 months (274 g). Patients without LV hypertrophy showed no statistical change in LV mass. In patients with LV hypertrophy, the decrease in LV mass correlated with the octreotide-induced decrease in growth hormone but not with BP. BP, LV dimensions, and percent of fractional shortening were not altered by therapy in either group. Hand volume decreased in both groups. Normalization of growth hormone secretion is associated with reduction of LV mass in acromegalic patients with LV hypertrophy within 1 week of initiating therapy with octreotide.

Myasthenia gravis

Myasthenia gravis is an autoimmune disorder with autoantibodies to acetylcholine receptors of skeletal muscle. Johannessen and associates[41] from Bergen, Norway, studied LV diastolic function with M-mode and Doppler echocardiography in 25 patients with myasthenia and in a group of age- and heart rate-matched control subjects. In the patients, diastolic peak filling rate was reduced by 37%, and Doppler peak early filling velocity (E) was reduced by 12% compared with the control subjects (2.7 ± 0.7 vs 4.2 ± 1.0 s^{-1}, and 76 ± 8 vs 85 ± 15 cm/s, respectively). Peak atrial filling velocity (A) was increased by 38% (68 ± 17 vs 48 ± 9 cm/s), and consequently the E:A ratio in the group of patients was reduced by 33% (1.22 ± 0.40 vs 1.81 ± 0.33). End-diastolic dimension was 5.0 ± 0.5 cm in both groups, heart rate was 70 ± 12 vs 68 ± 16 beats/min, M-mode EF was 76 ± 8 vs 79 ± 5%, M-mode peak ejection rate was −1.9 ± 0.4 vs −2.1 ± 0.3 s^{-1}, and peak aortic outflow velocity was 109 ± 18 vs 98 ± 13 cm/s. Twenty-three patients and 15 control subjects were studied before and after intake of the acetylcholine-esterase inhibitor pyridostigmine. Whereas diastolic measures were unaltered in the control group, peak filling rate in the patients increased by 23% (2.7 ± 0.7 to 3.3 ± 0.9 s^{-1}), E increased by 9% (76 ± 14 to 83 ± 15 cm/s), A decreased by 9% (68 ± 17 to 62 ± 17 cm/s) and the E:A ratio increased by 16% (1.22 ± 0.4 to 1.42 ± 0.4). Heart rate and systolic measures were unaltered in both groups after pyridostigmine. It is concluded that diastolic filling is impaired in some patients with myasthenia gravis and that pyridostigmine tends to normalize the diastolic function in these patients.

Primary antiphospholipid syndrome

To determine the prevalence of cardiac valvular involvement in patients with the primary antiphospholipid syndrome, Galve and associates[42] from Barcelona, Spain, studied 28 consecutive patients with mean follow-up of 21 months with the primary antiphospholipid syndrome during a 10-year period. Ten patients with the primary antiphospholipid syndrome had cardiac valvular involvement including 4 with mitral, 4 with aortic, and 2 with both mitral and aortic valve involvement. Eight of 10 patients had a regurgitant murmur. None of the 28 age- and sex-matched healthy controls had valvular disease. The mean mitral valve thickness determined by Doppler echocardiography in patients with mitral valve involvement was 7.0 ± 1.6 mm compared with 2.7 ± 0.8 mm in patients with normal valves and 3.2 ± 0.9 mm in the control group. The mean aortic valve thickness in patients with aortic valve involvement was 3.8 ± 0.5 mm compared with 1.4 ± 0.3 mm in patients with normal values and 1.4 ± 0.5 mm in the control group. Stenotic lesions were not found. Regurgitation was severe in 2 patients (1 required surgery), moderate in 3 patients, and mild in 3 patients. Valvular involvement is frequently found in patients with the primary antiphospholipid syndrome.

MISCELLANEOUS TOPICS

Complications of endomyocardial biopsy

Deckers and associates[43] in Baltimore, Maryland, determined the incidence, nature and subsequent management of complications occurring during RV endomyocardial biopsy in patients with cardiomyopathy. All events occurred during 546 procedures in 464 consecutive patients. The internal jugular vein was the primary site of introduction of the biopsy catheter in 96% of cases. There were 33 complications (6%). Fifteen (2.7%) occurred during catheter insertion, including 12 arterial punctures, 2 vasovagal reactions and 1 episode of prolonged bleeding, but all of these were without important complications. Eighteen (3.3%) occurred during the biopsy itself, including 6 arrhythmias, 5 conduction abnormalities, 4 possible perforations (0.7%) and 3 definite perforations (0.5%). Two of the three patients with a definite perforation died (0.4%). These complications were not associated with specific clinical or hemodynamic characteristics for the patients. Therefore, it is concluded that the overall rate of endomyocardial biopsy complications is low, but mortality may occur.

Restrictive cardiomyopathy in children

Lewis[44] from Los Angeles, California, reviewed the clinical profile and outcome of idiopathic restrictive cardiomyopathy in 8 children who presented at a mean age of 4 ± 3 years (range 1 to 10 years). All patients had CHF with systemic venous congestion. Right and/or left atrial enlargement were the most common electrocardiographic findings and were present in all patients. LV shortening fraction was normal in 5, increased in 2 and mildly reduced in 1. The most striking echocardiographic finding was severe biatrial dilatation in the presence of normal or near-normal ventricular cavity dimensions. Marked elevation of LV end-diastolic pressure was noted in all 7 patients undergoing catheterization (34 ± 7 mmHg; range 24 to 40 mmHg). RV end-diastolic pressure was elevated (18 ± 7 mmHg) but significantly different from LV pressure. A characteristic early diastolic dip with rapid rise to elevated plateau was present in 5 of 7. Median survival was 1.4 years. Six patients died .2 to 7 years after they were initially seen. The actuarial survival rate 1.5 years after presentation was 44%, decreasing to 29% at 4 years. Restrictive cardiomyopathy has a worse prognosis in children than in adults and consideration for early transplantation may be necessary. It is important to differentiate this diagnosis from constrictive pericarditis which can present without preceding signs of acute pericarditis.

References

1. Manolio TA, Baughman KL, Rodeheffer R, Pearson TA, Bristow JD, Michels VV, Abelmann WH, Harlan WR: Prevalence and etiology of idiopathic dilated cardiomyopathy (Summary of a National Heart, Lung, and Blood Institute workshop). Am J Cardiol 1992 (June 1); 69:1458–1466.

2. Surgrue DD, Rodeheffer RJ, Codd MB, Ballard DJ, Fuster V, Gersh BJ: The clinical course of idiopathic dilated cardiomyopathy: A population-based study. An Intern Med 1992 (July 15); 117:117–123.

3. Michels VV, Moll PP, Miller FA, Tajik AJ, Chu JS, Driscoll DJ, Burnett JC, Rodeheffer RJ, Chesebro JH, Tazelaar HD: The frequency of familial dilated cardiomyopathy in a series of patients with idiopathic dilated cardiomyopathy. N Engl J Med 1992 (Jan 9); 326:44–82.

4. Falk RH, Foster E, Coats MH: Ventricular thrombi and thromboembolism in dilated cardiomyopathy: A prospective follow-up study. Am Heart J 1992 (January); 123:136–142.

5. Dusleag J, Klein W, Eber B, Gasser R, Brussee H, Rotman B, Grisold M: Frequency of magnetic resonance signal abnormalities of the brain in patients aged <50 years with idiopathic dilated cardiomyopathy. Am J Cardiol 1992 (June 1); 69:1446–1450.

6. Denereaz D, Zimmermann M, Adamec R: Significance of ventricular late potentials in non-ischemic dilated cardiomyopathy. Euro Heart J 1992 (July);13:895–901.

7. Abramson SV, Burke JF, Kelly JJ Jr, Kitchen JG III, Dougherty MJ, Yih DF, McGeehin FC III, Shuck JW, Phiambolis TP: Pulmonary hypertension predicts mortality and morbidity in patients with dilated cardiomyopathy. An Intern Med 1992 (June 1); 116:888–895.

8. De Maria R, Gavazzi A, Caroli A, Ometto R, Biagini A, Camerini F: Ventricular arrhythmias in dilated cardiomyopathy as an independent prognostic hallmark. Am J Cardiol 1992 (June 1); 69:1451–1457.

9. Hochleitner M, Hortnagl H, Hortnagl H, Fridrich L, Gschnitzer F: Long-term efficacy of physiologic dual-chamber pacing in the treatment of end-stage idiopathic dilated cardiomyopathy. Am J Cardiol 1992 (Nov 15); 70:1320–1325.

10. Brecker SJD, Xiao HB, Sparrow J, Gibson DG: Effects of dual-chamber pacing with short atrioventricular delay in dilated cardiomyopathy. Lancet 1992 (Nov 28); 340:1308–1312.

11. Epstein ND, Fananapazir L, Lin HJ, Mulvihill, White R, Lalouel J-M, Lifton RP, Nienhuris AW, Leppert M: Evidence of Genetic Heterogeneity With Five Kindreds With Familial Hypertrophic Cardiomyopathy. Circulation 1992 (February); 85:635–647.

12. Watkins H, Rosenzweig A, Hwang DS, Levi T, McKenna W, Seidman CE, Seidman JG: Characteristics and prognostic implications of myosin missense mutations in familial hypertropic cardiomyopathy. N Engl J Med 1992 (Apr 23); 326:1108–1114.

13. Hecht GM, Panza JA, Maron BJ: Clinical course of middle-aged asymptomatic patients with hypertropic cardiomyopathy. Am J Cardiol 1992 (Apr 1); 69:935–940.

14. Chikamori T, Counihan PJ, Doi YL, Takata J, Stewart JT, Frenneaux MP, McKenna WJ: Mechanisms of exercise limitation in hypertrophic cardiomyopathy. J Am Coll Cardiol 1992 (March); 19:507–12.

15. Fananapazir L, Chang A, Epstein S, McAreavey D: Prognostic Determinants in Hypertrophic Cardiomyopathy, Prospective Evaluation of a Therapeutic Strategy Based on Clinical, Holter, Hemodynamic, and Electrophysiological Findings. Circulation 1992 (September); 86:730–740.

16. Spirito P, Lakatos E, Maron BJ: Degree of left ventricular hypertrophy in patients with hypertrophic cardiomyopathy and chronic atrial fibrillation. Am J Cardiol 1992 (May 1); 69:1217–1222.

17. Dritsas A, Gilligan D, Sbarouni E, Oakley CM, Nihoyannopoulos: Influence of left ventricular hypertrophy and function on the occurrence of ventricular tachycardia in hypertrophic cardiomyopathy. Am J Cardiol 1992 (Oct 1); 70:913–916.

18. Panza JA, Maris TJ, Maron BJ: Development and determinants of dynamic obstruction to left ventricular outflow in young patients with hypertrophic cardiomyopathy. Circulation (April) 1992;85:1398–1405.

19. Koga Y, Kihara K, Yamaguchi R, Wada T, Toshima H: Therapeutic effect of oral dipyridam-

ole on myocardial perfusion and cardiac performance in patients with hypertrophic cardiomyopathy. Am Heart J 1992 (February); 123:433–438.

20. Pretrone RK, Klues HG, Panza JA, Peterson EE, Maron BJ: Coexistence of mitral valve prolapse in a consecutive group of 528 patients with hypertrophic cardiomyopathy assessed with electrocardiography. J Am Coll Cardiol 1992 (July); 20:55–61.

21. Roberts WC, Kishel JC, McIntosh CL, Cannon RO, Maron BJ: Severe mitral or aortic valve regurgitation, or both, requiring valve replacement for infective endocarditis complicating hypertrophic cardiomyopathy. J Am Coll Cardiol 1992 (February); 19:365–71.

22. Lazzeroni E, Rolli A, Aurier E, Botti G: Clinical significance of coronary artery disease in hypertrophic cardiomyopathy. Am J Cardiol 1992 (Aug. 15); 70:499–501.

23. Klues H, Maron B, Dollar A, Roberts W: Diversity of Structural Mitral Valve Alterations in Hypertrophic Cardiomyopathy. Circulation 1992 (May); 85:1651–1660.

24. Maron BJ, Wolfson JK, Roberts WC: Relation between extent of cardiac muscle cell disorganization and left ventricular wall thickness in hypertrophic cardiomyopathy. Am J Cardiol 1992 (Sept 15); 70:785–790.

25. Jeanrenaud X, Goy JJ, Kappenberger L: Effects of dual-chamber pacing in hypertrophic obstructive cardiomyopathy. Lancet 1992 (May 30); 339:1318–1323.

26. Fananapazir L, Cannon R, Tripodi D, Panza J: Impact of Dual-Chamber Permanent Pacing in Patients With Obstructive Hypertrophic Cardiomyopathy With Symptoms Refractory to Verapamil and Beta-Adrenergic Blocker Therapy. Circulation 1992 (June); 85:2149–2161.

27. McAreavey D, Fananapazir L: Altered cardiac hemodynamic and electrical state in normal sinus rhythm after chronic dual-chamber pacing for relief of left ventricular outflow obstruction in hypertrophic cardiomyopathy. Am J Cardiol 1992 (Sept 1); 70:651–656.

28. Diodati JG, Schenke WH, Waclawiw MA, McIntosh CL, Cannon RO III: Predictors of exercise benefit after operative relief of left ventricular outflow obstruction by the myotomy-myectomy procedure in hypertrophic cardiomyopathy. Am J Cardiol 1992 (June 15); 69:1617–1622.

29. Cohn LH, Trehan H, Collins JJ Jr: Long-term follow-up of patients undergoing myotomy/myectomy for obstructive hypertrophic cardiomyopathy. Am J Cardiol 1992 (Sept 1); 70:657–660.

30. Grigg LE, Wigle ED, Williams WG, Daniel LB, Rakowski H: Transesophageal Doppler echocardiography in obstructive hypertrophic cardiomyopathy: Clarification of pathophysiology and importance of intraoperative decision making. J Am Coll Cardiol 1992 (July); 20:42–52.

31. Marwick TH, Stewart WJ, Lever HM, Lytle BW, Rosenkranz ER, Duffy CI, Salcedo EE: Benefits of intraoperative echocardiography in the surgical management of hypertrophic cardiomyopathy. J Am Coll Cardiol 1992 (November); 20:1066–72.

32. Dec GW Jr., Waldman H, Southern J, Fallon JT, Hutter AM Jr., Palacios I: Viral myocarditis mimicking acute myocardial infarction. J Am Coll Cardiol 1992 (July); 20:85–9.

33. Lipshultz SE, Orav EJ, Sanders SP, Hale AR, McIntosh K, Colan SD: Cardiac structure and function in children with human immunodeficiency virus infection treated with zidovudine. N Engl J Med 1992 (Oct 29); 327:1260–1265.

34. Castro SD, Migliau G, Silvestri A, D'Amati G, Giannantoni P, Cartoni D, Kol A, Vullos V, Cirelli A: Heart involvement in AIDS: A prospective study during various stages of the disease. Eur Heart J 1992 (Nov); 13:1452–1459.

35. Jacob AJ, Sutherland GR, Bird AG, Brettle RP, Ludlam CA, McMillan A, Boon NA: Myocardial dysfunction in patients infected with HIV: Prevalence and risk factors. Br Heart J 1992 (Dec); 68:549–553.

36. Sasson Z, Rasooly Y, Chow CW, Marshall S, Urowitz MB: Impairment of left ventricular diastolic function in systemic lupus erythematosus. Am J Cardiol 1992 (June 15); 69:1629–1634.

37. Sturfelt G, Eskilsson J, Nived O, Truedsson L, Valind S: Cardiovascular disease in systemic lupus erythematosus: A study of 75 patients from a defined population. Medicine 1992; 71:216–223.

38. Roldan CA, Shively BK, Lau CC, Gurule FT, Smith EA, Crawford MH: Systemic lupus erythematosus valve disease by transesophageal echocardiography and the role of antiphospholipid antibodies. J Am Coll Cardiol 1992 (November); 20:1127–34.

39. Rossi E, Zuppi P, Pennestri F, Biasucci LM, Lombardo A, De Marinis L, Loperfido F: Acromegalic cardiomyopathy: Left ventricular filling and hypertrophy in active and surgically treated disease. Chest 1992 (Oct); 102:1204–1208.

40. Lim MJ, Barkan AL, Buda AJ: Rapid reduction of left ventricular hypertrophy in acromegaly after suppression of growth hormone hypersecretion. An Intern Med 1992 (Nov 1); 117:719–726.

41. Johannessen KA, Mygland A, Gilhus NE, Aarli J, Vik-Mo H: Left ventricular function in myasthenia gravis. Am J Cardiol 1992 (Jan 1); 69:129–132.

42. Galve E, Ordi J, Barquinero J, Evangelista A, Vilardell M, Soler-Soler J: Valvular heart disease in the primary antiphospholipid syndrome. An Intern Med 1992 (Feb 15); 116:293–298.

43. Deckers JW, Hare JM, Baughman KL: Complications of transvenous right ventricular endomyocardial biopsy in adult patients with cardiomyopathy: a seven-year survey of 546 consecutive diagnostic procedures in a tertiary referral center. J Am Coll Cardiol 1992 (January); 19:43–7.

44. Lewis AB: Clinical profile and outcome of restrictive cardiomyopathy in children. Am Heart J (June) 1992; 1213:1589–1593.

Congenital Heart Disease

ATRIAL SEPTAL DEFECT

Mühler and associates[1] from Aachen, Germany, studied 10 patients with a mean age of 3.6 years with a sinus venosus ASD using two-dimensional echocardiography. The defects were easily visualized using a long axis vena cava superior-inferior plane with a subcostal approach, while the atrial septum seemed to be intact in the coronal plane conventionally used for ASDs of the primum or secundum type. Additional color flow mapping in 2 patients demonstrated shunting across the ASD. These authors show excellent anatomical detail of the sinus venosus ASD which has eluded detection in a number of past investigations using conventional echocardiographic imaging. These views, which have been described previously and are somewhat more difficult to obtain in older patients and adults than in children, are very useful for this defect.

ATRIOVENTRICULAR SEPTAL DEFECT

Echocardiographic observations

Minich and associates[2] from Ann Arbor, Michigan, used an en face view of the AV valve in 69 children undergoing repair of atrioventricular septal defect to evaluate leaflet anatomy and size. Adequate images were obtained in 63 of 69 who ranged from 1 day to 14 years and weighed from 1 to 55 kg. Echocardiographic results were compared with surgical observations in 62 patients and with autopsy findings in 1. With the echocardiographic technique 32 of 33 patients with a common orifice and 28 of 30 patients with 2 separate valve orifices were correctly identified. The methodology clearly differentiates patients with common orifices from patients with 2 separate orifices. This technique can be extremely useful in identifying orifice size in patients with unbalanced atrioventricular septal defects and can be useful in determining operability in patients with questionable hypoplastic left ventricles. This information can be useful in planning the surgical approach.

Operative repair

Capouya and associates[3] from Los Angeles, California, reported results from operative repair of complete AV canal in 105 patients between January, 1982 and December, 1990. Repair was performed with a single pericardial patch in 82% and intraoperative assessment of left AV valve competence was performed in all cases. Suturing of the cleft was required in 91% and 60% required annuloplasty to establish satisfactory competence. The early overall mortality rate was 11 of 105 or 10.5%. From 1986 to 1990, the early mortality rate decreased to 7.7%. In a mean follow-up of 39 months late survival was 96% for the 94 early survivors. Reoperation was performed in 11 patients, 6 for failure of AV valve repair, 3 for patch dehiscence and 2 for residual VSDs. These data demonstrate that routine approximation of the cleft and aggressive use of left AV valve annuloplasty is safe and results in an excellent outcome with a low prevalence of reoperation.

VENTRICULAR SEPTAL DEFECT

With aortic regurgitation

Trusler and associates[4] from Toronto, Canada, reported late results of 70 patients aged 2 to 36 years (mean 10) who had repair of VSD and AR from 1968 to 1988. The VSD was perimembranous in 50 and subpulmonary in 20. The VSDs were situated immediately below the right coronary leaflet with prolapse of that leaflet in 2/3 with most of the remainder below the right commissure or the anterior part of the noncoronary leaflet. Associated structural defects included some fusion of the commissure present in 18 of 70 and occurred more often with a VSD in or below the commissure between the right and noncoronary leaflets. Follow-up ranged from 2 to 20 years (mean 10). There were no early deaths or cases of atrioventricular block but there were 2 late deaths. Patient survival was 96% at 10 years and freedom from valvuloplasty failure and freedom from reoperation were 76 and 85% respectively at 10 years. The major predictor for failure was the presence of an associated structural defect. Age at repair and the position of the VSD were not significant risk factors. Aortic valvuloplasty produces good palliation in most children and should be undertaken early after appearance of this complication to prevent excessive deformity, stretching, or degenerative changes in the valve leaflet.

Bonhoeffer and associates[5] from Bergamo and Milan, Italy, and Monaco, presented a new surgical approach for AR associated with prolapse of an aortic cusp and infundibular VSD. Operation was performed in 5 children 3 to 16 years of age with the VSD closed by a patch anchored to another patch through the prolapsed cusp. The second patch was pulled up with the prolapsed cusp and then fixed in the aortic wall

(Figure 8-1). In all 5 patients, clinical signs of AR disappeared and only minimal AR could be detected by color flow Doppler mapping. In addition, there was significant decrease in LV diameter following operation. This new surgical approach may prove useful in this difficult patient group in whom avoidance of valve replacement is highly desirable.

Multiple defects

Seraff and associates[6] from Paris, France, reported surgical closure of isolated multiple VSDs in 130 children at a mean age of 14 ± 18 months, and a mean weight of 7 ± 4 kg. Sixty-one were <1 year of age. In addition, 61 had either pulmonary stenosis or PA banding. All others had severe pulmonary hypertension with a mean systolic pressure of 76 ± 21 mmHg and disabling CHF. The surgical management was based on the location of the defects and the ventricular dominance that was assessed pre- and intraoperatively. Midtrabecular VSDs were always centered by the moderator band and therefore divided into low trabecular, midtrabecular, and high trabecular defects. The perimembranous septum was involved in 102 patients, the trabecular in 121, the inlet septum in 12, and the infundibular septum in 9. The "Swiss cheese" form of the lesion was present in 50 patients. Closure of the VSDs included dacron patch and mattress sutures. The defects were first approached through a right atriotomy which was sufficient for complete repair in 82 patients. In midtrabecular VSDs section of the moderator band in 24 allowed closure of all defects with a single dacron patch. Right ventriculotomies in 32, left ventriculotomies in 4, or both right and left ventriculotomies in 2 were necessary to secure repair in 48 patients. The hospital mortality was 8%. The causes of death were residual VSD in 5, pulmonary hypertension in 2, hypoplastic right ventricle in 1, hypoplastic left ventricle in 1 and myocardial infarction in 1. Among 18 survivors with residual VSD, 6 were reoperated on, with 2 deaths. A permanent pacemaker was necessary in 4 patients. Low trabecular VSDs and left ventriculotomy were significant

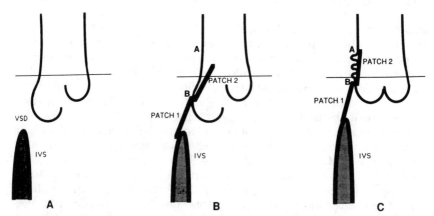

Fig. 8-1. The surgical technique. (A) Anatomy of the syndrome: prolapse of the aortic cusp, which occludes the ventricular septal defect (VSD) almost entirely. The horizontal line shows the level chosen to reconstruct the aortic annulus. (B) The first patch is positioned to close the VSD, and the inferior border of the second patch is anchored. (C) The cusp is lifted up, and the second patch is fixed in the aortic wall. Note the reduction in the distance between points A and B. (IVS = interventricular septum.) Reproduced with permission from Bonhoeffer, et al.[5]

risk factors for morbidity, including death and residual VSD. At 7 years of follow-up, 90% of survivors were in New York Heart Association class I. Actuarial survival and freedom from reoperation at 7 years was 90% and 88% respectively. These authors show good results from this difficult group of patients. The avoidance of left ventriculotomy is important, if possible. Use of an umbrella device at the time of surgery and the use of Dacron felt, soaked with biological glue, may also be helpful in some patients to close apical defects.

Trabecular defect

Hiraishi and associates[7] from Kanagawa, Japan, used 2-dimensional echocardiography and color Doppler imaging to determine the prevalence and course of trabecular VSDs. A total of 1,028 term newborns were examined with birthweights ranging from 2.4 to 4.4 kg. A trabecular VSD was found in 21 patients (2%) with 10 girls and 11 boys affected. A separate group of 21 neonates with isolated VSD from another population were also followed. The morphologic features of the defect were classified as 1 of 2 defects in 36 cases and as a mesh-like defect in 6 case. Reduction in size began from the RV side or from within the trabecular septum. Spontaneous closure occurred most commonly during the first 6 months of life and was observed in 32 cases (76%) by 12 months of age. The frequency of closure was not related to morphologic features and initial size of the defect but apical defects tended to have higher persistent patency than did defects in other locations. The authors concluded that the frequency of trabecular VSD in neonates is higher than previous estimates but that the frequency of spontaneous closure of these defects is also quite high.

SINGLE VENTRICLE

Bulboventricular size

Matitiau and associates[8] from Boston, Massachusetts, studied bulboventricular foramen size in 28 neonates and infants ≥5 months old who presented with single left ventricle and were followed for 2 to 5 years. All patients had their entire systemic outflow through the foramen. The foramen was measured in 2 planes by echocardiography and its area calculated and indexed to body surface area. One patient died before surgical treatment. The mean initial foramen area index was .94 cm^2/m^2 in 12 patients in whom the foramen was bypassed as the first procedure in early infancy. The remaining 15 patients underwent other palliative operations but the foramen continued to serve as the systemic outflow tract. There was 1 surgical death. Foramen obstruction occurred during followup in 6 of 14 survivors whose mean initial foramen area index was 1.75 cm^2/m^2. The remaining 8 patients did not develop obstruction at followup and had an initial foramen larger than the other 2 groups with an average area index of 3.95 cm^2/m^2. All patients with an initial area index <2 cm^2/m^2 who did not undergo early foramen bypass developed late obstruction. An excellent correlation was found between antemortem echocardiographic measurements of foramen size and autopsy size measurement. Aortic arch obstruction occurred in 16 patients who had mean initial foramen index significantly smaller than 12 patients who did not have obstruction. In addition, 8 patients without obstruction underwent PA banding and 4 patients developed foramen obstruction and 4 did not. The mean foramen index was significantly smaller in the group that developed obstruction. These authors show very interesting data in patients with bulboventricular foramen obstruction. It is clear that these measurements can be useful in planning operative strategy that should include early relief of obstruction to prevent massive hypertrophy which can render a patient high risk for subsequent Fontan procedure.

With subaortic obstruction

O'Leary and associates[9] from Rochester, Minnesota, reported results of a staged approach to Fontan operation for patients with double inlet left ventricle, anterior subaortic outlet chamber and subaortic obstruction. Thirty-two patients were divided by subaortic gradient into 3 groups: mild gradients (10 to 25 mmHg), intermediate gradient (26 to 40 mmHg) and more severe gradients (>40 mmHg). Patients with mild gradients who had a single staged operation had the best outcome with a mortality of only 6%. Staging improved the outcome from a previous report in 1984 from 67% to 17% for patients with more severe obstruction. Factors contributing to improved results included improved surgical techniques, better perioperative care, the appropriate application of staged repair. These authors recommend simultaneous relief of obstruction and modified Fontan operation for patients with subaortic gradients <25 mmHg. Those with gradients >40 mmHg should have repair in 2 stages and it is unclear whether the 1 stage or 2 stage approach is better for patients with an intermediate gradient. The problem of subaortic obstruction in patients with single ventricle anatomy continues to be an important one. Early relief of obstruction is extremely important and complete relief of obstruction at the time of Fontan operation is mandatory to achieving good early and late results.

Arterial switch operation

Lacour-Gayet and associates[10] from Paris, France, performed the arterial switch operation in 7 infants with univentricular hearts, ventriculoarterial discordance, and subaortic stenosis. The principle of the operation is to switch the subaortic obstruction into a subpulmonary obstruction and create a natural protection of the pulmonary vascular bed through a restrictive bulboventricular foramen. All 7 infants had associated aortic obstruction of various degrees including 1 with an interrupted aortic arch, 5 with coarctation with arch hypoplasia and 1 with isolated arch hypoplasia. There were 3 patients with double-inlet left ventricle, 3 with tricuspid atresia, and 1 with TGA, VSD and RV hypoplasia. The operation included arch repair with prosthetic material, atrial septectomy, and the arterial switch. An associated pulmonary shunt was required in 5 patients and PA banding in 1. There was 1 early and 1 late death. This palliative operation has several advantages: reconstruction of a harmonious aortic root, natural protection of the pulmonary bed, prevention of deleterious myocardial hypertrophy, and aortic arch reconstruction without the introduction of foreign material. This aggressive technique may provide satisfactory palliation when the bulbo ventricular foramen/aortic annulus ratio is <.8 or when the subaortic stenosis is severe enough to be associated with arch obstruction. This technique offers an alternative to PA banding and aortico-pulmonary connections for this condition.

PULMONIC VALVE STENOSIS

Balloon valvuloplasty

O'Connor and associates[11] from Ann Arbor, Michigan, compared results of 20 balloon valvuloplasty treated children and their age- and gradient-matched surgical control patients using prospective, noninvasive evaluation. The average age at intervention was 4.3 years for the valvuloplasty group versus 4.7 years for the surgical group. Before intervention the peak PS gradient was 76 ± 5 and 74 ± 4 for the valvuloplasty and surgery groups respectively. Late evaluation included exam, echocardiography, Holter monitoring, treadmill study, and chest radiography performed an average of 5.3 years after valvuloplasty and 11.7 years after surgery. There was no evidence of restenosis in the valvuloplasty group with residual gradient at follow-up 24 ± 3 mmHg versus 35 ± 4 mmHg immediately after valvuloplasty. Comparison of the late residual gradients between treatment groups showed no hemodynamically significant difference (24 ± 3 vs 16 ± 2 mmHg) for balloon versus surgery patients. There was a significant difference in the degree of severity of pulmonary insufficiency and ventricular ectopic activity between groups. In the valvuloplasty group 11 patients had no insufficiency and the remaining had mild insufficiency. In the surgery group 9 had mild and 9 had moderate insufficiency. Ventricular ectopic activity was absent in 19 of the valvuloplasty group with the remaining patient having Lown grade 1 activity. In contrast, 6 children in the surgery group had complex ventricular arrhythmia. These authors show similar results, in terms of relief of stenosis with balloon valvuloplasty versus surgical valvotomy. Patients with a dysplastic pulmonary valve, pulmonary annulus hypoplasia and complex RV outflow obstruction were excluded from this study. There was a slightly higher residual gradient in the balloon treated group but this is a small difference. There was a suggestion of deleterious effects of pulmonary insufficiency in terms of ventricular arrhythmia. Most patients followed for many years after surgical valvotomy have not shown progressive deterioration unless they have developed pulmonary hypertension.

TETRALOGY OF FALLOT

Operative outcomes

Marie and associates[12] from Nancy, France, studied 35 patients who had repair of TF. Sustained VT was obtained with ventricular stimulation in 10 (group 1) while 25 (group 2) had no sustained VT. Group 1 patients were significantly older at the time of surgery (7 ± 3 vs 4 ± 4 years) and had longer follow-up periods (12 ± 4 vs 5 ± 2 years). RV systolic pressure, end-systolic and end-diastolic normalized RV volumes were higher in group 1 while RV end-diastolic pressure, LV and RV EFs were similar in the 2 groups. Stepwise discriminant analysis was used to predict patients with inducible sustained VT; time period from surgery to follow-up, normalized RV end-systolic volume, and RV systolic pressure were higher in group 1 and allowed classification of 90% of patients in group 1 and 96% in group 2. These authors suggest that increased RV systolic wall stress may be a determinant of inducible VT in postoperative TF patients. Data are still unclear as to which postoperative TF patients require pharmacological treatment. It appears that those with frequent complex ventricular ectopy on ambulatory electrocardiographic monitoring, as well as those who have inducible sustained VT need careful consideration for pharmacological treatment.

Kirklin and associates[13] from Birmingham, Alabama, and Boston, Massachusetts, reviewed survival after entry and survival after repair in 196 consecutive patients with TF presenting at 2 institutions. Survival after repair was 94%, 91%, and 91% at 1 month, 1 year, and 5 years, respectively. Size and configuration of right and left PAs had no demonstrable effect on survival, prevalence of transannular patching, or postrepair RV-LV pressure ration. Small size of the pulmonary annulus and trunk were risk factors for death, transannular patching, and high postrepair pressure. High postrepair pressure ratio was a risk factor for death, as was very young age (<approximately 3 months), particularly when other risk factors co-existed, such as Down's syndrome, atrioventricular canal, multiple VSDs, or large aorticopulmonary collateral arteries. These authors show excellent results from early repair of TF with 2 slightly different protocols at 2 institutions. It does appear that infants <3 months can be repaired with an acceptable mortality if they do not have other risk factors, such as Down's syndrome, markedly small pulmonary annulus or multiple VSDs.

Waien and associates[14] from Toronto, Canada, followed a group of 151 adult patients with repaired TF for a mean of 3.2 years. Four patients died during follow-up but only 2 deaths can be attributed to TF repair. There were no sudden deaths. Clinically 94% of patients are symptom free. A subset of 36 patients were followed up for a mean of 6.7 years with serial testing at 3 year intervals consisting of right heart catheterization at initial study only, 24 hour ambulatory electrocardiographic monitoring, exercise electrocardiogram and rest and exercise radionuclide angiography. Exercise capacity assessed by serial testing remained stable whereas exercise-induced arrhythmias steadily decreased. Radionuclide angiography showed significant improvement in exercise RVEF over time with no change in resting RVEF and a decrease in both resting and exercise LVEF at the first 3 year follow-up which did not progress at 6 years. These authors show an excellent outcome for these patients who were operated on at an average age of 14 years and studied an average of 14 years after operation. It is of interest that despite resting RVEFs at the lower limit of normal and exercise RVEFs that were in general abnormal, these patients showed no progressive decrease in clinical or laboratory measurements of RV dysfunction.

PULMONIC VALVE ATRESIA

With right ventricular-coronary fistula

Giglia and associates[15] from Boston, Massachusetts, studied 82 patients with pulmonary atresia and intact ventricular septum and found 26 (32%)

who had right ventricle-to-coronary artery fistulas. Of these 26, 23 had adequate preoperative coronary angiograms for analysis. RV decompression was achieved in 16, 7 of 16 had fistulas and each survived decompression. Stenoses of a single coronary artery was present in 6 of 16 and 4 of 6 survived RV decompression. Stenoses and/or occlusion of both right coronary artery and left anterior descending was present in 3 of 16 and all 3 died shortly after RV decompression. These authors conclude that potential right ventricle steal does not preclude successful RV decompression. Fistulas with stenoses to a single coronary artery may not preclude successful RV decompression but RV decompression appears to be contraindicated in the presence of stenoses and/or occlusion involving both the right and left coronary systems. Nonsurvival after RV decompression seems to depend on the amount of LV myocardium at risk which is distal to coronary stenoses, especially when involvement of both arteries limit effective collateralization. This anomaly continues to be difficult to deal with in those patients with a small right ventricle and multiple coronary arterial abnormalities. Of particular interest in this study was the ability to decompress the right ventricle in the absence of stenoses with apparently no untoward effects on RV or LV function.

Balloon valvuloplasty

Leung and associates[16] from Aberdeen, Hong Kong, performed balloon valvuloplasty in 12 infants following initial transventricular closed pulmonary valvotomy for pulmonary atresia with an intact ventricular septum. All infants underwent early closed valvotomy when echocardiography revealed a tripartite right ventricle without sinusoidal-coronary arterial fistulae. After valvotomy the overall mortality rate was 25% (3 of 12). The only surgical death was due to failure to establish continuity between the RV cavity and the pulmonary trunk. The other infants died of neonatal complications after successful valvotomy. Angiography performed 5 to 18 months after valvotomy documented substantial growth of the RV inflow and outflow dimensions in the 9 survivors. Balloon dilatation procedures were performed in 7 infants on 12 occasions. All but 1 achieved a significant drop in the RV to LV peak systolic pressure ratio from .96 ± .4 to .56 ± .28. Valvuloplasty was not required in 1 infant and failed in the other who then underwent successful surgical RV outflow tract reconstruction. After these staged procedures, follow-up at 1 to 20 months (mean 14.8 months) revealed resting cyanosis in 3 infants related to severe infundibular stenosis in 1 and a subnormal tricuspid annulus in 2. The remaining 5 infants were active and pink with O_2 saturations >97% and a mean Doppler estimated gradient of 19 mmHg (range 8 to 36 mmHg) across the pulmonary valve. These authors indicate good results from an initial closed valvotomy followed by balloon valvuloplasty in patients with pulmonary atresia and intact septum who have adequate sized right ventricles without RV dependent coronary circulation.

Right ventricular outflow patch

Steinberger and associates[17] from Minneapolis, Minnesota, reported 19 newborns who underwent neonatal RV outflow tract patch for pulmonary atresia and intact ventricular septum. An aortopulmonary shunt proceeded the operation in 4 infants and coronary sinusoids were ligated in 3 newborns. Based on RV morphology the newborns were divided into 2 groups. Group 1 included 9 patients with a tripartite right ventricle and group 2 10 patients with bipartite or monopartite right ventricle. Before surgery group 1 had significantly larger RV volumes. Five-year survival was 79% for the entire group. There were 4 deaths all in group 2 who died within 12 months of their initial surgery. Fourteen of 15 survivors are acyanotic and without symptoms. A biventricular repair was achieved in 12 of 15 and the other 3 patients are awaiting evaluation. All survivors had significant RV and tricuspid annulus growth. These authors show excellent results for this very difficult group of patients. It appears that they operated on a group with somewhat larger and more favorable RV anatomy and less coronary sinusoids than the usual group of patients with this entity. Nevertheless, their results are impressive.

Biventricular "repair"

Laks and associates[18] from Los Angeles, California, performed repair of pulmonary atresia with intact ventricular septum in 19 patients ages 5 to 66 months with a mean age of 24 months. An adjustable ASD was used in 12 of 19 patients undergoing biventricular repair. The ASD snare was closed in the operating room after coming off bypass in 2 patients and in the other 10 patients closure could not be tolerated at the time of surgery as evidenced by elevation of right atrial pressure by >15 mmHg and decreased blood pressure. The ASD was closed in 7 patients by the snare device and 1 additional patient had the ASD narrowed in the early postoperative period. One patient underwent delayed closure 16 months after surgery at the time of cardiac catheterization. A snare-controlled adjustable ASD can be a helpful adjunct to partial biventricular repair of pulmonary atresia with intact ventricular septum by reducing the risk of low cardiac output and severe venous hypertension in the early postoperative period.

Bidirectional cavopulmonary anastomosis

Albanese and associates[19] from Rome, Italy, performed bidirectional cavopulmonary anastomosis in 27 patients younger than 2 years of age, including 12 patients with heterotaxia syndrome. Age and weight of patients averaged 14 months and 8 kg, respectively. Pulmonary atresia was found in 11 and 16 had pulmonary stenosis. The main pulmonary artery was ligated in 7 patients in the latter group, subsequently reopened in 1 and left open in 9 and subsequently ligated in 2. There were 4 hospital deaths (15%). All patients were discharged with anticoagulant/antithrombotic therapy for 6 months. There were 2 late deaths before further operations (8.7%). Two patients, 1 with acquired massive pulmonary arteriovenous fistulas and 1 with progressive common AV valve regurgitation subsequently underwent definitive repair and both died. Actuarial survival at 48 months was 72%. These authors present a fairly typical experience for the use of this procedure in patients with complex conditions. Heterotaxia syndrome, significant AV valve regurgitation, and preoperative mean pulmonary artery pressure >15 mmHg continue to be risk factors for overall morbidity and mortality.

Right ventricular size and function after repair

Schmidt and associates[20] from San Francisco, California, measured RV end-diastolic and stroke volumes from orthogonal subcostal echocardiographic images in 24 infants with pulmonary atresia (18) or critical pulmonary stenosis (6) and intact ventricular septum before and at an average of 5 days and then 19 days after pulmonary valvotomy. The preoperative echocardiographic volumes were compared with angiographic determinations. End-diastolic and stroke volumes calculated by the echocardiographic method correlated closely with those calculated by the angiographic method. All but 1 infant had RV hypoplasia before valvotomy with an end-diastolic volume of 17 ± 6 ml/m² (45 ± 17% of normal). RV to LV area ratio was 0.56 ± 0.09 (normal 0.95). RV end-diastolic volume decreased to 11 ± 5 ml/m² and stroke volume decreased from 8 ± 4 to 6 ± 3 ml/m² 5 days after valvotomy. At 19 days after valvotomy, RV end-diastolic volume and RV to LV area ratios had increased to their respective preoperative values and RV stroke volumes had increased to 10 ± 4 ml/m². These findings indicate that RV volume can be calculated by 2-dimensional echocardiography and these findings can be used serially in patients with pulmonary atresia and intact septum. RV volumes and stroke volumes decreased early after decompression of the outflow obstruction. Therefore, an additional temporary source of auxiliary pulmonary blood flow may be necessary. Echocardiographic studies may be useful as an aid in determining when the PGE infusion, used to maintain ductal patency, may be discontinued.

TRANSPOSITION OF THE GREAT ARTERIES

Mustard procedure

de Begona and associates[21] from Loma Linda, California, reported 34 infants <1 month of age who underwent a Mustard intraatrial procedure for repair of simple TGA. Weights ranged from 2.6 to 4.4 kg and 30 patients were <2 weeks of age. Mechanical ventilation was required in 8 patients preoperatively and PGE₁ in 117 patients. Deep hypothermic circulatory arrest averaging 53 minutes was used in all patients. The duration of postoperative intubation and ventilatory support average 1.7 ± 1 day with a range of 1 to 5 days. There were no hospital deaths and follow-up has extended from 1 month to 14 years with a mean of 3 years. One infant died 2 months postoperatively of aspiration and a second infant died at 1 year with RV and tricuspid valve dysfunction. Baffle complications occurred in 6 of 32 including superior caval stenosis in 4, inferior caval stenosis in 1 and pulmonary venous obstruction in 3. Reoperation for baffle obstruction was performed in 3 patients and balloon angioplasties in 2. One patient required permanent pacemaker implantation. Three patients had trivial and 2 moderate LV outflow tract obstruction after the procedure with 1 patient developing progressive obstruction. These authors show excellent results for the atrial repair of TGA at an early age which is similar but slightly older than the age most people perform arterial repair now. Follow-up of these patients in terms of late problems will be important to contrast with the follow-up of arterial switch patients.

Right ventricular failure after mustard or senning operation

Chang and associates[22] from Boston, Massachusetts, reported surgical management and outcome for 10 patients ages 3.6 to 23.5 years who developed symptomatic RV failure after prior arterial switch operation. Anatomic correction with either an arterial switch operation in 3 patients or PA to aorta anastomosis and right ventricle to PA conduit in 2 patients was performed. Before anatomic correction, 4 of 5 patients had a PA band to prepare the left ventricle. The interval between preparation and correction ranged from 8 days to 12 months with a median of 2 months. One patient died after an arterial switch operation and in the remaining 5 patients, co existing LV dysfunction precluded anatomic correction; all 5 survived cardiac transplantation. Survival for the entire group of 10 patients is 90% and a median postoperative hospital stay was 17 days. During follow-up 12 to 62 months (median of 27 months) there were no deaths. AF after anatomic correction was common and was moderate to severe in 3 patients, 1 of whom required AVR 4 months after surgery. The choice of operative intervention for patients who develop severe progressive CHF following atrial repair of TGA remains a difficult one. The two-stage arterial switch operation is feasible in some patients but a number have LV dysfunction and would preclude this option. The overall prevalence of this complication later after atrial repair is unclear but may be as high as 10 to 20% of survivors.

Rastelli procedure ± Lecompte modification

Vouhé and associates[23] from Paris, France, reported complete repair for TGA, VSD, and pulmonary outflow tract obstruction in 62 patients using either the Rastelli or Lecompte procedure. The Rastelli operation was used in 22 patients (35%) at a mean age of 8 years. The VSD was enlarged anteriorly in 8 patients and RV-PA continuity was established with an extra cardiac valve in 9 or nonvalved conduit in 13. Lecompte modification was used in 40 patients at a mean age of 3 years. The conal septum was extensively excised when present in 30 of 40, anterior translocation of pulmonary bifurcation was performed in 32 of 40, and RV-PA continuity was established by direct anastomosis without a prosthetic conduit. There were 7 early deaths, 2 after the Rastelli procedure (9%) and 5 after the Lecompte procedure (13%). Four patients were lost to follow-up, yielding 93% complete follow-up with a mean follow-up of 55 months. There were 2 late deaths, one in each group. Actuarial probability of survival at 5 years was 83 ± 9% after the Rastelli operation and 84 ± 6% after the Lecompte procedure. All long-term survivors except for 1 in the Rastelli group were in functional class I. Later operation for obstruction of the extracardiac conduit was required in 5 patients in the Rastelli group or 28%. Three late operations were required after the Lecompte operation, 1 for residual VSD and 2 for residual pulmonary outflow obstruction. At the most recent examination residual pulmonary outflow tract obstruction was present in 7 patients of the Rastelli group (39%) and 6 in the Lecompte group (19%). The combined likelihood of reoperation for residual pulmonary outflow obstruction was significantly higher in the Rastelli group (67% vs 27%). Both procedures provide satisfactory early and late results. The Lecompte allows complete repair in infancy and is feasible in some patients with anatomic contraindications to the Rastelli operation and may reduce the need for reoperation due to conduit or homograft problems. The Lecompte procedure does require extensive mobilization of the PA and anterior translocation at the point of bifurcation which necessitates division and generous resection of the ascending aorta. The Lecompte procedure has theoretical advantages, such as the decreased incidence for LV outflow tract obstruction and the lack of problems with conduits which may necessitate reoperation. Whether or not it will stand the test of time is not clear at present.

Arterial switch operation

Lupinetti and associates[24] from Ann Arbor, Michigan, described early and intermediate results in 126 patients with TGA who underwent arterial repair. Operation was performed at a median age of 6 days with 76 patients operated on within the first 7 days of life. Coronary artery anatomy differed from the usual arrangement in 37 patients. Simultaneous procedures included VSD closure in 35, repair of interrupted arch in 2, and coarctation repair in 5. Hospital mortality was 5.5% with 3 deaths among the most recent 100 patients. There was 1 late noncardiac death and 1 late death after reoperation. Reoperation for PA stenosis was required in 10 of the first 63 patients. Of the last 63 patients, all of whom had PA reconstruction with a single pericardial patch, only 1 required reoperation. Echocardiography performed in 115 of 119 surviving patients at a mean of 12 months after repair demonstrated qualitative normal LV function, minimal LV outflow gradients, and no more than trivial AR. Peak gradient across the RV outflow tract was 19 ± 3 mm in patients with separate PA patches and 5 ± 2 mm in those with a single patch used in the more recent patients. Follow-up is 96% complete with a mean of 2.5 years since surgery (range 1 month to 8 years). The actuarial survival rate at 5 years, including operative mortality, was 92%. All patients are in sinus rhythm and none requires antiarrhythmic medications. These authors show outstanding results from surgical survival and freedom from reoperation in this group of patients.

Baylen and associates[25] from Hershey, Pennsylvania, reviewed clinical records and echocardiographic findings of 23 infants with uncomplicated TGA. Fifteen infants did not undergo septostomy prior to arterial switch repair and 8 did have septostomy. Before PGE_1 infusion PO_2 in infants who did not undergo septostomy was 26 mmHg and did not differ from patients with septostomy. After PGE_1 infusion PO_2 increased significantly to 43 ± 8 mmHg in the group without septostomy but did not increase in patients with septostomy. Echocardiographic features generally demonstrated a nonrestrictive foramen ovale in patients without septostomy and a restrictive foramen ovale in patients with septostomy. Thus, the diameter of the foramen ovale was the primary factor influencing arterial oxygenation during PGE_1. These infants underwent the arterial switch operation at a mean age of 70 ± 65 hours with an overall survival rate of 96% with only 1 postoperative death. Absence of septostomy had no negative influence on any postoperative variable, including ventilatory and inotropic support, time to discharge, or mortality. Although there can be a marked improvement in cyanosis after institution of PGE_1 with what appears to be a sizable foramen ovale, some of these infants develop pulmonary edema with continued PGE infusion over a number of days while awaiting arterial switch repair. Thus, the decision as to whether or not to perform septostomy needs to be carefully evaluated in each patient. Many infants are not repaired for a week or more after diagnosis and thus may have changing requirements in regard to atrial septostomy in accordance with the degree of pulmonary flow.

Day and associates[26] from Los Angeles, California, reviewed the results of 70 newborn infants with TGA who had an arterial switch operation at a mean age of 5.6 days and a range of 2 to 26 days. The origin and distribution of coronary arteries were identified preoperatively, as well as intraoperatively. There were 4 early deaths and 5 surviving patients with symptoms of impaired cardiac function. No late deaths occurred in patients followed 2 to 50 months. Evidence of myocardial ischemia was present in 3 of 4 deaths and in 4 of the 5 patients with cardiovascular symptoms. Patients with commissural or intramural coronary origins between the great arteries had significantly greater cardiovascular morbidity and mortality because of coronary ischemia than patients with the most common coronary patterns. Coronary anatomy may influence surgical management and the postoperative course of newborn infants with TGA.

Kirklin and associates[27] from Birmingham, Alabama, reported a multi-institutional prospective study on 538 neonates with simple TGA or TGA and VSD entering for diagnosis and treatment at <15 days of age and undergoing an arterial switch repair. The 1 month and 1 and 5 year survivals were 84%, 82%, and 82% respectively. The hazard function for death had a rapidly declining single phase that approached 0 by 12 months after surgery. Among the 8 patients who died ≥ to 3 months after operation, 4 had severe ventricular dysfunction, probably related to imperfect coronary arterial transfer. Coexisting single VSD was not a risk factor for death. Origin of the left main coronary artery or only the left anterior descending or the circumflex artery from the right posterior sinus was a risk factor that was even stronger when an intramural course was present. Multiple VSDs were a risk factor as were longer global myocardial ischemic times and total circulatory arrest time. In addition, certain institutions were shown to be risk factors for death with the results in some improving with increasing experience and in some they did not. These authors present an enormous amount of data on this very important problem. It does appear that the arterial switch operation can be carried out in this unselected group of patients with a mortality of approximately 10% in the best institutions in this series. The details of the risk factors for poor outcome should be studied in detail by all physicians dealing with this problem.

Wernovsky and associates[28] from Boston, Massachusetts, reported results for 2-stage arterial switch consisting of preliminary PA banding and aortopulmonary shunt to prepare the left ventricle for an arterial switch operation in 28 patients with TGA. A successful arterial switch was performed at a median of 7 days following preparatory procedure in 24 of 27 survivors; 1 child had a Senning performed and 2 others died. During the interval between operation the LV to RV pressure ratio increased from 48 to 98% and LV mass increased from 46 ± 17 to 72 ± 23 g/m². After the preparatory procedure, the initial postoperative period was characterized by a low output syndrome. These authors show interesting data on this group of patients who because of low LV pressure and postnatal age require preliminary PA banding before arterial switch. Apparently these patients become extremely sick postoperatively and skilled ICU care is needed to care for them. It is of great interest that reoperation can be performed in approximately 1 week after banding and shunt procedure due to the rapid ability of the neonatal heart to hypertrophy.

DISCRETE SUBAORTIC STENOSIS

Echocardiographic features

Gewillig and associates[29] from Leuven, Belgium, studied flow characteristics of 26 patients with a mean age of 20 ± 10 years ≥6 months after operation for isolated discrete subvalvular AS. In addition, a control group between the ages of 17 ± 13 years was studied for comparison. The control subjects had laminar flow through systole in the LV outflow tract. By contrast, turbulence originating well below the site where the shelf had previously been resected was observed in 20 of 26 patients. In 16 of these 20, turbulence was caused by a ridge which in 13 could be identified as an offshoot of the ventricular band. In 4 patients the turbulence was caused by malalignment of the muscular and membranous septum, resulting in protrusion of the muscular septum into the outflow tract. Except for the latter 4 patients the aortic root diameter was 84 ± 10% of values predicted by body surface area, with values in 6 patients falling below the 3rd percentile. The mitral-aortic separation was 10 ± 4 mm with values in 21 patients falling above the 97th percentile. These data support the theory that discrete subvalvular AS may be caused by a chronic flow disturbance, preferably in a small and long outflow tract. LV bands, if reaching the outflow tract, may be a factor. These findings argue for careful echocardiographic and surgical exploration of the outflow tract well below the subvalvular stenosis to detect and resect structures that cause turbulence. This interesting study is thought provoking and although speculative, at best, at least lends a hypothesis to the postnatal development of subaortic stenosis, as well as to the frequent reoccurrence after surgical intervention.

Frommelt and associates[30] from Ann Arbor, Michigan, reviewed the clinical and echocardiographic data of 77 patients with subaortic stenosis diagnosed between 1983 and 1991. Isolated subaortic stenosis was present in 28 and associated cardiac lesions were present in 49. The most frequently encountered associated lesions were VSD in 19 and coarctation of the aorta/interrupted aortic arch in 14. Serial echocardiographic studies performed in 38 of 77 patients documented significant progression of the LV outflow tract gradient in 66% and development of AR in 66%. Surgical resection was performed in 36 patients with preoperative gradient of 63 ± 31 mmHg versus immediate postoperative gradient of 14 ± 14 mmHg. The immediate postoperative echocardiogram demonstrated no worsening of AR in any patient and regression of AR in 1 patient. Intermediate term follow-up studies were available in 13 at a mean of 4 years postoperatively. Recurrence of stenosis occurred in 2 of 13 but degree of AR did not increase in any patient. These authors conclude that two-dimensional and Doppler echocardiography are sensitive techniques in the diagnosis and management of patients with subaortic stenosis. Progression of gradient is prominent and occurs at a higher frequency in patients with associated lesions.

Management

de Vries and associates[31] from Rotterdam, The Netherlands, reviewed data from 57 patients with isolated fixed subaortic stenosis including 27 surgically treated patients, with special emphasis on the occurrence of AR during a mean follow-up period of 6.7 years. The number of patients with AR increased preoperatively in the total group from 23% at diagnosis to 54% after 3.7 years of follow-up. The prevalence of AR in the 27 surgically treated patients was higher at 81% than that in the nonsurgically treated group but remained unchanged after a mean postoperative period of 4.7 years. In all patients but 1, AR remained of minor hemodynamic significance. After surgery 15 patients (55%) showed a relapse; 11 redeveloped a subvalvular pressure gradient >30 mmHg and discrete subvalvular ridges from 6 months to 24 years after surgery. Follow-up did not reveal any benefit from early surgery. The unpredictable course and sometimes severe progression make frequent and careful follow-up necessary. These authors recommend surgical treatment only in patients with progressive disease and reject the hypothesis that operation on mild disease will prevent AR.

AORTIC ISTHMIC COARCTATION

With ventricular septal defect

Park and associates[32] from New York, New York, reviewed data from 39 infants with coarctation of the aorta and VSD to determining mortality, morbidity, outcome and factors that might predict survival or the need for VSD closure. Of the 8 patients who did not require surgery before 3 months of age, 7 underwent coarctation repair alone at a mean age of 2.3 years. Of the 23 infants managed with coarctation repair alone before 8 months of age, 9 needed no additional surgical treatment and 6 required early and 8 required late repair of VSD. Simultaneous PA banding with coarctation repair was performed in 7 patients and 1 eventually required debanding after spontaneous VSD closure. The overall mortality was 10% with a mean follow-up time of 5.7 years. Of 39 infants, 16 never required a second operation for VSD closure. For patients who had only coarctation repair or repair plus PA banding at <3 months of age, VSD size was categorized as small, moderate or large, on the basis of defect size at operative repair or echocardiographic or angiographic assessment. Defect size did not necessarily correlate with the need for operative VSD repair. Stepwise multiple regression analysis revealed that increased RV to LV peak systolic pressure and decreased systemic venous oxygen content were significantly predictive of the eventual need for VSD repair. These authors conclude that most infants with coarctation ad VSD do not require PA banding or open heart closure of VSD at the time of VSD repair and a significant number will not require a second operation. Early PA banding remains a good treatment strategy for patients with multiple VSDs, very large VSDs, and complex congenital heart disease such as TGA with VSD or AV canal defect.

Balloon dilatation

Minich and associates[33] from Ann Arbor, Michigan, reported clinical outcome in 11 children who underwent surgery after unsuccessful balloon angioplasty defined as a residual systolic gradient > 20 mmHg in 10 and a saccular aneurysm in 1. Data were compared with a control group of 7 children who had surgical repair without prior angioplasty during the same time. Angioplasty was performed at 4 ± 1 years of age and resulted in decreasing mean peak systolic gradient from 54 ± 3 to 27 ± 2. Follow-up angiography in 7 and MRI in 4 documented a discrete residual stenosis in 10 and a small saccular aneurysm in 1. Collateral circulation decreased in 3 patients. The subsequent surgical procedures and outcome were similar in the study and control groups. No paraplegia or mortality occurred. Pathological exam revealed irregular intimal surfaces with small flaps of intima in 5 of 10 resected specimens from the study group and in 2 of 6 from the control group. Follow-up evaluation 1.1 ± .2 years after operation for the subjects and .6 ± .3 years for the control group documented similar mild residual gradients and normal systolic blood pressures in both groups. Surgical repair appears to be safe and effective after unsuccessful balloon angioplasty of native coarctation. These authors, as well as a number of other groups, have continued to use balloon angioplasty for native coarctation. There is probably a slightly higher prevalence of aneurysm formation in these patients than in patients who undergo surgical repair, but the risk of aneurysm in the angioplasty group appears relatively small and some patients (parents) may choose this option despite knowing the potential for aneurysm formation and the need for subsequent surgery.

Anjos and associates[34] from London, United Kingdom, reported balloon dilation of aortic recoarctation in 27 patients. Dilation was not performed in 1 patient due to suspected perforation and the remaining 26 patients had 30 procedures. The age at first dilation ranged between 2.6 months and 18 years. After dilation, systolic gradient decreased from 49 ± 17 to 20 pm 17 mmHg. A reduction of gradient of ≤20 mmHg occurred after the first dilation in 65% of patients. Residual gradients between 25 and 80 mmHg were present in the remaining 9 patients. During follow-up of 2 months to 7 years, 5 of 17 patients with good initial result developed further recoarctation with 2 having successful redilation, 2 having reoperation and 1 awaiting repeat dilation. Of 9 patients with gradients >20 mmHg after the first dilation, 1 had successful redilation and 3 had reoperation. The remaining 5 patients are being managed conservatively. Aneurysms developed after dilation in 2 patients, 1 immediately and the other at 2 months. In all, 15 patients or 53% had a good, and 11 (42%) a poor late hemodynamic result. Aortic diameters at different levels of the aortic arch and at the reconstructed isthmus were significantly higher in the group with the good late result than in those with the poor result. This report of aneurysms after balloon dilation with recoarctation is disturbing, as it was felt that this would be a very rare occurrence in this particular group. Both patients with aneurysms had balloon/aortic diameter ratios at the diaphragm of 1.4 and 1.2 respectively. Although these ratios support oversized balloons as the cause of aneurysm formation, there are 3 other cases with balloon/aortic diameter ratios at diaphragm > 1.2 who did not develop aneurysm. It would appear prudent to try to avoid balloons larger than this ratio although some patients may require larger balloons to produce an effective hemodynamic result. As the authors point out, this can be effective management for some patients but is not without risk.

Effect of repair on aortic arch

Brouwer and associates[35] from Groningen and Rotterdam, The Netherlands, reviewed data from 15 consecutive infants <3 months of age who underwent coarctation repair and were evaluated echocardiographically. A Z-value was calculated, being the number of standard deviations the aortic arch differs from the expected derived from a control group. A hypoplastic aortic arch was present in 8 of 15 infants with a mean value of −7 ± 1. The other 7 infants had a normal arch with a mean Z-value of −2 ± 1. All infants underwent simple resection and end-to-end anastomosis. The mean Z-value increased significantly 6 months after operation in those with a hypoplastic arch to −1 ± 7 and in those with a normal arch to .1 ± 1. There were no deaths and recoarctation developed in 1 patient. These authors stress that simple resection and end-to-end anastomosis is the operation of choice for aortic coarctation associated with a hypoplastic arch and arch enlargement with a retrograde subclavian flap or carotid subclavian angioplasty is not necessary.

Myers and associates[36] from Hershey, Pennsylvania, studied growth of the transverse aortic arch in 17 patients undergoing subclavian flap angioplasty treatment for isolated coarctation. Preoperative and postoperative angiograms were reviewed and patients were divided into operation at 1 month or earlier and between 1 month and 1 year of age. The transverse aortic arch in both groups did grow when compared with control groups. The group repaired at <1 month of age achieved more growth than those repaired later. No aortic arch gradients were present at postoperative follow-up. These authors present good evidence for growth of the transverse aortic arch which normally is a relatively small structure when compared with ascending and descending aorta. In control subjects this area is about 60% of the transverse aortic arch. In patients with coarctation the average is 23% in the youngest infants and 29% in the older infants. The authors did not address the question of the severely hypoplastic transverse arch which usually is only 1 or 2 mm in diameter. In these patients most surgeons, including this group, favor a radical repair of coarctation with transverse aortic arch enlargement.

Consequences of patch aortoplasty

Mendelsohn and associates[37] from Ann Arbor, Michigan, followed 29 patients identified 5.6 years post-path aortoplasty for coarctation and classified them into 7 with aneurysm and 22 with no aneurysm. The presence of an aneurysm was defined angiographically as a ratio of the repair site diameter to diaphragmatic aortic diameter ≥1.5. One patient underwent semiemergency aneurysmectomy and 2 without aneurysm were lost to follow-up. The remaining 26 patients were evaluated 3 to 5 years later by exam and chest radiography. Progressive aneurysm dilatation was documented by an increase in aortic ratio from 1.6 to 2.0 in 5 of 6 patients in Group A. Only 1 of 20 patients without initial aneurysm showed aneurysmal dilation. These data indicate that patients with significant aortic dilation following patch aortoplasty repair of coarctation require close long-term follow-up for the possibility of progressive dilatation and the need for urgent repair.

Ambulatory blood pressure after repair

Leandro and associates[38] from Toronto, Canada, studied ambulatory BP and alterations in LV performance in 20 patients with normotension at rest after successful coarctation repair. Exercise testing, BP monitoring and echocardiographic studies were performed in 13 boys and 7 girls with a mean age of 14 ± 2 and 15 ± 3 years, respectively. There was no evidence of recoarctation and comparisons were made with 20 matched control subjects. No differences were found in systolic BP at rest or peak exercise between patients and controls. Male patients developed a significant arm/leg gradient at peak exercise. Systolic ambulatory BP was higher throughout the day in the male group but in the female group systolic BP was higher only during sleep. No differences were found in diastolic BP or heart rate between patients and controls. The transverse aortic arch was smaller and the LV mass greater in all patients and the relation of wall stress to rate-corrected velocity of shortening was above normal in 8 of 20 patients, indicating enhanced contractility. The mitral inflow E/A ratio on the atrial echocardiogram was significantly reduced in the patient group, suggesting LV hypertrophy and increased LA pressure in a compensated state. These studies demonstrate that patients with successfully treated aortic coarctation who are normotensive at rest and do not have an exaggerated BP response to exercise have evidence of cardiac target involvement, possibly secondary to mild systemic hypertension, documented by ambulatory BP monitoring.

AORTIC VALVE ATRESIA

Patterns of anomalous pulmonary venous connection/drainage

Seliem and associates[39] from Philadelphia, Pennsylvania, viewed preoperative echocardiographic Doppler color flow mapping studies of 317 patients with hypoplastic left heart who underwent stage I Norwood procedure. Anomalous connection or drainage, or both, of the pulmonary veins occurred in 20 patients or 6.3%. Subcostal and suprasternal scans showed the best anatomic details of the pulmonary veins. Total anomalous connection to a confluence behind the left atrium with persistent vertical vein occurred in 8 patients and 8 patients had normal connection to the left atrium but obstruction to flow out of the atrium. The final 4 patients had right pulmonary veins to the right or left superior vena cava (2) or right pulmonary veins that drained to the right of a deviated intraatrial septum (2). Although these abnormalities may not prevent satisfactory completion of the staged Norwood approach, they are vitally important to be delineated prior to proceeding with a Fontan operation. In addition, these abnormalities could make transplantation extremely difficult to accomplish and should be considered in any patient prior to management with either Norwood or transplantation strategies.

Operative management

Starnes and associates[40] from Stanford, California, reported the past 3 years experience in 35 newborn infants referred for surgical management of hypoplastic left heart. Surgical palliation by first-stage Norwood or cardiac transplantation was offered. Palliation was chosen by 24 families (68%) and transplantation by 11 families (32%). Of the 11 infants listed for transplantation, 5 underwent transplantation and because of a lack of donors, after an average wait of 25 days (range of 19 to 31 days) the remaining 6 underwent palliation with no perioperative deaths. Of the 30 infants undergoing palliation, including crossover, 20 (67%) survived the first operative stage. Among the last 19 infants undergoing palliation early survival was 84%. Risk factors for poor outcome were year of operation and circulatory arrest time >50 minutes. Among the 13 infants undergoing palliation with a circulatory arrest time of <50 minutes there were 12 survivors; among 12 having an arrest time of >50 minutes there were 4 survivors. At intermediate follow-up, 6 infants have undergone second-stage Glenn procedures with 5 survivors. There were 8 late deaths, 4 by respiratory infections and 4 by cardiac problems, including a thrombosed shunt in 1 infant. Cardiac transplantation was carried out in 5 infants with .3 survivors. Size of aorta, tricuspid regurgitation and ventricular wall thickness did not prove to be risk factors for poor outcome. These authors indicate that infants should be managed selectively on the basis of donor availability and family wishes. There was a 32% surgical mortality for the Stage I Norwood procedure plus 40% late deaths; this was followed by a 16% mortality at the time of the Glenn procedure. Transplantation provides better mid-term outcome if one refers to the Loma Linda experience. Further comparative studies such as this one will be useful to determine how effective the Norwood procedure is long-term in a number of centers and how many infants will need transplantation as the ultimate outcome after the Norwood procedure.

Farrell and associates[41] from Philadelphia, Pennsylvania, reviewed the outcome of 76 consecutive patients, ages 5 months to 6 years (median 19 months) who underwent a modified Fontan procedure after initial palliation for hypoplastic left heart. Modifications of the procedure included transatrial baffle of pulmonary venous return to the tricuspid valve in 10 and inferior vena cava baffle within the right atrium to the superior vena caval-PA anastomosis with PA augmentation in 66. Actuarial survival rates were 74% at 1 month, 58% at 12 months, 56% at 2 years, and 52% at 4 years. Of the 43 survivors, 25 have returned for postoperative catheterization at a median of 13 months after the initial procedure. Hemodynamic values were CI 2.8 ± 0.6 $1/min/m^2$; right atrial pressure 11 ± 2 mmHg; PA wedge pressure 6 ± 3 mmHg; and arterial O_2 saturation $94 \pm 3\%$. No patient had significant tricuspid or native pulmonary valve insufficiency. These authors show comparable survival after a Fontan procedure to other patients with complex lesions. See Table 1, page 120. Although there still is significant mortality for the first stage of the Norwood procedure, these investigators have made significant advances in the treatment of hypoplastic left heart syndrome. Continued follow-up and comparison with patients who are treated with transplantation is definitely needed.

TABLE 8-1. *Clinical and Morphologic Findings in 17 Patients with Anomalous Origin of the Left Main Coronary Artery from the Right Coronary Artery or the Right Aortic Sinus. Reproduced with permission from Roberts et al.*[49]

Case	Age (yr) & Sex	Origin of LMCA	Anomaly Group	Length of LMCA (cm)	AP	SD	Death Outside Hospital	Cause of Death	Length of RCA >LCCA	Slit-Like Ostium	No. of Major CAs >75% ↓ in CSA by Plaque	LV Scar (1 to 3+)	HW (g)
1	22 M	RAS	A	4.5	0	+	+	HC	+	0	0	0	870
2	44 F	RAS†	A	3.0	+	+	+	Trauma	+	0	0	0	255
3	13 F	RAS	B	1.1	0	+	+	Coronary anomaly	+	+	0	0	210
4	14 M	RAS	B	1.2	0	+	+	Coronary anomaly	+	+	0	0	370
5	14 M	RAS	B	—	0	+	+	Coronary anomaly	—	+	0	0	380
6	19 M	RAS	B	1.1	0	+	+	Coronary anomaly	+	+	0	0	325
7	29 M	RAS	B	—	+	+	+	Coronary anomaly	0	+	0	+	350
8	39 F	RAS	B	—	0	+	+	Coronary anomaly	0	+	0	0	220
9	64 F	RAS	B	2.4	+	0	0	Coronary anomaly	+	+	0	+++	510
10	81 M	RAS	B	2.0	0	+	+	Trauma	+	0	0	0	420
11	50 F	RAS†	B	—	0	+	+	Atherosclerotic CAD	+	0	3	+++	650
12	34 M	RAS	C	4.7	0	0	+	Trauma	+	0	0	0	330
13	48 M	RAS	C	4.5	0	+	+	Trauma	+	0	0	0	550
14	32 M	RAS	D	3.3	0	+	+	Trauma	0	0	0	0	325
15	45 M	RAS	D	4.5	+	+	+	Atherosclerotic CAD	+	0	1	+++	580
16	57 F	RAS	D	3.6	0	0	+	Opiate addiction‡	+	0	0	0	300
17	69 M	RCA	D	3.0	0	0	0	Forme fruste Marfan	+	0	0	0	685

†Common ostium of both RCA and LMCA.
‡Complications arising from the addiction.
AP = angina pectoris; CA = coronary artery; CAD = coronary artery disease; CSA = cross-sectional area; HC = hypertrophic cardiomyopathy; HW = heart weight; LCCA = left circumflex coronary artery; LMCA = left main coronary artery; LV = left ventricular; RAS = right aortic sinus; RCA = right coronary artery; SD = sudden death; + = present or positive; 0 = absent or negative; — = no information available.

EBSTEIN'S ANOMALY

Diagnosis in neonates

Gentles and associates[42] from Auckland, New Zealand, reviewed 48 patients with Ebstein's anomaly, 35% of whom presented in the first week of life. Duration of follow-up extended to 32 years (> 10 years in 35%). Twenty of the 48 patients (42%) died, 6 in the first week of life and 1 at age 5 months. Thirteen of the 41 patients surviving to age 6 months subsequently died with overall 50% survival reached at 47 years. Significant predictors of death were male sex, cardiothoracic ratio ≥.65, New York Heart Association Class III or IV, and breathlessness. Eight patients died suddenly and all but 1 had a history of AF or SVT. A cardiothoracic ≥.65 is a better predictor of sudden death than functional status. All who developed AF died within 5 years. These data indicate that patients with Ebstein's anomaly who have significant and/or increasing cardiomegaly, as well as a history of rhythm disorder do poorly. Cardiac surgery before massive cardiomegaly in mildly symptomatic patients appears indicated although neither mild disease nor successful surgery are totally protective against sudden death.

Celermajer and associates[43] from London and Cambridge, United Kingdom, reviewed presentation and outcome of 50 patients with neonatal Ebstein's anomaly seen from 1961 to 1990. The majority (88%) presented in the first 3 days of life with cyanosis in 80% as the most common presenting feature. Associated defects were present in 27 infants (54%) including PS in 11 and pulmonary atresia in 7. There were 9 deaths (18%) in the neonatal period and 15 late deaths due to hemodynamic deterioration in 9, sudden death in 5, and noncardiac cause in 1 at a mean age of 5 years (range 4 months to 19 years). Actuarial survival at 10 years was 61%. A new echocardiographic grade from 1 to 4 was devised with the use of the ratio of the area of the right atrium and atrialized right ventricle to the area of the functional right ventricle and left heart chambers. Severity of grades was established with grade 1 indicating a ratio of <.5 and grade 4 a ratio of ≤1.5. Cardiac death occurred in 0 of 4 infants with grade 1 and in 5 of 5 infants with grade 4 with intermediate mortality for the other grades. In a multivariate analysis of clinical and investigational features at presentation, echocardiographic grade of severity was the best independent predictor of death. These data suggest that infants with a grade 3 or 4 echocardiographic severity index may need consideration for transplant or conversation to a tricuspid atresia type anomaly.

In Wolff-Parkinson-White syndrome

Ebstein's anomaly is the most commonly occurring congenital abnormality associated with the WPW syndrome. However, the effects of Ebstein's anomaly on the risks and benefits of surgical ablation of accessory pathways in patients with WPW syndrome are unknown. Pressley and co-workers[44] in Durham, North Carolina, compared the long-term outcome of 38 WPW patients with Ebsteins' anomaly undergoing accessory pathway ablation to a reference population of 384 similarly treated patients without the anomaly. Ebstein's anomaly was mild in 21 patients and moderate-to-severe in 17 patients. Sixteen patients required tricuspid valve surgery, and 23 had an ASD or patent foramen ovale repaired. Baseline clinical characteristics and preoperative clinical arrhythmias were similar in both groups. Ten-year survival was 92% and 91% for patients with and without Ebstein's anomaly, respectively. During a mean follow-up of 6 and 5 years, 82% of patients with and 90% without Ebstein's anomaly had either clinically insignificant or no arrhythmias, and 18% versus 10% reported symptoms suggesting arrhythmias lasting longer than 1 minute, respectively. AF was reduced postoperatively to 9% in patients with and to 4% in those without the anomaly. Fewer hospitalizations were reported postoperatively by 90% versus 96% of patients with and without Ebstein's anomaly; 9% versus 6% of patients were disabled at follow-up, respectively. Patients with Ebstein's anomaly are improved significantly after accessory pathway ablation. The presence of this anomaly should not preclude accessory pathway ablation in these patients.

Operative treatment

Danielson and associates[45] from Rochester, Minnesota, reported results on 189 patients with Ebstein's anomaly who underwent repair. Ages ranged from 11 months to 64 years with a median of 16 years. Tricuspid valve reconstruction was possible in 58% and in 37% a prosthetic valve, usually a bioprosthesis, was inserted. In the remainder a modified Fontan or other procedure was performed. There 12 hospital deaths (6.3%). All patients who had accessory conduction paths underwent successful ablation of the pathways as a part of the operative treatment. Follow-up was obtained in 151 patients (85%). Of those patients with follow-up more than 1 year after operation, 93% were asymptomatic or only mildly symptomatic. There were 10 late deaths; 7 cardia, 2 noncardiac and 1 of unknown cause. Postoperative Doppler echocardiographic assessment showed the atrial septum was intact in all patients and tricuspid valve function was good to excellent in most patients. Valve reconstruction was required 1.4 to 14 years later in 4 of the 110 patients. Postoperative reduction in heart size was usual, atrial arrhythmias were reduced and late postoperative exercise testing showed a significant improvement in performance with maximal oxygen consumption increasing from a mean of 47% of predicted before operation to a mean of 72% after operation. There have been 12 successful pregnancies in 9 patients following operation. These authors show excellent results from a large group of patients with this unusual anomaly. Indications for operation appear to be cardiomegaly with cardio-thoracic ratio > .65 and symptoms that are more than mild or have recently progressed. The prognosis is poorest in those who have CHF, marked cyanosis, associated anomalies, a larger cardiac silhouette and diagnosis in infancy. Problems of both RV and LV dysfunction are common and the authors are attempting to operate at a younger age before symptoms develop.

CORONARY ANOMALY

Left main from pulmonary trunk

Karr and associates[46] from Boston, Massachusetts, reviewed echocardiographic and doppler data from 10 patients with anomalous left coronary artery arising from the PA in 27 patients with dilated cardiomyopathy. The direction of flow in the 3 main segments of the left coronary artery system was determined and in all 10 patients with anomalous left coronary artery, flow mapping demonstrated an abnormal jet from the left coronary into the pulmonary trunk and retrograde flow in at least 2 segments of the left coronary system. Doppler color mapping was performed in 19 of 27 patients with dilated cardiomyopathy and demonstrated antegrade flow in at least 1 segment of the left coronary system in 16 of the 19 patients but flow direction was not determined in the other 3 patients. Coronary anatomy was confirmed by aortic root or LV angiography in 14 patients and at autopsy in 1 patient and was not directly confirmed in 4 patients. The left coronary artery appeared to arise from the aortic root by 2-dimensional imaging alone in all patients with dilated cardiomyopathy and in 5 of 10 patients with anomalous left coronary artery (50% false negative diagnoses). These authors demonstrate detection of an abnormal jet in the pulmonary trunk and retrograde flow in the left coronary system by Doppler flow mapping in all 10 patients studied retrospectively with anomalous left coronary artery. Two-dimensional echocardiographic imaging is inconclusive and often misleading in this diagnosis. Determining flow direction of the left coronary system with dilated cardiomyopathy is useful for attempting to exclude anomalous left coronary artery but can be a technically difficult feat. Any patients whose Doppler flow mapping is not absolutely characteristic for anomalous left coronary should have aortic angiography if the diagnosis of anomalous left coronary is entertained.

Sauer and associates[47] from Munich, Germany, studied 33 children with a median age at initial cardiac catheterization of .4 years with anomalous origin of the left coronary artery from the PA without associated significant cardiovascular anomalies. A 2 coronary circulation was reestablished in 31 of 33 children. There was 1 death before the intended operation and 1 child had the left coronary artery ligated. There were 6 operative deaths, 5 intraoperative and 1 death 12 hours after operation. Preoperative factors associated with a higher perioperative mortality included young age at operation, left and balanced type of coronary artery circulation, electrocardiographic signs of extensive myocardial infarction including marked ST elevation in at least 2 leads. An extreme right dominant type of coronary circulation with left axis deviation on the electrocardiogram was linked with adequate perfusion of the posterolateral LV wall. At autopsy, severe increase of heart weight to 2 to 3 times normal was established in 6 of 7 children. Perioperative mortality was determined primarily by the extent of myocardial ischemia.

Vouhé and associates[48] from Paris, France, reported direct aortic reimplantation of the anomalous artery in 31 consecutive children with anomalous left coronary artery from the PA. There were 5 deaths (16%) with 3 hospital deaths and 2 early deaths within 3 months. The severity of preoperative LV dysfunction of the only incremental risk factor for mortality: 31% mortality among patients with LV shortening fraction <.2 versus 0% with LV shortening fraction ≥20%. There were no late deaths up to 6 years with a survival rate of 84 ± 7%. Late results were evaluated in 23 survivors having a follow-up longer than 12 months. LV function recovered to normal in all patients and 96% were free of symptoms. Moderate to severe MR decreased to minimal or no MR in 5 of 7 patients and the reimplanted anomalous artery was patent in all. These authors stress that direct aortic reimplantation is technically feasible in most patients with anomalous left coronary artery and yields a high rate of patency;

LV resection is unnecessary, the mitral valve should not be interfered with at initial operation and patients with moderate LV dysfunction should be operated on early. Those with severe LV dysfunction may have to be considered for transplantation.

Left main from right aortic sinus

Roberts and Shirani[49] from Bethesda, Maryland, studied 17 patients at necropsy in whom the LM coronary artery arose from either the right aortic sinus or the most proximal portion of the right coronary artery. After its origin, the LM coronary artery coursed to the left side of the heart by 1 of 4 routes, and the clinical consequences of such courses were described by the authors. The findings in the 17 patients are summarized in Table 8-1 and the 4 subtypes of anomalous origin of the left main are shown in the Figure 8-2. These findings indicate that if an anomalously arising LM coronary artery courses anterior (group A) to the RV outflow tract, behind the RV outflow tract (infracristal) (group C) or dorsal (group D) to the ascending aorta, symptoms of cardiac dysfunction or myocardial ischemia do not result. In contrast, if the anomalously arising LM coronary artery courses between (group B) the pulmonary trunk and ascending aorta, symptoms of myocardial ischemia usually occur, and death is a frequent consequence.

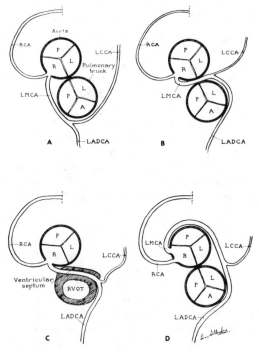

Fig. 8-2. Diagram showing the 4 subtypes of anomalous origin of the left main coronary artery (LMCA) from the right aortic sinus. A = anterior; L = left; LADCA = left anterior descending coronary artery; LCCA = left circumflex coronary artery; P = posterior; R = right; RCA = right coronary artery; RVOT = right ventricular outflow tract. Reproduced with permission from Roberts WC and Shirani.[49]

Hypoplasia of both right and left circumflex arteries

When the right coronary artery is dominant, i.e., it courses to the crux of the heart, the LC coronary artery is usually quite small and therefore may be considered hypoplastic (Figure 8-3). Conversely, when the LC is the dominant coronary artery, i.e., it courses to the crux of the heart, the right coronary artery is usually small and therefore may be considered hypoplastic. Hypoplasia of both right and LC coronary arteries in the same heart, however, is rare. Roberts and Glick[50] from Bethesda, Maryland, examined 3,400 hearts during the last 8 years and found that at least 8 had hypoplasia of both right and LC coronary arteries. The authors pointed out that hypoplasia of both right and LC coronary arteries has never been reported angiographically. In the 8 patients reported by Roberts and Glick, 3 had a coronary angiogram during life and bilateral hypoplasia of the right and LC coronary arteries were not suspected in any of them. Of the 8 necropsy patients described, it appears likely that the bilateral coronary hypoplasia was a functional significance in 2 patients.

Causing sudden death

Taylor and associates[51] in Washington, D.C., evaluated congenital coronary anomalies that are associated with sudden death and exercise-related death. The clinicopathologic records of 242 patients with isolated coronary artery anomalies were reviewed for information on mode of death and abnormalities of the initial segment angle takeoff, valvelike

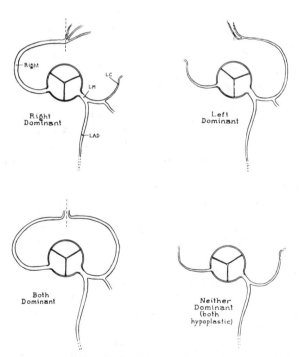

Fig. 8-3. Diagram showing graphic definitions of dominance and hypoplasia. The 8 patients described had right and left circumflex (LC) coronary arteries similar to these depicted in the bottom right diagram. LAD = left anterior descending; LM = left main coronary artery. Reproduced with permission from Roberts WC and Glick BN.[50]

ridges or aortic intramural segments and the course of the anomalous coronary artery. Cardiac death occurred in 142 patients (59%); 78 (32%) of these deaths occurred suddenly. Of sudden deaths, 45% occurred with exercise. Sudden death and exercise-related death were most common with origin of the LM coronary artery from the right coronary sinus. Anomalous origin of the right coronary artery from the left coronary sinus was also commonly associated with exercise-related sudden death. High risk anatomy involved abnormalities of the initial coronary artery segment or coursing of the anomalous artery between the pulmonary artery and the aorta. Younger patients ≤30 years old were significantly more likely than older patients ≥30 years to die suddenly (62% vs 12%) or during exercise (40% vs 2%) despite their low frequency of significant CAD. Thus, younger patients (≤30 years old) with an isolated coronary artery anomaly are at risk of dying suddenly with exercise.

PATENT DUCTUS ARTERIOSUS

Transcatheter occlusion

Rashkind's "double umbrella" technique for percutaneous transcatheter occlusion of patent arterial duct (ductus arteriosus) (PDA) has been used successfully in several centers. To assess its feasibility, safety, and efficacy in routine practice, a European registry was established and the results were reported.[52] In 642 of 686 patients entered in the study, the device was successfully implanted at the first attempt, and in a further 9 at a subsequent attempt. Four hundred and ninety-one patients (71% of all patients entered) had doppler-echocardiographic evidence of complete occlusion with a single device at the latest follow-up. Kaplan-Meier survival estimates indicated a complete occlusion rate of 82.5% at 1 year after implantation of a single device. A second device was implanted in 41 patients with residual flow, and 37 of these had complete occlusion, giving an overall latest follow-up occlusion rate of 77% and an actuarial complete occlusion rate for 1 or 2 devices of 94.8% at 30 months after implantation of the first device. Two early deaths occurred (9.3%), both in patients with associated ventricular septal defect. Complications included embolization of the device in 18 patients (2.4%), of whom 6 underwent catheter-retrieval of the device. Mechanical hemolysis occurred in a further 4 patients (0.5%). Transcatheter occlusion of the arterial duct is a safe and effective alternative to surgical closure. A second device is sometimes needed to achieve complete occlusion.

THE FONTAN OPERATION

Late follow-up

Driscoll and associates[53] from Rochester, Minnesota, studied 352 patients who had a Fontan operation prior to 1985. The overall 1, 5, and 10 year survivals were 77%, 70%, and 60% respectively. Factors associated with lower survival were univentricular heart or complex congenital anomaly other than tricuspid atresia, early calendar year of operation, heterotaxia syndrome, early age at operation, increased PA pressure, AV valve dysfunction, and higher New York Heart Association class. Reoperations were necessary for 103 of the 352 patients. At least 20% have or have had arrhythmias requiring medication or mechanical pacemaker. Between 7 and 10% have had protein-losing enteropathy/hypoproteinemia. At 5 years postoperatively, 35% were alive with a better functional classification than preoperatively, 17% were alive and in the same functional classification, 36% died or were in a worse functional classification. Of the surviving patients, 43% can do as much exercise as their peers, whereas 3% are incapable of exercise. These authors present excellent data regarding intermediate follow-up for a large group of patients who had Fontan operation. It is particularly worrisome that there is continued morbidity and mortality following apparently successful Fontan operation. Further data are needed on patients who undergo operation at an earlier age to determine if current patient selection criteria will result in improved long-term outcome.

In infants

Weber and associates[54] from Hershey, Pennsylvania, reported results for Fontan operation in 47 patients with early Fontan carried out at a mean age of 1.5 ± .5 years (range .6 to 2) in 17 children and compared that to results in 30 older patients, mean age 7.5 ± 5 years (range of 2.4 to 23). Preoperatively both groups had acceptable hemodynamic status for a successful Fontan result. Operative variables, including cardiopulmonary bypass time, aortic cross-clamp time and core temperature were similar between groups and did not affect mortality. The postoperative mortality rate including early surgical was 18% in the infant group versus 23% in the older group. Immediate postoperative arrhythmias were more frequent in the infant group (71% vs 25%) with no related mortality, while late arrhythmias occurred with equal frequency in both groups. The infant group required a longer hospital stay (22 ± 9 vs 14 ± 5 days). These authors add further information to the debate regarding Fontan operation in infancy. It should be pointed out that the younger patients were operated at a later date than the older patients and in addition more of the younger patients had the technique of total cavo-pulmonary connection used. It does appear that the Fontan can be performed safely in younger patients whose risk factors for successful Fontan are minimal.

In heterotaxy syndrome

Culbertson and associates[55] from Los Angeles, California, studied the medical records of 20 consecutive pediatric patients with asplenia (n = 12) and polysplenia (n = 8) who underwent the Fontan procedure at a mean age of 56 months for patients with asplenia and 39 months for patients with polysplenia. There were 2 early and 2 late deaths for a total mortality of 20% in patients with heterotaxy syndrome as compared with 8.5% for patients without this syndrome who underwent Fontan procedure during the same time period. Factors that significantly increased the risk of Fontan were preoperative > mild AV valve regurgitation, hypoplastic PAs, and mean PA pressure ≥15 mmHg after 6 months of age. In additional RV morphology with elevated end-diastolic pressure ≥10 mmHg was a possible risk factory for poor outcome. The entire mortality occurred in patients with asplenia but this group has a higher incidence of AV valve regurgitation, elevated PA pressure, and abnormal PA anatomy than those patients with polysplenia syndrome. These authors suggest that a decision as to the ultimate reparative procedure in these patients should be made early with adequate control of pulmonary blood flow. Both echocardiography and cardiac catheterization should be carried out 1 to 3 months after a palliative procedure and no later than 6 months of age if no procedure is performed to assess hemodynamic variables and the presence or absence of valvular regurgitation.

In single ventricle

Mayer and associates[56] from Boston, Massachusetts, studied the outcome of 225 modified Fontan operations carried out between 1984 and 190 for patients with defects other than tricuspid atresia. Overall 30 patients (13%) had failure of this operation defined as death or Fontan takedown. Results improved significantly during the period of the study with failure rates of 7% and 3% in the last two years of the review, respectively. Multivariate analysis showed that PA distortion, PA pressure, age <3 years, use of nonoxygenated cardioplegic solution, and cardiopulmonary bypass time > 180 minutes were associated with worse outcome, while "favorable" atrioventricular anatomy (non-left atrioventricular valve stenosis/atresia or common atrioventricular valve) and age > 9 years were associated with improved outcome. In the past 2 years, 31% of patients were < 3 years of age. In the last 2 years of the 2 study the operation failed on only 2 of 28 patients (7%) <3 years of age, compared with an overall failure rate of 4 of 90 patients (4%) during the same interval. Any potential increase in risk associated with younger age must be weighed against the deleterious effects of alternative additional palliative procedure such as PA distortion by shunts or depressed ventricular function resulting from longer period of pressure or volume overload. These considerations have influenced the authors to continue their policy of earlier Fontan operation rather than delaying this procedure. The suggestion is that because of recent trends future analysis will show that young age alone may not continue to be a risk factor for modified Fontan operation. The fenestrated ASD in these patients is used extensively by this group but the role of fenestration in the future is still not totally settled.

Akagi and associates[57] from Toronto, Canada, used radionuclide angiography and ventricular cineangiography to study ventricular function in patients with a univentricular or atrioventricular connection who underwent Fontan repair. There were 28 preoperative studies and 36 studies > 1 year after repair. Data were compared with the control population. Before operation end-diastolic volume and wall mass were significantly increased compared with those of control subjects; however, the mass/volume ratio was normal for the preoperative group. Although end-diastolic volume returned to normal after the procedure, wall mass remained elevated and contributed to an elevated mass/volume ratio post repair. Systemic vascular resistance was also significantly elevated compared with that prior to surgery and compared to control patients. Preoperative ejection fraction, peak ejection rate, end-diastolic volumes, and peak filling rate were all significantly reduced when compared with those of the control subjects and remained so after surgery. These data suggest that systolic and diastolic function are depressed preoperatively in these patients and remains unchanged after creation of an atrial-dependent circulation. Afterload reduction therapy in these patients who usually do not have significant symptoms would undoubtedly improve pump characteristics and possibly natural history. A prospective study is needed to evaluate this question.

Sluysmans and associates[58] from Boston, Massachusetts, used echocardiography to study ventricular dimensions, volume, shape, wall stress, and systolic function in 84 patients aged .2 to 35 years with double inlet single left ventricle or tricuspid atresia. Measurements were obtained in 67 patients after arterial shunt of PA band and in 47 patients a median of 4.4 years after a Glenn shunt in 9 patients or a Fontan operation in 38. Before the Fontan procedure, ventricular volumes were 2 to 3 times normal. Ventricular afterload became abnormal after 2 years of age and with age, LV shape changed progressively from ellipsoidal to spherical, as indicated by decrease in long axis:short axis ratio from normal of 1.9 toward unity. Concomitantly, the ratio of circumferential to meridional end-systolic walls tress fell from 1.3 to unity. The age related change in shape and load occurred in concert with progressive deterioration of LV systolic function and contractility. Aortic oxygen saturation, an indicator of pulmonary blood flow and therefore volume work was inversely and independently correlated with contractility. In the group of patients in whom a Glenn or a Fontan operation was performed at <10 years of age, ventricular dimensions, volumes, and wall stress diminished and LV function and contractility improved after surgery. In patients undergoing surgery after 10 years of age, few had improvements of LV function. These authors present additional evidence that there is progressive deterioration of ventricular function in patients with single left ventricle prior to a Fontan type procedure. In addition, early surgery is associated with a more favorable outcome on long-term ventricular contractility.

Previous pulmonary trunk banding

Malcic and associates[59] from Munich, Germany, studied 38 patients who underwent the Fontan operation who were classified into 2 groups. Group 1 consisted of 18 patients with previous PA banding at a mean age of 7 months and group 2 consisted of 20 patients with native PS. In group 1, 10 children had tricuspid atresia, 6 had double inlet left ventricle and 2 had complex malformations. Group 2 consisted of 12 patients with tricuspid atresia, 6 double inlet ventricle and 2 with complex malformations. The patients with PA banding had slightly lower hemoglobin and hematocrit values preoperatively but were not significantly different in terms of end-diastolic volume, EF, mass to body ratio, or PA size as assessed by Nakata index. Patients with banding did have a higher ventricular mass index and a higher prevalence of subaortic stenosis and AV valve insufficiency. Severe pericardial effusions in the early postoperative period were frequent in the group with pulmonary banding and particularly prevalent in patients with long-standing banding; banding was not associated with increased mortality. Significant increments in ventricular mass after PA banding may represent a risk for unfavorable morbidity after the Fontan operation.

With baffle fenestration

Kopf and associates[60] from New Haven, Connecticut, reported results in 10 patients who underwent fenestrated Fontan operation with a 4 to 6 mm circular fenestration because of 2 or more risk factors for morbidity and death following conventional Fontan operation. There were no deaths in the fenestration group but a similar group of recent high risk patients without fenestration had a mortality rate of 2 of 8. Patients with fenestration had significantly less drainage from the chest tube, less inotropic support and shorter intensive care and hospital stays than patients without fenestration. Comparison with a recent group of low risk patients undergoing the Fontan operation showed no statistical difference in postoperative parameters. Fenestrations were closed in all 10 patients at 9 days to 6 months after operation by means of a transcatheter clamshell occluder device. Two patients had left PA balloon angioplasty and 3 patients had other atrial communications closed with additional clamshell devices. During short-term follow-up periods averaging 18 months all patients were clinically well; however, 1 patient with mitral atresia required reoperation for obstruction between left atrium and tricuspid valve, not related to the clamshell device. These date suggest that fenestration may be 1 method for achieving lower morbidity and mortality rates among high risk patients undergoing the Fontan procedure. This remains a complex issue; there are no other comparative studies testing the hypothesis that fenestration does improve results in high risk patients. An alternative method for leaving an adjustable ASD following Fontan operation has been described previously by Laks, et al (Ann Thorac Surg, 1991; 52:1084–95). This latter method does not require postoperative catheterization for ASD closure and may yield similar results with less expense and inconvenience for the patient.

Mavroudis and associates[61] from Chicago, Illinois, performed the fenestrated Fontan operation in 17 high risk patients with univentricular hearts with a median age of 3 years and age range of 1.2 to 25 years. High risk characteristics were depressed ventricular function and/or hypertrophy in 12, AV valve insufficiency in 5, PA distortion in 6, elevated pulmonary resistance > 2 units $\cdot$ M^2 in 4, previously failed Fontan in 2 and associated WPW syndrome in 1. Mean baffle fenestration was 3.5 mm and ranged from 2.7 to 5 mm. Multiple regression analysis revealed cardiac index was greater with open than with closed fenestration during volume loading and oxygen delivery was also greater with open than with closed fenestration. Survival was 100% with a mean follow-up of 10 months; pleural drainage was high in 2 patients. Subsequent transcatheter fenestration closure resulted in increased oxygen saturation from 87 to 96%. This adjunct to Fontan operation can improve survival in high risk patients and subsequent transcatheter fenestration closure can be performed after hemodynamic assessment.

Bridges and associates[62] from Boston, Massachusetts, studied patients having a modified Fontan operation to compare 91 patients with baffle fenestration to 56 patients without baffle fenestration. Outcome variables were failure, as indicated by death or take-down of Fontan procedure, duration of postoperative pleural effusions and duration of hospitalization. Survival and clinical status after hospital discharge were ascertained. The 2 groups did not differ with respect to age or anatomic diagnosis. Patients having baffle fenestration were at significantly greater preoperative risk by univariate and multivariate analysis. Operative failure was low in both groups being 11% without and 7% with baffle fenestration, p = NS. Durations of pleural effusions and hospitalization were significantly shorter and postoperative systemic venous pressure lower in patients with baffle fenestration. Neither date of surgery nor a previous bi-directional cavopulmonary anastomosis appeared to contribute to improved outcome. There were no late deaths. Functional status in both groups was good with 82% in the New York Heart Association class I.

Arrhythmias afterwards

Gewillig and associates[63] from London, United Kingdom, studied the prevalence, predisposing factors, and clinical significance of arrhythmias early and late after the Fontan operation for congenital heart disease. All 104 consecutive patients undergoing Fontan repair from 1975 to 1988 were studied retrospectively and hospital records reviewed for perioperative arrhythmia. Clinical information and annual electrocardiograms were available for all 78 hospital survivors during a follow-up of up to 13 years (mean of 3.7). Ambulatory electrocardiographic monitoring was performed in 67 patients (81%). Perioperative tachycardia occurred in 11 patients (1%) with atrial flutter in 8 and His bundle tachycardia in 3. Multivariate analysis showed that increased preoperative mean PA pressure and low aortic oxygen saturation were significant risk factors for the development of atrial flutter but not for His bundle tachycardia. Despite intensive medical treatment, 10 of these 11 patients died. At the last visit, 72 of 78 (92%) were in sinus rhythm on their standard electrocardiogram. Junctional rhythm was present in 3, 2 patients had atrial flutter and 1 had a paced rhythm. Ambulatory monitoring did not show important bradycardia or ventricular arrhythmia. Actuarial survival free of SVT was 82% 8 years after operation. Multivariate analysis identified older age, increased right atrial size, and increased mean preoperative PA pressure as risk factors for arrhythmia during intermediate follow-up. Late tachycardias, in contrast to those occurring in the perioperative period, were not associated with increased mortality. These authors show a relatively low prevalence of important mid-term of late rhythm disturbances. Dysrhythmia can be a serious complication in these patients, related probably more to effects on systemic ventricular output than to changes in pulmonary blood flow.

Peters and Somerville[64] from London, United Kingdom, retrospectively analyzed data from 60 patients undergoing the Fontan procedure at a mean age of 12 ± 7 years. Postoperative arrhythmias occurred in 34 patients (57%) and 11 of 19 (58%) early deaths within 7 days of surgery were related to arrhythmias. All patients with AF and HIS bundle tachycardia died. There was a higher prevalence of early arrhythmias which were less well tolerated in double inlet ventricle (9 of 19) than in tricuspid atresia (8 of 37). There were no other preoperative determinants of early arrhythmias or deaths from early arrhythmia. Late arrhythmia (after 7 days) occurred in 37% of hospital survivors. These patients had higher RA pressures both early and late after operation and lower ventricular EFs late after operation. Of those with atrial arrhythmias 86% had RA obstruction and 57% had an RA thrombus or pulmonary embolism at presentation. The actuarial arrhythmia-free survival for hospital survivors was 60% at 10 years. These authors show poorly tolerated atrial arrhythmias in this group of patients. The arrhythmias probably mainly affect systemic ventricular output and then secondarily pulmonary blood flow. Late arrhythmias may be the first manifestation of RA obstruction and/ or thrombus.

Pulmonary venous obstruction

Fogel and Chin[65] from Philadelphia, Pennsylvania, retrospectively evaluated 12 cases of pulmonary venous pathway obstruction documented at 43 ± 28 months of age by autopsy in 3 cases and by catheterization in 9 cases following modified Fontan operation. Obstruction was defined as an A wave ≥4 mmHg and patients and mechanisms of obstruction included narrowed pulmonary vein ostia in 6 cases, narrowed left atria outlet in 4 and atrial baffle obstruction in 3. Two causes of obstruction were present in 1 patient. No patient has pulmonary venous congestion on chest x-ray. Pathway diameters were considerably smaller than those found in 11 age-matched controls who had undergone Fontan procedure and had no pulmonary venous obstruction. With Doppler ultrasound that was a relatively narrow range of velocities distal to the obstruction from 1.3 to 2.5 m/ms. These authors conclude that patients who have undergone a Fontan procedure and have pulmonary venous obstruction (1) chest roentgenography cannot be used as a screening tool; (2) distal velocities as low as 1.3 m/s occur, usually with nonphasic, continuous forward flow; and (3) pathway diameters may be used as an output-independent parameter to determine significant pulmonary venous pathway obstructions.

Therapy of subaortic stenosis afterwards

Razzouk and associates[66] from Toronto, Canada, studied 12 children who developed subaortic stenosis after Fontan operation. All had absent resting and isoproterenol-provoked pressure gradient before the Fontan procedure. Six had a univentricular heart of LV morphology, 3 had a single ventricle of RV morphology, 1 had tricuspid atresia with TGA, 1 had pulmonary atresia with intact septum, and 1 had corrected TGA with hypoplastic systemic ventricle. The median interval between Fontan operation and the recognition of subaortic stenosis was 2.5 years. Surgical treatment was undertaken in 10 patients after a prior Fontan procedure: 5 had myectomy and enlargement of VSD with 2 operative deaths; 2 had placement of a valved conduit from the ventricular apex to the descending aorta and both died postoperatively; 2 with single ventricle had subaortic myectomy and 1 had enlargement of VSD and pulmonary aortic connection. Complete heart block developed in only 1 patient. Postoperative testing with Doppler echocardiography demonstrated good relief of subaortic stenosis. All 6 children who survived the operation are well 4 months to 4 years later. Subaortic stenosis is a progressive lesion that may develop after a Fontan operation. Surgical treatment continues to carry a significant mortality and careful screening for this complications is extremely important following operation.

MISCELLANEOUS TOPICS

The Marfan syndrome ≤20 years of age

El Habbal[67] from Manchester, United Kingdom, evaluated the prevalence of serious cardiovascular manifestations in the first 20 years of life in a series of 186 patients with the Marfan syndrome. Age distribution upon entry to study ranged from <1 year to 20 years. Entry to the study was on referral for assessment of the cardiovascular system. Echocardiographic measurements of the aortic root diameter were obtained in 91 patients with Marfan's syndrome, age 1 month to 20 years, in whom the diagnosis of dilated aortic root was questioned. In this group 15 randomly selected patients, aged 4 to 10 years underwent yearly measurements and were compared with those who had serious cardiovascular manifestations. These data were compared to a control group of 150 normal subjects ages 3 weeks to 20 years. Serious cardiovascular complications occurred in 8 patients below 20 years of age with sudden rupture of the ascending aorta in two, aortic valve replacement for severe AR in 3, and emergency replacement of the ascending aorta for acute dissection in 2. There was 1 death at repeat cardiac surgery due to severe CHF. Most patients with the Marfan syndrome had aortic root diameters at or above 2 standard deviations above normal (see El Habbal, page 755, figure 1). Serial measurements in the randomly selected group of 15 patients showed similar aortic growth velocities as the normal group (see El Habbal, page 755, figure 2). In contrast, the 8 patients with serious cardiovascular manifestations showed marked deviation from normal growth velocity of the aortic root (see El Habbal, page 756, figure 3). Serious cardiovascular complications occurred more commonly in patients with a negative family history. These data lend further weight to the practice of regular measurement of the aortic root diameter in children with the Marfan syndrome. This author apparently did not have any experience with beta blockers in an attempt to ameliorate the serious complications that occurred in a small number of their patients.

Complications of cardiac catheterization

Cassidy and associates[68] from San Francisco, California, prospectively studied catheterization complications in 1,037 catheterizations including 885 diagnostic and 152 diagnostic/interventional procedures performed in 888 patients ages 1 day to 27 years with a median age of 16 months. There were 15 major complications (1.4%), 70 minor complications (6.8%) and 30 incidents (2.9%). Two patients died as a result of the procedure and 2 as a result of pericatheterization clinical deterioration caused by the cardiac abnormality. The majority of complications were successfully treated and the patients had no residua. Of the patients with 13 nonfatal major complications and 70 minor complications, residua were evident in 7 patients and 3 without evident residua had the potential for sequelae. A comparison of diagnostic and balloon atrial septostomy cases in the present study with similar cases in a 1974 study from the same institution shows that the prevalence of major complications decreased from 2.9% to 0.9%; minor complications and incidents have decreased from 11.7% to 7.9% and pericatheterization deaths not attributable to catheterization decreased from 2.8 to 0.2%. These authors show an excellent record in terms of safety of performing pediatric catheterization. The most disturbing problems continues to be vascular problems usually in association with arterial balloon dilatation procedures. Thrombolytic therapy has helped to reduce the incidence of decreased pulses after such procedure and newer, low profile catheters should help in the future.

Valvuloplasty for congenital mitral stenosis

Grifka and associates[69] from Houston, Texas, performed double transseptal, double-balloon valvuloplasty for 8 patients with severe congenital MS. Isolated congenital MS was present in 2 and 6 had additional defects. Ages ranged from .6 to 36 years (median 9 years). All procedures were tolerated well. After valvuloplasty the left atrial a wave minus LV end-diastolic pressure gradient was reduced from 25 ± 6 to 9 ± 3 mmHg. The mitral valve mean gradient was reduced from 18 ± 7 to 8 ± 3 mmHg and LV end-diastolic pressure was unchanged (see Grifka, figure 2, page 126). All patients had marked clinical improvement and only 1 patient developed significant MR. Repeat valvuloplasty was necessary in 2 of the first 4 patients 7 months later. Follow-up evaluation on 6 patients from 4 to 54 months revealed no recurrence of symptoms or increased MR. This approach results in less trauma to the atrial septum and femoral veins with potentially less left to right atrial shunt following valvuloplasty. Three patients with parachute mitral valve, which has been considered not amenable to this technique, were treated and 2 of the 3 had a good early result. This procedure can provide useful palliation to allow growth of these children until such time as valve replacement may be necessary and is feasible.

Intravascular stents

Hosking and associates[70] from Toronto, Canada, reported implantation of 24 intravascular stents in 17 patients in either branch pulmonary arteries (RV to PA conduits or an aorta pulmonary collateral vessel). Follow-up time ranged from 1 to 14 months and the mean age at implantation was 7 ± 6 years. Optimal stent position as obtained in 22 of 24 implantations. No embolization or thrombotic event has been documented. Among patients with conduit obstruction the gradient was immediately reduced from 85 ± 30 to 35 ± 20 mmHg. However, 3 patients required conduit replacement because of persistent obstruction elevated RV pressures. Clinical improvement was noted in 10 of 11 patients with PA stenosis in association with enlargement of vessel diameter by 92 ± 90% and gradient reduction by 22 ± 24 mmHg. These data indicate the usefulness of vascular stents in selected patients, particularly those with PA stenosis following repair of TF or pulmonary atresia. Early results are encouraging, as indicated by this report, as well as those from Mullins, et al (Circulation, 1998;77:188–199) and O'Laughlin, et al (Circulation, 1991;83:1923–1939.

Homografts in right-sided conduits

Cleveland and associates[71] from Toronto, Canada, reported results of 219 patients who had cryopreserved homograft extracardiac valved conduits placed in the pulmonary circuit. Average age at operation was 7 years and 132 patients had a pulmonary homograft and 87 had an aortic homograft. Mortality was 11% and hospital survivors have been followed for an average of 30 months. Fourteen patients died during follow-up, almost all related to the complexity of their original malformation. Reoperation for conduit-related problems was required in 32 patients or 15%. Actuarial freedom from conduit operation is 55% at 5 years. The most common indication for reoperation was calcific stenosis in 27 patients. Reoperation for aortic homografts was similar to that for pulmonary homografts. The long-term function of cryopreserved homograft valved conduits in the pulmonary circulation is disappointing. It was originally hoped that these conduits would provide a long-term durable prothesis which had previously been demonstrated for fresh homografts.

Aortoventriculoplasty

Frommelt and associates[72] from Ann Arbor, Michigan, reported AVR and aortoventriculoplasty results in 19 patients ages 1 day to 18 years (mean 6 years). Operative indications included complex LV outflow tract obstruction after aortic valvotomy and/or subaortic resection in 6, severe AR after valvotomy or AVR in 4, severe AR with bacterial endocarditis in 1, truncus arteriosus with truncal insufficiency in 3, failure of apical-aortic conduit in 3 and combined AS and MS in 2. In all patients, valve insertion was performed after patch enlargement of the annulus and septum. Associated procedures included coronary artery reimplantation in 5 and MVR in 2. Mechanical valve protheses were used in 15 patients and allografts in 4. There were 3 hospital deaths (16%), 2 in patients with severe pulmonary vascular disease and no late deaths. Actuarial survival was 84% at 1 month and beyond with a mean follow-up of 2.5 years. Complications have included complete heart block in 1, residual VSD in 1 and early postoperative peripheral embolus in 1. No late thromboembolic events have occurred. These are impressive results for a number of relatively small patients with severe LV outflow tract obstruction. Of interest will be follow-up with these patients when their next operation is required.

Aortic arch repair via sternotomy

Karl and associates[73] from Melbourne, Australia, reported repair of interrupted aortic arch and coarctation plus hypoplastic aortic arch in 55 consecutive infants with a median age at operation of 6 days and median weight 3.1 kg. All patients has significant CHF and the majority required prostaglandin E_1 resuscitation and inotropic support with or without ventilation before operation. All operations were performed via sternotomy with core cooling and circulatory arrest. Isolated myocardial perfusion was used in 13 patients during arch repair. A complete intracardiac biventricular repair was performed except in patients expected to require Fontan operation as definitive treatment. The overall operative mortality was 15% with a 9% mortality for arch repair plus biventricular intracardiac repair. When arch repair plus palliative intracardiac repair was performed the mortality was 40%. Actuarial survival was 75% at 12 months with no subsequent deaths over 1294 patient-months with a mean of 28 months follow-up. Actuarial freedom from recurrent arch obstruction was 69% at 46 months' follow-up. These authors show extremely impressive results for this difficult group of patients. In particular, 8 patients with interrupted arch plus truncus arteriosus were operated with no mortality. There are very few, if any, survivors of this combination of defects reported in the literature. It is hopeful that these results can be duplicated by other groups.

References

1. Mühler EG, Engelhardt W, von Bernuth G: Detection of sinus venosus atrial septal defect by two-dimensional echocardiography. Eur Heart J (April) 1992;13:453–456.
2. Minich LA, Snider AR, Bove EL, Luppineti FM, Vermilion RP: Echocardiographic Evaluation of Atrioventricular Orifice Anatomy in Children with Atrioventricular Septal Defect. J Am Coll Cardiol (January) 1992;19:149–153.
3. Capouya ER, Laks H, Drinkwater DC, Pearl JM, Milgalter E: Management of the left atrioventricular valve in the repair of complete atrioventricular septal defects. J Thorac Cardiovasc Surg (July) 1992;104:196–203.
4. Trusler GA, Williams WG, Smallhorn JF, Freedom RM: Late Results after Repair of Aortic Insufficiency Associated with Ventricular Septal Defect. J Thorac Cardiovasc Surg (February) 1992;103:276–281.

5. Bonhoeffer P, Fabbrocini M, Lecompte Y, Cifarelli A, Ballerini L, Frigiola A, Menicanti L, Festa P: Infundibular septal defect with severe aortic regurgitation: a new surgical approach. An Thorac Surg (May) 1992;53:851–853.

6. Seraff A, Lacour-Gayet F, Bruniaux J, Ouaknine R, Losay J, Petit J, Binet J-P, Planché C: Surgical Management of Isolated Multiple Ventricular Septal Defects. J Thorac Cardiovasc Surg (March) 1992;103:437–443.

7. Hiraishi S, Agata Y, Nowartari M, Oguchi K, Misawa H, Hirota H, Fujino N, Horiguchi Y, Yashiro K, Nakae S: Incidence and Natural Course of Trabecular Ventricular Septal Defect: Two-Dimensional Echocardiography and Color Doppler Flow Imaging Study. J Pediatri (March) 1992;120:409–415.

8. Matitiau A, Geva T, Colan SD, Sluysmans T, Parness IA, Spevak PJ, van der Velde M, Mayer JE Jr, Sanders SP: Bulboventricular Foramen Size in Infants with Double-Inlet Left Ventricle or Tricuspid Atresia with Transposed Great Arteries: Influence on Initial Palliative Operation and Rate of Growth. J Am Coll Cardiol (January) 19:142–148.

9. O'Leary PW, Driscoll DJ, Connor AR, Puga FJ, Danielson GK: Subaortic obstruction in hearts with univentricular connection to a dominant left ventricle and an anterior subaortic outlet chamber. J Thorac Cardiovasc Surg (November) 1992;104:1231–1237.

10. Lacour-Gayet F, Seraff A. Fermont L, Bruniaux J, Rey C, Touchot A, Petit J, Planche C: Early palliation of univentricular hearts with subaortic stenosis and ventriculoarterial discordance. The arterial switch option. J Thorac Cardiovasc Surg (November) 1992;104:1238–1245.

11. O'Connor BK, Beekman RH, Lindauer A, Rocchini A: Intermediate-term outcome after pulmonary balloon valvuloplasty: comparison with a matched surgical control group. J Am Col Cardiol (July) 1992;20:169–173.

12. Marie PY, Marçon F, Brunotte F, Briançon S, Danchin N, Worms AM, Robert J, Pernot C: Right Ventricular Overload and Induced Sustained Ventricular Tachycardia in Operatively "Repaired" Tetralogy of Fallot, Am J Cardiol (March 15) 1992;69:785–789.

13. Kirklin JW, Blackstone EH, Jonas RA, Shimazaki Y, Kirklin JK, Mayer JE Jr, Pacifico AD, Castaneda AR: Morphologic and surgical determinants of outcome events after repair of tetralogy of Fallot and pulmonary stenosis. J Thorac Cardiovasc Surg (April) 1992;103:706–723.

14. Walen SA, Liu PP, Ross BL, Williams WG, Webb GD, McLaughlin PR: Serial follow-up of adults with repaired tetralogy of Fallot. J Am Coll Cardiol (August) 1992;20:295–300.

15. Giglia TM, Mandell VS, Connor AR, Mayer Jr JE, Lock JE: Diagnosis and management of right ventricle-dependent coronary circulation in pulmonary atresia with intact ventricular septum. Circulation (November) 1992;86:1516–1528.

16. Leung MP, Lo RNS, Cheung H, Lee J, Mok CK: Balloon valvuloplasty after pulmonary atresia and intact ventricular septum. Ann Thorac Surg (May) 1992; 53:864–870.

17. Steinberger J, Berry JM, Bass JL, Fokes JE, Braunlin EA, Krabill KA, Rocchini AP: Results of a right ventricular outflow patch for pulmonary atresia with intact ventricular septum. Circulation (November) 1992;86 (suppl II):II–167–II–175.

18. Laks H, Pearl JM, Drinkwater DC, Jarmakani J, Isabel-Jones J, George BL, Williams RG: Partial biventricular repair of pulmonary atresia with intact ventricular septum. Use of an adjustable atrial septal defect. Circulation (November) 1992;86 (Suppl II); II–159–II–166.

19. Albanese SB, Carotti A, Di Donata RM, Mazzera E, Troconis CJ, Giannico S, Picardo S, Marcelletti C: Bidirectional cavopulmonary anastomosis in patients under two years of age. J Thorac Cardiovasc Surg (October) 1992;104:904–909.

20. Schmidt KG, Cloez J-L, Silverman NH: Changes of right ventricular size and function in neonates after valvotomy for pulmonary atresia or critical pulmonary stenosis and intact ventricular septum. J Am Coll Cardiol (April) 1992;19:1032–1037.

21. de Begona JA, Kawaushi M, Fullerton D, Razzouk AJ, Gundry SR, Bailey LL: The Mustard procedure for correction of simple transposition of the great arteries before 1 month of age. J Thorac Cardiovasc Surg (November) 1992;104:1218–1224.

22. Chang AC, Wernovsky G, Wessel DL, Freed MD, Parness IA, Perry SB, O'Brien P, van Praagh R, Hanley FL, Jonas RA, Castaneda AR, Mayer Jr, JE: Surgical management of later right ventricular failure after Mustard or Senning Repair. Circulation (November) 1992;86 (suppl II);II–140–II–149.

23. Vouhé PR, Tamisier D, Leca F, Ouaknine R, Vernant F, Neveux J-Y: Transposition of the

Great Arteries, Ventricular Septal Defect, and Pulmonary Outflow Tract Obstruction. J. Thorac Cardiovasc Surg (March) 1992; 103:428–436.

24. Lupinetti FM, Bove EL, Minich L, Snider AR, Callow LB, Meliones JN, Crowley DC, Beekman RH, Serwer G, Dick II M, Vermilion R, Rosenthal A: Intermediate-term Survival and Functional Results after Arterial Repair for Transposition of the Great Arteries. J Thorac Cardiovasc Surg (March) 1992;103:421–427.

25. Baylen BG, Grzeszcak M, Gleason ME, Cyran SE, Weber HS, Myers J. Waldhausen J: Role of balloon atrial septostomy before early arterial switch repair of transposition of the great arteries. J Am Coll Cardiol (April) 1992;19:1025–1031.

26. Day RW, Laks H, Drinkwater DC: The influence of coronary anatomy on the arterial switch operation in neonates. J Thorac Cardiovasc Surg (September) 1992;104:706–712.

27. Kirklin JW, Blackstone EH, Tchervernkov CI, Castaneda AR, Congenital Heart Surgeons Society: Clinical outcomes after the arterial switch operation for transposition. Patient, support, procedural and institutional risk factors. Circulation (November) 1992;86:1501–1515.

28. Wernovsy G, Giglia TM, Jonas RA, Mone SM, Colan SD, Wessel DL: Course in the intensive care unit after "preparatory" pulmonary artery banding and aortopulmonary shunt placement for transposition of the great arteries with low left ventricular pressure. Circulation (November) 1992;86 (suppl II):II–133–II–139.

29. Gewillig M, Daenen W, Dumoulin M, de Hauwaert LV: Rheologic Genesis of Discrete Subvalvular Aortic Stenosis: A Doppler Echocardiographic Study. J Am Coll Cardiol (March 15) 1992;19:818–824.

30. Frommelt MA, Snider AR, Bove EL, Lupinetti F: Echocardiographic assessment of subvalvular aortic stenosis before and after operation. J Am Coll Cardiol (April) 1992;19:1018–1023.

31. De Vries AG, Hess J. Witsenburg M, Frohn-Mulder IME, Bogers AJJC, Bos E: Management of fixed subaortic stenosis: a retrospective study of 57 cases. J Am Coll Cardiol (April) 1992;19:1013-1017.

32. Park JK, Bell RD, Ellis K, Gersony WM: Surgical management of the infant with coarctation of the aorta and ventricular septal defect. J Am Coll Cardiol (July) 1992;20:176–180.

33. Minich LA, Beekman RH III, Rocchini AP, Heidelberger K, Bove EL: Surgical Repair is Safe and Effective after Unsuccessful Balloon Angioplasty of Native Coarctation of the Aorta. J Am Col Cardiol (February) 1992;19:389–393.

34. Anjos R, Qureshi SA, Rosenthal R, Murdoch I, Hayes A, Parsons J, Baker EJ, Tynan M: Determinants of Hemodynamic Results of Balloon Dilation of Aortic Recoarctation. Am J Cardiol (March 1) 1992;69:665–671.

35. Brouwer MHJ, Cromme-Dijkhuis AH, Ebels T, Eijgelaar A: Growth of the hypoplastic aortic arch after simple coarctation resection and end-to-end anastomosis. J Thorac Cardiovasc Surg (August) 1992;104:426–433.

36. Myers JL, McConnell BA, Waldhausen JA: Coarctation of the Aorta in Infants: Does the aortic arch grow after repair? Ann Thorac Surg (November) 1992;54:869–875.

37. Mendelsohn AM, Crowley DC, Lindauer A, Beekman III RH: Rapid progression of aortic aneurysms after patch aortoplasty repair of coarctation of the aorta. J Am Coll Cardiol (August) 1992;20:381–385.

38. Leandro J, Smallhorn, JR, Benson L, Musewe N, Balfe JW, Dyck JD, West L, Freedom R: Ambulatory blood pressure monitoring and left ventricular mass and function after successful surgical repair of coarctation of the aorta. J. Am Col Cardiol (July) 1992;20:197–204.

39. Seliem MA, Chin AJ, Norwood WI: Patterns of Anomalous Pulmonary Venous Connection/Drainage in Hypoplastic Left Heart Syndrome: Diagnostic Role of Doppler Color Flow Mapping and Surgical Implications. J Am Coll Cardiol (January) 1992;19:135–141.

40. Starnes VA, Griffin ML, Pitlick PT, Bernstein D, Baum D, Ivens K, Shumway NE: Current approach to hypoplastic left heart syndrome. Palliation, transplantation, or both? J Thorac Cardiovasc Surg (July) 1992;104:189–195.

41. Farrell PE Jr, Change AC, Murdison KA, Baffa JM, Norwood WI, Murphy JD: Outcome and Assessment after the Modified Fontan Procedure for Hypoplastic Left Heart Syndrome. Circulation (January) 85:16–122.

42. Gentles TL, Calder AL, Clarkson PM, Neutze M: Predictors of Long-Term Survival with Ebstein's Anomaly of the Tricuspid Valve. Am J Cardiol (February 1) 1992;69:377–381.

43. Celermajer DS, Cullen S, Sullivan ID, Spiegelhalter DJ, Wyse RKH, Deanfield JE: Outcome in neonates with Ebstein's anomaly. J Am Coll Cardiol (April) 1992;19:1041–1046.

44. Pressley JC, Wharton JM, Tang ASL, Lowe JE, Gallagher JJ, Prystowsky EN: Effect of Ebstein's Anomaly on Short- and Long-term Outcome of Surgically Treated Patients With Wolff-Parkinson-White Syndrome. Circulation 1992 (October);86:1147–1155.

45. Danielson GK, Driscoll DJ, Mair DD, Warnes CA, Oliver Jr WC: Operative treatment of Ebstein's anomaly. J Thorac Cardiovasc Surg (November) 1992;104:1195–1202.

46. Karr SS, Parness IA, Spevak PJ, van de Velde ME, Colan SD, Sanders SP: Diagnosis of anomalous left coronary artery by Doppler color flow mapping: distinction from other causes of dilated cardiomyopathy. J Am Coll Cardiol (May) 1992;19:1271–1275.

47. Sauer U, Stern H, Meisner H. Buhlmeyer K, Sebening F: Risk factors for perioperative mortality in children with anomalous origin of the left coronary artery from the pulmonary artery. J Thorac Cardiovasc Surg (September) 1992;104:696–705.

48. Vouhé PR, Tamisier D, Sidi D, Vernant F, Mauriat P, Pouard P, Leca F: Anomalous left coronary artery from the pulmonary artery: results of isolated aortic reimplantation. Ann Thorac Surg (October) 1992;54:621–627.

49. Roberts WC, Shirani J: The four subtypes of anomalous origin of the left main coronary artery from the right aortic sinus (or from the right coronary artery). Am J Cardiol 1992 (Jul 1); 70:119–121.

50. Roberts WC, Glick BN: Congenital hypoplasia of both right and left circumflex coronary arteries. Am J Cardiol 1992 (Jul 1);70:121–123.

51. Taylor AJ, Rogan KM, Virmani R. Sudden cardiac death associated with isolated congenital coronary artery anomalies. J Am Coll Cardiol 1992 (September);20:640–7.

52. European Registry: Transcatheter occlusion of persistent arterial duct. Lancet 1992 (Oct 31);340:1062–1066.

53. Driscoll DJ, Offord KP, Feldt RH, Schaff HV, Puga FJ, Danielson GK: Five- to Fifteen-Year Follow-up after Fontan Operation. Circulation (February) 1992;85:469–496.

54. Weber HS, Gleason MM, Myers JL, Waldhausen JA, Cryan SE, Baylen BG: The Fontan Operation in Infants Less than 2 Years of Age. J Am Coll Cardiol (March 15) 1992;19:828–833.

55. Culbertson CB, George BL, Day RW, Laks H, Williams RG: Factors influencing survival of patients with heterotaxy syndrome undergoing the Fontan procedure. J Am Coll Cardiol (September) 1992;20:678–684.

56. Mayer JE Jr, Bridges ND, Lock JE, Hanley FL, Jonas RA, Castaneda AR: Factors Associated with Marked Reduction in Mortality for Fontan Operations in Patients with Single Ventricle. J Thorac Cardiovasc Surg (March) 1992;103:444–452.

57. Akagi T, Benson LN, Green M, Ash J, Gilday DL, Williams WG, Freedom RM: Ventricular performance before and after Fontan repair for univentricular atrioventricular connection: angiographic and radionuclide assessment. J Am Coll Cardiol (October) 1992;20:920–926.

58. Sluysmans T, Sanders SP, van der Velde M, Matitiau A, Parness IA, Spevak PJ, Mayer JE Jr, Colan SD: Natural history and patterns of recovery of contractile function in single left ventricle after Fontan operation. Circulation (December) 1992;86:1753–1761.

59. Malcic I, Sauer U, Stern H, Kellerer M, Kuhlein B, Locher D, Buhlmeyer K, Sebening F: The influence of pulmonary artery banding on outcome after the Fontan operation. J Thorac Cardiovasc Surg (September) 1992;104:743–747.

60. Kopf GS, Kleinman CS, Hijazi ZM, Fahey JT, Dewar ML, Hellenbrand WE: Fenestrated Fontan operation with delayed transcatheter closure of atrial septal defect. J Thorac Cardiovasc Surg (June) 1992;103:1039–1048.

61. Mavroudis C, Zales VR, Backer CL, Muster AJ, Latson LA: Fenestrated Fontan with delayed catheter closure. Effects of volume loading and baffle fenestration on cardiac index and oxygen delivery. Circulation (November) 1992; 86 (suppl II): II–85–II–92.

62. Bridges ND, Mayer JE Jr, Lock JE, Jonas RA, Hanley FL, Keane JF, Perry SB, Castaneda AR: Effect of baffle fenestration on outcome of the modified Fontan operation. Circulation (December) 1992;86:1762–1769.

63. Gewillig M, Wyse RK, de Leval MR, Deanfield JE: Early and Late Arrhythmias after the Fontan Operation: Predisposing Factors and Clinical Consequences. Br Heart J (January) 1992;67:72–79.

64. Peters NS and Somerville J: Arrhythmias after the Fontan procedure. Br Heart J (August);68:199–204.

65. Fogel MA, Chin AJ: Imaging of pulmonary venous pathway obstruction in patients after the modified Fontan procedure. J Am Coll Cardiol (July) 1992;20:181–190.

66. Razzouk AJ, Freedom RM, Cohen AJ, Williams WG, Trusler GA, Coles JG, Burrows PE, Rebeyka IM: The recognition, identification of morphologic substrate, and treatment of subaortic stenosis after Fontan operation. J Thorac Cardiovasc Surg (October) 1992;104:938–944.

67. El Habbal MH: Cardiovascular manifestations of Marfan's Syndrome in the Young. Am Heart J (March) 1992;123:752–757.

68. Cassidy SC, Schmidt KG, van Hare GF, Stanger P, Teitel DF: Complications of pediatric cardiac catheterization: a 3-year study. J Am Col Cardiol (May) 1992;19:1285–1983.

69. Grifka RG, O'Laughlin MP, Nihill MR, Mullins CE: Double-Transseptal, Double-Balloon Valvuloplasty for Congenital Mitral Stenosis. Circulation (January) 1992;85:123–129.

70. Hosking MCK, Benson LN, Nakanishi T. Burrows PE, Williams WG, Freedom RM: Intravascular stent prothesis for right ventricular outflow obstruction. J Am Coll Cardiol (August) 1992;20:373–380.

71. Cleveland DC, Williams WG, Razzouk AJ, Trusler GA, Rebeyka IM, Duffy L, Kan Z, Coles JG, Freedom RM: Failure of cyropreserved homograft valved conduits in the pulmonary circulation. Circulation (November 1992);86 (suppl II);II–150–II–153.

72. Frommelt PC, Lupinetti FM, Bove EL: Aortoventriculoplasty in infants and children. Circulation (November) 1992;86 (suppl II);II–176–II–180.

73. Karl TR, Sano S, Brawn W, Mee RBB: Repair of hypoplastic or interrupted aortic arch via sternotomy. J Thorac Cardiovasc Surg (September) 1992;104:688–695.

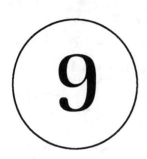

Congestive Heart Failure

Prevalence in the USA

Schocken and associates[1] in Tampa, Florida, studied the prevalence and mortality rate of patients with CHF in noninstitutionalized men and women in the USA. CHF data were collected from the National Health and Nutrition Examination Survey from 1971 to 1975 and were used to determine the prevalence of CHF on the basis of both self-reported and clinical definitions. Mortality data were derived from the National Health and Nutrition Examination Survey Epidemiologic Follow-up Study conducted from 1982 to 1986. The prevalence of self-reported CHF approximated 1% of the noninstitutionalized U.S. adult population. The prevalence of CHF based on clinical criteria was 2%. Thus, these estimates suggest that between 1 and 2 million adults are affected. Mortality at 10 and 15 years for those with CHF increases in gradual fashion with increasing age, with men more likely to die than women (Figure 9-1). In the group ≥55 years of age, the 15-year total mortality rate was 39% for women and 72% for men. Thus, CHF is a common problem in the USA with significant prevalence and mortality, both of which increase with advancing age.

Prognostic indicators

In an investigation by Parameshwar and associates[2] from London, UK, 127 patients with chronic CHF were studied to identify parameters predictive of prognosis. Patients were followed for a mean of 15 months. The group as a whole had severe ventricular dysfunction with a median EF of 17% and a median peak rate of oxygen consumption of 14 ml/kg/min. During the follow-up period 23 patients (18%) died and 18 (14%) underwent cardiac transplantation. The effect of the following variables

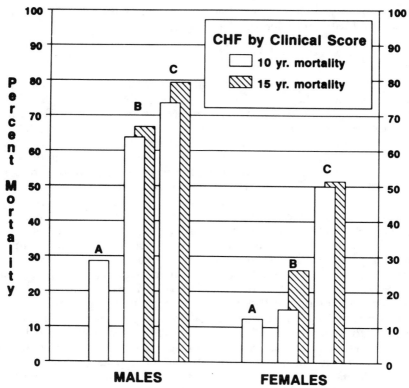

Fig. 9-1. Ten- and fifteen-year mortality of congestive heart failure (CHF) assessed by score (≥3). A = 25 to 54 years, B = 55 to 64 years, C = 65 to 74 years. Reproduced with permission from Schocken, et al.[1]

on outcome (death or transplantation) were examined: age, cause of heart failure, cardiothoracic ratio on chest radiography, LV end-systolic dimension on echocardiography, LVEF on radionuclide ventriculography, mean dose of diuretic, plasma sodium and urea concentrations, and peak oxygen consumption during exercise. Although all variables except cause of CHF affected outcome on univariate analysis, multivariate analysis identified 3 variables that were statistically significant and independent predictors of outcome. In order of importance these were plasma sodium level, LVEF and peak oxygen consumption. Even in this group of patients with severe CHF, these variables were predictive of outcome.

To determine the prognostic significance of asymptomatic LV dilatation and LV dysfunction, Lauer and associates[3] from Boston and Framingham, Massachusetts, followed 1,493 men who were free of symptomatic cardiovascular disease by M-mode echocardiography for a mean of 4.15 years. At baseline examination, 170 men (11.4%) had an abnormally high end-diastolic LV internal dimension (≥56 mm) and 76 (5.1%) had an abnormally low fractional shortening (≤30%). During the follow-up period, 68 men experienced 92 cardiovascular disease events. After adjusting for age and traditional cardiovascular disease risk factors in proportional-hazards analyses, fractional shortening was a significant independent predictor of cardiovascular risk. Increased risk was also associated with combinations of low fractional shortening and high end-diastolic internal dimension and with low percent fractional shortening with LV hypertrophy. In conclusion, subclinical LV dilatation and LV systolic dysfunction, although uncommon in men free of overt cardiovascular disease, are associated with increased risk for new cardiovascular disease events.

Cardiac arrest

Cardiac arrest in patients with CHF may be the result of remediable factors such as pulmonary edema, drug toxicity, or electrolyte abnormalities, or it may be due to primary arrhythmias. The relation of prior aborted cardiac arrest or sustained VT to subsequent prognosis was assessed in 458 consecutive patients referred for management of advanced CHF (LVEF 0.2 ± 0.07) in an investigation carried out by Stevenson and associates[4] from Los Angeles, California. All patients received tailored vasodilator and diuretic therapy and were then followed as outpatients. Patients were divided into 4 groups: 388 patients (85%) with no prior cardiac arrest or sustained VT, 31 patients (7%) with a primary arrhythmia cardiac arrest, 22 patients (5%) with a secondary cardiac arrest, and 27 patients (4%) with sustained VT without cardiac arrest. Patients with cardiac arrest resulting from a primary arrhythmia were usually treated with antiarrhythmic drugs (25 patients), and 5 patients received an implantable defibrillator. After hospital discharge actuarial 1-year sudden death risk (17%) and total mortality (24%) rates for the group with primary arrhythmia were similar to corresponding values in patients with no history of cardiac arrest or sustained VT (17% and 30%, respectively). In patients with a secondary cardiac arrest as a result of exacerbation of CHF (11 patients), torsade de pointes (10 patients), or hypokalemia (1 patient), therapy focused on removal of aggravating factors. Actuarial 1-year sudden death (39%) and total mortality (54%) rates for the group with secondary arrest were higher than for patients without a history of cardiac arrest. Patients with sustained VT without cardiac arrest tended to have less severe heart failure, and only 1 of these 17 patients died suddenly for an actuarial 1-year mortality rate of 6%. Multivariate analysis identified a history of secondary cardiac arrest as a predictor of sudden death and total mortality independent of LVEF, PA wedge pressure, AF, type of vasodilator, and serum sodium level. Thus the prognosis for survivors of life-threatening arrhythmias who have advanced CHF varies. Patients who have had primary arrhythmias treated with available therapies have a prognosis similar to that in patients without prior cardiac arrest who have a comparable severity of CHF. Cardiac arrest as a result of remediable factors is indicative of a high risk despite attempts to control the precipitating factors. Patients with CHF who have sustained VT without cardiac arrest have a relatively favorable outcome.

Atrial natriuretic factor

To develop a noninvasive clinical predictive model for acute CHF in a frail elderly cohort using bedise clinical assessment (history and physical examination) and venous atrial natriuretic peptide (ANP) levels, Davis and associates[5] from Boston, Massachusetts, performed a 1-year prospective blinded cohort study involving 331 frail elderly volunteers free of acute illness at study entry. Their mean age was 88 ± 7 years and 23% were men. The main outcome measure was clinical episodes of CHF with confirmation of acute pulmonary edema by chest roentgenogram. Fifteen percent of the elderly cohort developed at least 1 episode of CHF during the 1-year follow-up period. Those developing CHF had significantly higher mean ± SE ANP values at study entry: 493 ± 55 vs 207 ± 15 pmol/

L. The risk for development of CHF rose progressively with increasing ANP levels at study entry. In multivariate analysis, only 2 independent variables significantly predicted CHF: ANP value greater than 200 pmol/ L and history of CHF in the previous year. Stratifying the cohort by these 2 variables results in 3 CHF risk groups: 55% of the population at 3% annual risk of CHF, 37% of the population at 20% to 24% annual risk of CHF, and 8% of the population at 66% annual risk of CHF. This simple clinical prediction model identifies elderly subjects at risk for CHF and allows appropriate focusing of medical resources for prevention, early detection, and treatment of this highly morbid clinical syndrome.

Semigran and associates[6] in Boston, Massachusetts, assessed the direct effects of atrial natriuretic peptide on myocardial function in 10 patients with CHF. Mean arterial pressure decreased with atrial natriuretic peptide from 89 ± 3 to 80 ± 2 mm Hg. LV end diastolic pressure also decreased with atrial natriuretic peptide from 24 ± 2 to 16 ± 3 mm Hg. Cardiac index increased during infusion of atrial natriuretic peptide from 2.0 ± 0.2 to 2.4 ± 0.2 liters/min per m² whereas heart rate did not change. In comparison, mean arterial pressure decreased by a greater amount with nitroprusside 90 ± 4 to 73 ± 3 mm Hg, as did left ventricular end diastolic pressure while heart rate increased slightly. Cardiac index increased following nitroprusside by an amount similar to that seen with atrial natriuretic factor. Peak positive first derivative of LV pressure, ejection fraction, and stroke work index were unchanged by both agents. Both atrial natriuretic peptide and nitroprusside shortened the time constant of isovolumetric relaxation, but only nitroprusside shortened the time constant calculated by the derivative method. Atrial natriuretic peptide did not shift the end diastolic pressure-volume point away from the relation constructed from baseline and nitroprusside points. The relationship between end systolic pressure and volume during atrial natriuretic peptide administration was shifted slightly leftward from the baseline value in four patients, slightly rightward in 4, and not at all in 1 patient, indicating no consistent inotropic effect. These data suggest that atrial natriuretic peptide has no direct effect on myocardial contractile or diastolic function in patients with CHF.

In an investigation by Lewis and associates[7] from Haifa, Israel, atrial natriuretic peptide levels were measured in 17 patients with severe CHF (New York Heart Association functional class IV) and the response of the peptide was studied during changes in cardiac filling pressures induced by a 24-hour infusion of nitroglycerin. In the control state plasma atrial natriuretic peptide levels (687 ± 551 pg/ml) were 10-fold normal. During the administration of nitroglycerin, natriuretic peptide levels decreased with changes matching very closely the decreases in PA wedge pressure and RA pressure, a 1% mean decrease in the peptide level for every 1.5 to 2% mean change in atrial filling pressures. In patients with hemodynamic tolerance to constant-dose nitroglycerin infusion, the resulting increase in atrial pressures was accompanied by an appropriate secondary increase in the plasma atrial natriuretic peptide level. During the 24-hour study period there was a direct linear relationship between both PA wedge pressure and RA pressure and the plasma atrial natriuretic peptide level, with a zero-pressure atrial natriuretic peptide intercept near normal. The findings were no different in a subgroup of 5 patients receiving simultaneous treatment with captopril, except that plasma renin activity was higher and the aldosterone level lower than in the control group by a factor of approximately 2.5. The close relationship and tracking of atrial pressure and natriuretic peptide curves suggested that the sensitivity of the atrial stretch response to changes in atrial filling pressures was maintained in severe CHF.

With normal systolic function

CHF is typically associated with impaired LV systolic function. Few reports exist describing the long-term outcome in patients with CHF and normal LV systolic function. Setaro and associates[8] from New Haven, Connecticut, followed 52 patients initially hospitalized with CHF and intact LV function (EF >45%) for 7 years. Mean age when initially identified was 71 ± 11 years (range 36 to 96), and average LVEF was 61 ± 11%. CHF was graded by a clinicoradiographic index, with a mean of 7.0 ± 2.3 (range 3 to 12, 13 indicates worst CHF). A third heart sound was present in 19 patients (37%), and 17 (33%) had presented with acute pulmonary edema. Principal cardiovascular diagnoses were CAD in 27 (52%), hypertensive heart disease in 16 (31%) and restrictive cardiomyopathy in 7 (13%). At 7 years, cardiovascular mortality was 46% (24 of 52), and noncardiovascular mortality was 10% (5 of 52). Survival was not correlated with age, principal diagnosis, third heart sound, pulmonary edema at presentation, LVEF, or presence or degree of LV diastolic dysfunction. Cardiovascular morbidity, consisting of nonfatal recurrent CHF, AMI, unstable angina or other cardiovascular events occurred in 29% (15 of 52). Combined cardiovascular mortality and morbidity was 75% (39 of 52). In patients with CHF, intact LV systolic function does not confer the same favorable prognosis it defines in other clinical situations. For such patients, the risk of future cardiovascular events is high, a finding that should be considered when designing therapeutic strategies in this group.

TREATMENT

Review

An excellent review of both the pathophysiology[9] and treatment[10] of chronic CHF was provided by Milton Packer and it appeared in the July 11, 1992, issue of *Lancet* (Table 9-1).

Captopril

Neurohormonal activation has major impact on the pathophysiology of CHF. The Munich Mild Heart Failure Trial was designed to test the hypothesis that interference with the reninangiotensin system by antiotensin converting enzyme inhibition favorably influences the natural history of CHF.[11] A total of 170 patients, median New York Heart Association class II, were randomized to double blind treatment with 25 mg captopril twice a day or placebo in addition to standard treatment for a median observation period of 2.7 years. The main outcome measures were progression of CHF to New York Heart Association class IV on an optimally adjusted standard treatment, death due to progressive CHF and sudden death (Figure 9-2). CHF progressed to class IV in 9 patients (10.8%) treated with captopril and in 23 patients (26.4%) treated with placebo. The mean survival time until this end point was 223 days longer in the captopril group (Kaplan-Meier life table analysis). Also, progressive deterioration

TABLE 9-1. *Effects of Therapeutic Interventions on Symptoms and Survival. Reproduced with permission from Packer.*[10]

Agent	Effect on symptoms	Effect on survival
Diuretics		
Thiazide/loop diuretics	Favourable	Unknown
Atriopeptidase inhibitors	Unknown	Unknown
Direct-acting vasodilators		
Nitrates+hydralazine	Equivocal	Probably favourable
Minoxidil	Adverse	Probably adverse
Calcium channel blockers	Adverse	Adverse
Flosequinan	Favourable	Unknown
Amlodipine/felodipine	Favourable	Unknown
Positive inotropic agents		
Beta-adrenergic agonists	No effect	Adverse
Phosphodiesterase inhibitors	Equivocal	Adverse
Digitalis	Favourable	Unknown
Pimobendan	Favourable	Unknown
Neurohormonal antagonists		
Converting-enzyme inhibitors	Favourable	Favourable
Alpha-adrenergic blockers	No effect	No effect
Beta-adrenergic blockers	Favourable	Possibly favourable

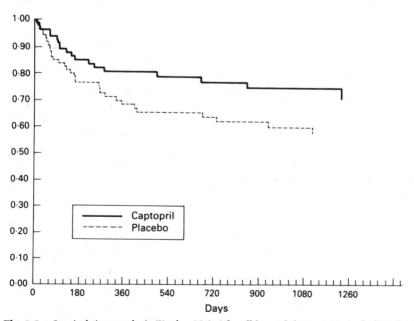

Fig. 9-2. Survival time analysis (Kaplan-Meier) for all heart failure events including death due to progressive heart failure, sudden death, and progression of heart failure to NYHA class IV. Reproduced with permission from Kleber, et. al.[11]

to severe CHF was a powerful predictor of total mortality and death from CHF; 80% of deaths due to progressive CHF occurred after this end point. There were fewer deaths caused by progressive CHF in the captopril group than in the placebo group (4 v 11) but similar numbers of sudden deaths (11 v 10). Progressive CHF was the cause of death in 18.2% of all deaths in the captopril group and 50% in the placebo group. Total CHF events (the end point on which power calculation was based) were also more common in the placebo group (19 v 32 events) but not significantly so. Total mortality was similar to both groups (22 of 83 v 22 of 87). Angiotensin converting enzyme inhibition in conjunction with standard therapy early in the course of CHF slowed the progress of CHF and thus favorably altered the natural history of the disease.

Enalapril

All surviving patients in a double-blind study comparing the effects of enalapril and placebo on survival and severe CHF were recommended to be treated with active drug after stopping the trial. Kjekshus and associates[12] for the Consensus Trial Group analyzed 2-year follow-up from the end of the blinded trial and found that among 77 survivors of 127 patients originally allocated to the group with enalapril that 38 were still alive. Of 126 patients allegated to the group with placebo, 58 survived the blinded study, and after 2-year follow-up 26 were still alive. Thus, the difference between the original treatment groups remained, despite that treatment with enalapril was made available to all surviving patients and that those in the group with enalapril were sicker at baseline than those in the group with placebo. If enalapril was prescribed, the mortality was 47% compared with 75% if it was not. Life-table analysis suggests a marked carry-over effect of treatment in the group with enalapril that lasted for up to 15 months before mortality rates became comparable in the 2 treatment groups. This strongly suggests that enalapril confers structural protection to the failing myocardium.

Kinstam and associates[13] for the SOLVD Investigators examined hemodynamic determinants of clinical status in patients with LV systolic dysfunction. Preload reserve—LV distension during exercise—was related to clinical status, and the effect of enalapril was examined in 97 patients with EF <0.35 who were enrolled in the trial, Studies of Left Ventricular Dysfunction (SOLVD). Sixty-one asymptomatic patients (group I) were compared with 36 patients with symptomatic heart failure (group II). Radionuclide LV volumes were measured at rest and during maximal cycle exercise. Group II patients had higher resting heart rates, end-diastolic and end-systolic volumes, and lower EF. During exercise, only patients in group I had increased stroke volume (from 35 ± 8 to 39 ± 11 ml/m² [mean $\pm$ SD]) due to an increase in end-diastolic volume (from 119 ± 29 to 126 ± 29 ml/m²), contributing to a greater increase in LV minute output. After administration of intravenous enalapril (1.25 mg), LV end-diastolic volume response to exercise was augmented in group II (rest, 140 ± 42; exercise, 148 ± 43 ml/m²) and LV output response increased slightly. Thus, in patients with asymptomatic systolic dysfunction, recruitment of preload during exercise is responsible for maintaining a stroke volume contribution to the cardiac output response. In patients with symptomatic CHF preload reserve is absent, and the cardiac output response depends solely on heart rate. Enalapril may augment preload reserve.

In patients with CHF, activation of the renin-angiotensin system is common and has been postulated to provide a stimulus for further LV structural and functional derangement. Konstam and SOLVD investigators[14] in Boston, Massachusetts tested the hypothesis that chronic administration of the angiotensin converting enzyme inhibitor enalapril prevents or reverses LV dilatation and systolic dysfunction among patients with depressed EF and symptomatic CHF. The investigators examined subsets of patients enrolled in the Treatment Trail of Studies of Left Ventricular Dysfunction (SOLVD). Fifty-six patients with mild to moderate CHF underwent serial radionuclide ventriculograms, and 16 underwent serial left heart catheterizations, before and after randomization to enalapril (2.5-20 mg per day) or placebo. At 1 year, there were significant treatment differences in LV end-diastolic volume, end-systolic volume, and EF. These effects resulted from increases in end-diastolic volume and end-systolic volume in the placebo group and decreases in end-diastolic volume and end-systolic volume in the enalapril group (Figure 9-3). Mean LVEF increased in enalapril patients from 0.25 to 0.29. There was a significant treatment difference in LV end-diastolic pressure at 1

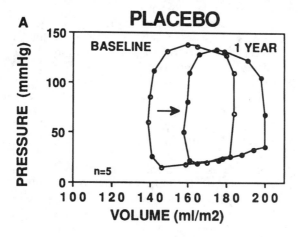

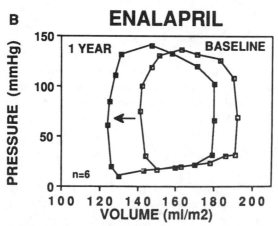

Fig. 9-3. Mean left ventricular pressure-volume loops at baseline and 1 year in patients randomized to placebo (panel A) and to enalapril (panel B). At 1 year, the entire curve was shifted to the right for the placebo group and to the left for the enalapril group. Reproduced with permission from Konstam, et al.[14]

year, with changes paralleling those of end-diastolic volume. The time constant of LV relaxation changed only in the placebo group. Serial radio-nuclide studies over a period of 33 months showed increases in LV volumes only in the placebo group. Two weeks after withdrawal of enalapril, end-diastolic volume and end-systolic volume increased to baseline levels but not to the higher levels observed with placebo. In patients with CHF and reduced LVEF, chronic angiotensin converting enzyme inhibition with enalapril prevents progressive LV dilatation and systolic dysfunction. These effects probably result from a combination of altered remodeling and sustained reduction in preload and afterload.

Ljungman and associates[15] for the CONSENSUS Trial Group studied the effect on renal function of long-term treatment with either enalapril (n = 123) or placebo (n = 120) in addition to conventional therapy in a randomized trial in patients with severe CHF (New York Heart Association functional class IV; the Cooperative North Scandinavian Enalapril Survival Study). Enalapril was administered in a dose of 2.5 to 40 mg/day. The analysis was restricted to the first 6 months of treatment. There was an average initial increase of 10 to 15% (10 to 20 umol/liter) irrespective of baseline serum creatinine within the first 3 weeks of enalapril treatment, whereafter mean serum creatinine remained on a similar level during the first 6 months. Enalapril was well-tolerated by most patients, and serum creatinine was reduced in 24%. Serum creatinine increased by 100% in 13 patients (11%) in the enalapril group (mainly as a consequence of intercurrent disease or severe hypotension, and usually transiently) and in 4 (3%) in the placebo group. The maximal increase in serum creatinine in the enalapril group was inversely correlated to the diastolic BP at baseline and to the mean diastolic and systolic BP measured at the time of the maximal increase in serum creatinine. According to multivariate regression analysis, the maximal increase in serum creatinine was also slightly influenced by the dose of furosemide taken. The development of hypotension emerged as the strongest factor explaining an abnormal increase in serum creatinine. Patients with marked reduction of baseline glomerular filtration rate had an increased risk of developing hypotension. Therefore, low beginning doses of enalapril and monitoring of BP and serum creatinine are recommended in patients with severe heart failure, especially in those with marked reduction of glomerular filtration rate and in those expected to have an excessive stimulation of the renin-angiotensin system.

It is not known whether the treatment of patients with asymptomatic LV dysfunction reduces mortality and morbidity. The SOLVD Investigators[16] studied the effect of enalapril on total mortality and mortality from cardiovascular causes, the development of CHF, and hospitalization for CHF among patients with an EF of 0.35 or less and who were not receiving drug treatment for CHF. Patients were randomly assigned to receive either placebo (n = 2,117) or enalapril (n = 2,111) at doses of 2.5 to 20 mg per day in a double-blind trial. Follow-up averaged 37.4 months. There were 334 deaths in the placebo group, as compared with 313 in the enalapril group (reduction in risk, 8%) (Figure 9-4). The reduction in mortality from cardiovascular causes was larger but was not statistically significant (298 deaths in the placebo group vs 265 in the enalapril group; risk reduction, 12%) (Figure 9-5). When the authors combined patients in whom CHF developed and those who died, the total number of deaths and cases of CHF was lower in the enalapril group than in the placebo group (630 vs 818; risk reduction, 29%). In addition, fewer patients given enalapril died or were hospitalized for CHF (434 in the enalapril group vs 518 in the

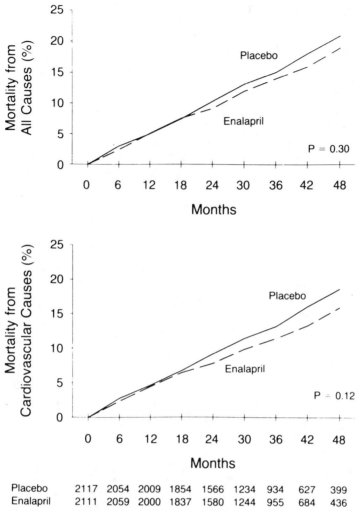

Placebo	2117	2054	2009	1854	1566	1234	934	627	399
Enalapril	2111	2059	2000	1837	1580	1244	955	684	436

Fig. 9-4. Total Mortality (Upper Panel) and Mortality from Cardiovascular Causes (Lower Panel) in the Prevention Trial. The numbers at the bottom of the figure are the numbers of patients in each group who were alive at base line and after each six-month period. Reproduced with permission from SOLVD Investigators.[16]

placebo group; risk reduction 20%) (Figure 9-6). The angiotensin-converting-enzyme inhibitor enalapril significantly reduced the incidence of CHF and the rate of related hospitalizations, as compared with the rates in the group given placebo, among patients with asymptomatic LV dysfunction. There was also a trend toward fewer deaths due to cardiovascular causes among the patients who received enalapril.

Angioedema with ACE inhibitors

To evaluate and describe the clinical course of angioedema reactions induced by angiotensin converting enzyme (ACE) inhibitors, Hedner and associates[17] from Goteborg, Sweden, reviewed all reports of angioedema reactions associated with ACE inhibitors submitted to Swedish Adverse Reactions Advisory Committee. The numbers of cases judged to be in-

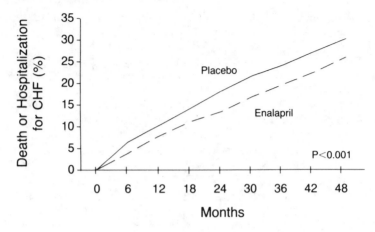

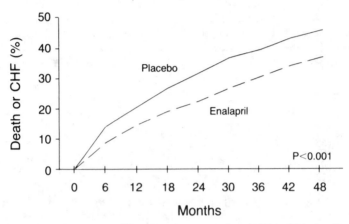

Fig. 9-5. Death or Hospitalization for Congestive Heart Failure (CHF) and Death or Development of Heart Failure in the Prevention Trial. See Figure 9-4 for the numbers of patients at risk at each time point. Reproduced with permission from SOLVD Investigators.[16]

duced by ACE inhibitors were related to their annual usage, estimated from total sales of defined daily doses, as well as to the estimated number of new patients. All cases of angioedema associated with ACE inhibitors reported to the World Health Organization's international drug information system also were summarized. Of the 38 reported cases in Sweden between 1981 and 1990, 36 were judged to be related to ACE inhibitors. During 1981 through 1990, altogether 1,309 cases of angioedema associated with ACE inhibitors were registered with the international drug information system. The incidence of reported cases of angioedema increased largely in parallel with the increased sales (usage) of ACE inhibitors. Of the 36 Swedish patients, 77% experienced the reaction within the first 3 weeks after starting treatment. Ten patients needed hospitalization, 2 of whom had life threatening laryngeal obstruction. With 1 exception all 36 patients were free of symptoms within 1 week after discontinuing the drug. Angioedema induced by antiotensin converting enzyme inhibitors is a rare but potentially life threatening reaction, which in most instances occurs shortly after the start of treatment. Any patient in whom the reaction is suspected should have the treatment interrupted and, if necessary, be admitted for observation.

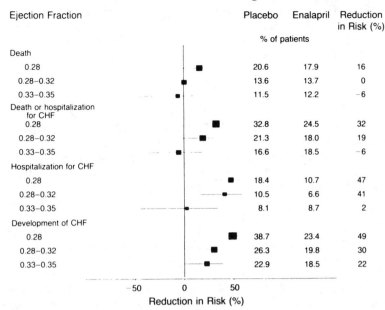

Fig. 9-6. Effect of Enalapril on Mortality, Incidence of Congestive Heart Failure (CHF), and Hospitalization for Heart Failure in Various Subgroups Defined According to the Ejection Fraction. Each subgroup composes one third of the study population. For each subgroup, the reduction in risk with enalapril is shown as a percentage (squares). (A negative value for risk reduction indicates an increase in risk.) The horizontal lines indicate the 95 percent confidence intervals. The size of each square is proportional to the number of events in the subgroup. The vertical line corresponds to a finding of no effect. The chi-square statistic for the interaction of the ejection fraction with the effect of enalapril on the risk of death was 2.16 (P = 0.34); that for the interaction of the effect of enalapril on the combined end point of death or hospitalization for CHF was 9.30 (P = 0.009); that for the interaction with its effect on hospitalization for CHF alone, 8.76 (P = 0.012); and that for the interaction with its effect on the development of CHF, 9.87 (P = 0.007). Reproduced with permission from SOLVD Investigators.[16]

Nitrates

To evaluate the therapeutic potential of organic nitrates in patients with chronic CHF already treated with angiotensin-converting enzyme (ACE) inhibitors, Mehra and associates[18] from Los Angeles, California, studied the temporal hemodynamic effects of oral isosorbide dinitrate, 40-120 mg administered every 6 hours to 11 nitrate responders who had been treated with captopril 89 ± 32 mg/day. The administration of isosorbide dinitrate resulted in a significant decline in mean right atrial pressure, from 13 cant decline in mean right atrial pressure, from 13 ± 6 mm Hg at baseline (mean value of measurements performed every 2 hours for 24 hours with captopril therapy) to 9 ± 4 mm Hg at 1 hour with persistent effect for most of the study period. Mean pulmonary artery pressure decreased from 38 ± 7 mm Hg at baseline to 29 ± 9 mm Hg at 1 hour, with effect persisting for 24 hours. Mean pulmonary artery wedge pressure also decreased from 24 ± 6 to 15 ± 7 mm Hg at 1 hour and remained significantly reduced for 20 hours. Systemic BP demonstrated a transient decrease lasting 2 hours after initiation of therapy which was asymptomatic in all patients. The results of this study demonstrate a preserved vasodilatory effect of organic nitrates in patients already treated with ACE inhibitors. Nitrates mediated improvement in right and left ventricular filling pressures, and reduction of pulmonary hypertension demonstrates a rationale for the use of these therapeutic methods in combination and suggest the need for long-term evaluation of the effect of nitrate therapy in patients with chronic CHF already treated with ACE inhibitors.

Metoprolol

In an investigation carried out by Paolisso and colleagues[19] from Naples, Italy, 10 patients with CHF were given metoprolol (50 mg/day) or placebo during a double-blind, crossover, randomized study. After a run-in period of 4 weeks, metoprolol and placebo were administered over a period of 3 months, which was separated by a washout period of 4 weeks. At the end of the run-in, metoprolol, and placebo periods, all patients underwent metabolic (oral glucose tolerance and hyperinsulinemic glucose clamp tests) and noninvasive cardiologic (New York Heart Association classification, bimodal echocardiographic LV end-diastolic determination, maximal oxygen consumption, LV radionuclide EF) tests. The results show that beta-adrenergic blockade significantly enhances insulin-mediated suppression of hepatic glucose output and increase in glucose uptake with a concurrent improvement in New York Heart Association functional class and the multistage exercise treadmill test score. After administration of metoprolol all changes in glucose turnover parameters were found to correlate with the decrease in basal plasma free fatty acid levels. In conclusions, these findings confirm the beneficial cardiologic effects of beta-adrenergic blockade in CHF and demonstrate that metoprolol is also useful for reversing the metabolic damage caused by exaggerated plasma norepinephrine levels.

Methoxamine

Bronchial hyperresponsiveness to cholinergic stimuli such as the inhalation of methacholine is common in patients with impaired LV function. Such hyperresponsiveness is best explained by cholinergic vasodilation of blood vessels in the small airways, with extravasation of plasma due to high LV filling pressure. Because this vasodilation may be prevented by the inhalation of the vasoconstrictor agent methoxamine, Cabanes and associates[20] from Paris, France, studied the effect of methoxamine on exercise performance in patients with chronic LV dysfunction. The authors studied 19 patients with a mean LVEF of $22 \pm 4\%$ and moderate exertional dyspnea. In the first part of the study, the authors performed treadmill exercise tests in 10 patients (group 1) at a constant maximal workload to assess the effects of 10 mg of inhaled methoxamine on the duration of exercise (a measure of endurance). In the second part of the study, the authors used a graded exercise protocol in 9 additional patients (group 2) to assess the effects of inhaled methoxamine on maximal exercise capacity and oxygen consumption. Both studies were carried out after the patients inhaled methoxamine or placebo given according to a randomized, double-blind, crossover design. In group 1, the mean duration of exercise increased from 293 ± 136 seconds after the inhalation of placebo to 612 ± 257 seconds after the inhalation of methoxamine. In group 2, exercise time (a measure of maximal exercise capacity) increased from 526 ± 236 seconds after placebo administration to 578 ± 255 seconds after methoxamine, and peak oxygen consumption increased from 18.5 ± 6.0 to 20.0 ± 6.0 ml per minute per kilogram of body weight. The inhalation of methoxamine enhanced exercise performance in patients with chronic LV dysfunction. However, the improvement in the duration of exercise at a constant workload (endurance) was much more than the improvement in maximal exercise capacity assessed with a progressive workload. These data suggest that exercise-induced vasodilation of airway vessels may contribute to exertional dyspnea in such patients.

Pimobendan

Pimobendan, a new oral cardiotonic and vasodilator agent, increases myocardial contractile force through specific inhibition of phosphodiesterase type III and increased calcium sensitivity of the myocardial contractile elements. Katz and associates[21] from Bronx, New York, Minneapolis, Minnesota, Philadelphia, Pennsylvania, and Ridgefield, Connecticut, studied the effects of pimobendan on LV performance and maximal exercise capacity in a multicenter, randomized, double-blind, placebo-controlled trial involving 52 patients with severe CHF despite diuretics, digoxin, and angiotensin-converting enzyme inhibitors. The acute hemodynamic evaluation included 3 single doses of 2.5, 5.0 and 10.0 mg of oral pimobendan, which was subsequently administered at a daily dose of 5 or 10 mg for 4 weeks. Acute administration of pimobendan significantly increased the resting cardiac index and lowered pulmonary capillary wedge pressure in a dose-dependent manner, whereas heart rate and systemic arterial pressure were not substantially altered. Patients receiving pimobendan, 5 and 10 mg daily, had a significantly greater increase in maximal exercise duration than those receiving placebo, that is, 144 ± 30 and 124 ± 33 seconds versus 58 ± 25 seconds. Peak oxygen uptake increased by 1.7 ± 0.8 and 2.2 ± 1.3 mg/kg/min in patients receiving pimobendan at a daily dose of 1 and 10 mg, respectively, whereas it decreased by 0.1 ± 0.6 ml/kg/min in patients receiving placebo. Thus pimobendan acutely improves resting LV performance and chronically increases exercise duration and peak oxygen uptake in patients with severe CHF concomitantly treated with digoxin, diuretics, and angiotensin-converting enzyme inhibitors.

References

1. Shocken DD, Arrieta MI, Leaverton PE, Ross EA. Prevalence and mortality rate of congestive heart failure in the United States. J Am Coll Cardiol 1992; 20:301–6.
2. Parameshwar J, Keegan J, Sparrow J, Sutton CG, Poole-Wilson PA: Predictors of prognosis in severe chronic heart failure. Am Heart J 1992 (February); 123:421–426.
3. Lauer MS, Evans JC, Levy D: Prognostic implications of subclinical left ventricular dilatation and systolic dysfunction in men free of overt cardiovascular disease (the Framingham Heart Study). Am J Cardiol 1992 (Nov 1); 70:1180–1184.
4. Stevenson WG, Middlekauff HR, Stevenson LW, Saxon LA, Woo MA, Moser D: Significance of aborted cardiac arrest and sustained ventricular tachycardia in patients referred for treatment therapy of advanced heart failure. Am Heart J 1992 (July); 124:123–130.
5. Davis KM, Fish LC, Elahi D, Clark BA, Minaker KL: Atrial natriuretic peptide levels in the prediction of congestive heart failure risk in frail elderly. JAMA 1992 (May 20); 267:2625–2629.
6. Semigran MJ, Aroney CN, Herrmann HC, Dec GW, Boucher CA, Fifer MA. Effects of atrial natriuretic peptide on myocardial contractile and diastolic function in patients with heart failure. J Am Coll Cardiol 1992 (July); 20:98–106.
7. Lewis BS, Makhoul N, Dakak N, Flugelman MY, Yechiely H, Halon DA, Kahana L: Atrial

natriuretic peptide in severe heart failure: Response to controlled changes in atrial pressure during intravenous nitroglycerin therapy. Am Heart J 1992 (October); 124:1009–1016.

8. Setaro JF, Soufer R, Remetz MS, Perlmutter RA, Zaret BL: Long-term outcome in patients with congestive heart failure and intact systolic left ventricular performance. Am J Cardiol 1992 (May 1); 69:1212–1216.

9. Packer M: Pathophysiology of chronic heart failure. Lancet 1992 (July 11); 340:88–92.

10. Packer M: Treatment of chronic heart failure. Lancet 1992 (July 11); 340:92–95.

11. Kleber FX, Niemoller L, Doering W: Impact of converting enzyme inhibition on progression of chronic heart failure: Results of the Munich Mild Heart Failure Trial. Br Heart J 1992 (Apr); 67:289–296.

12. Kjekshus J, Swedberg K, Snapinn S: Effects of enalapril on long-term mortality in severe congestive heart failure. Am J Cardiol 1992 (Jan 1); 69:103–107.

13. Konstam MA, Kronenberg MW, Udelson JE, Kinan D, Metherall J, Dolan N, Edens T, Howe D, Kilcoyne L, Benedict C, Youngblood M, Barrett J, Yusuf S: Effectiveness of preload reserve as a determinant of clinical status in patients with left ventricular systolic dysfunction. Am J Cardiol 1992 (June 15); 69:1591–1595.

14. Konstam M, Rousseau M, Kronenberg M, Udelson J, Melin J, Stewart D, Dolan N, Edens T, Ahn S, Kinan D, Howe D, Kilcoyne L, Metherall J, Benedict C, Yusuf S, Pouleur H, for the SOLVD Investigators: Effects of the Angiotensin Converting Enzyme Inhibitor Enalapril on the Long-term Progression of Left Ventricular Dysfunction in Patients With Heart Failure. Circulation 1992 (August); 86:431–438.

15. Ljungman S, Kjekshus J, Swedberg K: Renal function in severe congestive heart failure during treatment with enalapril (the Cooperative North Scandinavian Enalapril Survival Study [CONSENSUS] Trial). Am J Cardiol 1992 (Aug 15); 70:479–487.

16. SOLVD Investigators: Effect of enalapril on mortality and the development of heart failure in asymptomatic patients with reduced left ventricular ejection fractions. N Engl J Med 1992 (Sept 3); 327:685–691.

17. Hedner T, Samuelsson O, Lunde H, Lindholm L, Andren L, Wiholm BE: Angio-oedema in relation to treatment with angiotensin converting enzyme inhibitors. Br Med J 1992 (Apr 11); 304:941–946.

18. Mehra A, Ostrzega E, Shotan A, Johnson JV, Elkayam U: Persistent hemodynamic improvement with short-term nitrate therapy in patients with chronic congestive heart failure already treated with captopril. Am J Cardiol 1992 (Nov 15); 70:1310–1314.

19. Paolisso G, Gambardella A, Marrazzo G, Verza M, Teasuro P, Varricchio M, D'Onofrio F: Metabolic and cardiovascular benefits deriving from B-adrenergic blockade in chronic congestive heart failure. Am Heart J 1992 (January); 123:103–110.

20. Cabanes L, Costes F, Weber S, Regnard J, Benvenuti C, Castaigne A, Guerin F, Lockhart A: Improvement in exercise performance by inhalation of methoxamine in patients with impaired left ventricular function. N Engl J Med 1992 (June 18); 326:1661–1665.

21. Katz SD, Kubo SH, Jessup M, Brozena S, Troha JM, Wahl J, Cohn JN, Sonneblick EH, LeJemtel TH: A multicenter, randomized, double-blind, placebo-controlled trial of pimobendan, a new cardiotonic and vasodilator agent, in patients with severe congestive heart failure. Am Heart J 1992 (January); 123:95–103.

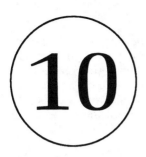

Miscellaneous Topics

Tamponade

To determine the clinical features, course and outcome of patients with cardiac tamponade, Wall and associates[1] from Durham, North Carolina, prospectively studied 57 consecutive patients with new, large pericardial effusions. Twenty-five patients (44%) developed cardiac tamponade with venous hypertension and a pulsus paradoxus >10 mmHg. Electrocardiography, radiographic studies and echocardiography did not differentiate patients with and without tamponade. All 57 patients underwent thorough diagnostic evaluation followed by subxiphoid pericardial biopsy and drainage. A diagnosis was obtained in 53 patients (93%). Collagen vascular disease was significantly more frequent in the 25 patients with than in the 32 without cardiac tamponade (24 vs 3%). The frequency of malignant and uremic effusions was equal in both groups, whereas radiation-induced effusions seldom produced tamponade. At 1-year follow-up, 3 patients (12%) with tamponade had recurrent effusions, and 1 needed reoperation. This was not significantly different from the 32 patients without tamponade. Twelve-month mortality was also similar in both groups (36 vs 44%). This prospective series disclosed several unexpected findings: (1) Cardiac tamponade occurred in almost 50% of patients with new large pericardial effusions; (2) both malignancy and collagen vascular disease occurred with equal frequency as etiologies, whereas radiation-induced tamponade was unusual; (3) thorough clinical evaluation resulted in few idiopathic etiologies; and (4) subxiphoid pericardiotomy was effective for both diagnosis and therapy of tamponade.

In cardiac tamponade cardiac output falls, but peripheral vascular resistance increases, so that systemic BP may be maintained at normal or near-normal levels. Brown and associates[2] from New York, New York, observed a patient with cardiac tamponade whose BP was markedly elevated. To determine the frequency of elevated BP in patients with cardiac tamponade and their hemodynamic characteristics, they studied 18 consecutive patients with tamponade from a variety of causes using right-sided cardiac catheterization. Six of the 18 consecutive patients had systolic arterial BP ranging from 150 to 210 mm Hg (mean [±SD]; 176 ± 26) and diastolic pressures ranging from 100 to 130 mm Hg (mean, 113 ± 14). All 6 had previously been hypertensive. After pericardiocentesis there was a significant decrease in BP (to 139 ± 13 mm Hg systolic, and 83 ± 6 mm Hg diastolic) and peripheral vascular resistance (from 2,150 ± 588 to 1207 ± 345 dyn · sec · cm^{-5}). Cardiac output increased in all 6. The other 12 patients, 3 of whom had a history of hypertension, had significant increases in cardiac output and systolic BP (from 119 ± 13 to 127 ± 7 mm Hg) after pericardiocentesis, whereas peripheral vascular resistance decreased. Both groups had similar degrees of cardiac tamponade, as indicated by measurements of cardiac output and intrapericardial, right atrial, and pulmonary-artery wedge pressures. Elevated BP may occur in some patients with cardiac tamponade who have preexisting hypertension. Moreover, BP may fall after pericardiocentesis in patients who have elevated BP associated with tamponade.

Doppler vs 2-dimensional echocardiography

Respiratory changes in LV inflow velocities by Doppler echocardiography have been used to assess cardiac tamponade. Doppler echocardiography, however, has not been compared to RA or RV collapse. Schutzman and associates[3] from Cleveland, Ohio, performed pulsed Doppler echocardiography of LV inflow velocities with respiratory monitoring in 28 patients with small to large pericardial effusions. Ten of the 17 patients (59%) with large effusions had equalization of right-sided diastolic pressures before pericardial drainage. The measurements performed included percent change in LV inflow peak early velocity, isovolumic relaxation time, change in inferior vena cava diameter from apnea to inspiration, and the presence of RA and RV collapse. Percent change in early LV inflow velocities significantly correlated with pericardial effusion size and RV collapse, and showed a trend with RA collapse. Pericardial effusions with a LV inflow velocity change >22% were found to have right-sided equalization at a 95% confidence interval. The data indicate that the respiratory changes in Doppler echocardiographic parameters are useful in the assessment of pericardial effusion and tamponade. This study concurs with the hypothesis that there is a continuum of hemodynamic compromise in pericardial effusion that is easily detected by Doppler echocardiography.

Pericardioscopy

In cases of malignant pericardial effusion, surgical subxiphoid biopsy sometimes fails to prove malignancy. In an investigation by Millaire and associates[4] from Lille, France, to assess the usefulness of pericardioscopy, which allows an endoscopic investigation of the pericardial cavity, this technique was systematically performed during surgical drainage procedures that were performed on 40 patients who had pericardial effusion of suspected malignant origin. Twenty-six patients had a history of neoplasm, 10 had a history of hematologic malignancy, and 4 had recent tumors or lymphadenopathies that were suspected to be of malignant origin. Classical tests that are usually performed during a conventional surgical drainage procedure (fluid studies and subxiphoid biopsy) were combined with direct visualization of the pericardial surfaces and guided biopsies of suspicious areas. The follow-up period after pericardioscopy was at least 12 months. Two early deaths occurred after pericardioscopy, but no death was directly related to the endoscopy. According to all of the tests that were performed, diagnoses were malignant pericardial effusion in 15 of 40 patients (group I, 37%) and nonmalignant pericardial effusion in 25 of 40 patients (group II, 73%). In 3 of 13 patients (23%) in group I, the diagnosis was obtained only by pericardioscopy (results of cytologic studies and subxiphoid biopsy were negative). In 2 patients in group I, pericardioscopy could not be completed, but the diagnosis of malignant pericardial effusion was obtained by pericardiocentesis. In group II, effusion was considered to be postradiation pericarditis in 5 cases, infectious pericarditis in 3 cases (bacterial in 1 and tuberculous in 2), hemopericardium induced by coagulation disturbances in 3 cases, and idiopathic pericarditis in 14 cases. Mid- and long-term follow-up (mean duration 35 months; range 12 to 72 months) showed that in group I the median survival time was 42 days, whereas in group II it was 1 year. The difference between the 2 life curves was significant. Thus pericardioscopy appears to be a technique that does not increase the risk of the surgical drainage procedure. Its main benefit is a greater diagnostic sensitivity as a result of direct visualization of the pericardial surfaces and guided biopsies. It should be available as the time that the surgical drainage procedure is performed, since the diagnosis of malignant pericardial effusion has significant prognostic consequences.

CARDIAC AND/OR PULMONARY TRANSPLANTATION

Organ procurement

To estimate the potential supply of organ donors and to measure the efficiency of organ procurement efforts in the USA, Evans and associates[5] from Seattle, Washington, and San Francisco, California, developed a geographic data base consisting of multiple cause of death and sociodemographic data compiled by the National Center for Health Statistics. All deaths are evaluated as to their potential for organ donation. Two classes of potential donors are identified: class 1 estimates are restricted to causes of death involving significant head trauma only, and class 2 estimates include class 1 estimates as well as deaths in which brain death was less probable. Over 23,000 people are currently awaiting a kidney, heart, liver, heart-lung, pancreas, or lung transplantation. Donor supply is inadequate, and the number of donors remained unchanged at approximately 4,000 annually for 1986 through 1989, with a modest 9.1% increase in 1990. Between 6900 and 10,700 potential donors are available annually (e.g., 28.5 to 43.7 per million population). Depending on the class of donor considered, organ procurement efforts are between 37% and 59% efficient. Efficiency greatly varies by state and organ procurement organization. Many more organ donors are available than are being accessed through existing organ procurement efforts. Realistically, it may be possible to increase by 80% the number of donors available in the United States (up to 7,300 annually). It is conceivable, although unlikely, that the supply of donor organs could achieve a level to meet demand.

Waiting times

As the number of heart transplants and the number of transplant programs has increased, so has the waiting time for a suitable organ. To more accurately assess the magnitude of this increase and the influence of recipient size, Sekela and associates[6] from Houston, Texas, reviewed waiting times for large (body surface area ≥ 1.95 m²) and small (body surface area < 1.95 m²) patients with respect to era of transplantation. Patients who underwent transplantation early (1984 to December 31, 1986) waited 35 ± 47 days (mean $\pm$ standard deviation), whereas patients who underwent transplantation in the late era (1987 to September 30, 1989) waited 83 ± 102 days. Large patients waited longer (130 ± 142 days) in the late era than did small patients (60 ± 67 days). During the heterotopic era (October 1, 1989 to June 30, 1990), waiting times for large patients who received a heterotopic transplant (67 ± 46 days) were significantly shorter than those for patients who received an orthotopic transplant (166 ± 157 days). Waiting times for small patients remained unchanged. In addition, waiting time mortality decreased from 24% to 9%. Comparison of orthotopic and heterotopic procedures performed during the same era revealed no significant differences in recipient age, preoperative status, graft ischemic time, donor age, early and midterm survival, or early postoperative functional status. Heterotopic heart transplantation may effectively increase the size of the donor pool, decrease the waiting time, and decrease waiting time mortality without increasing the morbidity of the procedure.

Relation between experience and outcome

Policies related to organ transplantation in the USA are designed to ensure that centers and physicians with experience in transplantation perform these procedures. It is essential to confirm the validity of such policies, since they may limit access to transplantation services. To determine the relation between experience with heart transplantation and mortality after the procedure, Laffel and associates[7] from Boston, Massachusetts, and San Diego, California, merged data from the registry of the International Society for Heart and Lung Transplantation with data from a survey that provided additional information about patients and transplantation centers. The study included 1,123 patients who received a heart transplant at 1 of 56 hospitals in the US from 1984 through 1986. The authors used univariate and bivariate techniques, as well as logistic regression, to analyze our data. They observed an institutional learning curve for heart transplantation. Patients who received 1 of a center's first 5 transplants had higher mortality rates than patients who received a subsequent transplant (20% vs 12%). In addition, a correlation between the training of key personnel on the transplantation team and mortality at new transplantation centers was found. For example, new centers staffed by cardiologists with previous training in heart transplantation had lower mortality rates among heart-transplant recipients than centers without experienced cardiologists (7% vs 16%). By contrast, the previous training of the surgeons who performed transplantations was not related to the mortality rate associated with the procedure. Experience with heart transplantation is associated with a better outcome for patients after that procedure.

In the first year of life

Starnes and associates[8] from Stanford, California, reported 17 infants < 1 year of age who have undergone heart (12), heart-lung (3) and lung (2) transplantation for end-stage cardiopulmonary disease. Infants undergoing heart transplantation had a mean age of 4.5 months (range 19 days to 12 months), with the diagnosis of cardiomyopathy in 4 and congenital heart disease in 8, with 4 of 8 having hypoplastic left heart syndrome. Actuarial survival at 1 and 2 years was 74% and compares favorably with the survival of older children at 1 and 2 years of 82 and 69%. The lineraized rejection rate was less in infants as compared with children more than 1 year of age. In intermediate follow-up, no graft atherosclerosis has been noted. Using a 3 drug protocol with steroid taper to alternate day steroids or off completely by 6 months, is the goal which has been accomplished in 6 of 12 infants. Heart-lung and lung transplantation has been performed in 5 infants with 1 death in each group. A pulmonary lobe from a larger and older donor was transplanted into a 4 week old infant as a single-lung transplant with good outcome. The 3 surviving infants are well 24, 18, and 2 months after transplantation. Obliterative bronchiolitis has not been clinically apparent in this group. These authors show excellent short term results from transplantation in infancy. The use of pulmonary lobe transplantation potentially expands considerably the donor pool.

Pulmonary hypertension before

Costard-Jäckle and colleagues[9] in Stanford, California, determined whether patients with pulmonary hypertension are at risk of developing fatal right sided heart failure after heart transplantation. To evaluate the risk potential, candidates for heart transplantation were screened by measuring rest right heart pressures and the response to nitroprusside. To test the validity of this approach, the influence of pretransplantation right heart catheterization data on outcome after transplantation was analyzed in 293 of 301 consecutive patients. Patients with a pulmonary vascular resistance >2.5 Wood units measured at baseline had a 3-month mortality rate of 17.9% compared with 6.9% in patients with pulmonary vascular resistances ≤2.5 units. Patients with pulmonary vascular resistances >2.5 units at baseline were differentiated further according to their hemodynamic responses to nitroprusside. Patients in whom resistances could be reduced to ≤2.5 units with a stable systemic systolic pressure ≥85 mmHg had a 3-month mortality rate of 3.8%. However, patients whose pulmonary vascular resistances could not be reduced to < 2.5 units, and those in whom resistances could be reduced to ≤2.5 units but only at the expense of systemic hypotension had a 3-month mortality rates of 40.6% and 27.5%, respectively. The 10 patients dying of right heart failure belong to the latter 2 groups. Thus, right heart hemodynamic measurements and the response to nitroprusside are useful in predicting early mortality after heart transplantation.

Hypercholesterolemia afterwards

Although hypercholesterolemia is a frequent complication in cardiac transplant recipients, the exact mechanism contributing to its development is unknown. Kubo and associates[10] from Minneapolis, Minnesota, retrospectively examined cholesterol levels in 151 thoracic transplant patients treated with cyclosporine, azathioprine and prednisone to evaluate the factors influencing the heterogeneity of changes after the first year after transplantation in patients on a standard 3-drug immunosuppression regimen. Three groups were compared including ischemic heart transplant (n = 72), nonischemic heart transplant (n = 64) and heart-lung/lung transplant (n = 15) recipients. After the first year, 64 patients

(43%) developed consistent hypercholesterolemia (>240 mg/dl) for which pharmacologic treatment was initiated. Forty-eight patients (67%) in the ischemic heart transplant group required treatment, significantly greater than both the nonischemic (n = 14; 22%) and heart-lung/lung transplant (n = 2; 13%) group. Univariate and forward stepwise multivariate regression analysis identified 4 factors that were all significantly and independently correlated with follow-up cholesterol including prednisone dose, baseline cholesterol, glucose and weight gain. Changes in triglycerides in the 3 groups of patients were similar to changes in cholesterol. Furthermore, the increase in cholesterol in patients requiring treatment was primarily due to an increase in LDL cholesterol. These data demonstrate that hypercholesterolemia is common in heart transplant recipients treated with standard 3-drug immunosuppression and generally develops within the first 2 years after transplantation. However, this complication is not uniform and appears to be most strongly related to previous CAD. Finally, this complication is a multifactorial process that is related to several risk factors, including prednisone dose, glucose levels and weight gain.

In an open, randomized study, Barbir and associates[11] from London, and Edinburgh, UK, compared the efficacy and safety of bezafibrate (400/mg/day) and fish oil (Maxepa) (10 g/day) for 3 months in 87 cardiac transplant recipients with serum total cholesterol >6.5 or triglycerides > 2.8 mmol/l, or both. After 1 month, bezafibrate reduced total cholesterol by 13%, LDL cholesterol by 20% and apolipoprotein B by 13%. It also increased apolipoprotein A1 and HDL cholesterol by 12 and 20%, respectively, and significantly reduced fibrinogen at 3 months. Mexepa had no significant effect on these variables, but was as effective as bezafibrate in reducing triglycerides (36 and 31%, respectively). Both drugs increased lipoprotein (a) to a similar extent, and bezafibrate significantly increased serum creatinine. These results suggest that bezafibrate has better lipid-, apolipoprotein- and hemostatic modifying properties than does Mexepa, but its potentially adverse adverse effect on renal function needs further investigation.

High concentrations of serum lipoprotein (a) (Lp(a)) are associated with an increased risk of atherosclerotic vascular disease in the nontransplanted population. Its relation with accelerated CAD in cardiac transplant recipients has not been studied until Barbir and associates[12] from London and Brighton, UK, measured serum LP (a) in 130 cardiac transplant recipients undergoing routine follow-up, which included annual coronary angiography. The median LP(a) concentration in 33 patients with CAD was 71 mg/dl, which was significantly higher than the corresponding value of 22 mg/dL in the 97 patients without CAD. Multivariant analysis showed the serum Lp (a) value to be a higher significant risk factor for CAD irrespective of the other factors included in the regression analysis. Thus a high concentration of serum Lp(a) is an important, independent risk factor for the development of accelerated CAD in transplant recipients.

Coronary artery disease afterwards

Accelerated coronary atherosclerosis is a major factor limiting allograft longevity in cardiac transplant recipients. Histopathology studies have demonstrated the insensitivity of coronary angiography for detecting early atheromatous disease in this patient population. Intracoronary ultrasound is a new imaging technique that provides characterization of vessel wall morphology. St. Goar and co-workers[13] in Stanford, California compared in vivo intracoronary ultrasound with angiography in cardiac transplant recipients. The LAD coronary was studied with intracoronary ultrasound in 80 cardiac transplant recipients at the time of routine screening coronary angiography 2 weeks to 13 years after transplantation. A mean and index of intimal thickening were obtained at four coronary sites. Intimal proliferation was classified as minimal, mild, moderate, or severe according to thickness and degree of vessel circumference involved. Twenty patients were studied within 1 month of transplantation and had no angiographic evidence of coronary disease. An intimal layer was visualized by ultrasound in only 13 of these 20 presumably normal hearts. The 60 patients studied 1 year or more after transplantation all had at least minimal intimal thickening. Twenty-one patients showed minimal or mild, 17 moderate, and 21 severe thickening. Forty-two of these 60 patients had angiographically normal coronary arteries, 21 of whom had either moderate or severe thickening (Figure 10-1). All 18 patients with angiographic evidence of coronary disease had moderate or severe intimal thickening, but there was no statistically significant difference in intimal thickness or index when compared with the patients with moderate or severe proliferation and normal angiograms. The majority of patients 1 or more years after cardiac transplantation have ultrasound evidence of intimal thickening not apparent by angiography. Intracoronary ultrasound offers early detection and quantitative of transplant coronary disease and provides characterization of vessel wall morphology, which may prove to be a prognostic marker of disease.

Accelerated CAD is the most serious complication after cardiac trans-

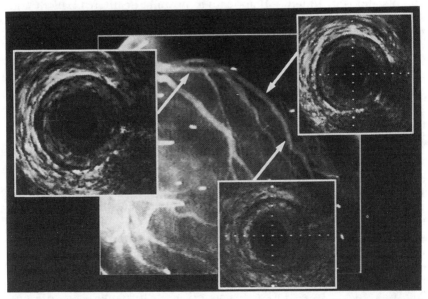

Fig. 10-1. Angiogram with ultrasound images from three representative sites in the left anterior descending coronary artery (LAD) of a 37-year-old man 3 years after transplantation. Although the angiogram is without evidence of coronary disease, the ultrasound images demonstrate severe concentric intimal thickening throughout the proximal and mid LAD. Echodensity in the vessel wall in the left ultrasound image at the 3 o'clock position and in the upper right image at the 4 o'clock position are examples of acoustic artifact produced by the coronary guide wire and mechanical support strut. Reproduced with permission from St. Goar, et al.[13]

plantation. Its ideology is unclear. Dunn and associates[14] from London, UK, investigated the frequency of antiendothelial antibodies against human umbilical vein subendothelial cells by 1-dimensional sodium dodecyl sulphate polyacrylamide gel electrophoresis and western blotting. Peptide-specific antiendothelial antibodies were found in 15/21 heart transplant recipients with accelerated CAD and 1/20 transplant patients who had not developed the disease. Positive immunofluorescence of patients' serum on frozen sections of coronary vessels confirmed the endothelial specificity of antibodies. These results provide evidence of an immune etiology for transplant-associated CAD and could have important implications for its diagnosis and therapy.

Accelerated allograft atherosclerosis is the main cause of death of cardiac transplant recipients after the first year after transplantation. Because no medical therapy is known to prevent or retard graft atherosclerosis and retransplantation is associated with a shortened allograft survival, alternative, palliative therapy with PTCA has been attempted. Because no single medical center has performed PTCA in a large number of cardiac transplant recipients, Halle and colleagues[15] in Richmond, Virginia retrospectively analyzed their complete experience of PTCA in cardiac transplant patients to determine the safety, efficacy, limitations, and long-term outcome of PTCA in allograft coronary vascular disease at 11 medical centers. Thirty-five patients underwent 50 PTCA procedures for 95 lesions after transplantation. The primary indications for PTCA included angiographic coronary disease in 22 cases and noninvasive evidence of ischemia in 18 procedures. Angiographic success, defined as ≤50% post-PTCA stenosis, occurred in 88 of 95 lesions. Mean pre-PTCA stenosis was 83%; mean post-PTCA stenosis was 29%. Periprocedural complications included AMI and late in-hospital death in 1 patient and 3 groin hematomas. Twenty-three of the 35 patients had no severe adverse outcome such as death, retransplantation, or AMI at 13 months after PTCA. Four patients died less than 6 months after PTCA, and 4 died more than 6 months after PTCA. Two patients had retransplantation 2 months after PTCA, and 1 patient had retransplantation 18 months after PTCA. PTCA may be applied in selected cardiac transplant recipients with comparable success and complication rates to routine angioplasty. Whether angioplasty prolongs allograft survival remains to be determined by a prospective, controlled trial.

Mullins and associates[16] from Cambridge, UK, reviewed their experience with CAD late after cardiac transplantation. Of a population of 383 orthotopic cardiac transplant recipients operated upon between January 1979 and June 1990, 447 coronary angiograms were available for review in 193 patients. Thirteen of a possible 18 results of post mortem examinations from patients dying from CAD were available. CAD was defined as any evidence of disease on coronary angiography. Post mortem examinations were performed with standard techniques. The angiographic prevalence of CAD was 3% (1/32 patients) and 40% (19/47 patients) at 1 and 5 years respectively. Twenty-six grafts failed due to CAD compared with 132 graft failures from all causes during this period. Acute thrombosis was present in a large vessel in 7 of 13 fatal cases undergoing necropsy (54%). Noticeable large vessel involvement with disease in smaller distal arteries was present in 4 patients (31%). The remaining 2 patients (15%) had small artery disease alone. Twelve of the 13 patients had significant cardiomegaly (cardiac weight ≥400 g) with a mean weight of 510 (range 370–740) g. CAD is the main late complication after cardiac transplantation (Table 10-1). A combination of coronary thrombosis, ischemia from stenoses of

TABLE 10-1. *Causes of death in cardiac transplant patients between January 1979 and June 1990. Reproduced with permission from Mullins.*[16]

Causes of death	Time from transplantation		
	0–90 days	90 days–1 year	> 1 year
Rejection	23	9	1
Infection	21	8	3
Coronary occlusive disease	0	2	26
Sudden cardiac death	1	1	3
Donor heart failure	6	0	0
Stroke	4	1	0
High pulmonary resistance	4	0	0
Multifactorial	4	0	0
Lymphoma	1	0	2
Malignancy	0	1	5
Abdominal complications	2	0	0
Operative bleeding	1	0	0
Unknown	1	1	1
Total	68	23	41

large and small coronary vessels, and cardiomegaly contribute to the graft failure of these patients.

Vasomotor responses to nitroglycerin, acetylcholine or adenosine afterwards

Coronary artery vasomotion is altered after cardiac transplantation. The impact of accelerated transplant coronary atherosclerosis and myocardial rejection on vasomotion is not well understood. Intravascular ultrasound is a new imaging method with the ability to study real-time changes in coronary artery dimensions. Pinto and colleagues[17] in Stanford, California, studied epicardial coronary artery response to nitroglycerin in 32 cardiac transplant recipients, 3 weeks to 10 years after transplantation with intracoronary ultrasound. Cross-sectional luminal area and diameter were measured at a fixed position in the LAD coronary artery immediately before and every 30 seconds for 5 minutes after 0.4 mg of sublingual nitroglycerin. Cross-sectional area increased from a baseline of 13.1 mm^2 to 15.8 mm^2 at maximal vasodilation; luminal diameter increased from 4.0 to 4.5 mm. This increase reached statistical significance at 1.5 minutes after administration of nitroglycerin; mean maximum increase occurred at 4.5 minutes. Patients with biopsy-proven mild or moderate concurrent rejection had a significantly blunted vasodilatory response versus the nonrejection group, although a vasodilatory effect was still present. Nitroglycerin response was well preserved in patients up to 10 years after transplantation; however, there was a trend toward a decreased response in patients studied immediately after transplantation. Coronary intimal thickness, as measured by ultrasound, had no impact on the vasodilatory response. Vasodilatory response to nitroglycerin in cardiac transplant recipients is attenuated during episodes of cardiac rejection. This response is preserved in long-term survivors and is independent of the degree of intimal thickening. Intravascular ultrasound provides a new method to document real-time epicardial coronary vasomotion.

The coronary arteries of transplanted hearts frequently develop accelerated diffuse arteriosclerosis. The effects of this disease on resistance vessel function are unknown. To investigate the integrity of endothelium-dependent small-vessel vasodilation in transplanted hearts, Treasure and co-workers[18] in Boston, Massachusetts, assessed coronary blood flow responses to the endothelium-dependent dilator adenosine in 40 studies of 29 transplant patients 1–3 years after transplantation and in 7 nontransplanted controls. Coronary blood flow was measured at constant arterial pressure with a Doppler catheter in the LAD. Controls, years 1 transplant patients, and year 2 transplant patients had similar increases in coronary blood flow in response to acetylcholine (232%, 200%, and 201%), whereas year 3 transplant patients had increased coronary blood flow of only 100%. An index of the proportion of coronary blood flow reserve attributable to endothelium-dependent dilation was obtained by normalizing each patient's peak acetylcholine flow response by the peak adenosine flow response. In patients receiving both acetylcholine and adenosine, endothelium-dependent flow responses declined over time (57% in controls, 56% for year 1, 47% for year 2, and 29% for year 3). An increased mean cyclosporine level and increased transplant recipient age predicted a preserved endothelium-dependent microvascular response. Thus, microvascular endothelium-dependent dilation deteriorates over time in the transplanted heart, which may reflect underlying graft arteriosclerosis and contribute to ischemic damage of the myocardium.

Allograft vasculopathy after heart transplantation is thought to represent a response to endothelial injury in the graft vessels. To assess endothelial function before the onset of anatomic disease, Mills and co-investigators[19] in Gainesville, Florida, evaluated coronary vasomotor responses to adenosine, acetylcholine, and nitroglycerin in transplant recipients by intravascular ultrasound imaging and Doppler flow studies. Nine patients were studied 1 year after heart transplantation. Acetylcholine provoked significant vasoconstriction to 82% of maximal coronary artery diameter but was associated with an increase in mean coronary blood flow from 63 to 204 ml/min. Coronary blood flow increased fivefold in response to adenosine, a normal response. The vasomotor response to acetylcholine at 1 year after heart transplantation is consistent with endothelial dysfunction in the epicardial conduit vessels. Microvascular function as judged by coronary flow reserve appears to be normal.

Circadian rhythm of blood pressure afterwards

van de Borne and associates[20] from Brussels, Belgium, recorded 24-hour BP and heart rate profiles in 19 patients 1 and 7 months after cardiac transplantation using noninvasive ambulatory monitors using the periodogram method. These recordings were compared with those of control subjects matched for age, sex and daytime ambulatory BP. One month after transplantation, the nighttime decrease in systolic and diastolic BPs were attenuated in the patients as compared to the control subjects. The daily oral dose of prednisolone was inversely correlated with the magnitude of the nighttime decreases in systolic and diastolic BP. In contrast, 7 months after transplantation, the nighttime decrease in systolic and diastolic BPs reappeared in the patients and was of similar magnitude as that in the control subjects. When the immunosuppressive regimens during the 2 periods of recordings were compared, the reduction in the daily oral dose of prednisolone administered to the patients 7 months after transplantation was correlated with the observed increase in the day-night systolic and diastolic BP difference. Thus, data show the reappearance of normal circadian BP profiles in patients with long-term heart transplants, and suggest that glucocorticoid administration may contribute to the abnormal nocturnal BP profiles observed 1 month after transplantation.

Effect on ventilatory response to exercise

Patients with CHF frequently exhibit an excessive ventilatory response to exercise, which is acutely unaltered by therapeutic interventions. To investigate whether these ventilatory responses resolve after cardiac transplantation, Marzo and associates[21] from Philadelphia, Pennsylvania, performed exercise testing with measurement of respiratory gases before and 1.4 ± 0.6 months after cardiac transplantation in 15 ambulatory patients with severe CHF. Ventilatory response was also measured in 7 age-matched, sedentary control subjects. LVEF at rest and hemodynamic measurements were obtained before and after transplantation in all patients. After transplantation, EF at rest increased from 16 ± 6 to 56 ± 10%, pulmonary capillary wedge pressure declined from 26 ± 8 to 12 ± 5 mmHg, and cardiac index increased from 1.7 ± 0.5 to 2.8 ± 0.5 L/min/m^2. Peak oxygen consumption increased from 12 ± 2 to 19 ± 3 ml/kg/min, but remained significantly lower than that in control subjects (33.4 ± 6.9 ml/kg/min). Minute ventilation (V_E) was significantly reduced after transplantation, but excessive compared with normal values. Ventilation at a carbon dioxide production of 1 liter/min decreased significantly after cardiac transplantation (52 ± 8 to 39 ± 4 L), but remained elevated when contrasted to that in control subjects (31.4 ± 3.4 liters). Ventilatory response to exercise is significantly improved after cardiac transplantation; however, V_E remains excessive. This may reflect an attenuated cardiac output response to exercise, abnormal intrapulmonary pressures or persistent deconditioning.

Monoclonal antimyosin antibody

Detection and treatment for rejection after transplantation are based on the identification of myocyte damage upon endomyocardial biopsy. Noninvasive detection of such damage is possible with ^{111}In-labeled monoclonal antimyosin antibodies. Although the presence and degree of monoclonal antimyosin antibody uptake parallels the rejection activity detected by biopsy, the relation between the degree of uptake and the occupance of severe rejection-related complications has not been previously assessed. Ballester and co-investigators[22] in Barcelona, Spain, performed 247 monoclonal antimyosin antibody studies coinciding with biopsies in 52 patients 1–71 months after transplantation. A heart-to-lung ratio was used as a measure of relative monoclonal antimyosin antibody uptake with a heart lung ratio of 1.55 discriminating normal from abnormal studies. Of the 247 antimyosin studies, 149 coincided with absent, 38 with mild, and 60 with moderate rejection at biopsy. Heart lung ratio was 1.7, 1.8 and 1.9 in the three biopsy groups respectively. Two hundred thirty-eight of 247 antimyosin studies coexisted with absent rejection-related complications; in 9 of 247 patients, such complications were detected (5 CHF episodes due to rejection and four episodes of vascular occlusion, which resulted in 5 deaths), and mean heart lung ratio was 1.7 and 2.1 in the two groups, respectively. No complications were noted in 193 studies of patients with heart lung ratios less than 2.0 whereas in 9 of 45 with heart lung ratio of 2.0 or greater, complications, occurred. None of the 23 patients prospectively followed since surgery who had a gradual decrease in monoclonal antimyosin antibody uptake during the first 3 months showed rejection-related complications, whereas persistent uptake was associated with complications in 5 of 9 patients. No rejection-related complications are seen coinciding with heart lung ratio of less than 2.0, whereas patients who have complications have a heart lung ratio of more than 2.0. The early 3-month pattern of decreasing monoclonal antimyosin antibody uptake is associated with a clinical course free of rejection-related complications, whereas a persistent pattern is a signal of the possibility of such complications.

Transesophageal echocardiography afterwards

Polanco and associates[23] from Detroit, Michigan, performed both transesophageal echocardiography and transthoracic echocardiography in 30 patients with orthotopic heart transplantation. Transesophageal echocardiography identified LA appendage and flow across the atrial septum, but neither was identified by transthoracic echocardiography. In addition, pronounced bulging of the atrial septum was seen in 6 patients by transesophageal but not by transthoracic echocardiography. Spontaneous echo contrast in the atria was detected by transesophageal echocardiography in 14 patients, but in only 1 patient by transthoracic echocardiography. Abnormal geometry of the atria and donor-recipient atrial anastomotic sites were identified in all patients by both transthoracic and transesophageal echocardiography.

Hyperuricemia and gout afterwards

To determine the frequency and characteristics of hyperuricemia and gouty arthritis among cyclosporine-treated heart transplant recipients, Burack and associates[24] from Pittsburgh, Pennsylvania, evaluated 196 surviving adult heart or heart/lung transplant recipients. Medical records were reviewed to determine peak serum uric acid levels after transplantation, and to evaluate potential risk factors for hyperuricemia. Patients were surveyed by postal questionnaire for a history of gouty arthritis, with positive responses evaluated by telephone interview and/or examination of the patient. Hyperuricemia occurred in 72% of male and 81% of female patients and was not correlated with cyclosporine level, presence of hypertension, or degree of renal insufficiency. Eleven (6%) patients had gout prior to transplantation; 14 (8%) had onset of definite gout and 7 (4%) had probable gout a mean of 17 months after transplantation. Polyarticular arthritis and/or tophi developed in 6 (43%) of the posttransplant-onset definite gout group within a mean of 31 months. Both hyperuricemia and gouty arthritis occur with increased frequency among cyclosporine-treated heart or heart/lung transplant recipients. The clinical course of gout in these patients is often accelerated, with management complicated by the patients' renal insufficiency and interaction with transplant-related medications.

Arrhythmias afterwards

The etiology and clinical significance of sustained arrhythmias, and atrial and ventricular premature complexes (APCs and VPCs, respectively) after cardiac transplantation are controversial. Scott and associates[25] from New Castle upon Tyne, United Kingdom, studied 50 adult recipients surviving 2 weeks by continuous telemetry while in the hospital and by ambulatory electrocardiographic monitoring at 2, 4, 6, 12 and 24 weeks after transplantation. The median APC frequency was greater among subjects who experienced allograft rejection in the early postoperative period (0.7/hour, range 0 to 23) than among those who did not (0.2/hour, range

0 to 10.4). The APC frequency in all subjects decreased from 0.25/hour (range 0 to 23) early to 0/hour (0 to 14) later. Atrial flutter was the most frequent sustained arrhythmia; it was recorded in 5 of 21 rejectors and in 1 of 29 nonrejectors, and 11 of 16 episodes (69%) were related to acute rejection temporally. VPCs were recorded in all patients early after transplantation, but the median frequency subsequently decreased from 4.6/hour (range 0.5 to 470) early to 1.25/hour (range 0 to 225) later. VPC frequency was unrelated to rejection. Sustained VT was recorded once and was caused by the proarrhythmic effect of flecainide. Thus, APCs and VPCs occur frequently after transplantation. Frequent APCs are associated with rejection, whereas the main determinant of VPC frequency is time after transplantation. Atrial flutter is closely associated with rejection and should be regarded as an indication for endomyocardial biopsy. VT occurs seldom, and in this study was due to proarrhythmic drug effects.

Causes of death

Rose and associates[26] from Cape Town, South Africa, investigated the principal and contributory causes of death in 81 autopsied heart transplant patients who died at a single hospital in Cape Town, South Africa. They subdivided the patients according to the immunosuppressive regimen used as well as the postoperative survival period. Mean graft survival was 488 days. Chronic rejection (30%), infection (23%), and acute rejection (20%) were the most common principal causes of death (Table 10-2). Both fatal and nonfatal infections involved the lung predominantly. A review of the literature revealed 198 other autopsied heart transplant patients whose principal cause of death could be analyzed; infection accounted for almost half of these latter deaths, followed by acute and chronic

TABLE 10-2. *Principal Cause of Death Following Heart Transplantation Related to Postoperative Survival in 81 Patients. Reproduced with permission from Rose.*[26]

Cause	Days, No. (%)			Total (N=81)
	0-90 (N=32)	91-365 (N=20)	>365 (N=29)	
Chronic rejection	0	4 (20)	20 (69)	**24** (30)
Infection	11 (34)	8 (40)	0	**19** (23)
Acute rejection	7 (22)	5 (25)	4 (14)	**16** (19)
Miscellaneous	4 (13)	3 (15)	2 (3.5)	**9** (11)
Defective donor liver	5 (16)	0	0	**5** (6)
Operative	3 (9)	0	0	**3** (4)
Unknown	1 (3)	0	1	**2** (2.5)
Malignancy	0	0	2 (7)	**2** (2.5)
Metabolic	1 (3)	0	0	**1** (1)

rejection (Figure 10-2). Contributory causes of death in the 81 patients were as follows: infection (17%), acute rejection (16%), chronic rejection (14%), miscellaneous conditions (14%), embolism (14%), pancreatitis (11%), peptic ulcer (9%), inadequate donor heart (3%), and malignancy (1%). The authors concluded that infection, together with acute and/or chronic rejection, are still the major causes of death in heart transplant patients.

VENOUS DISEASE

Risk of pulmonary embolism

A superb review of the risk of and prophylaxis for venous thromboembolism in hospital patients was provided by the Thromboembolic Risk Factors (THRIFT) Consensus Group and published in the 5 September 1992 *British Medical Journal.*[27]

Monreal and associates[28] from Barcelona, Spain, analyzed prospectively the influence of several diseases and clinical conditions on the presence of pulmonary embolism (PE) in a large series of patients with deep venus thrombosis (DVT) in the lower extremities. Lung scan findings from a series of 434 consecutive patients with DVT (with and without symptoms of PE) were studied and then correlated to 4 clinical variables: age, sex, elapsed time since clinical symptoms had appeared in the leg to diagnosis, degree of proximity of venous thrombus, and the presence or not of several risk factors that could have predisposed to thrombus development. According to scintigraphic findings, 164 patients were considered to have PE (asymptomatic in 76 of them), while 200 patients were classified as having only DVT. Lung scan was considered to be

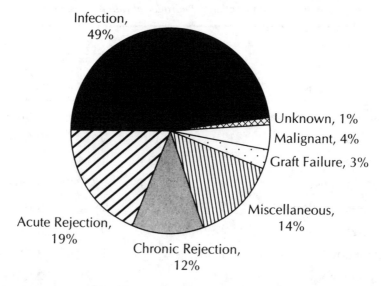

Fig. 10-2. Principal cause of death derived from review of 198 published heart transplant autopsies. Reproduced with permission from Rose, et al.[26]

indeterminate for PE in 70 patients, and they were not included in the study. No differences were found in terms of age, sex, interval of time elapsed since onset of symptoms to diagnosis, or in the degree of proximity of the thrombus. However, several differences between groups were found when comparing the presence or absence of several predisposing factors for thrombosis: DVT developing in immobilized patients was associated with a significantly lower incidence of PE as compared with non-immobilized patients. Conversely, patients with a history of venous thromboembolism had a significantly higher rate of embolism (31/51 vs 133/313). On logistic regression analysis, a history of venous thromboembolism showed a statistically significant association with more than a 2-fold higher risk of having PE for patients with such an antecedent.

Heparin

Low-molecular-weight heparin has a high bioavailability and a prolonged half-life in comparison with conventional unfractionated heparin. Limited data are available for low-molecular-weight heparin as compared with unfractionated heparin for the treatment of deep-vein thrombosis. In a multicenter, double-blind clinical trial, Hull and associates[29] compared fixed-dose subcutaneous low-molecular-weight heparin given once daily with adjusted-dose intravenous heparin given by continuous infusion for the initial treatment of patients with proximal-vein thrombosis, using objective documentation of clinical outcomes. Six of 213 patients who received low-molecular-weight heparin (2.8%) and 15 of 219 patients who received intravenous heparin (6.9%) had new episodes of venous thromboembolism (95% confidence interval for the difference, 0.02% to 8.1%. Major bleeding associated with initial therapy occurred in 1 patient receiving low-molecular-weight heparin (0.5%) and in 11 patients receiving intravenous heparin (5.0%), a reduction in risk of 91%). This apparent protection against major bleeding was lost during long-term therapy. Minor hemorrhagic complications were infrequent. Ten patients receiving low-molecular-weight heparin (4.7%) died, as compared with 21 patients receiving intravenous heparin (9.6%), a risk reduction of 51%. Low-molecular-weight heparin is at least as effective and as safe as classic intravenous heparin therapy under the conditions of this study and more convenient to administer. The simplified therapy provided by low-molecular-weight heparin may allow patients with uncomplicated proximal deep-vein thrombosis to be cared for in an outpatient setting.

Warfarin

The Research Committee of the British Thoracic Society chaired by M. F. Sudlow[30] carried out a multicenter comparison of 4 weeks' and 3 months' anticoagulation in patients admitted to hospital with acute deep vein thrombosis (DVT), pulmonary embolism (PE), or both. Of 712 patients enrolled, 358 were assigned 4 weeks' treatment and 354 3 months'. Objective confirmation of the diagnosis was obtained in 71%. PE caused or contributed to death in 7 patients (3 treated for 4 weeks, 4 for 3 months). Adverse effects were uncommon, although 1 patient (4-week group) died of hemorrhage. The numbers of patients whose thromboembolism failed to resolve on treatment was lower in the 3-month group than in the 4-week group (13 [3.7%] vs 24 [6.7%]), as was the number who had recurrences (14 [4.9%] vs 28 [7.8%]). Among patients with postoperative DVT or PE the rate of treatment failure and recurrence was low (1.6%) and there was little difference between the treatment groups. By contrast, among medical patients the rate was 12.85, with a clear difference in favor of 3 months' treatment. If venous thromboembolism arises after surgery, 4 weeks of anticoagulation should be adequate. In other settings, patients with new DVT, PE, or both, who do not have a persisting underlying cause of risk factor should receive anticoagulants for 3 months.

Central venous and pulmonary artery catheters

The incidence of infection increases with the prolonged use of central venous catheters, but it is unclear whether changing catheters every 3 days, as some recommend, will reduce the rate of infection. It is also unclear whether it is safer to change a catheter over a guide wire or insert it at a new site. Cobb and associates[31] form Charlottesville, Virginia, conducted a controlled trial in adult patients in intensive care units who required central venous or PA catheters for more than 3 days. Patients were assigned randomly to undergo 1 of 4 methods of catheter exchange: replacement every 3 days either by insertion at a new site (group 1) or by exchange over a guide wire (group 2), or replacement when clinically indicated either by insertion at a new site (group 3) or by exchange over a guide wire (group 4). Of the 160 patients, 5% had catheter-related bloodstream infections, 16% had catheters that became colonized, and 9% had major mechanical complications. The incidence rates (per 1000 days of catheter use) of bloodstream infection were 3 in group 1, 6 in group 2, 2 in group 3, and 3 in group 4; the incidence rates of mechanical complications were 14, 4, 8, and 3, respectively. Patients randomly assigned to guide-wire-assisted exchange were more likely to have bloodstream infection after the first 3 days of catheterization. Insertions at new sites were associated with more mechanical complications. Routine replacement of central vascular catheters every 3 days does not prevent infection. Exchanging catheters with the use of a guide wire increases the risk of bloodstream infection, but replacement involving insertion of catheters at new sites increases the risk of mechanical complications.

PULMONARY EMBOLISM

Clinical course

Pulmonary embolism is a potentially fatal disorder. Information about the outcome of clinically recognized pulmonary embolism is sparse, particularly given that new treatments for more seriously ill patients are not available. Carson and associates[32] from multiple USA medical centers prospectively followed 399 patients with pulmonary embolism diagnosed by lung scanning and pulmonary angiography, who were enrolled in a multicenter diagnostic trial. The authors reviewed all hospitalizations, all new investigations of pulmonary embolism, and all deaths among the patients within 1 year of diagnosis. Of the 339 patients, 375 (94%) received treatment for pulmonary embolism usually conventional anticoagulation. Only 10 patients (2.5%) died of pulmonary embolism; 9 of them had clinically suspected recurrent pulmonary embolism. Clinically apparent pulmonary embolism recurred in 33 patients (8.3%), of whom 45% died during follow-up. Ninety-five patients with pulmonary embolism (23.8%)

died within 1 year. The conditions associated with these deaths were cancer (relative risk, 3.8), left-sided CHF (relative risk, 2.7), and chronic lung disease (relative risk, 2.2). The most frequent causes of death in patients with pulmonary embolism were cancer (in 34.7%), infection (22.1%), and cardiac disease (16.8%). When properly diagnosed and treated, clinically apparent pulmonary embolism was an uncommon cause of death, and it recurred in only a small minority of patients. Most deaths were due to underlying diseases. Patients with pulmonary embolism who had cancer, CHF, or chronic lung disease had a higher risk of dying within 1 year than did other patients with pulmonary embolism.

Report of a task force

To assess the state of the art of venous thrombosis and pulmonary embolism for the medical and other health-related professions, the World Health Organization (WHO) and the International Society and Federation of Cardiology (ISFC) convened a task force in Geneva, Switzerland. Members of the task force prepared position papers and presented brief oral presentations. A report was subsequently prepared by the task force members, who contributed sections in their areas of expertise. Revisions of the report occurred during the task force meeting itself in Geneva and during the ensuing months. The final report authored by Goldhaber and Morpurgo[33] was approved by the WHO-ISFC Task Force on Pulmonary Embolism Steering Committee. They concluded that more quantitative information was needed on the frequency of venous thrombosis and pulmonary embolism in hospitalized medical patients as well as in outpatients at high risk. They urged that population studies should focus on incidence, survival, and long-term complications in different parts of the world with respect to gender and race.

In men vs women

Quinn and associates[34] from Boston, Massachusetts, Baltimore, Maryland, and Detroit, Michigan, compared in women and men suspected of pulmonary embolism the frequency, risk factors, diagnosis, and presentation of pulmonary embolism as well as the accuracy of the ventilation/perfusion scan (V/Q scan) as a diagnostic tool (Figure 10-3). Data were collected during a prospective study (the Prospective Investigation of Pulmonary Embolism Diagnosis) to establish the accuracy of the V/Q scan compared with pulmonary angiograms. Patients suspected of pulmonary embolism for whom a request was made for a V/Q scan or pulmonary angiogram (496 women and 406 men) were studied. Women 50 years old and under had a decreased frequency of pulmonary embolism compared with men of that age (16% vs 32%), but there was no difference in patients over 50 years old (Breslow-Day test) (Figure 10-4). Risk factors for pulmonary embolism, the usefulness of the V/Q scan, and 1-year mortality were not different for women and men. Estrogen use in women was not associated with an increased frequency of pulmonary embolism, except in women using oral contraceptives who had undergone surgery within 3 months; 4 of 5 (80%) had emboli compared with 4 of 28 (14%) age-matched surgical patients not using estrogens. Women 50 years old and under (even young women using oral contraceptives) who were suspected of having pulmonary emboli and were enrolled in the Prospective Investigation of Pulmonary Embolism Diagnosis study had a smaller frequency of pulmonary embolism than men of that age. The risk factors for pulmonary

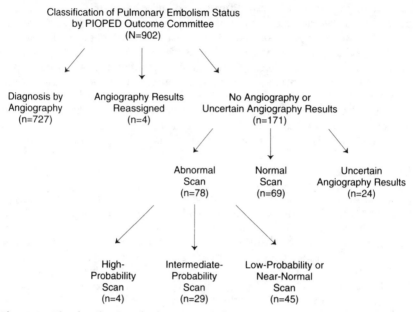

Fig. 10-3. The classification of pulmonary embolism status by the Prospective Investigation of Pulmonary Embolism Diagnosis (PIOPED) Outcome Committee, consisting of senior investigators, from angiography finding and/or considerations of clinical status. Reproduced with permission from Quinn, et al.[34]

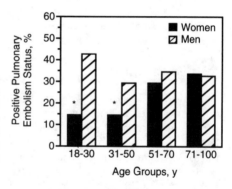

Fig. 10-4. The prevalence of pulmonary embolism in women and men as broken down by age. The asterisks indicate that P<.05 for the difference in the age distribution between women and men for the 18-to-30-year and the 31-to-50-year age groups. Reproduced with permission from Quinn, et al.[34]

embolism were the same for women and men, except that women using oral contraceptives had an increased risk of pulmonary embolism following surgery. Although the V/Q scan was a useful tool in the preliminary evaluation for pulmonary embolism in these women, a pulmonary angiogram was often needed for accurate diagnosis.

Patent foramen ovale

The prevalence of a patent foramen ovale is about 25%. In cases with venous thromboembolism and raised right-sided heart pressures, a patent foramen ovale may permit paradoxical emboli, which could complicate the course of pulmonary embolism. Echocardiography enables detection of a patent foramen ovale during life. Kasper and associates[35] from Freiburg, Germany, studied 85 patients who presented with hemodynamically significant pulmonary embolism as judged by clinical, echocardiographic, or hemodynamic indices and who had an echocardiographic evaluation for patent foramen ovale. Thirty-three patients (39%) had a patent foramen ovale. Clinical symptoms suggestive of paradoxical embolism were more likely in patients with than in those without a patent foramen ovale (39% vs 6%), with new neurological deficits occurring in 11 patients (9 vs 3) and a vascular occlusion in 8 (7 vs 1). Arterial oxygen tension was lower in patients with a patent foramen ovale (mean 55 [SD 14] vs 62 [16] mmHg). Mortality was not different between the 2 groups (27% vs 19%). Cardiopulmonary complications in terms of resuscitation, intubation, or the use of catecholamines were more frequently observed in patients with a patent foramen ovale (48% vs 23%). Patients with a patent foramen ovale and hemodynamically significant pulmonary embolism are more likely to have arterial hypoxemia and vascular occlusions, possibly due to paradoxical emboli.

Pulmonary arteriography

The Prospective Investigation of Pulmonary Embolism Diagnosis addressed the value of ventilation/perfusion scans in acute pulmonary embolism. Stein and coworkers[36] in Detroit, Michigan, evaluated the risks and diagnostic validity of pulmonary angiography in the 1,111 patients who underwent angiography in the pulmonary embolism study. Complications were death in 5, nonfatal complications in 9, and less significant or minor in 60. More fatal or major nonfatal complications occurred in patients from the medical intensive care unit than elsewhere: 5 of 22 versus 9 of 989. Pulmonary artery pressure, volume of contrast material, and presence of pulmonary embolism did not significantly alter the frequency of complication. Renal dysfunction, either major (requiring dialysis) or less severe, occurred in 13 of 1,111. Patients who developed renal dysfunction after angiography were older than those who did not have renal dysfunction, 74 years vs. 57 years. Angiograms were nondiagnostic in 35 patients, and studies were incomplete in 12, usually because of a complication. Surveillance after negative angiogram showed pulmonary embolism in 4 of 675 patients. Angiograms, interpreted on the basis of consensus readings, resulted in a unchallenged diagnosis in 96%. The risks of pulmonary angiography were sufficiently low to justify it as a diagnostic tool in the appropriate clinical setting. Clinical judgment is probably the most important consideration in the assessment of risk.

During endomyocardial biopsy

Kreher and associates[37] in Minneapolis, Minnesota, determined the frequency of occult right heart thromboembolism during endomyocardial biopsy in 51 cardiac transplant recipients undergoing endomyocardial biopsy who were studied echocardiographically. Patients were randomized into 2 groups. In Group 1, the venous sheath was flushed between each biopsy attempt and in Group 2, it was flushed only at the time of initial placement. Right heart thromboemboli were identified in 18 (35%) of 51 patients. Seventeen (94%) of these 18 patients were in Group 2. Patients requiring more than six biopsy attempts had a significantly higher incidence of embolism. Other variables, such as antiplatelet therapy, operator experience and total time of the procedure did not correlate with thrombus development and thromboemboli. All right sided heart emboli were asymptomatic. Therefore, these data demonstrate a high incidence

of occult pulmonary embolism during uncomplicated routine endomyocardial biopsy.

Recombinant tissue-type plasminogen vs urokinase

Goldhaber and associates[38] in Boston, Brookline, and West Roxbury,
Massachusetts; Washington, D.C.; Rochester, Minnesota; Salt Lake City,
Utah; Marshfield, Wisconsin; Akron, Ohio; and Kansas City, Kansas, have
conducted a trial in which 90 patients were enrolled to determine the
influence of a novel dosing regimen of urokinase in patients with pulmonary embolism. Patients were randomized to receive either 100 mg in 2
hours of tissue plasminogen activator or a novel dosing regimen of urokinase: 3 million units in 2 hours with the initial 1 million units given as
a bolus injection over 10 minutes. Both drugs were delivered through a
peripheral vein. To determine the efficacy after initiation of therapy, repeat
pulmonary angiograms were performed at 2 hours in 87 patients and
graded in a blinded manner by six investigators. Among the 42 patients
given tissue plasminogen activator, 79% showed angiographic improvement in 2 hours compared with 67% of the 45 patients randomized to
urokinase therapy. The mean change in perfusion lung scans between
baseline and 24 hours was similar for both treatments. Three patients
had intracranial hemorrhages which was fatal in one. These data indicate
that a 2 hour infusion of tissue plasminogen activator and a new dosing
regimen for urokinase exhibit relatively similar efficacy and safety in the
treatment of patients with acute pulmonary embolism.

Alteplase + heparin vs heparin

Dalla-Volta and colleagues[39] in Padova, Italy, evaluated the efficacy
and safety of alteplase followed by heparin as compared to heparin alone
in 36 patients with angiographically documented pulmonary emboli.
Twenty patients were allocated randomly to a 2 hour infusion of alteplase
(10 mg bolus, then 90 mg over 2 hours) followed by heparin. The other
16 patients were given intravenous heparin at a continuous infusion rate
of 1,750 IU/h. The vascular obstruction assessed at pulmonary angiography decreased significantly in alteplase-treated patients from a baseline
of 28 ± 3 to a value of 25 ± 5 2 hours after the start of the infusion, but
in the heparin group there was no change in the degree of vascular
obstruction. Mean PA pressures decreased significantly from a baseline
of 30 ± 7.8 mmHg to 21 ± 6.7 in the alteplase group and increased in
the heparin group. Lung scans were performed at baseline and on days
7 and 30. There were no differences between the two groups in the follow-
up lung scans, but there were significant decreases from the baseline
values. Bleeding occurred in 14 of 20 alteplase-treated patients and in 6
of 16 in the heparin group. There were 3 major bleeding episodes in the
alteplase group and 2 in the heparin group. Two patients died after
fibrinolysis and one patient in the heparin group died of recurrent pulmonary embolism. These data suggest that alteplase results in a greater
and faster improvement of the angiographic and hemodynamic variables
compared with heparin. The high frequency of bleeding observed with
alteplase in this trial suggests that patients should be selected carefully
before thrombolytic therapy is given.

Alteplase vs urokinase

Meyer and associates[40] in Paris, Tours and Besancon, France; Freiburg, Germany; London, England; and Leuven, Belgium in a twelve center double-blind study evaluated the ability of either urokinase as an intravenous bolus, then infusion or alteplase as a bolus followed by heparin to lyse angiographically documented acute massive pulmonary emboli in 63 patients. The primary objective was to compare the resolution of pulmonary embolism as judged by the change in total pulmonary resistance during the subsequent two hours. Further objectives were to evaluate the change in total pulmonary resistance over the next ten hours and the degree of angiographic resolution at 12 to 18 hours. By 2 hours, total pulmonary vascular resistance decreased by $18 \pm 22\%$ in the urokinase-treated patients and by $36 \pm 17\%$ in the alteplase-treated patients. Continuous monitoring of pulmonary artery mean pressures, cardiac indexes and total pulmonary resistances revealed that these variables improved faster in the alteplase group with consistently significant differences from 30 minutes to 3 to 4 hours in the treatment groups. After 12 hours, the decrease in total pulmonary resistance was $53 \pm 19\%$ in the urokinase-treated patients compared with $48 \pm 17\%$ in the alteplase-treated patients and the reductions in the angiographic severity score were $30 \pm 25\%$ and $24 \pm 18\%$, respectively. Bleeding was equally frequent in the two treatment groups except that more urokinase-treated patients developed hematomas at puncture sites. Thus, thrombolytic therapy may be useful in selected patients in the treatment of massive pulmonary emboli.

AORTIC DISEASE

Expansion rates of aneurysms

The risk of rupture of an aortic aneurysm increases with size and rapid expansion rate. Masuda and associates[41] from Chiba, Japan, studied the expansion rate, and compared the results with those of abdominal aortic aneurysm. Forty thoracic aortic aneurysms and 25 abdominal aortic aneurysms were serially examined with enhanced and nonenhanced computed tomography. The mean expansion rate of thoracic aortic aneurysms was 1.3 ± 1.2 mm/yr and was significantly lower than 3.9 ± 3.2 mm/yr of abdominal aortic aneurysms. The factors increasing expansion rate of thoracic aortic aneurysms were initial size of aneurysms, diastolic BP, and presence of renal failure by univariate analysis. Multivariate analysis concerning the entire aortic aneurysms also revealed that the large size of the aneurysm and the presence of the aortic aneurysm in the abdomen increased expansion rate of aneurysms.

Aortic root aneurysms

Bentall's technique for repair of annuloaortic ectasia has been associated with postoperative bleeding and with false aneurysms of the anastomotic site between the coronary orifices and valve-containing graft. To reduce the incidence of these complications, Lewis and associates[42] from Houston, Texas, modified the Bentall procedure, using a simplified technique to implant the graft and to create a fistula between the closed perigraft space and right atrium to control bleeding. A continuous suture of monofilament polypropylene was used to implant the prosthetic valve ring and to anastomose the coronary orifices to the Dacron fabric. In some instances, a brief period of hypothermic circulatory arrest was needed to perform the distal aortic anastomosis. Among 562 patients undergoing operation for aneurysm of the ascending aorta between January 1, 1980, and February 28, 1990, 280 underwent graft replacement with a valve-containing composite conduit. Most (82%) had annuloaortic ectasia. In 267, the authors performed a classic Bentall procedure with direct anastomosis between the coronary orifices and fabric graft. The remaining 13 patients underwent other procedures for coronary connection. Early mortality was 5.0%. Reoperation for bleeding was needed in 13.2% of patients who underwent operation before the right atrial fistula technique was used and in 4.4% after the technique was used. Actuarial survival was 71% at 5 years and 65% at 7 years. For hospital survivors, it was 76% at 5 years and 70% at 7 years. During follow-up, only 9 patients have required reoperation. A false aneurysm at the coronary anastomosis, which was associated with prosthetic valve endocarditis, developed in 1 patient. No permanent fistulas have developed. Thus, by using simplified methods to implant the graft and to control postoperative bleeding, the Bentall technique can be performed successfully with excellent early and late results.

Aortic dissection

Aortic dissection requires prompt and reliable diagnosis to reduce the high mortality. Nienaber and coworkers[43] in Hamburg, Germany, assessed the reliability of both electrocardiographic-triggered magnetic resonance imaging and transesophageal two-dimensional echocardiography, combined with color-coded Doppler flow imaging for the diagnosis of thoracic aortic dissection and associated epiphenomena. Fifty-three consecutive patients with clinically suspected aortic dissection were subjected to a dual non-invasive imaging protocol in random order. Imaging results were compared and validated against the independent morphologic "gold standard" of intraoperative findings in 27, necropsy in 7, and/or contrast angiography in 53 patients. No serious side effects were encountered with either imaging method. In contrast to a precursory screening transthoracic echogram, the sensitivities of both magnetic imaging and esophageal imaging were 100% for detecting a dissection of the thoracic aorta, irrespective of its location. The specificity of esophageal echocardiography was lower than the specificity of magnetic imaging for a dissection, which resulted mainly from false-positive esophageal echocardiographic findings confined to the ascending segment of the aorta. In addition, magnetic imaging proved to be more sensitive than esophageal echocardiography in detecting the formation of thrombus in the false lumen of both the aortic arch and the descending segment of the aorta. There were no discrepancies between the two imaging techniques in detecting the site of entry to a dissection, aortic regurgitation, or pericardial effusion. Both magnetic imaging and esophageal echocardiography are atraumatic, safe, and highly sensitive methods to identify and classify acute and subacute dissections of the entire thoracic aorta. Esophageal echocardiography is associated with lower specificity for lesions in the ascending aorta. These results may still favor esophageal echocardiography as a semi-invasive diagnostic procedure after a precursory screening transthoracic echogram in suspected aortic dissection, but they establish magnetic imaging as an excellent method to avoid false-positive findings. Anatomic mapping by magnetic resonance may emerge as the most comprehensive approach and morphological standard to guide surgical interventions.

Elefteriades and associates[44] from New Haven, Connecticut, analyzed long-term results in 71 patients (45 men and 26 women) treated over 17 years for documented descending aortic dissection. Forty-nine patients were treated medically and 22, surgically. Actuarial survival was 65% at 1 year, 57% at 3 years, 50% at 5 years, and 28% at 10 years for the whole group. For the group treated medically, survival was 73%, 63%, 58%, and 25% at 1 year, 3 years, 5 years, and 10 years, respectively, and for the group treated surgically, 47%, 40%, and 28% at 1 year, 3 years, and 5 years, respectively. Ten (20.4%) of the 49 medically treated patients died early (5 of rupture), and 14 (28.6%) died late (8 of dissection). Five medically treated patients crossed over to surgical management for complications of dissection. Among the surgically treated patients, 6 underwent standard graft replacement of the proximal descending aorta, 8 underwent the fenestration procedure (with a standardized retroperitoneal abdominal approach), and 4 underwent the thromboexclusion operation. Specific analysis of fenestration in 14 patients (including some with persistent descending aortic dissection after replacement of the ascending aorta for dissection) found it to be safe and effective. Actuarial survival after fenestration was 77%, 77%, and 53% at 1 year, 3 years, and 5 years, respectively. Thromboexclusion was found effective, and postoperative studies confirmed thrombosis of the descending aorta with preservation of the lowest intercostal arteries. Fifteen of the 21 surviving medically treated patients agreed to return for follow-up imaging. Nine had thrombosis of the false lumen. An interesting radiographic finding was that 4 of the 15 restudied patients had a saccular aneurysm in the aorta at the level of the left subclavian artery. The authors recommend a complication-specific approach to the management of descending aortic dissection. Uncomplicated dissection is treated medically, whereas complicated dissection is treated surgically, with realized rupture treated by standard graft replacement, limb ischemia treated by fenestration, and enlargement or impending rupture treated by thromboexclusion.

Aortic arch plaques by echocardiography

The cause of cerebral infarction is obscure in up to 40% of patients with this disorder who are studied prospectively. Amarenco and associates[45] from Villejuif, France, determined the frequency of ulcerated plaques in the aortic arch and explored the part they may play in the formation of cerebral emboli. Using an autopsy data bank, the authors studied the prevalence of ulcerated plaques in the aortic arch in 500 consecutive patients with cerebrovascular and other neurologic diseases who were studied at autopsy. Ulcerated plaques were present in 26% of the 239 patients with cerebrovascular disease but in only 5% of the 261 patients with other neurologic diseases. After the authors controlled for age and heart weight, the adjusted rates were 16.9% and 5.1%, respectively. Among the patients with cerebrovascular disease, the prevalence of ulcerated plaques in the aortic arch was 28% in the 183 patients with cerebral infarcts and 20% in the 56 patients with brain hemorrhage. The prevalence of ulcerated plaques was 61% among the 28 patients with no known cause of cerebral infarction, as compared with 22% among the 155 patients with a known cause of cerebral infarction. After adjustment for covariates, the prevalence was 57.8% among patients with no known cause of cerebral infarction and 20.2% among those with a known cause (adjusted odds ratio, 5.7; 95% confidence interval, 2.4 to 13.6). The presence of ulcerated plaques in the aortic arch was not correlated with the presence of extracranial internal-carotid-artery stenosis, suggesting that these were two independent risk factors for stroke. Ulcerated plaques in the aortic arch may play a part in causing cerebral infarction, especially in patients in whom cerebral infarction has no known cause.

Stroke is a serious complication of cardiopulmonary bypass with a frequency of 2–5%. Ribakove and associates[46] from New York, New York, prospectively used transesophageal echocardiography (TEE) in 97 patients >65 years of age (mean age, 73 years) to identify those at high risk for aortic atheroemboli. The atheromatous disease of the aorta was graded by TEE: grade I = minimal intimal thickening (n = 29); II = extensive intimal thickening (n = 33); III = sessile atheroma (n = 15); IV = protruding atheroma (n = 10); V = mobile atheroma (n = 10). Clinical evaluation was also performed by intraoperative aortic palpation. Four patients who were graded as having normal aortas by palpation had intraoperative strokes. In contrast, 3 of these 4 patients were in grade V on TEE. The relationship of TEE to incidence of stroke was statistically significant, whereas there was no significant correlation between clinical grade and stroke incidence. Four of 10 TEE grade V patients were treated with hypothermic circulatory arrest and aortic arch debridement, and none suffered strokes. The other 6 patients were treated with standard techniques, and 3 had strokes. These results suggest that patients with mobile atheromatous disease are at high risk for embolic strokes that are not predicted by routine clinical evaluation. Selective use of circulatory arrest in the presence of TEE-detected mobile arch atheromas may reduce the risk of intraoperative stroke.

Katz and associates[47] in New York, New York, evaluated 130 patients ≥65 years of age with intraoperative transesophageal echocardiography to detect the aortic arch protruding atheromas and determine if these patients were at high risk for perioperative stroke. Protruding atheromas were found in 23 (18%) of 130 patients. In 19 (83%) of these 23 patients, palpation of the aortic arch at operation did not identify significant abnormalities. Five patients (4%) had perioperative strokes. Logistic regression identified aortic arch atheroma as the only historical or procedural variable predictive of stroke. A history of peripheral or cerebrovascular disease, presence of aortic calcification, cardiac risk factors, age and duration of cardiopulmonary bypass did not predict stroke. In contrast, patients with protruding atheromas with mobile components were at highest risk. There were 3 (25%) of 12 patients with a mobile atheroma who had a stroke versus 2 (2%) of 118 patients without a mobile atheroma. Displacement and detachment of the frail, protruding atheromas by aortic arch cannulation or the high pressure jet emanating from the cannula tip may play an important role in the development of embolization and stroke.

Management of small abdominal aortic aneurysm

Katz and associates[48] from Lebanon, New Hampshire, reviewed data from an earlier longitudinal study of patients with small abdominal aortic aneurysms (AAAs) less than 5 cm in diameter to estimate incidence rates of rupture or acute expansion. The authors constructed a Markov decision tree to compare early surgery with watchful waiting in patients with asymptomatic AAAs less than 5 cm in diameter, with respect to long-term survival in quality-adjusted life years. The average annual rates of rupture or acute expansion for AAAs with a maximal transverse diameter of < 4.0, 4.0 to 4.9, and at least 5.0 cm, are 0, 3.3, and 14.4 events per 100 patient-years of observation, respectively. At an average rupture rate of 3.3 events per 100 patient-years and an average operative risk for elective surgery of 4.6% at 30-days. The benefit of early surgery decreases with increased age at presentation. If the average rupture rate for AAAs less than 5 cm is assumed to be low (e.g., 0.4 event per 100 patient-years), watchful waiting is favored, particularly as operative risk increases. The decision in this subgroup, however, is sensitive to possible future increases in operative risk. In the majority of scenarios that were examined, early surgery is preferred to watchful waiting for patients with AAAs less than 5 cm in diameter. Watchful waiting is generally favored, however, for patients with a low risk of AAA rupture or acute expansion, including those patients who present with very small AAAs (e.g., <4 cm). More accurate data concerning the rupture risk of AAAs less than 5 cm would improve clinical decision making.

Coronary narrowing with abdominal aortic aneurysm

Mautner and associates[49] from Bethesda, Maryland, determined in 27 patients (mean age at death 72 ± 9 years) with abdominal aortic aneurysm ≥5.0 cm in its widest transverse diameter, the amounts of narrowing at necropsy in the 4 major (left main, left anterior descending, left circumflex, and right) epicardial coronary arteries were determined. During life, 12 of the 27 patients (44%) had symptoms of myocardial ischemia: angina pectoris alone in 2, AMI alone in 3, angina pectoris and AMI in 5, and sudden coronary death in 2. Ten of the 27 patients (37%) died from consequences of myocardial ischemia. Six (22%) died from rupture of the AAA. Grossly visible LV necrosis or fibrosis, or both, was present in 15 patients (56%). Of the 27 patients, 23 (85%) had narrowing 76 to 100% in cross-sectional area of 1 or more major coronary arteries by atherosclerotic plaque. The mean number of coronary arteries per patient severely (>75%) narrowed was 2.0 ± 1.3/4.0. Of the 108 major coronary arteries in the 27 patients were divided into 5-mm segments and a histologic section, stained by the Movat method, was prepared from each segment. The mean percentages of the resulting 1,475 5-mm segments narrowed in cross-sectional area 0 to 25%, 26 to 50%, 51 to 75%, 76 to 95% and 96 to 100% were 17, 37, 28, 15 and 3%, respectively. The percentages of 5-mm coronary segments narrowed >75% in cross-sectional area were similar in the right, left anterior descending, and left circumflex coronary arteries. Thus, patients with AAA nearly always have diffuse and severe coronary atherosclerosis.

PERIPHERAL ARTERIAL DISEASE

Aspirin

In the US Physicians' Health Study the early termination of the aspirin arm has provided the opportunity to test the hypothesis that low-dose aspirin (325 mg on alternate days) might affect the subsequent occurrence of peripheral arterial surgery. In the study, a randomized double-blind placebo-controlled trial among 22,071 healthy US male physicians aged 40-84 years, there were, during an average of 60 months of treatment and follow-up, 56 participants who underwent arterial surgery (20 aspirin, 36 placebo) and this data was reported by Goldhaber and associates[50] from Boston, Massachusetts. The relative risk of peripheral arterial surgery in the aspirin group was .54 and highly significant. These data indicate that chronic administration of low-dose aspirin to apparently healthy men reduces the need for peripheral arterial surgery.

Angioplasty

Previous studies regarding the mechanism by which PTCA increases luminal patency have generally used animal models or postmortem specimens from occasional fatal cases of PTCA performed in human patients. In either case, conclusions regarding participatory mechanisms have relied exclusively on nonserial, PTCA histopathological examination. Losordo and co-workers[51] in Boston, Massachusetts, performed intravascular ultrasound examination before and after balloon PTCA in 40 consecutive patients with iliac artery stenoses. The areas of the arterial wall, plaque, lumen, and areas resulting from PTCA-induced plaque fractures were measured immediately after PTCA in vivo and compared with findings recorded immediately before PTCA. PTCA increased luminal cross-sectional area from 11.5 mm^2 before PTCA to 25.4 mm^2 after PTCA. Cross-sectional area of the portion of the post-PTCA neolumen contained within PTCA-induced plaque fractures measured 10.0 mm^2; the neolumen excluding the area contributed by these plaque fractures measured 15.4 mm^2. Thus, the area contained within plaque fractures accounted for 10.0 mm^2 of the 13.9-mm^2 increase in luminal cross-sectional area after PTCA. Analysis of cross-sectional area occupied by atherosclerotic plaque disclosed that plaque cross-sectional area decreased from 34 mm^2 before PTCA to 22 mm^2 after PTCA. Plaque cross-sectional area was thus reduced ("compressed") by 11 mm^2. Total artery cross-sectional area increased ("stretched") slightly from 45 mm^2 before PTCA to 48 mm^2 after PTCA. In vivo analysis of iliac stenoses by intravascular ultrasound immediately before and after PTCA demonstrated that plaque fractures and "compression" of atherosclerotic plaque are the principal factors responsible for increased luminal patency resulting from balloon PTCA. "Stretching" of the arterial wall provides an additional, but minor, contribution.

Ten-year mortality

Several investigators have observed a doubling of the mortality rate among patients with intermittent claudication, and Criqui and associates[52] from La Jolla, California, had reported previously a 4-fold increase in the overall mortality rate among subjects with large-vessel peripheral arterial disease as diagnosed by noninvasive study. In the present study, Criqui and associates investigated the association of large-vessel peripheral arterial disease with rates of mortality from all cardiovascular diseases and from CAD. They examined 565 men and women (average age, 66 years) for the presence of large-vessel peripheral arterial disease by means of 2 noninvasive techniques—measurement of segmental BP and determination of flow velocity by Doppler ultrasound. The authors identified 67 subjects with the disease (12%), whom they followed prospectively for 10 years. Twenty-one of the 34 men (62%) and 11 of the 33 women (33%) with large-vessel peripheral arterial disease died during follow-up, as compared with 31 of the 183 men (17%) and 26 of the 225 women (12%) without evidence of peripheral arterial disease (Figures 10-5 and 10-6). After multivariate adjustment for age, sex, and other risk factors for cardiovascular disease, the relative risk of dying among subjects with large-vessel peripheral arterial disease as compared with those with no evidence of such disease was 3.1 for deaths from all causes, 5.9 for all deaths from cardiovascular disease, and 6.6 for deaths from CAD. The relative risk of death from causes other than cardiovascular disease was not significantly increased among the subjects with large-vessel peripheral arterial disease. After the exclusion of subjects who had a history of cardiovascular disease at base line, the relative risks among those with large-vessel peripheral

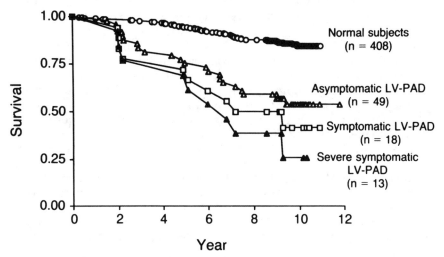

Fig. 10-5. Kaplan-Meier Survival Curves Based on Mortality from All Causes among Normal Subjects and Subjects with Symptomatic or Asymptomatic Large-Vessel Peripheral Arterial Disease (LV-PAD). Reproduced with permission from Criqui, et al.[52]

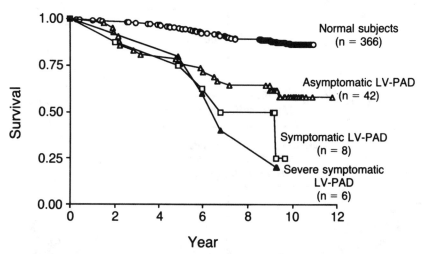

Fig. 10-6. Kaplan-Meier Survival Curves Based on Mortality from All Causes among Normal Subjects and Subjects with Symptomatic or Asymptomatic Large-Vessel Peripheral Arterial Disease (LV-PAD), after the Exclusion of Subjects with Evidence of Cardiovascular Disease at Base Line. Reproduced with permission from Criqui, et al.[52]

arterial disease remained significantly elevated. Additional analyses revealed a 15-fold increase in rates of mortality due to cardiovascular disease and CAD among subjects with large-vessel peripheral arterial disease that was both severe and symptomatic. Patients with large-vessel peripheral arterial disease have a high risk of death from cardiovascular causes.

Associated coronary narrowing

Mautner and associates[53] from Bethesda, Maryland, determined in 26 patients (mean age at death 68 ± 9 years) who had undergone amputation (at mean age 63 ± 12 years) of 1 or both lower extremities due to severe peripheral arterial atherosclerosis, the amounts of narrowing at necropsy in the 4 major (LM, LAD, LC, and right) epicardial coronary arteries. During life, 15 of the 26 patients (58%) had symptoms of myocardial ischemia: angina pectoris alone in 1, AMI alone in 5, and angina and/or infarction plus CHF or sudden coronary death in 9. Twelve of the 26 patients (42%) died from consequences of myocardial ischemia: AMI in 5, sudden coronary death in 3, chronic CHF in 3, and shortly after CABG in 1. Grossly visible LV necrosis or fibrosis, or both, was present in 21 patients (81%). Of the 26 patients, 24 (92%) had narrowing 76 to 100% in cross-sectional area of 1 or more major coronary arteries by atherosclerotic plaque (Figure 10-7). The mean number of coronary arteries per patient severely (>75%) narrowed was 2.3 ± 1.0/4.0. Of the 104 major coronary arteries in the 26 patients were divided into 5-mm segments and a histologic section, stained by the Movat method, was prepared from each segment. The mean percentages of the resulting 1,322 five-mm segments narrowed in cross-sectional area 0 to 25%, 26 to 50%, 51 to 75%, 76 to 95% and 96 to 100% were 17, 20, 35, 19 and 9%, respectively (Figure 10-8). The percentages of 5-mm coronary segments narrowed >75% in cross-sectional area were

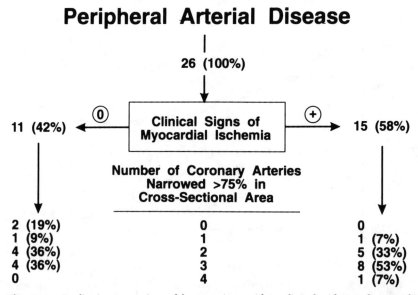

Fig. 10-7. Qualitative comparison of the 11 patients *without* clinical evidence of myocardial ischemia (cases 1 to 11, Table I) with the 15 patients *with* clinical evidence of myocardial ischemia (cases 12 to 26, Table I). Reproduced with permission from Mautner, et al.[53]

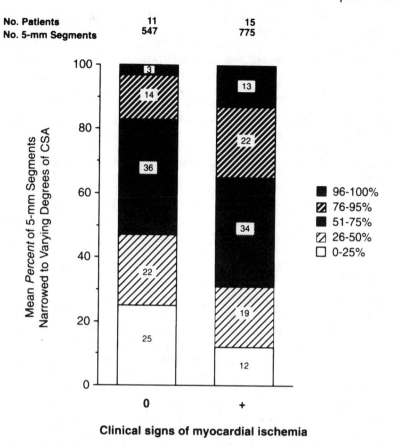

Fig. 10-8. Mean percentages of 5-mm segments of the sum of the 4 major coronary arteries narrowed to varying degrees in cross-sectional area (CSA) in 26 amputees: comparison of 11 patients *without* (cases 1 to 11, Table I) with 15 patients *with* (cases 12 to 26, Table I) clinical evidence of myocardial ischemia. Reproduced with permission from Mautner, et al.[53]

similar in the left anterior descending, left circumflex and right coronary arteries. Thus, patients with peripheral arterial atherosclerosis severe enough to warrant amputation nearly always have diffuse and severe coronary atherosclerosis at the time of necropsy.

STROKE

Patent foramen ovale

To determine and compare the prevalence of patent foramen ovale in patients with stroke of undetermined origin (cryptogenic) and in patients with stroke of determined origin to assess the possible role of patent foramen ovale as a risk factor for cryptogenic stroke, Tullio and associates[54] from New York, New York, studied 146 patients (73 men, 73 women) with acute ischemic stroke referred to the echocardiographic laboratory for evaluation. The patients were considered to have strokes of determined origin or cryptogenic strokes according to the National

Institute of Neurologic Disorders and Stroke Databank Criteria. The presence of patent foramen ovale was assessed by contrast echocardiography, performed blinded for type of stroke. The overall prevalence of patent foramen ovale was 26 of 146 patients (18%). Patients with cryptogenic stroke (31%) had a significantly higher prevalence of patent foramen ovale than did patients with an identifiable cause of stroke (69%) in both the younger (<55 years; 48% compared with 4%) and the older (≥55 years; 38% compared with 8%) age groups. Multiple logistic regression analysis was used to identify the presence of a patent foramen ovale as strongly associated with the diagnosis of cryptogenic stroke (odds ratio, 7.2), irrespective of patient age and other stroke risk factors. Patients with cryptogenic stroke have a higher prevalence of patent foramen ovale than patients with stroke of determined cause in all age groups, even after correcting for the presence of recognized stroke risk factors. This identifies patent foramen ovale as a risk factor for cryptogenic stroke. Regardless of patient age, contrast echocardiography should be considered when the cause of stroke is unknown.

Risk of coronary event afterwards

Proposed guidelines for the diagnosis of transient ischemic attack (TIA) involve interpretation of symptoms, so it can be difficult to distinguish a TIA from other disorders, such as migraine, epilepsy, syncope, or neurosis. Atypical cerebral and visual events also may be classified as TIA. To see whether TIA or stroke patients with atypical cerebral or visual symptoms are at high or low risk of cardiac complications, Koudstaal and associates[55] for the Dutch TIA Study Group from several European centers prospectively followed 572 patients with a diagnosis of TIA or minor ischemic stroke, but whose symptoms did not fully accord with internationally accepted criteria. The authors compared their outcome with that of 2,555 other TIA or stroke patients in the Dutch TIA Study Group trial who had unequivocal symptoms. All patients were treated with aspirin. During mean follow-up of 2.6 years the risk of a major vascular event did not differ between the groups (14.5% in patients with atypical symptoms vs 15.1% of patients with typical attacks). Patients with atypical attacks had a lower risk of stroke (5.6% vs 9.4%, hazard ratio 0.6, 95% confidence interval 0.4–0.9) and a higher risk of a major cardiac event (8.4% vs 5.9%, 1.4, 1.0–2.0) than did patients with typical attacks. These differences could not be explained by differences in cardiac risk factors, and were independent of minor discrepancies in baseline characteristics between the groups. A heavy or tired feeling in 1 or 2 limbs was the only atypical symptom associated with cerebral rather than cardiac events (ratio cardiac/cerebral events 0.8). For all other atypical symptoms cardiac events were about twice as common as cerebral events (range 1.3–2.5). The findings suggest that TIA or minor stroke patients with atypical symptoms may have symptomatic heart disease, especially cardiac arrhythmia.

ODDS AND ENDS

Calcium antagonist for primary pulmonary hypertension

Primary pulmonary hypertension is a progressive, fatal disease of unknown cause. Vasodilator drugs have been used as a treatment, but their efficacy is uncertain. Rich and associates[56] from Chicago, Illinois, treated 64 patients with primary pulmonary hypertension with high doses of either nifedipine (20 mg) or diltiazem (60 mg). If they had a resting tachycardia, and the doses were repeated every hour until a favorable response was achieved (defined as a more than 20% decrease in PA pressure and pulmonary vascular resistance) unless systemic hypotension or other intolerable side effects precluded further drug testing. The patients were treated for up to 5 years. Their survival was compared with that of the patients who did not respond and with patients enrolled in the National Institutes of Health Registry on Primary Pulmonary hypertension. Warfarin was given to 55% of the patients as concurrent therapy, on the basis of a lung scan showing nonuniformity of PA blood flow (47% of patients who responded and 57% of those who did not respond). Seventeen patients (26%) responded to treatment, as indicated by a 39% fall in PA pressure and a 53% fall in the pulmonary-vascular-resistance index. Nifedipine (mean daily dose, 172 ± 41 mg) was given to 13 patients, and diltiazem (mean daily dose, 720 ± 208 mg) was given to 4 patients. After 5 years, 94% of the patients who responded (16 of 17) were alive, as compared with 55% of the patients who did not respond (26 of 47). The survival of the patients who responded was also significantly better than that of the NIH registry cohort and patients from the NIH registry who were treated at the University of Illinois. The use of warfarin was associated with improved survival, particularly in the patients who did not respond. This study suggests that high doses of calcium-antagonists in patients with primary pulmonary hypertension who respond with reductions in PA pressure and pulmonary vascular resistance may improve survival over a 5-year period.

Predicting pulmonary artery wedge pressure

The noninvasive prediction of PA wedge pressure is important for the recognition and treatment of a variety of cardiovascular disorders. The response of the arterial pressure to the Valsalva maneuver has been shown to correlate with the PA wedge pressure. McIntyre and associates[57] from Boston, Massachusetts, and Portland, Maine, devised a noninvasive method to measure PA wedge pressure response at the bedside and correlated these measurements with the PA wedge pressure measured directly with a PA catheter. Simultaneous, blinded, noninvasive measurements of the ratio of the final amplitude to the initial amplitude of the pulse wave form during the stress phase of the Valsalva maneuver (pulse-amplitude ratio) and direct measurements of the PA wedge pressure were obtained in 20 clinically stable patients and in 14 clinically unstable patients who were receiving vasoactive agents, 12 of whom also had endotracheal tubes in place. Using linear regression analysis, the authors found that the pulse-amplitude ratio strongly correlated with the measured PA wedge pressure over a range of baseline values from 4 to 32 mmHg for the 20 clinically stable patients and the 14 clinically unstable patients. The method also correctly predicted changes in the PA wedge pressure after the administration of nitroglycerin or furosemide and after expansion of the intravascular volume. These preliminary data indicate that a simple noninvasive method can accurately predict the PA wedge pressure and changes in the PA wedge pressure in response to medical therapy.

Effects of intranasal cocaine

Boehrer and associates[58] in Dallas, Texas, assessed the hemodynamic effects of intranasal cocaine, 2 mg/kg, in 15 patients, including 8 men and 7 women, ages 30 to 70 years referred for cardiac catheterization. Heart rate, systemic arterial pressure, cardiac index, pulmonary capillary wedge and PA pressures and LV pressures and first derivative (dP/dt) were measured before and 15, 30, and 45 minutes after intranasal administration of saline (n = 5) or cocaine 2 mg/kg (n = 10). In the patients given cocaine, there was an increase in heart rate, mean systemic arterial pressure, cardiac index, and positive and negative dP/dt. These data indicate that intranasal cocaine in a dose similar to that used "recreationally" does not exert a deleterious influence on intracardiac pressures and LV performance.

Valvular operations in carcinoid heart disease

Between 1982 and 1989, 10 patients with carcinoid heart disease underwent tricuspid valve replacement with a mechanical prosthesis and pulmonary velvectomy in 9 patients and pulmonary valve replacement in 1 patient at the Mayo Clinic and the results were reported by Knott-Craig and associates[59] from Rochester, Minnesota. Two patients had carcinoid tumor metastatic to the heart, involving the right atrium in 1 case and both ventricles in the other. One patient had concomitant coronary artery bypass with the saphenous vein, and 1 patient had a quadruple valve replacement for histologically proved carcinoid disease of all 4 valves. The 30-day mortality was 10% and the late mortality was 30%. The remaining 6 patients were alive 4, 4, 4, 7, 24 and 46 months postoperatively. A review of the English literature identified 28 additional patients who underwent tricuspid valve replacement for carcinoid heart disease. There was no significant difference in the survival of patients with a bioprosthesis versus a mechanical valve in the tricuspid position. The 4-year survival for the 38 patients undergoing tricuspid valve replacement for carcinoid heart disease was 48% ± 13%. Symptomatic patients who have carcinoid heart disease and whose metastic malignant disease is not an imminent threat to life should be offered valve replacement. Operating soon after the onset of increasing cardiac symptoms, before disease and whose metastic malignant disease is not an imminent threat to life should be offered valve replacement.

Open heart surgery in Europe

The European Academy of Sciences and Arts founded in 1990 an Institute for Cardiac Survey with the specific task of monitoring the development of cardiac interventions. The first European survey on cardiac surgery set up in 1990 was accomplished in 1991. All cardio-surgical units in Europe were contacted directly and 63% responded. All national health authorities, the ministries, the national societies for cardiac surgery and the national academies of sciences were asked for support so that finally the data is a compilation from the whole of Europe, including the former Soviet Union, and covers 704,000,000 people.[60] In Europe in 1990 414 cardio-surgical units covered the 704,000,000 people operating on an average of 462 cases a year. Thus, each unit covered a population of 1.70 million. In 1990, 191,299 open heart procedures were performed (Figures

10-9 and 10-10). This number represents a mean of 354 cases per million population.

Acronyms of major cardiologic trials

Cheng[61] from Washington, D.C., listed alphabetically acronyms of major cardiologic trials (Table 10-3).

Cardiologic books published in 1992

GENERAL CARDIOLOGY

*1. Willerson JT, editor, with 8 associate editors (Baim DS, Cooley DA, Frazier OH, Grundy SM, Kaplan NM, Packer M, Sweeney MS, Zipes DP). *Treatment of Heart Diseases.* New York: Gower Medical Publishing, 1992:528, $159.50.

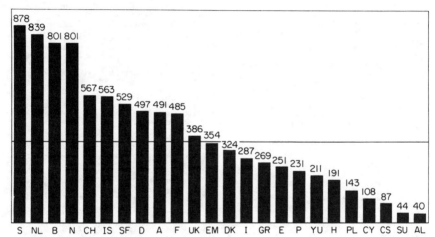

Fig. 10-9. Open heart procedures per million population. EM = European mean. Reproduced with permission from Unger F and Hutler J.[60]

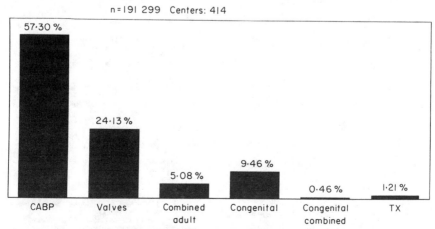

Fig. 10-10. Subsets of the total open heart load. CABP = coronary artery bypass surgery, TX = heart replacement, heart-lung replacement, by means of transplantation and artificial heart. Reproduced with permission from Unger F and Hutler J.[60]

TABLE 10-3. *Acronyms of Major Cardiologic Trials. Reproduced with permission from Cheng, et al.*[61]

ACME (Angioplasty Compared to Medicine)
AFASAK (Atrial Fibrillation, Aspirin, Antikoagulation)
AFTER (Antistreplase Following Thrombolysis Effect on Reocclusion)
AICLA (Accidents Ischémiques Cérebraux Liés a l'Atherosclérose)
AIMS (APSAC Intervention Mortality Study)
AIRE (Acute Infarction Remipril Efficacy)
AITIA (Aspirin in Transient Ischemic Attacks)
AMIS (Aspirin in Myocardial Infarction Study)
AMPI (APSAC in Acute Myocardial Infarction Placebo-Controlled Investigation)
ANBP (Australian National Blood Pressure Trial)
APRICOT (Antithrombotics in Prevention of Reocclusion in Coronary Thrombolysis)
APRICOT (Aspirin vs Coumadin Trial)
APSI (Acebutalol Prevention Secondaire del'Infarctus)
APSIM (APSAC dans l'Infarctus du Myocarde)
APSIS (Angina Prognosis Study with Isoptin and Seloken Trial)
ARIC (Atherosclerosis Risk in Communities Study)
ARIS (Antyrane Reinfarction Italian Study)
ARMS (APSAC Reocclusion Multicenter Study)
ART (Anturane Reinfarction Trial)
ASK (Australian SK Trial in Stroke)
ASPECT (Anticoagulants in Secondary Prevention of Events in Coronary Thrombosis)
ASPS (Australian Swedish Pindolol Study)
ASSET (Anglo-Scandinavian Study of Early Thrombolysis)
ATACS (Antithrombotic Therapy in Acute Coronary Syndromes)
ATEST (Atenolol and Streptokinase Trial)
ATIAIS (Auturane Transient Ischemic Attack Italian Study)
BAATAF (Boston Area Anticoagulation Trial for Atrial Fibrillation)
BARI (Bypass Angioplasty Revascularization Investigation)
BEST (Beta-Blocker Stroke Trial)
BHAT (Beta-Blocker Heart Attack Trial)
BIRNH (Belgian Interuniversity Research on Nutrition and Health)
BRHS (British Regional Heart Study)
BWIS (Baltimore Washington Infant Study)
CABRI (Coronary Artery Bypass Revascularization Investigation)
CAFA (Canadian Atrial Fibrillation Anticoagulation Study)
CAMIAT (Canadian Amiodarone Myocardial Infarction Arrhythmia Trial)
CAPPHY (Captopril Primary Prevention in Hypertension)
CAPRIE (Clopidogrel vs Aspirin in Patients at Risk of Ischemic Events)
CAPS (Cardiac Arrhythmia Pilot Study)
CARDIA (Coronary Artery Risk Development in Young Adults)
CARPORT (Coronary Artery Restenosis Prevention On Repeated Thromboxane-Antagonism)
CASH (Cardiac Arrest Study Hamburg)
CASIS (Canadian Amlodipine-Atelenolol in Silent Ischemia Study)
CASS (Coronary Artery Surgery Study)
CAST (Cardiac Arrhythmia Suppression Trial)
CATS (Canadian American Ticlopidine Study)
CATS (Captopril and Thrombolysis in Myocardial Infarction Study)
CDP (Coronary Drug Project)
CECCC (Confidential Enquiry into Cardiac Catheterization Complications)
CEDIM (Italian Study on 1-Carnitine and Digital Echocardiography in Myocardial Infarction)
CITO (Collaboratione Italiana par la Thrombosi in Ortopedia)
CLAS (Cholesterol Lowering Atherosclerosis Study)
CLIP (Cholesterol Lowering Intervention Program)
CONSENSUS (Cooperative North Scandinavian Enalapril Survival Study)
CORIS (Coronary RIsk Factor Study)
CRAFT (Catheterization Rescue Angioplasty Following Thrombolysis)
DART (Diet and Reinfarction Trial)
DAVIT (Danish Verapamil in Myocardial Infarction Trial)
DIMT (Dutch Ilopamine Multicenter Trial)
DRS (Diltiazem Reinfarction Study)
DUCCS (Duke University Clinical Cardiology Studies)
Dutch IRS (Dutch Invasive Reperfusion Study)
DVT (Danish Verapamil Trial)
EARS (European Atherosclerosis Research Study)
EAST (Emory Angioplasty Surgery Trial)
ECCOMAC (European Concerted CoMmunity Action Programmes)
ECAT (European Concerted Action on Thrombosis and Disabilities)
ECATAP Trial (ECAT Angina Pectoris Trial)
ECTIM (Etude Cas-Témoins sur l'Infarctus du Myocarde)
ECSG (European Cooperative Study Group)
ECSS (European Coronary Surgery Study)
ECST (European Carotid Surgery Trial)
EIS (European Infarction Study)
ELCA Registry (Excimer Laser Coronary Angioplasty Registry)
EMERAS (Estudio Multicenter Estreptoquinasa Republicas Americas Sud)
EMIAT (European Myocardial Infarction Amiodarone Trial)
EMIP (European Myocardial Infarction Project)
EMPAR (Enoxaparine Maxipa Prevention of Angioplasty Restenosis)
EMS (European Multicenter Study)
EPPI (Etude de Prescription Post Infarctus)
EPSIM (Enquete de Prevention Secondaire de l'Infarctus du Myocarde)
ERICA (European Risk and Incidence, a Coordinated Analysis)
ESPS (European Stroke Prevention Study)
ESVEM (Electrophysiologic Study vs Electrocardiographic Monitoring)
ETDRS (Early Treatment Diabetic Retinopathy Study)
EVA (European Vascular Agency)

EVAS-IM (Etude Vaudois APSAC vs Streptokinase dans Infarctus du Myo carde)
EXCEL (Expanded Clinical Evaluation of Lovastatin)
EWPHE (European Working Party on Hypertension in the Elderly)
FACET (Flosequinan ACE-Inhibitor Trial)
FATS (Familial Atherosclerosis Treatment Study)
FHS (Framingham Heart Study)
FIPS (Frankfurt Isoptin Progression Study)
FRESH (Food Reeducation Elementary School Health Study)
GABI (German Angioplasty Bypass Investigation)
GAMIS (German Austrian Myocardial Infarction Study)
GAUS (German Activator Urokinase Study)
GCP (German Cardiovascular Prevention Study)
GEMT (German Eminase Multicenter Trial)
GISSI (Gruppo Italiano per lo Studio della Streptochinasi nell'Infarto Miocardico)
GMT (Göteborg Metoprolol Trial)
GPP (Göteborg Primary Prevention Trial)
GRASP (Glaxo Restenosis and Symptoms Project)
GREAT (Grampian Region Early Antistreplase Trial)
GRECO (German Study with Recombinant t-PA in Coronary Conclusion)
GUIDE Trial (Guidance by Ultrasound Imaging for Decision Endpoints Trial)
GUSTO (Global Utilization of Streptokinase and t-PA for Occluded Arteries)
HALS (Heart Attacks in London Study)
HAPPHY (Heart Attack Prevention in Primary Hypertension)
HART (Heparin Aspirin Reperfusion Trial)
HDFP (Hypertension Detection and Follow-Up Program)
HHS (Helsinki Heart Study)
HINT (Holland Interuniversity Nifedipine/Metoprolol Trial)
HYNON (Hypertension Non-Drug Treatment Cooperative Study)
ICIN (Intracoronary Streptokinase Trial of the Interuniversity Cardiology Institute of the Netherlands)
IMAGE (International Metoprolol/Nifedipine Angina Exercise Trial)
IMPACT (International Mexiletine & Placebo Antiarrhythmic Coronary Trial)
INCLEN (International Clinical Epidemiology Network)
INTACT (International Nifedipine Trial on Antiatherosclerotic Therapy)
INTERSALT (International Studies of Salt and Blood Pressure)
iPPPSH (International Prospective Primary Prevention Study on Hypertension)
IRS (Invasive Reperfusion Study)
ISAM (Intravenous Streptokinase in Acute Myocardial Infarction)
ISIS (International Study of Infarct Survival)
KAMIT (Kentucky Acute Myocardial Infarction Trial)
LAPIS (Late Potentials in Myocardial Infarction Study)
LATE (Late Assessment of Thrombolytic Efficacy)
LIMIT (Leicester Intravenous Magnesium Intervention Trial)
LIMITS (Liquemin in Myocardial infarction During Thrombolysis with Saruplase)
LIT (Lopressor Intervention Trial)
LRC-CPPT (Lipid Research Clinics-Coronary Primary Prevention Trial)
MAPHY (Metoprolol Atherosclerosis Prevention in Hypertension)
MARCATOR (Multicenter American Research Trial with Cilazapril After Angioplasty to Prevent Transluminal Coronary Obstruction & Restenosis)
MARS (Monitored Atherosclerosis Regression Study)
MAST-I (Multicenter Acute Stroke Trial—Italy)
MDPIT (Multicenter Diltiazem Post Infarction Trial)
MEHP (Metoprolol in Elderly Hypertensive Patients)
MELODHY (Metoprolol Low Dose in Hypertension)
MERCATOR (Multicenter European Research Trial with Cilazapril After Angioplasty to Prevent Transluminal Coronary Obstruction & Restenosis)
M-HEART (Multi-Hospital Eastern Atlantic Restenosis Trial)
MIAMI (Metoprolol in Acute Myocardial Infarction)
MIDAS (Myocardial Infarction Data Acquisition System)
MILESTONE (Multicenter Iloprost European Study on Endangeitis)
MILIS (Multicenter Investigation of the Limitation of Infarct Size)
MITI (Myocardial Infarction Triage and Intervention)
MONICA (Monitoring Trends and Determinants in Cardiovascular Disease)
MPRG (Multicenter Postinfarction Research Group)
MRFIT (Multiple Risk Factor Intervention Trial)
NACI Registry (New Approaches to Coronary Intervention Registry)
NAMIS (Nifedipine Angina Myocardial Infarction Study)
NASCET (North American Symptomatic Carotid Endarterectomy Trial)
NCEP (National Cholesterol Education Program)
NGHS (NHLBI Growth and Health Study)
NHANES (National Health and Nutrition Examination Survey)
OCSP (Oxfordshire Community Stroke Project)
OSIRIS (Optimization Study of Infarct Reperfusion Investigated by ST-Monitoring)
PACK (Prevention of Atherosclerotic Complications with Ketanserin)
PACT (Pre-Hospital Application of Coronary Thrombolysis)
PACT (Pro-Urokinase in Acute Coronary Thrombosis)
PACTE (Prevention des Accidents Thrombo-Emboliques Chez les Porteurs de Protheses Valvulaires Cardiaques)
PAIMS (Plasminogen Activator Italian Multicenter Study)
PAMI (Primary Angioplasty Myocardial Infarction Trial)
PARIS (Persantine Aspirin Reinfarction Trial)

TABLE 10-3. *(continued)*

PARK (Prevention of Angioplasty Reocclusion with Ketanserin)
PARTNER (Peripheral Arterial Disease Response to Taprostene with New Established Response Criteria)
PASS (Practical Applicability of Saruplase Study)
PATS (Prehospital Administration of t-PA Study)
PDAY (Pathobiological Determinants of Atherosclerosis in Youth)
PIOPED (Prospective Investigation of Pulmonary Embolism Diagnosis)
PLAC (Pravastatin Limitation of Atherosclerosis in Coronary Arteries)
POSCH (Program on Surgical Control of Hyperlipidemia)
PREMIS (Prehospital Myocardial Infarction Study)
PRIMI (Prourokinase in Myocardial Infarction)
PROCAM Study (Prospective Cardiovascular Münster Study)
PROFILE (Prospective Randomized Flosequinan Longevity Evaluation)
PROMISE (Prospective Randomized Milrinone Survival Evaluation)
QUIET (Quinapril Ischemic Events Trial)
RADIANCE (Randomized Assessment of Digoxin and Inhibitors of Angiotensin Converting Enzyme)
RAAMI (Rapid Administration of Alteplase in Myocardial Infarction)
REPAIR (Reperfusion in Acute Infarction, Rotterdam)
RESCUE (Randomized Evaluation of Salvage Angioplasty with Combined Utilization of Endpoints)
RISK (Regional Study av Instabil Kranskärlssjukdom)
RITA (Randomized Intervention Treatment of Angina)
ROBUST (Recanalization of Occluded Bypass Graft, Urokinase Study Trial)
ROCKET (Regionally Organized Cardiac Key European Trial)
SAFE (Safety After Fifty Evaluation)
SALT (Swedish Aspirin Low-Dose Trial)
SAMIT (Streptokinase Angioplasty Myocardial Infarction Trial)
SAVE (Survival and Ventricular Enlargement)
SCATI (Studio sulla Calciparina nell'Angina e nella Trombosi Ventricolare nell'Infarto)
SCRIP (Stanford Coronary Risk Intervention Project)
SEPIVAC (Studio Epidemiologica sull'Incidenza delle Vasculopatie Acute Cerebrali)
SESAM (Study in Europe of Saruplase and Alteplase in Myocardial Infarction)
SHAVE (Steerable Housing for Atherovascular Excision)
SHEP (Systolic Hypertension in the Elderly Program)
SIAM (Streptokinase in Acute Myocardial Infarction)
SMISS (Silent Myocardial Ischemia Stress Study)
SMT (Stockholm Metroprolol Trial)
SOLVD (Studies of Left Ventricular Dysfunction)
SPAF (Stroke Prevention in Atrial Fibrillation)
SPINAF (Stroke Prevention in Nonrheumatic Atrial Fibrillation)
SPRINT (Secondary Prevention Reinfarction Israeli Nifedipine Trial)
SRT (Sorbinil Retinopathy Trial)

SSSS (Scandinavian Simvastatin Survival Study)
STAI (Study Ticlopidine in Angor Instable)
STAMP (Systemic Thrombolysis in Acute Myocardial Infarction with Prourokinase)
STARS (St. Thomas' Atherosclerosis Regression Study)
STEP (Study of Taprostene in Elective PTCA)
STIMS (Swedish Ticlopidine Multicentre Study in Patients with Intermittent Claudication)
STOP Hypertension (Swedish Trial in Old Patients with Hypertension)
SWIFT (Should We Intervene Following Thrombolysis)
TACS (Thrombolysis and Angioplasty in Cardiogenic Shock)
TACT (Ticlopidine vs Placebo for Prevention of Acute Closure Trial)
TAMI (Thrombolysis and Angioplasty in Myocardial Infarction)
TAPS (t-PA APSAC Patency Study)
TASS (Ticlopidine Aspirin Stroke Study)
TAUSA (Thrombolysis and Angioplasty in Unstable Angina)
TEAHAT (Thrombolysis Early in Acute Heart Attack Trial)
TEAM (Trial of Eminase vs Alteplase in Myocardial Infarction)
TIARA (Timolol en Infarcto Agudo, Republica Argentina)
TIBET (Total Ischemic Burden European Trial)
TICO (Thrombolysis in Coronary Occlusion)
TIMAD (Ticlopidine in Micro-Angiopathy of Diabetes)
TIMI (Thrombolysis in Myocardial Infarction)
TIPE (Thrombolysis in Pulmonary Embolism Study)
TIPE (Thrombolysis in Peripheral Embolism Patient Study)
TOHMS (Trial of Hypertensive Medications Study)
TOHP (Trials of Hypertension Prevention)
TOMHS (Treatment of Mild Hypertension Study)
TOP (Thrombolysis in Old Patients)
TPAT (Tissue Plasminogen Activator, Toronto)
TPT (Thrombosis Prevention Trial)
TRENT (Trial of Early Nifedipine Treatment in Acute Myocardial Infarction)
TRUST (Trial of United Kingdom for Stroke Treatment)
UNASEM (Unstable Angina Study Using Eminase)
UNSA (Unstable Angina Study)
UPET (Urokinase Pulmonary Embolism Trial)
URALMI (Urokinase and Alteplase in Myocardial Infarction)
USIM (Urochinasi per via Sistemica nell'Infarto Miocardico)
VACA Registry (Valvuloplasty and Angioplasty of Congenital Anomalies Registry)
V-HeFT (Veterans Heart Failure Trial)
WARIS (Warfarin Reinfarction Study)
WHA Study (Worcester Heart Attack Study)
WWICT (Western Washington Intracoronary Streptokinase Trial)
WWIST (Western Washington Intravenous Streptokinase Trial)

Colorful and good.

*2. Loscalzo J, Creager MA, Dzau VJ, editors. *Vascular Medicine. A Textbook of Vascular Biology and Diseases.* Boston: Little, Brown and Company, 1992:1211, $165.00.

Excellent.

3. Cooke JP, Frohlich ED, editors. *Current Management of Hypertensive and Vascular Diseases.* St. Louis: B.C. Decker (An Imprint of Mosby Year Book), 1992:380, $79.00.

Good.

*4. Kapoor AS, Singh BN, editors. *Prognosis and Risk Assessment in Cardiovascular Disease.* New York: Churchill Livingstone, 1993:578, $79.95.

This book was designed to provide an authoritative source of current information for determining prognosis in major cardiovascular diseases. It appears to fulfill this mission. This is a very good book.

5. Marriott HJL. *Bedside Cardiac Diagnosis.* Philadelphia: JB Lippincott Company, 1993:291, $49.95.

Marriott makes the point in his preface that about 80% of cardiovascular diagnoses are made by history alone, another 10% require the physical examination, and only the remaining 10% are dependent on laboratory investigation. This good book of 40 relatively short chapters focuses on physical signs of cardiovascular disease. Good reading.

6. Chesler E. *Clinical Cardiology.* Fifth Edition. New York: Springer-Verlag, 1993:451, $89.00.

A bedside approach to cardiology. I would vote for the Marriott one.

7. Lilly LS, editor. *Pathophysiology of Heart Disease. A Collaborative Project of Medical Students and Faculty.* Philadelphia: Lea & Febiger, 1993:325, $24.50.

This book is a collaborative project of 38 Harvard Medical Students with faculty. The students, i.e., potential consumers, dissatisfied with currently available textbooks of cardiology, made their needs known. A useful book, particularly for the price.

8. Hillis LD, Lange RA, Wells PJ, Winniford MD. *Manual of Clinical Problems in Cardiology With Annotated Key References. Fourth Edition.* Boston: Little, Brown and Company, 1992:553, $28.00.

A useful book, particularly for house officers and cardiology fellows, and the price is right.

LIPIDS AND OTHER RISK FACTORS

9. Frishman WH, editor and coauthor. *Medical Management of Lipid Disorders: Focus on Prevention of Coronary Artery Disease.* Mount Kisco, NY: Futura Publishing Company, Inc., 1992:328, $60.00.

A very practical book.

10. Kreisberg RA, Segrest J, editors. *Plasma Lipoproteins and Coronary Artery Disease.* Boston: Blackwell Scientific Publications, 1992:390, $74.95.

Very good.

11. Thompson GR, Wilson PW. *Coronary Risk Factors and their Assessment.* London: Science Press, 1992: approximately 150, $60.00.

A colorful book. I prefer the Frishman one.

12. Goor R, Goor N. *Eater's Choice. A Food Lover's Guide to Lower Cholesterol. Third Edition.* Boston: Houghton Mifflin Company, 1992:571, $12.95.

This husband and wife team are cholesterol and nutrition experts. They have written several "best sellers" on this subject. I have liked all their books for adults (They have also written 7 childrens' books), and this one is no exception.

MEDICAL THERAPY

13. Ewy GA, Bressler R, editors. *Cardiovascular Drugs and the Management of Heart Disease. Second Edition.* New York: Raven Press, 1992:496, $105.00.

Fine book.

14. Taylor GJ. *Thrombolytic Therapy for Acute Myocardial Infarction.* Boston: Blackwell Scientific Publications, 1992:240, $24.95.

The price is right.

15. Opie LH. *Angiotensin-Converting Enzyme Inhibitors: Scientific Basis for Clinical Use.* New York: Wiley-Liss, 1992:266, $34.95.

Covers this topic well.

INTERVENTIONAL CARDIOLOGY

16. Vogel JHK, King SB III, editors. *The Practice of Interventional Cardiology, Second Edition.* St. Louis: Mosby Year Book, 1993:718, $95.00.

Good book.

17. Schwartz RS, editor. *Coronary Restenosis.* Boston: Blackwell Scientific Publications, 1993:387, $84.95.

Good book.

18. Serruys PW, Strauss BH, King SB III, editors. *Restenosis after Inter-*

vention with New Mechanical Devices. Dordrecht: Kluwer Academic Publishers, 1992:504, $215.00.

A comprehensive assessment of restenosis from the perspective of new technologies including stenting, atherectomy, rotational abrasion, and lasers. At 42 cents a page, it is hardly worth it.

19. Ginsburg R, Geschwind HJ, editors. *Primer on Laser Angioplasty, Second Edition.* Mount Kisco, NY: Futura Publishing Company, Inc., 1992:520, $80.00.

For those interested in lasers, this is the book to have.

SYSTEMIC HYPERTENSION

20. Brunner HR, Waeber B, editors. *Ambulatory Blood Pressure Recording.* New York: Raven Press, 1992:192, $55.00.

Non-invasive ambulatory blood pressure recording is receiving progressively more attention since its beginning in about 1975. Over 300 publications on this subject appeared in 1990. This good small book nicely presents some of the problems and some benefits of ambulatory blood pressure monitoring.

*21. Loggie JMH, editor. *Pediatric and Adolescent Hypertension.* Boston: Blackwell Scientific Publications, 1992:416, $149.95.

Good.

22. Martinez-Maldonado M, editor. *Hypertension and Renal Disease in the Elderly.* Boston: Blackwell Scientific Publications, 1992:358, $79.95.

Nice book by outstanding contributors.

23. Cruickshank JM, Messerli FH. *Left Ventricular Hypertrophy and its Regression.* London: Science Press, 1992:107, $89.95.

In color. Not a lot of information. Almost a dollar a page!

CONGENITAL HEART DISEASE

*24. Freedom RM, Benson LN, Smallhorn JF, editors. *Neonatal Heart Disease.* London: Springer-Verlag, 1992:881, $180.00.

This book will probably be the bible for information on the newborn with heart disease. Although an edited book, one or more of the editors are authors of nearly all chapters.

25. Rao PS, editor. *Tricuspid Atresia. Second Edition.* Mount Kisco, NY: Futura Publishing Company, Inc., 1992:458, $98.00.

The first edition appeared just over 10 years ago. I like these comprehensive books on a single topic and that is what this one is.

26. Hess J, Sutherland GR, editors. *Congenital Heart Disease in Adolescents and Adults.* Dordrecht: Kluwer Academic Publishers, 1992:201, $100.00.

There are better ones on this subject.

ARRHYTHMIAS, ELECTROCARDIOGRAPHY, ELECTROPHYSIOLOGY, PACING, DEFIBRILLATORS

*27. Josephson ME, Second Edition. *Clinical Cardiac Electrophysiology: Techniques and Interpretations.* Philadelphia: Lea & Febiger, 1993:839, $95.00.

A must for students of this field. Josephson wrote every word. Outstanding.

28. Singer I, Kupersmith J, editors. *Clinical Manual of Electrophysiology.* Baltimore: Williams & Wilkins, 1993:453, $60.00.

Very few illustrations. Josephson a winner hands down.

29. Wit AL, Janse MJ. *The Ventricular Arrhythmias of Ischemia and Infarction. Electrophysiological Mechanisms.* Mount Kisco, NY: Futura Publishing Company, Inc., 1993:648, $150.00.

A fine book BUT the Josephson one is 37% less expensive and contains 23% more pages which are also larger.

30. Seelig CB. *Simplified EKG Analysis. A Sequential Guide to Interpretation and Diagnosis.* Philadelphia: Hanley & Belfus, Inc., 1992:119, $14.95.

31. Stein E. *Rapid Analysis of Electrocardiograms. A Self-Study Program. Second Edition.* Philadelphia: Lea & Febiger, 1992:404, $26.95.

32. Stein E. *Rapid Analysis of Arrhythmias. A Self-Study Program. Second Edition.* Philadelphia: Lea & Febiger, 1992:229, $24.95.

33. Kingma JH, van Hemel NM, Lie KI, editors. *Atrial Fibrillation, a Treatable Disease?* Dordrecht: Kluwer Academic Publishers, 1992:297, $99.00.

A hot topic. Content per page could have been more.

34. Luceri RM, editor. *Sudden Cardiac Death: Strategies for the 1990s.* Miami Lakes, Florida: Peritus Corporation, 1992:194, $60.00.

This book represents a collection of manuscripts concerning primarily implantable cardioverter-defibrillators and both the symposium and this publication are underwritten by Telectronics Pacing Systems. Not recommended.

35. Ellenbogen KA, editor. *Cardiac Pacing.* Boston: Blackwell Scientific Publications, 1992:464, $29.95.

A very good book for the money. Highly recommended.

ECHOCARDIOGRAPHY

*36. Silverman NH. *Pediatric Echocardiography.* Baltimore: Williams & Wilkins, 1993:628, $140.00.

Superb book. Loaded with fine illustrations.

37. Obeid AI. *Echocardiography in Clinical Practice.* Philadelphia: JB Lippincott Company, 1992:383, $125.00

A large book loaded with 2-dimensional, Doppler, and transesophageal images. The images should have been cropped and then they could have been reproduced much larger. Nevertheless, the reproductions are excellent. A useful book.

*38. Nanda NC, editor. *Doppler Echocardiography. Second Edition.* Philadelphia: Lea & Febiger, 1993:466, $129.00.

Beautiful book. Illustrations are splendid. Probably the best so far on this subject.

39. Labovitz AJ, Williams GA. *Doppler Echocardiography. The Quantitative Approach. Third Edition.* Philadelphia: Lea & Febiger, 1992:131, $29.95.

This third edition appears only 5 years after the first edition. It incorporates real-time flow mapping techniques into the text. The illustrations are superb.

40. Oka Y, Goldiner PL, editors. *Transesophageal Echocardiography.* Philadelphia: JB Lippincott Company, 1992:338, $150.00

Nice book but a good bit of wasted space. Photographs could have been cropped.

41. Missri J. *Transesophageal Echocardiography. Clinical and Intraoperative Applications.* New York: Churchill Livingstone, 1993:248, $124.95.

Good.

42. Dittrich HC, editor. *Clinical Transesophageal Echocardiography.* St. Louis: Mosby Year Book, 1992:178, $95.00.

An edited book with 22 contributors.

43. Labovitz AJ, Pearson AC. *Transesophageal Echocardiography: Basic Principles and Clinical Applications.* Philadelphia: Lea & Febiger, 1993:157, $39.50.

Good.

INTRAVASCULAR ULTRASOUND IMAGING

44. Tobis JM, Yock PG, editors. *Intravascular Ultrasound Imaging.* New York: Churchill Livingstone, 1992:262, $89.95.

Probably the best so far on this subject.

45. Cavaye DM, White RA. *Intravascular Ultrasound Imaging.* New York: Raven Press, 1993:119, $59.00.

Good but short and relatively expensive. Good reproductions.

CARDIAC IMAGING

46. Jay ME, *Plain Film in Heart Disease.* Boston: Blackwell Scientific Publications, 1992:207, $34.95.

This book is loaded with chest roentgenograms with brief case presentations. The space on the pages is poorly utilized. The book which is already relatively small could have been much smaller.

47. van der Wall E, Sochor H, Righetti A, Niemeyer MG. *What's New in Cardiac Imaging? SPECT, PET, and MRI.* Dordrecht: Kluwer Academic Publishers, 1992:544, $149.00.

48. van der Wall EE. *Nuclear Cardiology and Cardiac Magnetic Resonance. Physiology, Techniques and Applications.* Leiden, The Netherlands: Hans Soto Productions, 1992:285, $115.00.

49. Wagner M, Lawson TL. *Atlas of Chest Imaging. Correlated Anatomy with MRI and CT.* New York: Raven Press, 1992:134, $80.00.

The use of abbreviations in titles is not ideal. Over half of the pages utilize only a half of the page. The book could have been much smaller and that would have made it better. The reader is not getting his/her money's worth here.

50. Stanford W, Rumberger JA, editors. *Ultrafast Computed Tomography in Cardiac Imaging: Principles and Practice.* Mount Kisco, NY: Futura Publishing Company, Inc., 1992:351, $80.00.

A useful book.

*51. Bregmann SR, Sobel BE, editors. *Positron Emission Tomography of the Heart.* Mount Kisco, NY: Futura Publishing Company, Inc., 1992:313, $98.00.

I suspect that this book is the best one on this subject.

CARDIOVASCULAR SURGERY

*52. Kirklin JW, Barratt-Boyes BG, with the collaboration of Blackstone EH, Jonas RA, Kouchoukos NT. *Cardiac Surgery. Morphology, Diagnostic Criteria, Natural History, Techniques, Results, and Indications. Second Edition. Volumes 1 and 2.* New York: Churchill Livingstone, 1993:1860, $250.00.

This book is by far the best on this subject.

53. Bojar RM. *Adult Cardiac Surgery.* Boston: Blackwell Scientific Publications, 1992:562, $99.95.

This book does not include congenital heart lesions except for the congenitally malformed aortic valve, mitral valve prolapse, hypertrophic cardiomyopathy, and the Marfan syndrome seen in adulthood. This book by a single author is both good and useful, but can hardly compete with the Kirklin-Barratt-Boyes one!

54. Bharati S, Lev M, Kirklin JW. *Cardiac Surgery and the Conduction System. Second Revised Edition.* Mount Kisco, NY: Futura Publishing Company, Inc., 1992:159, $75.00.

This book primarily presents drawings and some gross pictures of views of the heart as might be seen at operation with delineation of courses of the conduction system in various types of congenital anomalies of the heart. The text is brief. Much empty space is present on the pages. The book is important because of the authors.

55. Kotler MN, Alfieri A, editors. *Cardiac and Noncardiac Complications of Open Heart Surgery: Prevention, Diagnosis, and Treatment.* Mount Kisco, NY: Futura Publishing Company, Inc., 1992:418, $62.00.

A useful book, interestingly edited by 2 cardiologists. Very little emphasis is given to mechanical or anatomic complications of cardiac surgery. Certainly they are not as important in the 1990s as they were in the 1960s but they remain important.

56. Engelman RM, Levitsky S, editors. *A Textbook of Cardioplegia for Difficult Clinical Problems.* Mount Kisco, NY: Futura Publishing Company, Inc., 1992:334, $75.00.

As Frank C. Spencer states in the Preface: ". . . the book is an excellent description of the wide variety of methods of cardioplegia used for the most difficult clinical problems throughout the world. This wide variation indicates that no one method has evolved as superior to another."

57. Kay PH, editor. *Techniques in Extracorporeal Circulation, Third Edition.* Oxford, UK: Butterworth–Heinemann Ltd., 1992:336, $195.00.

The first edition of this book appeared 16 years ago, and the second edition 11 years ago. Thus, it is time for an update and this was nicely accomplished by 45 authors.

58. Ross DN, English TAH, McKay R. *Principles of Cardiac Diagnosis and Treatment. A Surgeon's Guide. Second Edition.* London: Springer-Verlag, 1992:269, $129.00.

The first edition appeared in 1962, thirty years earlier. This book is pleasant reading but at nearly 50 cents a page, it's not worth it.

PERIPHERAL VASCULAR DISEASE

59. Polak JF. *Peripheral Vascular Sonography. A Practical Guide.* Baltimore: Williams & Wilkins, 1993:364, $78.00.

Good for this subject.

60. Dorros G. *Peripheral Vascular Interventions 1992. A Bibliographic Reference Manual.* Mount Kisco, NY: Futura Publishing Company, Inc., 1992:438, $80.00.

What it says it is, it is, a bibliography with some summaries. For those in this field, it may be useful.

61. Clement DL, Shepherd JT, editors. *Vascular Diseases in the Limbs. Mechanisms and Principles of Treatment.* St. Louis: Mosby Year Book, 1993:319, $79.00.

Well done.

MOLECULAR CARDIOLOGY

*62. Roberts R, editor. *Molecular Basis of Cardiology.* Boston: Blackwell Scientific Publications, 1993:518, $39.95.

As Eugene Braunwald states in the foreword, *Molecular Basis of Cardiology* is the best exposition of this new paradigm (the shift in cardiovascular science from organ physiology to molecular biology) currently available and will be of enormous value to cardiovascular scientists, scholarly cardiologists, and to new entrants in the field. The publisher provided the book in soft cover to keep the price reasonable.

63. Gotto AM, Jr, editor. *Cellular and Molecular Biology of Atherosclerosis.* London: Springer-Verlag, 1992:180, $83.00.

This book represents presentations at the 1991 Princess Lillian Symposium, which I attended. The presentations were good and their publication is better.

MISCELLANEOUS

*64. Katz AM. *Physiology of the Heart. Second Edition.* New York: Raven Press, 1992:687, $55.00.

The first edition was 1977. Thus, this second one is long overdue. This second edition is essentially an entirely new text.

65. Pashkow FJ, Dafoe WA, editors. *Clinical Cardiac Rehabilitation: A Cardiologist's Guide.* Baltimore: Williams & Wilkins, 1993:391, $59.00.

Good.

66. Anderson RH, Becker AE. *The Heart. Structure in Health and Disease.* London: Gower Medical Publishing, 1992:266, $165.00.

This book is a consolidation and expansion of their 2 previous books with Gower Medical Publishing, namely *Cardiac Anatomy* (1980) and *Cardiac Pathology* (1983). The pictures are in color. A beautiful book.

67. Yellon DM, Jennings RB, editors. *Myocardial Protection. The Pathophysiology of Reperfusion and Reperfusion Injury.* New York: Raven Press, 1992:214 $99.00.

This concise book on an important subject will be useful. The cost, however, is nearly 50 cents a page.

68. Fowles RE, editor. *Cardiac Biopsy.* Mount Kisco, NY: Futura Publishing Company, Inc., 1992:211, $47.00.

For anyone performing or examining biopsies of the heart, this is a good book to have.

69. Kaye D, editor. *Infective Endocarditis, Second Edition.* New York: Raven Press, 1992:497, $85.00.

This book is a follow-up of Kaye's first edition in 1976. The first edition emphasized the effects of antibiotics on infective endocarditis. The present edition, a considerable expansion from the first, continues to emphasize further changes in the disease including an older age of patients, less rheumatic heart disease, less pneumococcal and gonococcal endocarditis, more staphylococcal endocarditis, the increasing frequency in intravenous drug abusers, the problems of prosthetic and bioprosthetic endocarditis, the usefulness of echocardiography, and many management changes. This book is highly recommended.

CARDIOLOGIC ANNUALS

70. Roberts WC, Willerson JT, Mason DT, Rackley CE, Graham TP Jr. *Cardiology 1992.* Boston: Butterworth–Heinemann, 1992:480, $80.00.

71. Schlant RC (editor in chief), Collins JJ Jr, Engle MA, Frye RL, Kaplan NM, O'Rourke RA (editors). *Year Book of Cardiology 1992.* St. Louis: Mosby Year Book, 1992:441, $59.95.

The Schlant book, the thirty-second in the series, contains summaries and comments on 318 articles plus 111 figures and 5 tables. The Roberts book, the twelfth in the series, contains summaries of 740 articles plus 116 figures and 32 tables. The Roberts book provides 58% more summaries of articles than does the Schlant book on only 8% more pages because each page contains far more content. The cost of the Roberts book, however, is 30% higher than the Schlant book, and it lacks editorial comments from the editors on each article summarized.

COMMENTS

More and more cardiologic books! The first column I wrote on cardiologic books summarized those appearing in 1985 and it briefly discussed 16 books,[1] and the column in 1991 described 49 books.[2] The present piece discusses 71 books, 53 (75%) of which have a 1992 publication date and 18 (25%) of which have a 1993 publication date. The books marked with asterisks are those which I consider noteworthy either because of extremely high quality or uniqueness.

The costs of books continue to increase. The prices of the 71 books appearing in 1992 ranged from $12.95 to $250.00 (mean $88.39). The number of pages in the 71 books ranged from 119 to 1860 (mean 405). There was an insignificant relation between the number of pages a book contained and its cost. The total cost of the 71 books was $6,275.50 and the total numbers of pages in the 71 books was 28,835. Therefore, the average cost of each page was 22 cents.

Of the 71 books, 38 (55%) were edited with multiple contributors, and 33 (45%) were by 1 to 6 authors. Only 15 books (21%) had a single author.

Most books unfortunately continue to be published on acid paper.[3] Of the 71 books, only 9 (13%) were published on acid-free paper, i.e., permanent paper. The remaining 62 books (87%) will vanish into dust within 50 years. Congratulations to Butterworth–Heinemann, Kluwer Academic, and Springer-Verlag for publishing all of their books on acid-free paper, and to Futura for publishing some of their books on alkaline paper. I encourage all authors to require in their book contracts that the paper used for their books be acid-free. It is time for American book publishers to use permanent paper!

Reprinted with permission from Roberts, WC, American Journal of Cardiology Vol. 71 January 1, 1993, pp. 126-130.

References

1. Wall TC, Campbell PT, O'Connor CM, Van Trigt P, Kenney RT, Sheikh KH, Kisslo JA, Corey GR: Diagnosis and management (by subxiphoid pericardiotomy) of large pericardial effusions causing cardiac tamponade. Am J Cardiol 1992 (Apr 15); 69:1075–1078.

2. Brown J, MacKinnon D, King A, Vanderbush E: Elevated arterial blood pressure in cardiac tamponade. N Engl J Med 1992 (Aug 13);327:463–466.

3. Schutzman JJ, Obarski TP, Pearce GL, Klein AL: Comparison of Doppler and two-dimensional echocardiography for assessment of pericardial effusion. Am J Cardiol 1992 (Nov 15);70:1353–1357.

4. Millaire A, Wurtz A, deGroote P, Saudemont A, Chambon A, Ducloux G: Malignant pericardial effusions: Usefulness of pericardioscopy. Am Heart J 1992 (October);124:1030–1034.

5. Evans RW, Orians CE, Ashcer NL: The potential supply of organ donors: An assessment of the efficiency of organ procurement efforts in the United States. JAMA 1992 (Jan 8);267:239–246.

6. Sekela ME, Smart FW, Noon GP, Young JB: Attenuation of waiting time mortality with heterotopic heart transplantation. An Thorac Surg 1992 (Sept);54:547–551.

7. Laffel GL, Barnett AI, Finkelstein S, Kaye MP: The relation between experience and outcome in heart transplantation. N Engl J Med 1992 (Oct 22);327:1220–1225.

8. Starnes VA, Oyer PE, Bernstein D, Baum D, Gamberg P, Miller J, Shumway NE: Heart, Heart-Lung, and Lung Transplantation in the First Year of Life. Ann Thorac Surg (February) 1992;53:306–310.

9. Costard-Jäckle A, Fowler MB. Influence of preoperative pulmonary artery pressure on mortality after heart transplantation: Testing of potential reversibility of pulmonary hypertension with nitroprusside is useful in defining a high risk group. J Am Coll Cardiol 1992 (January);19:48–54.

10. Kubo SH, Peters JR, Knutson KR, Hertz MI, Olivari MT, Bolman RM, Hunninghake DB: Factors influencing the development of hypercholesterolemia after cardiac transplantation. Am J Cardiol 1992 (Aug 15);70:520–526.

11. Barbir M, Hunt B, Kushwaha S, Kehely A, Prescot R, Thompson GR, Mitchell A, Yacoub M: Maxepa versus bezafibrate in hyperlipidemic cardiac transplant recipients. Am J Cardiol 1992 (Dec 15);70:1596–1601.

12. Barbir M, Kushwaha S, Hunt B, Macken A, Thompson GR, Mitchell A, Robinson D, Yacoub M: Lipoprotein(a) and accelerated coronary artery disease in cardiac transplant recipients. Lancet 1992 (Dec. 19/26);340:1500–1502.

13. St. Goar FG, Pinto FJ, Alderman EL, Valantine HA, Schroeder JS, Gao SZ, Stinson EB, and Popp RL: Intracoronary Ultrasound in Cardiac Transplant Recipients In Vivo Evidence of "Angiographically Silent" Intimal Thickening. Circulation 1992 (March);85:979–987.

14. Dunn MJ, Crisp SJ, Rose ML, Taylor PM, Yacoub MH: Anti-endothelial antibodies and coronary artery disease after cardiac transplantation. Lancet 1992 (June 27);338:1566–1570.

15. Halle A, Wilson R, Massin E, Bourge R, Stadius M, Johnson M, Wray R, Young J, Davies R, Walford G, Miller L, Deligonul U, Rincon G, Kubo S, DiSciascio G, Crandall C, Cowley M, Vetrovec G: Coronary Angioplasty in Cardiac Transplant Patients, Results of a Multicenter Study. Circulation 1992 (August);86:458–462.

16. Mullins PA, Cary NR, Sharples L, Scott J, Aravot D, Large SR, Wallwork J, Schofield PM: Coronary occlusive disease and late graft failure after cardiac transplantation. Br Heart J 1992 (Sept);68:260–265.

17. Pinto FJ, St. Goar FG, Fischell TA, Stadius ML, Valantine HA, Alderman EL, and Popp RL: Nitroglycerin-Induced Coronary Vasodilation in Cardiac Transplant Recipients Evaluation With In Vivo Intracoronary Ultrasound. Circulation 1992 (January);85:69–77.

18. Treasure CB, Vita JA, Ganz P, Ryan TJ, Schoen FJ, Vekshtein VI, Yeung AC, Mudge GH, Alexander RW, Selwyn AP, Fish RD: Loss of the Coronary Microvascular Response to Acetylcholine in Cardiac Transplant Patients. Circulation 1992 (October);86:1156–1164.

19. Mills RM Jr, Billett JM, Nichols WW: Endothelial Dysfunction Early After Heart Transplantation, Assessment With Intravascular Ultrasound and Doppler. Circulation 1992 (October);86:1171–1174.

20. Van de Borne P, Leeman M, Primo G, Degaute JP: Reappearance of a normal circadian rhythm of blood pressure after cardiac transplantation. Am J Cardiol 1992 (Mar 15);69:794–801.

21. Marzo KP, Wilson JR, Mancini DM: Effects of cardiac transplantation on ventilatory response to exercise. Am J Cardiol 1992 (Feb 15);69:547–553.

22. Ballester M, Obrador D, Carrio I, Moya C, Auge JM, Bordes R, Marti V, Bosch I, Berna-Roqueta L, Estorch M, Pons-Llado G, Camara ML, Padro JM, Aris A, and Caralps-Riera JM: Early Postoperative Reduction of Monoclonal Antimyosin Antibody Uptake Is Associated With Absent Rejection-Related Complications After Heart Transplantation. Circulation 1992 (January);85:61–68.

23. Polanco G, Jafri SM, Alam M, Levine TB: Transesophageal echocardiographic findings in patients with orthotopic heart transplantation. Chest 1992 (Mar);101:599–602.

24. Burack DA, Griffith BP, Thompson ME, Kahl LE: Hyperuricemia and gout among heart transplant recipients receiving cyclosporine. Am J Med 1992 (Feb);92:141–146.

25. Scott CD, Dark JH, McComb JM: Arrhythmias after cardiac transplantation. Am J Cardiol 1992 (Oct 22);70:1061–1063.

26. Rose AG, Viviers L, Odell JA: Autopsy-determined causes of death following cardiac

transplantation: A study of 81 patients and literature review. Arch Pathol Lab Med 1992 (Nov);116:1137–1141.

27. Thromboembolic Risk Factors (THRIFT) Consensus Group: Risk of and prophylaxis for venous thromboembolism in hospital patients. Br Med J 1992 (Sept 5);305:567–574.

28. Monreal M. Ruiz J, Olazabal A, Arias A, Roca J: Deep Venous thrombosis and the risk of pulmonary embolism: A systematic study. Chest 1992 (Sept);102:677–681.

29. Hull RD, Raskob GE, Pineo GF, Green D, Trowbridge AA, Elliott G, Lerner RG, Hall J, Sparling T, Brettell HR, Norton J, Carter CJ, George R, Merli G, Ward J, Mayo W, Rosenbloom D, Brant R: Subcutaneous low-molecular-weight heparin compared with continuous intravenous heparin in the treatment of proximal-vein thrombosis. N Engl J Med 1992 (Apr 9);326:975–982.

30. Research Committee of the British Thoracic Society: Optimum duration of anticoagulation for deep-vein thrombosis and pulmonary embolism. Lancet 1992 (Oct 19);340:873–876.

31. Cobb DK, High KP, Sawyer RG, Sable CA, Adams RB, Lindley DA, Pruett TL, Schwenzer KJ, Farr BM: A controlled trial of scheduled replacement of central venous and pulmonary-artery catheters. N Engl J Med 1992 (Oct 8):327:1062–1068.

32. Carson JL, Kelley MA, Duff A, Weg JG, Fulkerson WJ, Palevsky HI, Schwartz JS, Thompson BT, Popovich J Jr, Hobbins TE, Spera MA, Alavi A, Terrin ML: The clinical course of pulmonary embolism. N Engl J Med 1992 (May 7);326:1240–1245.

33. Goldhaber SZ, Morpurgo M: Diagnosis, treatment, and prevention of pulmonary embolism: Report of the WHO/International Society and Federation of Cardiology Task Force. JAMA 1992 (Oct 7);268:1727–1733.

34. Quinn DA, Thompson BT, Terrin ML, Thrall JH, Athanasoulis CA, McKusick KA, Stein PD, Hales CA: A prospective investigation of pulmonary embolism in women and men. JAMA 1992 (Oct 7);268:1689–1696.

35. Kasper W, Geibel A, Tiede N, Just H: Patent foramen ovale in patients with hemodynamically significant pulmonary embolism. Lancet 1992 (Sept 5);340:561–564.

36. Stein PD, Athanasoulise, Alavi A, Greenspan RH, Hales CA, Saltzman HA, Vreim CE, Terrin ML, and Weg JG. Complications and validity of pulmonary angiography in acute pulmonary embolism. Circulation 1992 (February);85:462–468.

37. Kreher SK, Ulstad VK, Dick CD, DeGroff R, Olivari MT, Homans DC. Frequent occurrence of occult pulmonary embolism from venous sheaths during endomyocardial biopsy. J Am Coll Cardiol 1992 (March);19:581–5.

38. Goldhaber SZ, Kessler CM, Heit JA, Elliott CG, Friedenberg WR, Heiselman DE, Wilson DB, Parker JA, Bennett D, Feldstein ML, Selwyn AP, Kim D, Sharma GVRK, Nagel JS, Meyerovitz MF. Recombinant tissue-type plasminogen activator versus a novel dosing regimen of urokinase in acute pulmonary embolism: A randomized controlled multicenter trial. J Am Coll Cardiol 1992 (July);20:24–30.

39. Dalla-Volta S, Palla A, Santolicandro A, Giuntini C, Pengo V, Visioli O, Zonzin P, Zanuttini D, Barberesi F, Agnelli G, Morpurgo M, Marini MG, Visani L. PAIMS 2: Alteplase combined with heparin versus heparin in the treatment of acute pulmonary embolism. Plasminogen Activator Italian Multicenter Study 2. J Am Coll Cardiol 1992 (September);20:520–6.

40. Meyer G, Sors H, Charbonner B, Kasper W, Bassand J-P, Kerr IH, Lesaffre E, Vanhove P, Verstraete M on behalf of the European Cooperative Study for Pulmonary Embolism. Effects of intravenous urokinase versus alteplase on total pulmonary resistance in acute massive pulmonary embolism: A European multicenter double-blind trial. J Am Coll Cardiol 1992 (February);19:239–45.

41. Masuda Yoshiaki, Takanashi K, Takasu J, Morroka N, Inagaki Y: Expansion rate of thoracic aortic aneurysms and influencing factors. Chest 1992 (Aug);102:461–466.

42. Lewis CTP, Cooley DA, Murphy MC, Talledo O, Vega D: Surgical repair of aortic root aneurysms in 280 patients. Ann Thorac Surg 1992 (Jan);53:38–46.

43. Nienaber CA, Spielmann RP, vonKodolitsch Y, Siglow V, Piepho A, Jaup Tilman, Nicolas V, Weber P, Triebel HJ, and Bleifeld W: Diagnosis of Thoracic Aortic Dissection Magnetic Resonance Imaging Versus Transesophageal Echocardiography. Circulation 1992 (February);85:434–447.

44. Elefteriades JA, Hartleroad J, Gusberg RJ, Salazar AM, Black HR, Kopf GS, Baldwin JC, Hammond GL: Long-term experience with descending aortic dissection: The complication-specific approach. Ann Thorac Surg 1992 (Jan);53:11–21.

45. Amarenco P, Duyckaerts C, Tzourio C, Henin D, Bousser MG, Hauw JJ: The prevalence of ulcerated plaques in the aortic arch in patients with stroke. N Engl J Med 1992 (Jan 23);326:221–225.

46. Ribakove GH, Katz ES, Galloway AC, Grossi EA, Esposito RA, Baumann FG, Kronzon I, Spencer FC: Surgical implications of transesophageal echocardiography to grade the atheromatous aortic arch. Ann Thorac Surg 1992 (May);53:758–763.

47. Katz ES, Tunick PA, Rusinek H, Ribakove G, Spencer FC, Kronzon I. Protruding aortic atheromas predict stroke in elderly patients undergoing cardiopulmonary bypass: Experience with intraoperative transesophageal echocardiography. J Am Coll Cardiol 1992 (July);20:70–7.

48. Katz DA, Littenberg B, Cronenwett JL: Management of small abdominal aortic aneurysms: Early surgery vs watchful waiting. JAMA 1992 (Nov 18);268:2678–2686.

49. Mautner GC, Berezowski K, Mautner SL, Roberts WC: Degrees of coronary arterial narrowing at necropsy in men with large fusiform abdominal aortic aneurysm. Am J Cardiol 1992 (Nov 1);70:1143–1146.

50. Goldhaber SZ, Manson JE, Stampfer MJ, Lamotte F, Rosner B, Buring JE, Hennekens CH: Low-dose aspirin and subsequent peripheral arterial surgery in the Physician's Health Study. Lancet 1992 (July 18);340:143–145.

51. Losordo DW, Rosenfield K, Pieczek A, Baker K, Harding M, Isner JM: How Does Angioplasty Work? Serial Analysis of Human Iliac Arteries Using Intravascular Ultrasound. Circulation 1992 (December);86:1845–1858.

52. Criqui MH, Langer RD, Fronek A, Feigelson HS, Klauber MR, McCann TJ, Browner D: Mortality over a period of 10 years in patients with peripheral arterial disease. N Engl J Med 1992 (Feb 6);326:381–386.

53. Mautner GC, Mautner SL, Roberts WC: Amounts of coronary arterial narrowing by atherosclerotic plaque at necropsy in patients with lower extremity amputation. Am J Cardiol 1992 (Nov 1) 70:1147–1151.

54. Di Tullio M, Sacco RL, Gopal A, Mohr JP, Homma S: Patent foramen ovale as a risk factor for cryptogenic stroke. An Intern Med 1992 (Sept 15);117:461–465.

55. Koudstaal PJ, Algra A, Pop GAM, Kappelle LJ, Van Latum JC, Van Gijn J: Risk of cardiac events in atypical transient ischemic attack or minor stroke. Lancet 1992 (Sept 12);340:630–633.

56. Rich S, Kaufmann E, Levy PS: The effect of high doses of calcium-channel blockers on survival in primary pulmonary hypertension. N Engl J Med 1992 (July 9);327:76–81.

57. McIntyre KM, Vita JA, Lambrew CT, Freeman J, Loscalzo J: A noninvasive method of predicting pulmonary-capillary wedge pressure. N Engl J Med 1992 (Dec 10);327:1715–1720.

58. Boehrer JD, Moliterno DJ, Willard JE, Snyder RW, Horton RP, Glamann DB, Lange RA, Hillis LD. Hemodynamic effects of intranasal cocaine in humans. J Am Coll Cardiol 1992 (July);20:90–3.

59. Knott-Craig CJ, Schaff HV, Mullany CJ, Kvols LK, Moertel CG, Edwards WD, Danielson GK: Carcinoid disease of the heart: Surgical management of ten patients. J Thorac Cardiovasc Surg 1992 (Aug);104:475–581.

60. Unger F, Hutter J: Open heart surgery in Europe 1990. Eur Heart J 1992 (Oct);13:1345–1347.

61. Cheng TO: Acronyms of major cardiologic trials. Am J Cardiol 1992 (Dec 1);70:1512–1514.

Author Index

Note: Page numbers in italic indicate figures. Page numbers followed by t indicate tables.

Subject Index

Note: Page numbers in italic indicate figures. Page numbers followed by t indicate tables.